BRAIN DISEASE
THERAPEUTIC STRATEGIES AND REPAIR

Edited by

ODED ABRAMSKY MD, PhD
Professor, Department of Neurology
Hadassah University Hospital
Jerusalem
Israel

D ALASTAIR S COMPSTON PhD, FRCP
Professor and Head, Neurology Unit
University of Cambridge
Addenbrooke's Hospital
Cambridge
UK

ARIEL MILLER MD, PhD
Head, Division of Neuroimmunology
The Lady Davis Carmel Medical Center
Department of Neurology
Technion-Israel Institute of Technology
Haifa
Israel

GÉRARD SAID MD
Professor and Head of the Department of
Neurology
Hôpital Kremlin Bicêtre
Le Kremlin Bicêtre
France

MARTIN DUNITZ

© 2002 Martin Dunitz Ltd, a member of the Taylor & Francis Group

First published in the United Kingdom in 2002
by Martin Dunitz Ltd, The Livery House, 7–9 Pratt Street, London NW1 0AE

Tel: +44 (0) 20 7482 2202
Fax: +44 (0) 20 7267 0159
E-mail: info@dunitz.co.uk
Website: http://www.dunitz.co.uk

Although every effort has been made to ensure that all owners of copyright
material have been acknowledged in this publication, we would be glad to
acknowledge in subsequent reprints or editions any omissions brought to our
attention.

Although every effort has been made to ensure that drug doses and other
information are presented accurately in this publication, the ultimate
responsibility rests with the prescribing physician. Neither the publishers nor
the authors can be held responsible for errors or for any consequences arising
from the use of information contained herein. For detailed prescribing
information or instructions on the use of any product or procedure discussed
herein, please consult the prescribing information or instructional material
issued by the manufacturer.

A CIP record for this book is available from the British Library.

ISBN 1 84184 040 8

Distributed in the USA by
Fulfilment Center
Taylor & Francis
7625 Empire Drive
Florence, KY 41042, USA
Toll Free Tel.: +1 800 634 7064
E-mail: cserve@routledge_ny.com

Distributed in Canada by
Taylor & Francis
74 Rolark Drive
Scarborough, Ontario M1R 4G2, Canada
Toll Free Tel.: +1 877 226 2237
E-mail: tal_fran@istar.ca

Distributed in the rest of the world by
ITPS Limited
Cheriton House
North Way
Andover, Hampshire SP10 5BE, UK
Tel.: +44 (0) 1264 332424
E-mail: reception@itps.co.uk

Composition by Scribe Design, Gillingham, Kent, UK
Printed and bound in Great Britain by Biddles Ltd, Guildford and King's Lynn

Contents

Preface

We have brought together some of the world's leading scientists to review the latest insights and concepts that are the result of recent research into brain disease. Focusing on the conclusions of research carried out during DECADE OF THE BRAIN (1990–2000), the book encompasses the latest clinical and experimental findings on how the central nervous system responds to injury caused by inflammation, vascular accidents, trauma, and degenerative disorders such as multiple sclerosis, Alzheimer's disease, stroke and head injury. Particular attention is devoted to the role of genetic and environmental factors, apoptotic mechanisms, cytokines, chemokines, matrix metalloproteinases (MMPs), and free radicals in the acquisition of brain diseases and CNS response.

Based on the newly gained insights into such mechanisms of injury and response, novel therapeutic interventions, both experimental and clinical, aimed at promoting functional recovery are presented. These include the use of growth factors, anti-inflammatory agents, anti-oxidants and gene-based therapies, as well as that of stem cells for CNS remyelination and neuro-regeneration.

The editors wish to thank the many contributors to this book for their hard work, as well as Alan Burgess at Martin Dunitz for his help and guidance.

Ariel Miller

Contributors

†Author deceased

Oded Abramsky MD, PhD
Department of Neurology
Hadassah University Hospital
Jerusalem 91120
Israel

Jack P Antel MD
Neuroimmunology Unit
Montreal Neurological Institute
McGill University
3801 University Street
Montreal QC H3A 2B4
Canada

Juan J Archelos MD
Department of Neurology
Karl-Franzens-University
Auenbruggerplatz 22
8036 Graz
Austria

Zohar Argov MD
Department of Neurology and the
Agnes Ginges Center for
Neurogenetics
Hadassah University Hospital
and the Hebrew University-
Hadassah Medical School
Ein Kerem, Jerusalem 91120
Israel

**Peter O Behan DSc, MD, FACP,
FRCP(Lond)(Glas)(Ire)**
Department of Neurology
Institute of Neurological Sciences
University of Glasgow
1341 Govan Road
Glasgow G51 4TF
UK

Tamir Ben-Hur MD, PhD
Department of Neurology
The Agnes Ginges Center for
Human Neurogenetics
Hadassah University Hospital,
Jerusalem
Israel

Avraham Ben-Nun PhD
Department of Immunology
The Weizmann Institute of
Science
Rehovot 76100
Israel

Alessandra Bergami
Department of Neuroscience
San Raffaele Scientific Institute
Via Olgettina 60
20132 Milan
Italy

Isabelle Berry MD, PhD
Department of Nuclear Medicine
CHU Rangueil
31403 Toulouse
France

Monique Bessou
CHU Rangueil
31403 Toulouse
France

Allan J Bieber PhD
Department of Neurology and
Program in Molecular
Neuroscience
Mayo Medical and Graduate
Schools
200 First St SW
Rochester, MN 55905
USA

Julien Bogousslavsky MD
Department of Neurology
Centre Hospitalier Universitaire
Vaudois (CHUV)
CH-1011 Lausanne
Switzerland

Françoise Bouhour MD
Neurology Service A
Hôpital Neurologique
59 Boulevard Pinel
69003 Lyon
France

Abdalla Bowirrat MD
Department of Neurology
Sackler Faculty of Medicine
Tel-Aviv University Medical
School
Ramat-Aviv 69978
Israel

Elena Brambilla BS
Department of Neuroscience
San Raffaele Scientific Institute
Via Olgettina 60
20132 Milan
Italy

Thomas Brandt MD FRCP
Department of Neurology
Klinikum Grosshadern
Ludwig-Maximilians University
Marchioninstrasse 15
81377 Munich
Germany

Jill R Breen MD
Department of Neurology
University of Colorado Health
Sciences Center
4200 E 9th Avenue
Mail Stop B182
Denver, CO 80262
USA

Ligong Cao MD
Department of Neurology
The University of Alabama at
Birmingham
619 19th Street South
Birmingham AL, 35249–2402
USA

Joab Chapman MD
Department of Medicine B
Sheba Medical Center
Tel Hashomer 52621
Israel

**Abhijit Chaudhuri DM, MD,
MRCP(UK)**
Department of Neurology
Institute of Neurological Sciences
University of Glasgow
1341 Govan Road
Glasgow G51 4TF
UK

Bogoljub Ciric PhD
Department of Immunology
Mayo Medical and Graduate
Schools
200 First St SW
Rochester, MN 55905
USA

Michel Clanet MD
CHU Rangueil
31403 Toulouse
France

Giancarlo Comi MD
Department of Neuroscience
San Raffaele Scientific Institute
Via Olgettina 60
20132 Milan
Italy

Alastair Compston PhD, FRCP
Neurology Department
University of Cambridge Clinical
School
Addenbrooke's Hospital
Hills Road
Cambridge CB2 2QQ
UK

Christian Confavreux MD
Neurology Service A
Hôpital Neurologique
59 Boulevard Pinel
69003 Lyon
France

Frédéric Courbon
CHU Rangueil
31403 Toulouse
France

Lori Coward MD
Department of Pharmacology
The University of Alabama at
Birmingham
619 19th Street South
Birmingham AL, 35249–2402
USA

Armin Curt MD
ParaCare
Swiss Paraplegic Centre
University Hospital Balgrist
Forchstrasse 340
CH-8008 Zürich
Switzerland

Volker Dietz MD, FRCP
ParaCare
Swiss Paraplegic Centre
University Hospital Balgrist
Forchstrasse 340
CH-8008 Zürich
Switzerland

Pierre Duthil
CHU Rangueil
31403 Toulouse
France

Giora Z Feuerstein MD, MSc
Cardiovascular Diseases Research
DuPont Pharmaceuticals
Company
Experimental Station E400/3257
Rt 141 & Henry Clay Roads
Wilmington, DE 19880–0400
USA

Massimo Filippi MD
Neuroimaging Research Unit
Department of Neuroscience
Scientific Institute Ospedale San
Raffaele
Milan
Italy

Robert P Friedland MD
Laboratory of Neurogeriatrics
Case Western Reserve University
Cleveland OH
USA

Alon Friedman
Department of Neurosurgery
Ben-Gurion University
Beersheva
Israel

Peter Fuhr MD
Department of Neurology
School of Medicine
University of Basel
Basel
Switzerland

Roberto Furlan MD
Department of Neuroscience
San Raffaele Scientific Institute
Via Olgettina 60
20132 Milan
Italy

Yanina Galboiz MD
The Center for Multiple Sclerosis
& Brain Research
Department of Neurology
Carmel Medical Center
7 Michal Street
Haifa 34362
Israel

Nir Giladi
Movement Disorders Unit
Department of Neurology
Tel-Aviv Sourasky Medical
Center
6 Weizmann Street
Tel Aviv 64239
Israel

Donald H Gilden MD
Department of Neurology
University of Colorado Health
Sciences Center
4200 E 9th Avenue
Mail Stop B182
Denver, CO 80262
USA

David Glick
The Institute of Life Sciences
The Hebrew University of
Jerusalem
Israel

Haim Golan
Department of Nuclear Medicine
Ben-Gurion University
Beersheva
Israel

John Gow PhD
Department of Neurology
Institute of Neurological Sciences
University of Glasgow
1341 Govan Road
Glasgow G51 4TF
UK

Edna Grünblatt PhD
Department of Pharmacology
Technion-Faculty of Medicine
Eve Topf and US NPF Centers for
Neurodegenerative Diseases
Research
31096 Haifa
Israel

Peter Hagell
Section of Restorative Neurology
Wallenberg Neuroscience Center
University Hospital
SW-221 85 Lund
Sweden

Hans-Peter Hartung MD
Department of Neurology
Karl-Franzens-University
Auenbruggerplatz 22
8036 Graz
Austria

Sharon Hassin-Baer
Parkinson's Disease and
Movement Disorders Clinic
Department of Neurology
Chaim Sheba Medical Center
Tel Hashomer 52621
Israel

† Lea Averbuch-Heller MD
Neuro-Opthalmology Service
Departments of Neurology and
Opthalmology
Rabin Medical Center
Tel Aviv University
Petah Tikva 49100
Israel

Michael Hennerici MD
Universitätsklinikum Mannheim
University of Heidelberg
D-68135 Mannheim
Theodor-Kutzer-Ufer 1–3
Germany

Lutz-Peter Hiersemenzel MD
ParaCare
Swiss Paraplegic Centre
University Hospital Balgrist
Forchstrasse 340
CH-8008 Zürich
Switzerland

Patricia Jackson MD
Department of Chemistry
The University of Alabama at
Birmingham
619 19th Street South
Birmingham AL, 35249–2402
USA

Svein I Johannessen PhD
The National Center for Epilepsy
N-1303 Sandvika
Norway

Nathan Karin PhD
Department of Immunology
Rappaport Faculty of Medicine &
Rappaport Institute for Medical
Sciences
Technion-Israel Institute of
Technology
Haifa
Israel

Arnon Karni
Center for Neurologic Diseases
Brigham and Women's Hospital
Harvard Medical School
77 Avenue Louis Pasteur, HIM
730
Boston, MA 02115
USA

Dimitrios M Karussis MD, PhD
Department of Neurology
Hadassah University Hospital
Jerusalem 91120
Israel

Daniela Kaufer
The Institute of Life Sciences
The Hebrew University of
Jerusalem
Israel

Jürg Kesselring MD, PhD
Department of Neurology
Rehabilitation Centre
CH-7317 Valens
Switzerland

Samia J Khoury MD
Center for Neurologic Diseases
Brigham and Women's Hospital
Harvard Medical School
77 Avenue Louis Pasteur, HIM
730
Boston, MA 02115
USA

Bernd C Kieseier MD
Department of Neurology
Karl-Franzens-University
Auenbruggerplatz 22
8036 Graz
Austria

Marion Kirk MD
Department of Pharmacology
The University of Alabama at
Birmingham
619 19th Street South
Birmingham AL, 35249–2402
USA

Ulrike Klement Dipl. Psych
Department of Neurology
Rehabilitation Centre
CH-7317 Valens
Switzerland

Uwe Koedel MD
Department of Neurology
Ludwig-Maximilians-University
Marchioninistrasse 15
Munich 81377
Germany

Amos D Korczyn MD, MSc
Department of Neurology
Sackler Faculty of Medicine
Tel-Aviv University Medical
School
Ramat-Aviv
Tel-Aviv 69978
Israel

Nitza Lahat PhD
The Center for Multiple Sclerosis
& Brain Research
Department of Neurology
Carmel Medical Center
7 Michal Street
Haifa 34362
Israel

Ronen R Leker MD
Department of Neurology and the
Agnes Ginges Center for Human
Neurogenetics
Hadassah University Hospital
Ein Kerem
Jerusalem 91120
Israel

Letizia Leocani MD
Multiple Sclerosis Centre
San Raffaele Hospital
University of Milan
Milan 20132
Italy

David Leppert MD
Department of Neurology and
Neurobiology
School of Medicine
University of Basel
Basel
Switzerland

Yona Levites MSc
Department of Pharmacology
Technion-Faculty of Medicine
Eve Topf and US NPF Centers for
Neurodegenerative Diseases
Research
31096 Haifa
Israel

Olle Lindvall MD, PhD
Section of Restorative Neurology
Wallenberg Neuroscience Center
University Hospital
SW-221 85 Lund
Sweden

Alexander Lossos MD
Department of Neurology
Hadassah University Hospital
Jerusalem
Israel

Karim Makhlouf MD
Center for Neurologic Diseases
Brigham and Women's Hospital
Harvard Medical School
77 Avenue Louis Pasteur, HIM
730
Boston, MA 02115
USA

Silvia Mandel PhD
Department of Pharmacology
Technion-Faculty of Medicine
Eve Topf and US NPF Centers for
Neurodegenerative Diseases
Research
31096 Haifa
Israel

Claude Manelfe
CHU Rangueil
31403 Toulouse
France

Gila Maor PhD
Department of Cell Biology
Bruce Rappaport Family Research
Institute
Department of Pharmacology
31906 Haifa
Israel

Peggy M Marconi BS
Department of Microbiology
Faculty of Pharmacy
University of Ferrara
Ferrara
Italy

Gianvito Martino MD
Department of Neuroscience
San Raffaele Scientific Institute
Via Olgettina 60
20132 Milan
Italy

Stephen Meairs MD
Universitätsklinikum Mannheim
University of Heidelberg
D-68135 Mannheim
Theodor-Kutzer-Ufer 1–3
Germany

Eldad Melamed MD
Department of Neurology
Rabin Medical Center
The Sackler Faculty of Medicine
Tel Aviv University
Tel Aviv 69978
Israel

Ofer Merimsky MD
Department of Oncology
Tel-Aviv Sourasky Medical
Center
Tel-Aviv
Israel

Ariel Miller MD, PhD
The Center for Multiple Sclerosis
& Brain Research
Department of Neurology
Carmel Medical Center
7 Michal Street
Haifa 34362
Israel

Jorge Moncayo Gaete MD
Department of Neurology
Eugenio Espejo Hospital
Quito
Ecuador

Ronit Mosberg-Galili MD
Department of Neurology
Rabin Medical Center
The Sackler Faculty of Medicine
Tel Aviv University
Tel Aviv 69978
Israel

Miri Y Neufeld MD
EEG and Epilepsy Unit
Department of Neurology
Tel-Aviv Sourasky Medical
Center and
The Sackler Faculty of Medicine
Tel-Aviv University
Tel Aviv
Israel

JP Newman PhD
Department of Neurology
Hadassah Medical Organization
Hadassah University hospital
Kiryat Hadassah
Jerusalem
Israel

Daniel Offen PhD
Felsenstein Medical Research
Center
Rabin Medical Center
The Sackler Faculty of Medicine
Tel Aviv University
Tel Aviv 69978
Israel

Larry R Pease PhD
Department of Immunology
Mayo Medical and Graduate
Schools
200 First St SW
Rochester, MN 55905
USA

Hans-Walter Pfister MD
Department of Neurology
Ludwig-Maximilians-University
Marchioninistrasse 15
Munich 81377
Germany

Pietro L Poliani MD
Department of Neuroscience
San Raffaele Scientific Institute
Via Olgettina 60
20132 Milan
Italy

Jose Martin Rabey MD
Department of Neurology
Assaf Harofe Medical Center
Sackler School of Medicine
Tel Aviv University
Zerifin 70300
Israel

Alexander J Radziwill MD
Department of Neurology
School of Medicine
University of Basel
Basel
Switzerland

Lubica Rauova MD
Department of Medicine B
Center for Autoimmune Diseases
Sheba Medical Center
Tel Hashomer
Israel 52621

Eli Reichenthal
Department of Neurosurgery
Ben-Gurion University
Beersheva
Israel

Susanne Renaud MD
Department of Neurology
School of Medicine
University of Basel
Basel
Switzerland

Moses Rodriguez MD
Departments of Neurology,
Immunology and Program in
Molecular Neuroscience
Mayo Medical and Graduate
Schools
200 First St SW
Rochester, MN 55905
USA

Nicole Kerlero de Rosbo PhD
Department of Immunology
The Weizmann Institute of
Science
Rehovot 76100
Israel

Marco Rovaris MD
Neuroimaging Research Unit
Department of Neuroscience
Scientific Institute Ospedale San
Raffaele
Milan
Italy

Francesca Ruffini BS
Department of Neuroscience
San Raffaele Scientific Institute
Via Olgettina 60
20132 Milan
Italy

Gérard Said MD
Service de Neurologie
Hôpital de Bicêtre (Université
Paris XI)
94275 Le Kremlin Bicêtre
France

Nicole Schaeren-Wiemers PhD
Department of Neurology and
Neurobiology
School of Medicine
University of Basel
Basel
Switzerland

Yitzhak Schiller MD, PhD
Department of Neurology
Rambam Medical Center
Haifa
Israel 31096

Michal Schwartz MD
Department of Neurobiology
The Weizmann Institute of
Science
76100 Rehovot
Israel

Rosanne Seguin PhD
Neuroimmunology Unit
Montreal Neurological Institute
McGill University
3801 University Street
Montreal QC H3A 2B4
Canada

Sarah Shapiro PhD
The Center for Multiple Sclerosis
& Brain Research
Department of Neurology
Carmel Medical Center
7 Michal Street
Haifa 34362
Israel

Ilan Shelef
Dept of Radiology
Ben-Gurion University
Beersheva
Israel

Yehuda Shoenfeld MD
Department of Medicine B
Sheba Medical Center
Tel Hashomer
Israel 52621

Esther Shohami PhD
Department of Pharmacology
The Hebrew University
School of Pharmacy
Jerusalem, 91120
Israel

Tali Siegal MD
Neuro-Oncology Center
Hadassah University Hospital
Jerusalem
Israel

Aksel Siva MD
Department of Neurology
Cerrahpaşa School of Medicine
University of Istanbul
Istanbul
Turkey

Kenneth J Smith PhD
Neuroinflammation Research
Group
Department of
Neuroimmunology
Guy's, King's and St Thomas'
School of Medicine
Guy's Campus, King's College
St Thomas Street
London SE1 9RT
UK

Hermona Soreq PhD
The Institute of Life Sciences
The Hebrew University of
Jerusalem
Israel

Andreas J Steck MD
Department of Neurology
School of Medicine
University of Basel
Basel
Switzerland

Austin J Sumner MD
Department of Neurology
Louisiana State University Health
Sciences Center
1542 Tulane Avenue
New Orleans
Louisiana 70112
USA

Oren Tomkins
Department of Neurosurgery
Ben-Gurion University
Beersheva
Israel

Torbjörn Tomson MD, PhD
Department of Neurology
Karolinska Hospital
Stockholm
Sweden

Virginia Van Keulen
Department of Immunology
Mayo Medical and Graduate
Schools
200 First St SW
Rochester, MN 55905
USA

John Vissing MD
Department of Neurology and the
Copenhagen Muscle Research
Center
The National University Hospital,
Rigshospitalet
Blegdamsvej 9
DK-2100 Copenhagen
Denmark

Sandra Vukusic MD
Neurology Service A
Hôpital Neurologique
59 Boulevard Pinel
69003 Lyon
France

Xinkang Wang PhD
Cardiovascular Diseases Research
DuPont Pharmaceuticals
Company
Experimental Station E400/3257
Rt 141 & Henry Clay Roads
Wilmington, DE 19880–0400
USA

Arthur E Warrington PhD
Department of Neurology
Mayo Medical and Graduate
Schools
200 First St SW
Rochester, MN 55905
USA

Howard L Weiner MD
Center for Neurologic Diseases
Brigham and Women's Hospital
Harvard Medical School
77 Avenue Louis Pasteur, HIM
730
Boston, MA 02115
USA

John Whitaker MD, PhD
Department of Neurology
The University of Alabama at
Birmingham
619 19th Street South
Birmingham AL, 35249–2402
USA

Moussa BH Youdim PhD
Department of Pharmacology
Technion-Faculty of Medicine
Eve Topf and US NPF Centers for
Neurodegenerative Diseases
Research
31096 Haifa
Israel

Slimane Zerdoud
CHU Rangueil
31403 Toulouse
France

Part 1

Neuroimmunology and immune-mediated demyelination

1

The spectrum of neuroimmunologic diseases

Dimitrios M Karussis and Oded Abramsky

INTRODUCTION

Neurologic diseases in which the immune system plays a crucial role in their pathogenesis are defined as neuroimmune diseases. In most of them, the pathogenetic mechanism is that of an autoimmune attack against neuronal antigens, similar to that involved in organ-specific and systemic autoimmunity. In others, the immune system involvement is not clearly associated with or responsible for the pathogenesis of the disease.

AUTOIMMUNE DISEASES IN GENERAL

Generally, in autoimmune diseases the inflammatory process is initiated after the presumed auto-antigen is presented to lymphocytes by macrophages that act as antigen-presenting cells (APCs). For full activation/immunization, the lymphocyte has to receive two signals: (1) one provided by the MHC–antigen complex, which binds to the specific TCR (T-cell receptor); and the second (2) supplied by the B7-CD28 (adhesion molecule) complex. In the absence of the secondary costimulatory signal, the lymphocytes fail to produce the T-cell growth factor interleukin-2 (IL-2) and, therefore, antigen presentation leads to anergy of the lymphocytes towards the specific antigen.[1] There are also other accessory molecules, like the LFA1/ICAM-1, the CD40/CD40L (ligand) and the LFA3/CD2 complexes, which enhance lymphocyte reactivity in a non-specific manner. The latter represent a second pathway (independent of the TCR pathway) for T-cell activation.

Following activation by macrophages/APCs, lymphocytes (mainly of the helper CD4 subtype) expressing the specific TCR proliferate and expand. In parallel, they begin to express on their cell surface adhesion molecules/markers of activation (LFA1,3, ICAM-1, VLA-4) which help them to invade the vessel endothelium at the site of inflammation.[2-4] T-helper cells differentiate, becoming either Th1 cells, which stimulate cytotoxic, or CD4 T-cells (positive feedback) by producing IL-2, IL-12, TNF-α and IFN-γ (pro-inflammatory cytokines), or Th2 cells, that help mainly B-cells (producing auto-antibodies) and secrete IL-4, IL-6 and IL-10.[5-7] There is a 'balance' between the Th1 and Th2 subpopulations; in T-cell-mediated autoimmune diseases like multiple sclerosis (MS), the lymphocytes involved in the inflammatory process are mainly of the Th1 phenotype. However, the acquisition of a specific phenotype (Th1 or Th2) is rather transient, and the status of lymphocytes can be changed according to the immunologic milieu. It seems, therefore, that there are no 'good' and 'bad' cells, but the same cell can be differentiated in both directions. We believe that the Th1 to Th2 shift is a transient event and is not universally helpful in autoimmunity. Actually, such a shift may be harmful in antibody-mediated autoimmunity, as was recently shown in MOG (membrane oligodendrocyte glycoprotein)-induced EAE,[8] whereas it may be helpful in T-cell-mediated autoimmune diseases, like MS, but such a shift should not be permanent and it may be associated with increased danger for induction of antibody-mediated autoimmunity.

CD4 lymphocytes are also functionally and phenotypically divided into two subpopulations. The first population comprises 'memory' cells, which, after the initial encounter with the antigen, are rapidly induced to react/proliferate following a second exposure. These cells express the CD45 RO surface marker on their membranes. The second subpopulation is of the CD45 RA phenotype, and consists of cells which function as 'suppressor–

inducers'.[5,9] There is probably a cyclic relationship between CD4+ subpopulations: naive CD45Ra+ cells convert to CD45Ro+ memory cells upon antigen stimulation, but without continuous antigen stimulation they lose their CD45Ro expression and revert to being long-lived CD45Ra+ cells.[10,11] These CD45Ro+ lymphocytes represent activated memory cells and they are probably identical to the CD29+ lymphocytes expressing on their surface the b-chain of the VLA antigens (b1 integrins),[12] which is upregulated to facilitate adhesion to endothelial cells and subsequent passage into sites of inflammation. In MS and in other autoimmune diseases, like rheumatoid arthritis, autoimmune hemolytic anemia, Guillain-Barré Syndrome (GBS) and systemic lupus erythematosous (SLE),[13–18] the CD45Ra+ cells are usually downregulated, especially during the active phases (relapses) of the disease. In a longitudinal study, it was shown that newly diagnosed cases with SLE initially have a higher proportion of CD45Ra+ cells, which, as the disease progresses, reduces as a shift towards the CD45Ro phenotype takes place. This shift seems to be the result of conversion of resting cells into activated memory lymphocytes. However, since the CD45Ra+ cells are found in lower numbers in patients with autoimmune diseases as compared to age-matched healthy individuals, this finding may also indicate that loss of suppressor function could be, at least partially, related to the immunopathogenesis of autoimmunity in general; a low proportion of suppressor–inducer cells could permit autoreactive clones to carry out an autoimmune attack.

The basic concepts for self/non-self-discrimination and autoimmunity seem to be in a process of revision. Actually, it has been shown that even naive neonatal thymocytes can proliferate and react to any antigenic stimulation, depending on the 'conditions' provided. The potential for autoimmunity may exist in almost any individual with the suitable genetic background. What prevents autoimmunity is an immune network fully equipped with several immunoregulatory populations which—when they function properly—do not allow the outburst of autoreactivity. In support of this theory, several studies have reported immunologic defects observed in patients with neuroimmunologic diseases, thus indicating that malfunction of immunoregulatory mechanisms may be involved in the pathogenesis of these diseases. The most documented include defective suppressor cell activity, reduced NK cell activity and reduced proportions of suppressor–inducer cells,[13–15,18–20] all of which correlate reciprocally (negatively) with disease activity.

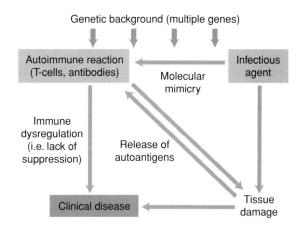

Figure 1.1 Interplay of multiple factors in the pathogenesis of autoimmunity.

Thus, for autoimmunity to develop, several events have to take place in a complicated interplay: (1) there has to be a specific (autoimmune-prone) genetic background (specific HLA subtypes); (2) there must be a 'trigger', usually an infectious agent; and (3) a dysregulation of the immune system has to occur, namely a defect in the normally existing suppressor/downregulatory immune mechanisms mentioned above. A schematic representation of this interplay between the components of this setting in autoimmune diseases is shown in Figure 1.1.

NEUROIMMUNE DISEASES

Only a few neurologic disorders fulfill the criteria of an autoimmune disease, that is: (1) the presence of specific immune (T- or B-cell-mediated) reactivity against a well-defined autoantigen; (2) the existence of a known pathogenic mechanism by which these antibodies or T-cells induce clinical and/or histopathologic features of the disease; and (3) the feasibility of inducing a similar disease in laboratory animals by immunization with the putative auto-antigen. Such definite neuro-autoimmune diseases include myasthenia gravis, Lambert–Eaton myasthenic syndrome (LEMS) and anti-MAG (myelin associated glycoprotein) demyelinating polyneuropathy (Table 1.1). In these diseases, the rationale for immunosuppressive therapy is obvious, and the results of treatment with plasmapheresis, IVIG, corticosteroids and azathioprine and cyclophosphamide have usually been very satisfactory.

A larger group of neuroimmunologic disorders includes diseases which can be characterized as a probable autoimmune pathogenesis (Table 1.1). They

Table 1.1 The spectrum of neuroimmune disorders	
Diseases with definite autoimmune pathogenesis	**Diseases with a probable autoimmune basis**
Myasthenia gravis	Guillain–Barré syndrome (acute inflammatory demyelinating polyneuropathy)
LEMS	Chronic inflammatory demyelinating polyneuropathy
Anti-MAG polyneuropathy	Multifocal neuropathy with anti-GM1 antibodies
	Multiple sclerosis
	'Stiff-person' syndrome
	Isaac's disease
	Paraneoplastic disorders
	Polymyositis/dermatomyositis inclusion body myositis
	Systemic vasculitis (SLE, polyarteritis nodosa, Sjögren's etc.)
	Rasmussen's encephalitis and some forms of pediatric epilepsy with anti-glutamate receptor antibodies

share common features with other autoimmune diseases, namely the increased incidence in women, a tendency for non-mendelian familial clustering (HLA susceptibility) and a relapsing–remitting course. Such diseases are rather loosely described as 'immune-mediated,' and include Guillain–Barré syndrome (acute inflammatory demyelinating polyneuropathy (AIDP)), chronic inflammatory demyelinating polyneuropathy (CIDP), multifocal neuropathy with anti-GM1 antibodies, MS, 'stiff-person' syndrome, Isaac's disease, paraneoplastic cerebellar degeneration, opsoclonus and neuropathy, polymyositis/dermatomyositis and systemic vaculitis (SLE, Sjögren's etc.). In the latter group, although inflammatory features are described and putative animal models exist,[21–24] there is no clear evidence of an autoimmune mechanism directed against a well-defined auto-antigen which is responsible for the pathogenic process. Moreover, several investigators claim that in these immune-mediated diseases, the inflammatory process may be an epiphenomenon of nervous tissue destruction or of a viral attack.[25] Supporting the uncertainty in these diseases are conflicting and controversial data on the effect of immunosuppressive treatments in halting the clinical progression.

Interestingly, the first group includes diseases affecting the peripheral nervous system or the muscles, whereas the second includes mostly diseases affecting the central nervous system (CNS). This may be explained by the fact that the CNS is considered to be an immunologically privileged site, and under normal conditions/circumstances no immune reactivity is observed in it.

However, even in the latter group, several clinical trials have shown some efficacy of steroids, plasmapheresis and immunosuppressive medications.

An attempt at a more detailed classification of the neuroimmune disorders, based on the pathogenetic mechanisms, is presented in Table 1.2. The first group includes the so-called 'idiopathic' autoimmune neurologic diseases, i.e. in which no defined etiologic factor has been isolated. This group is subdivided into (a) disorders primarily—and exclusively—affecting the central and peripheral nervous system (PNS) or the muscles, namely MS, myasthenia gravis, AIDP and CIDP, polymyositis, multifocal neuropathy with anti-GM1 antibodies, anti-MAG antibody-associated polyneuropathy, Rasmussen's encephalitis and some forms of pediatric epilepsy with anti-glutamate receptor antibodies, 'stiff-person' syndrome, Isaac's disease and isolated vasculitis of the CNS or of the PNS; and (b) diseases in which the neurologic involvement is a part of a systemic autoimmune syndrome, such as CNS and PNS involvement in systemic vasculitis (Table 1.3), SLE, polyarteritis nodosa, scleroderma, Sjögren's disease, Behçet's disease, Wegener's disease, giant cell arteritis (temporal arteritis and Takayasu), and sarcoidosis and dermatomyositis.

The second group includes neuroimmune diseases in which, following an infection, an immune-mediated process targeting neuroantigens is initiated, due to similarities between epitopes of the infectious agent and peptidic components of neuronal proteins. Such a pathogenetic mechanism, characterized as 'molecular mimicry', is assumed to be responsible for diseases such as post-polio

Table 1.2 Classification of neuroimmune disorders according to the pathogenetic mechanisms

Groups of neuroimmune diseases	Diseases or syndromes

A. **Idiopathic neuroimmune disorders**
  i. Primarily affecting the CNS, PNS or the
    muscles
	Multiple sclerosis
	AIDP
	CIDP
	Myasthenia gravis
	Polymyositis
	Stiff-person syndrome
	Isaac's disease
	Anti-GM1 polyneuropathies
	Anti-MAG polyneuropathy
	Isolated CNS vasculitis
	Isolated PNS vasculitis
	Rasmussen's encephalitis and some forms of pediatric epilepsy
	with anti-glutamate receptor antibodies

ii. Systemic autoimmune diseases secondarily affecting the CNS or PNS and muscles	Dermatomyositis SLE Behçet's disease Giant cell arteries (temporal arteries and Takayasu) Wegener's granulomatosis Polyarteritis nodosa Sjögren's Scleroderma Other systemic vasculitis

B. **Neuroimmune diseases following an immune trigger**
  i. Post-infectious disorders following a
    distinct immune trigger/stimulus
    (mechanism of molecular mimicry)
	Post-polio syndrome?
	Chronic neuroborreliosis
	Post-Campylobacter AIDP
	HIV-related polyneuropathy and MS-like disease?
	Sydenham's chorea
	PANDAS (tics, obsessive-compulsive disorder)

ii. Paraneoplastic disorders	Paraneoplastic cerebellar degeneration Paraneoplastic neuronopathy Limbic encephalitis Retinal degeneration Opsoclonus–myoclonus Cases of LEMS Cases of 'stiff-person' syndrome

C. **Unclassified neuroimmune disorders of**
  unknown origin with an inflammatory
  mechanism involved in their pathogenesis
	Neurosarcoidosis
	Tolosa–Hunt syndrome, and other granulomatous CNS disorders

D. **Neurologic diseases of primarily 'degenerative'**
  or genetic origin with evidence of additional
  inflammatory lesions
	Alzheimer's disease
	Muscular dystrophies
	Amyotrophic lateral sclerosis
	Stroke?

Table 1.3 Neurological involvement in systemic vasculitis

	CNS involvement	PNS and muscle involvement
SLE	Seizures, psychosis, multifocal vascular (ischemic) disease, meningitis	Peripheral neuropathy (overlapping symmetric or mononeuritis multiplex)
Polyarteritis nodosa	Seizures, psychosis, multifocal vascular (ischemic) disease, meningitis	Peripheral neuropathy (overlapping symmetric or mononeuritis multiplex)
Churg–Strauss angiitis	Encephalopathy, seizures, psychosis, multifocal vascular (ischemic) disease, meningitis	Peripheral neuropathy (overlapping symmetric or mononeuritis multiplex)
Hypersensitivity vasculitis		Plexopathies
Wegener's	Cranial polyneuropathy, basal meningitis, focal granulomatous disease	
Giant cell arteritis		
Temporal arteritis	Optic neuropathy, cranial neuropathies, strokes?	Polymyalgia rheumatica
Takayasu	Stroke, transient ischemic accidents, syncope	
Behçet's	Meningoencephalitis, multifocal white matter disease	

syndrome, chronic neuroborreliosis, *Campylobacter jejuni*-associated AIDP and β-hemolytic *Streptococcus* infection-related diseases (usually pediatric), namely Sydenham's chorea, obsessive-compulsive disorder (OCD) and other basal ganglia abnormalities (generally described as PANDAS: pediatric autoimmune neuropsychiatric disorders associated with streptococcal infection) (Tables 1.4 and 1.5). HIV infection-related demyelinating polyneuropathy or MS-like disease may also be included in the latter group.

A similar mechanism (of molecular mimicry) is presumed to be involved in the paraneoplastic neurologic syndromes; in this case, the molecular/epitope similarity is that of neuronal antigens with proteins on the surface of neoplastic cells. The latter subgroup includes paraneoplastic cerebellar degeneration (PCD), paraneoplastic limbic encephalopathy, paraneoplastic retinal degeneration, most of the cases of LEMS, paraneoplastic sensory neuronopathy and paraneoplastic opsoclonus/myoclonus.

Table 1.4 PANDAS: diagnostic criteria

1. Onset between the age of 3 years and puberty
2. Presence of tics and/or OCD
3. Episodic clinical course
4. Symptom exacerbations may be associated with a β-hemolytic *Streptococcus* infection
5. During exacerbations: motor hyperactivity and/or chorea

Table 1.5 PANDAS versus Sydenham's chorea

Clinical features	Sydenham's chorea	PANDAS
OCD	+	+++
Involuntary movements	+++	+
Inattention	+++	+++
Emotional lability	+++	+++
Carditis	++	–
Arthritis	+	+

+ = mild; ++ = moderate; +++ = severe

Table 1.6   Classification of neuroimmune disorders and the neuroantigen involved

Disease	Antigen	Comments
Guillain–Barré syndrome (AIDP)	Peripheral nerve myelin	Multiple specificities
	GM1	*Campylobacter*-associated
	GQ1b	Fisher variant
Chronic inflammatory demyelinating polyneuropathy (CIPD)	Beta-tubulin	Microtubules
	GM1	Myelin
	P_0	Myelin
Neuropathy with monoclonal gammopathy	Myeline-associated glycoprotein (MAG)	Especially IgM
	P_0	Myelin
	PMP22	Myelin
	Glycolopids GLPGS	Nerve membrane
	GM1	Myelin
	Sulfatides	Myelin
	Chondroitin sulfate C	Nerve membrane
Myasthenia gravis	AcHR α-subunit	Motor endplate
Lambert–Eaton myasthenic syndrome	Voltage-gated calcium channels	Nerve ending
Paraneoplastic CNS syndromes		
Encephalomyelitis	Hu	
Cerebellar degeneration	Yo	Purkinje cells
Opsoclonus–myoclonus	Ri	Neuron nuclei
Retinal degeneration	CAR	Retinal antigen
Stiff-person syndrome	Amyphyphisine	Vesicle protein
Multiple sclerosis	Myelin basic proteins?	Myelin/cellular immunity
	PLP?	
	MOG?	
Rasmussen's encephalitis	Glu R3	Glutamate receptor

The third group of neuroimmune diseases includes unclassified neurologic syndromes where an immune mechanism is strongly involved in their pathogenesis, but the precise mechanism is still obscure. This group includes diseases like neurosarcoidosis and granulomatous disease of the eye orbits and the CNS (Tolosa–Hunt syndrome).

Finally, there are neurologic diseases in which the primary pathogenic mechanism is degenerative or genetic, such as inclusion body myositis, Alzheimer's disease,[26–32] cases of muscular dystrophy[33,34] and even amyotrophic lateral sclerosis[35–37] and even stroke (cerebrovascular accidents),[38–42] where inflammatory changes have been observed but their significance for the disease pathogenesis is still unknown.

In recent years an extensive effort has been made to define the neuronal antigens which are the targets of the immune insult in neuroimmune disorders. Table 1.6 depicts an update of the current knowledge in this field.

CONCLUSION

It seems that the spectrum of neuroimmune disorders is greatly expanding. As the list of these diseases is extended and our knowledge concerning the specific mechanisms and auto-antigens involved in these diseases grows, the neurologic indications for therapeutic immune intervention (immunotherapies) are also expanded. However, we should always remember that immunotherapy should not become a 'panacea' for most of the neurologic syndromes with an unknown pathogenesis, and that we must develop more strict criteria for the definition of neuroimmune disorders. Otherwise, syndromes loosely defined as neuroimmune may include a variety of diseases with sometimes similar clinical and laboratory features but different pathogenesis; in this case, the response to immunotherapy may vary from good to total unresponsiveness, and potentially useful therapies for a subgroup of the patients may be neglected due to this 'dilution' of the clinical effect of a treatment in a non-homogeneous group of patients.

REFERENCES

1. Janeway CA. How the immune system recognizes invaders. *Sci Am* 1993; **269**: 73–79.
2. Washington R, Burton J, Todd RR, Newman W, Dragovic L, Dore-Duffy P. Expression of immunologically relevant endothelial cell activation antigens on isolated central nervous system microvessels from patients with multiple sclerosis. *Ann Neurol* 1994; **35**(1): 89–97.
3. Svenningsson A, Hansson GK, Andersen O, Andersson R, Patarroyo M, Stemme S. Adhesion molecule expression on cerebrospinal fluid T lymphocytes: evidence for common recruitment mechanisms in multiple sclerosis, aseptic meningitis, and normal controls. *Ann Neurol* 1993; **34**(2): 155–161
4. Dore DP, Newman W, Balabanov R et al. Circulating, soluble adhesion proteins in cerebrospinal fluid and serum of patients with multiple sclerosis: correlation with clinical activity. *Ann Neurol* 1995; **37**(1): 55–62.
5. Bradley LM, Duncan DD, Tonkonogy S, Swin SL. Characterization of antigen-specific CD4+ effector T cells in vivo: immunization results in a transient population of MEL-14–, CD45RB– helper cells that secrete interleukin 2 (IL-2), IL-3, IL-4 and interferon gamma. *J Exp Med* 1991; **174**: 547–559.
6. Bottomly K. A functional dichotomy in CD4+ T lymphocytes. *Immunol Today* 1988; **9**: 268–274.
7. Erb P, Troxler M, Fluri M, Grogg D, Alkan SS. Functional heterogeneity of CD-4 positive T cell subsets: the correlation between effector function and lymphokine is limited. *Cell Immunol* 1991; **135**: 232–244.
8. Genain CP, Abel K, Belmar N et al. Late complications of immune deviation therapy in a nonhuman primate. *Science* 1996; **274**(5295): 2054–2057.
9. Qin Y, Van Den Noort S, Kurt J et al. Dual expression of CD45RA and CD45RO isoforms on myelin basic protein-specific CD4+ T-cell lines in multiple sclerosis. *J Clin Immunol* 1993; **13**(2): 152–161.
10. Rothstein DM, Sohen S, Daley JF, Schlossman SF, Morimoto C. CD4+CD45RA+ and CD4+CD45RA– T cell subsets in man maintain distinct function and CD45RA expression persists on a subpopulation of CD45RA+ cells after activation with Con A. *Cell Immunol* 1990; **129**(2): 449–467.
11. Yamada A, Kaneyuki T, Hara A, Rothstein DM, Yokoyama MM. CD45 isoform expression on human neonatal T cells: expression and turnover of CD45 isoforms on neonatal versus adult T cells after activation. *Cell Immunol* 1992; **142**(1): 114–124.
12. Pilarski LM, Yacyshyn BR, Jensen GS, Pruski E, Pabst HF. Beta 1 integrin (CD29) expression on human postnatal T cell subsets defined by selective CD45 isoform expression. *J Immunol* 1991; **147**(3): 830–837.
13. Bongioanni P, Fioretti C, Vanacore R et al. Lymphocyte subsets in multiple sclerosis. A study with two-colour fluorescence analysis. *J Neurol Sci* 1996; **139**(1): 71–77.
14. Calopa M, Bas J, Mestre M, Arbizu T, Peres J, Buendia E. T cell subsets in multiple sclerosis: a serial study. *Acta Neurol Scand* 1995; **92**(5): 361–368.
15. Chofflon M, Weiner HL, Morimoto C, Hafler DA. Decrease of suppressor inducer (CD4+2H4+) T cells in multiple sclerosis cerebrospinal fluid. *Ann Neurol* 1989; **25**(5): 494–499.
16. Crucian B, Dunne P, Friedman H, Ragsdale R, Pross S, Widen R. Alterations in levels of CD28–/CD8+ suppressor cell precursor and CD45RO+/CD4+ memory T lymphocytes in the peripheral blood of multiple sclerosis patients. *Clin Diagn Lab Immunol* 1995; **2**(2): 249–252.
17. Rose LM, Ginsberg AH, Rothstein TL, Ledbetter JA, Clark EA. Fluctuations of CD4+ T-cell subsets in remitting-relapsing multiple sclerosis. *Ann Neurol* 1988; **24**(2): 192–199.
18. Zaffaroni M, Gallo L, Ghezzi A, Cazzullo CL. CD4+ lymphocyte subsets in the cerebrospinal fluid of multiple sclerosis and non-inflammatory neurological diseases. *J Neurol* 1991; **238**(4): 209–211.
19. Ilonen J, Surcel HM, Jagerroos H, Nurmi T, Reunanen M. T-lymphocyte subsets defined by double immunofluorescence in multiple sclerosis. *Acta Neurol Scand* 1990; **81**(2): 128–130.
20. Neighbour PA, Grayzel AI, Miller AE. Endogenous and interferon-augmented NK cell activity of human peripheral blood mononuclear cells in vitro. Studies of patients with multiple sclerosis, systemic lupus erythematosus or rheumatoid arthritis. *Clin Exp Immunol* 1982; **49**: 11–21.
21. Bernard CCA, Carnegie PR. Experimental autoimmune encephalomyelitis in mice: immunological response to mouse spinal cord and myelin basic protein. *J Immunol* 1975; **114**: 1537–1540.
22. Lublin FD, Maurer PH, Berry RG, Tippett D. Delayed relapsing EAE in mice. *J Immunol* 1981; **126**: 819–822.
23. Saeki Y, Mima T, Sakoda S et al. Transfer of multiple sclerosis into severe combined immunodeficiency mice by mononuclear cells from cerebrospinal fluid of the patients. *Proc Natl Acad Sci USA* 1992; **89**: 6157–6161.
24. Saida T, Saida K, Dorfman SH et al. Experimental allergic neuritis induced by sensitization with galactocerebroside. *Science* 1979; **204**: 1103–1106.
25. Kennedy PG, Steiner I. On the possible viral aetiology of multiple sclerosis. *J Med* 1994; **87**(9): 523–528.
26. Aisen PS. Inflammation and Alzheimer disease. *Mol Chem Neuropathol* 1996; **28**(1): 83–88.
27. Combs CK, Johnson DE, Karlo JC, Cannady SB, Landreth GE. Inflammatory mechanisms in Alzheimer's disease: inhibition of beta-amyloid-stimulated proinflammatory responses and neurotoxicity by PPARgamma agonists. *J Neurosci* 2000; **20**(2): 558–567.
28. Eikelenboom P, Rozemuller JM, van Muiswinkel FL. Inflammation and Alzheimer's disease: relationships between pathogenic mechanisms and clinical expression. *Exp Neurol* 1998; **154**(1): 89–98.

29. Gahtan E, Overmier JB. Inflammatory pathogenesis in Alzheimer's disease: biological mechanisms and cognitive sequeli. *Neurosci Biobehav Rev* 1999; **23**(5): 615–633.

30. Halliday G, Robinson SR, Shepherd C, Kril J. Alzheimer's disease and inflammation: a review of cellular and therapeutic mechanisms. *Clin Exp Pharmacol Physiol* 2000; **27**(1–2): 1–8.

31. McGeer EG, McGeer PL. Brain inflammation in Alzheimer disease and the therapeutic implications. *Curr Pharm Des* 1999; **5**(10): 821–836.

32. Rogers J, Webster S, Lue LF et al. Inflammation and Alzheimer's disease pathogenesis. *Neurobiol Aging* 1996; **17**(5): 681–686.

33. Fitzsimons RB. Facioscapulohumeral dystrophy: the role of inflammation. *Lancet* 1994; **344**(8927): 902–903.

34. Fitzsimons RB. Facioscapulohumeral muscular dystrophy. *Curr Opin Neurol* 1999; **12**(5): 501–511.

35. Drachman DB, Kuncl RW. Amyotrophic lateral sclerosis: an unconventional autoimmune disease? *Ann Neurol* 1989; **26**(2): 269–274.

36. Sekizawa T, Openshaw H, Ohbo K, Sugamura K, Itoyama Y, Niland JC. Cerebrospinal fluid interleukin 6 in amyotrophic lateral sclerosis: immunological parameter and comparison with inflammatory and noninflammatory central nervous system diseases. *J Neurol Sci* 1998; **154**(2): 194–199.

37. Appel SH, Smith RG, Alexianu MF, Engelhardt JI, Stefani E. Autoimmunity as an etiological factor in sporadic amyotrophic lateral sclerosis. *Adv Neurol* 1995; **68**: 47–57.

38. Arvin B, Neville LF, Barone FC, Feuerstein GZ. The role of inflammation and cytokines in brain injury. *Neurosci Biobehav Rev* 1996; **20**(3): 445–452.

39. Becker KJ. Inflammation and acute stroke. *Curr Opin Neurol* 1998; **11**(1): 45–49.

40. DeGraba TJ. The role of inflammation after acute stroke: utility of pursuing anti-adhesion molecule therapy. *Neurology* 1998; **51**(3 Suppl 3): S62–S68.

41. Kogure K, Yamasaki Y, Matsuo Y, Kato H, Onodera H. Inflammation of the brain after ischemia. *Acta Neurochir Suppl* 1996; **66**: 40–43.

42. del Zoppo G, Ginis I, Hallenbeck JM, Iadecola C, Wang X, Feuerstein GZ. Inflammation and stroke: putative role for cytokines, adhesion molecules and iNOS in brain response to ischemia. *Brain Pathol* 2000; **10**(1): 95–112.

2

Heterogeneity in multiple sclerosis

Alastair Compston

INTRODUCTION

The traditional view that any disease has one cause, mechanism and phenotype fits uncomfortably with contemporary knowledge concerning many of the common neurological disorders. Not only do these complex traits arise from the interplay of several susceptibility genes but, in many instances, the disease process must also be triggered by (mostly as yet unidentified) environmental factors. Furthermore, within the context of a specific condition, tissue injury may involve a cascade of interacting but specifically different events; and, conversely, an identical set of pathological processes may be expressed as entirely different clinical phenotypes. In short, these disorders are characterized by complexity and heterogeneity, but these terms convey different meanings. Complexity defines interrelated events which are nevertheless part of the same core process. Heterogeneity implies a specifically different sequence of events, determined by variations in the interplay of aetiological factors and expressed as shared or distinct phenotypes. Alternatively, genetic or environmental conditions may modify a core process to produce both complexity and/or heterogeneity. These principles are well illustrated by reference to neurodegenerative disorders characterized by impaired memory.

COMPLEXITY AND HETEROGENEITY IN NEURODEGENERATION

Focal or generalized impairment of memory is the defining feature of many disorders which are clinically distinguishable on the basis of associated features within a complex phenotype. Thus, while confusion may arise between normal ageing, early Alzheimer's, and frontotemporal dementia or Pick's disease, few clinicians would have difficulty in distinguishing these conditions from Down's

syndrome or familial prion disease. Equally, parkinsonism, progressive supranuclear palsy, corticobasal degeneration, familial multisystem atrophy and pallidopontonigral degeneration have many features in common, but each is a distinct clinical entity recognizable by its specific phenotype. And yet, each of these disorders shares the accumulation of phosphorylated tau as the central pathological process—albeit with subtle molecular differences distinguishing the underlying type I, II or III tauopathy.[1] It takes an experienced neuropathologist reliably to unravel these various tangles containing phosphorylated tau or, at the ultrastructural level, the associated straight and curved paired helical filaments. This example illustrates that a shared pathological process may be expressed as a variety of clinical phenotypes owing to chance or stochastic events and selective tissue vulnerability arising from conditioning factors.[2] But it redirects attention to the underlying cause of diseases which must necessarily be considered as part of syndromes. Here too, it may be difficult to achieve a unitary position, and the frontotemporal dementias provide a clear example of allelic heterogeneity.[3] The phenotype is known to be associated with one of 11 mutations mainly involving exon 10 of the three tau isoforms containing four microtubule-binding repeats.[4,5]

The situation is further complicated by the fact that neurofibrillary tangles are also a core feature of Alzheimer's disease when this occurs in families with mutations of presenilin 1 or 2, in the context of amyloid precursor protein mutations, and when increased sporadic susceptibility is conferred by the ApoE4 genotype.[2] Therefore, a shared core neuropathological process (which may be associated with other specific histological features) can result from both locus and allelic heterogeneity. To add another layer of difficulty with respect to aetiology, mechanism and phenotype, some familial forms of Alzheimer's disease (often associated with mutations of presenilin 1 or 2) are associated with intracytoplasmic inclusions of α-synuclein—indistinguishable at the molecular level from the Lewy bodies typically associated with Parkinson's disease.[6,7] In this situation, a single genetic mutation (presenilin 1 or 2) is associated with more than one pathological process (tauopathy with neurofibrillary tangles and α-synucleinopathy) but with a relatively faithful clinical phenotype—at least within individual families.[2]

It is therefore clear that a number of genes, acting independently or epistatically and perhaps modified by environmental events, can confer susceptibility to several distinct pathological processes expressed as specifically different clinical phenotypes. It therefore follows that variations in clinical expression of disease (or laboratory surrogates) may indicate complexity but they do not prove heterogeneity. Since specifically different pathological features can be the expression of a single gene mutation, they also do no more than suggest heterogeneity.

COMPLEXITY AND HETEROGENEITY IN MULTIPLE SCLEROSIS

Self-evidently, the clinical phenotype of multiple sclerosis is variable with respect both to clinical features present in any one affected individual and disease patterns among groups. Clearly, the suggestion that a patient with brainstem involvement has a different disease from the individual with spinal cord involvement is not necessarily logical—these differences more probably reflect the random involvement of different sites by the same pathological process. Furthermore, there is no evidence that the patient with infrequent episodes and full recovery enjoying prolonged periods of disease inactivity necessarily has a different disease from one in whom events move quickly through the relapsing, persistent and progressive phases of the disease. That is not to say that these two extremes of clinical course are definitely expressions of the same pathological sequence; more that such variations are only evidence for complexity which may or may not indicate heterogeneity.

The clinical phenotype of multiple sclerosis

The concept of a unitary clinical phenotype for multiple sclerosis becomes more difficult when considering the minority of patients who present with primary progressive disease. The later age of onset, unusual sex distribution with a predominance of males and more severe clinical course suggest

differences which are consistent with the pathologic and T1-weighted gadolinium-enhanced magnetic resonance demonstration of fewer inflammatory lesions.[8]

One good example does exist in which a specific clinical phenotype almost certainly does represent the expression of a genuinely different pathological process, reflecting, in turn, a specific genetic background. An occasional patient who meets the clinical criteria for definite multiple sclerosis and in whom there are associated magnetic resonance imaging abnormalities and cerebrospinal fluid oligoclonal bands has an illness in which there is disproportionate involvement of the anterior visual pathway. These are commonly women with male relatives already known to be affected by Leber's hereditary optic neuropathy and they have pathological mutations of mitochondrial DNA.[9] Harding's disease therefore represents true heterogeneity in that a specific genotype determines a characteristic phenotype. What remains unresolved is whether the mutation of mitochondrial DNA focuses the non-specific process of brain inflammation onto a particular site—constituting selective tissue vulnerability—or (as some have suggested) the condition is nothing more than a chance occurrence of relatively mild multiple sclerosis and coincident Leber's hereditary optic neuropathy. The latter interpretation seems highly improbable, given the number of cases of Harding's disease already described and the rarity of isolated Leber's hereditary optic neuropathy in women.

Another probable example of true heterogeneity is the distinct phenotype of demyelinating disease seen in Orientals and Africans. In Japan, multiple sclerosis shows either a so-called Western phenotype, in which a number of sites are involved, or an opticospinal pattern in which the clinical picture is dominated by involvement of visual and spinal cord pathways.[10] In its extreme form this mimics Devic's disease—a disorder which also occurs in Europeans, albeit rarely. Demyelinating disease is considered to be extremely rare in Africans but a number of cases have been described and clinical experience suggests that the phenotype is typically a severe illness dominated by one or more episodes usually affecting the anterior visual pathway and spinal cord—again combining the anatomical features of Devic's disease with the clinical course of moderately severe relapsing—remitting multiple sclerosis.[11] Unlike for Harding's disease, the evidence that this represents disease heterogeneity, arising from specific genetic or environmental modification of a core pathological process, remains circumstantial.

The pathogenesis of multiple sclerosis

The patient with multiple sclerosis faces an uncertain future, typically characterized by a course which is initially intermittent, leading to episodes with incomplete recovery, and finally slow progression. This pattern raises fundamental questions concerning the aetiology of inflammatory brain disease, the basis for symptom onset and recovery, and the nature of injury and repair of the central nervous system.

Perivascular inflammation leads to oligodendrocyte depletion, demyelination, remyelination, astrocytosis and axon degeneration. The precise sequence and relationship of these components is debated. Endothelial cells entangle inflammatory cells as they pass along the vessel wall. Infiltrating lymphocytes not activated against brain antigen return to the circulation or die by apoptosis. Chemokines interacting with specific receptors on migrating cells promote the outward migration of immune cells from the inflammatory nidus, and metalloproteases degrade tissue barriers. Proinflammatory cytokines amplify the immune response. Activated microglia degrade the oligodendrocyte–myelin unit if this is opsonized with ligands for (Fc and complement) receptors through release of cell-surface-bound tumour necrosis factor alpha (TNF-α). There may be contributions to recovery from removal of proinflammatory cytokines restoring conduction through myelinated axons which were never structurally damaged, rearrangement of sodium channels providing a variety of alternative patterns of conduction, and remyelination which is inhibited by astrocyte reactivity.

Much emphasis has been placed on the contribution of axon degeneration in both acute and chronic phases of the disease. Immunohistochemical staining for the amyloid precursor protein shows that axonal injury is initiated as part of the acute demyelinating episode.[12,13] Transection appears early and the circumstantial evidence suggests vulnerability of recently demyelinated axons to the inflammatory environment of acute lesions.[14] But there is also a chronic attrition which may be degenerative and secondary to loss of the trophic support normally provided by myelin. Acute lesions sometimes show an increase in the number of oligodendrocytes, indicating recruitment of new progenitors which then undergo differentiation.[15]

Axons in acute shadow plaques have undergone remyelination. Experimentally, remyelination can restore structure and function[16] but—in a clinical context—new myelin may not survive repeated injury. The source of remyelinating cells is presumed to be the oligodendrocyte progenitor which is found in the lesions of multiple sclerosis.[17,18] These and related clinical observations[19] indicate that inflammation is necessary for new lesion formation and conditions axon degeneration. Remyelination is associated with active inflammation and reactive astrocytosis, which deliver cytokines and growth factors to the lesion so that anti-inflammatory treatment need not to compromise the repair of demyelinated axons.

Variations in imaging protocol can be used to delineate some but not all features of the pathological process leading to demyelination and astrocytosis. There is preliminary evidence for differences in the regional distribution of lesions defined by T2-weighted imaging (which essentially depicts water accumulation in association with astrocytosis) and T1-weighted gadolinium enhancement, which images the inflammatory component.[20] The fact that these two principal types of lesion show significant differences in their anatomical clustering is at least consistent with the hypothesis that inflammation, demyelination and astrocytosis do not invariably follow in an orderly sequence but may arise independently as the expression of specifically different sequences of events. The same interpretation arises from histological comparison of the distribution of inflammation and axon injury.[13]

The concept of pathogenic heterogeneity is further developed in the recent pathological studies using biopsy and autopsy material, in which four distinct types of disease process are proposed.[21] Type 1 constitutes perivenous inflammation with a sharp definition to the edge of the lesion and significant remyelination; this occurs in patients with clinically definite multiple sclerosis usually in the relapsing phase and in only a small number of progressive cases. Type 2 consists of perivenous demyelination with local deposition of immunoglobulin and terminal complement components within sharply defined lesions also having remyelination; these patients have clinically definite multiple sclerosis with an equal distribution of relapsing and progressive cases. Type 3 lacks perivenous inflammation and the lesions are ill-defined with evidence for oligodendrocyte apoptosis; these features are also seen in areas of tissue ischaemia, and the clinical course is usually an acute monophasic illness with fewer cases of relapsing–remitting definite multiple sclerosis. Type 4 consists of perivenous inflammation with sharply defined lesions but oligodendrocyte loss in the normal-appearing white matter; these cases typically have primary progressive involvement of the cerebrum, cerebellum or brainstem. As with variations in the clinical phenotype, these histopathological patterns per se are better described as complexity rather than heterogeneity, unless and until specifically different aetiological factors can be linked to each type. In these preliminary assessments, types 3 and 4 are considered to represent a primary viral or ischaemic pathogenesis, whereas the hypothesis is that types 1 and 2 depend on specifically different combinations of genetic predisposing factors. This is of course entirely speculative but indicates the need to link aetiology to pathogenesis and phenotype before patterns of true heterogeneity can reliably be defined. More compelling is the evidence that these histopathological lesions cluster within patients. Each lesion from a given case offers the same histological features, arguing against the interpretation that these types represent phases in the temporal evolution of tissue injury and not aetiologically determined heterogeneity.

It is therefore necessary to consider the evidence for differences in aetiological factors which orchestrate the sequence of pathological events in multiple sclerosis.

The genetics of multiple sclerosis

Population studies
Multiple sclerosis has a familial recurrence rate of about 20%. The highest risk is for siblings, but within this category different recurrence rates are observed for identical twins (1:3), dizygotic twins (1:20), other siblings (1:20), half-siblings (1:50) and non-biological relatives adopted into families (1:400). The risk for children of a conjugal pair (1:5) is much higher than for the offspring of a single affected parent (1:50) and adoptees (1:400). Because multiple sclerosis usually manifests in early adult life, all these recurrence rates show age-specific differences, with a substantial reduction for family members remaining unaffected beyond the age of 50 years.[22]

Strategies for genetic analysis: case–control studies
Unlike in monogenic disorders, the genes responsible for complex traits are not mutations which code for aberrant gene products but normal polymorphisms. They are several, acting independently or through epistasis, and each may exert a very small contributory effect on some as yet undefined structure or physiological function.

Originally, the search for genes determining susceptibility to complex disease was organized by comparing the frequency of polymorphisms at a given genetic locus in groups of unrelated individuals with and without the trait. These population-based association studies were limited by the number of polymorphic systems which could be explored, the paucity of the hypotheses which directed the search to a particular region of interest, and the confounding effects of inappropriate choice of controls. However, an important principle to emerge was that (to a varying extent) alleles encoded at neighbouring loci tend to cosegregate. It seems that many adjacent markers are not yet randomly distributed by genetic recombinations, either because the number of generations over which mitoses have occurred is still too few to establish genetic equilibrium, or because there is evolutionary pressure to maintain these linkage disequilibria. From the practical point of view, this means that association studies can be informative even when the marker is up to 0.5 centiMorgans (cM) distant from the disease susceptibility locus. But the corollary is that identification of an associated allele provides no information on the identity of the functional polymorphism encoded in that region which is influencing susceptibility or some aspect of the disease course.

The probability of locus heterogeneity is suggested by detailed analysis of the most secure finding with respect to genetic susceptibility in multiple sclerosis—association with alleles of the major histocompatibility complex. The primary association in most northern European populations is with the DR15/DQ6 phenotype and its associated DRB1*1501–DRB5*0101–DQA1*0102–DQB1*0602 genotype.[23] There is a subsidiary association with DR3 (DR17)–DQ2 and its associated DRB1*0301–DRB5*0101–DQA1*0501–DQB1*0201 genotype. In some Mediterranean populations, notably Sardinian, there is an increased frequency of DR3 (DR17) but the main association is with DR4 and its associated DRB1*0405–DQA1*0301–DQB1*0302 genotype.[24] Although DR4 is also associated with multiple sclerosis in patients from the Canary Islands and Turkey, this DR4 haplotype is different from that found in Sardinians. Here, there is evidence for specifically different HLA associations which cannot be explained by site-specific similarities in sequence of the crucial elements binding peptide. The implication must be that either these polymorphisms are in linkage disequilibrium with a ubiquitous gene encoded within the major histocompatibility complex (which may or may not have a primary immunological function) or that the environmental trigger which initiates the disease process in multiple sclerosis varies and so selects specifically different genetic populations as maximally at risk.

This evidence for genetic heterogeneity is strengthened by the probability that the primary progressive form of multiple sclerosis seen in northern Europeans is also DR4-associated. The evidence is not entirely secure and the original finding from Scandinavia[25] was not easily replicated. There is support from a more recent study of primary progressive multiple sclerosis in Spain,[26] although a definitive study is needed. The best present position would be that the primary progressive phenotype does have an individual pathological profile (less inflammation and more focal axon degeneration) and occurs on a specifically different genetic background. Furthermore, only the opticospinal type of multiple sclerosis is associated with DPB1*0501 in northern and southern Japan, whereas the western type is DRB1*1501-associated.[27]

Strategies for genetic analysis: family-based linkage studies

Laboratory methods for distinguishing short sections of DNA, accurate mapping of the many available microsatellites and single nucleotide polymorphisms (SNPs) across the genome, availability of extended pedigrees in which affected status can reliably be determined, and deployment of appropriate statistical methods for assessing genome-wide significance, have collectively made it possible to tackle the genetics of complex traits in more detail.[28] Linkage analysis in affected family members either selects candidates based on a priori considerations of disease pathogenesis or performs systematic screens of the whole genome, using evenly spaced microsatellite markers or (in the future) SNPs. Six genome screens have now been completed using microsatellites, but none has reliably identified a chromosomal region which is certain to encode a susceptibility gene for multiple sclerosis.[29–34] Nevertheless, the degree of overlap between two or more screens allows certain regions of interest to be identified with reasonable confidence and, from this selection, allows the opportunity for studying new positional candidates based on mechanistic hypotheses and genetic mapping—an exercise which has gathered momentum with the availability of a first full map of the human genome.

Since the power of a linkage genome screen is critically dependent on the frequency of susceptibility alleles in the population studied, and is thus expected to vary between populations, linkage analysis may still be worth pursuing in a population where the frequency of susceptibility alleles is more favourable for historical reasons. When a small family population expands numerically in relative isolation, genetic drift can dramatically influence the frequency of mutant and polymorphic alleles. As a consequence, some genetically determined diseases may occur at higher than expected frequency. Isolated populations such as Finns, Sardinians, Icelanders and Tasmanians could provide special opportunities for resolving the issue of genetic susceptibility to complex traits such as multiple sclerosis. However, a recent genome-wide linkage screen in the largest available sample of Sardinian families with multiple sclerosis, while identifying three regions of interest (1q31, 10q23 and 11p15), nevertheless continues to show only modest evidence for linkage and fails to confirm the hypothesis that susceptibility genes might more easily be identified by family-based linkage in a small but genetically informative isolated population.[33]

This failure to identify with confidence regions of interest conferring disease susceptibility both in mixed and isolated European populations, each having a high prevalence of multiple sclerosis, has obvious implications for future genetic analyses of complex traits. Linkage data should be added from new populations with the aim of confirming and excluding regions of interest but, meanwhile, continued scrutiny of the human genome map for positional candidates may shorten the search for genes that determine susceptibility and influence the course of multiple sclerosis.

Meta-analysis has been explored in the expectation that this will reduce the evidence for false-positive peaks and strengthen the candidature of those which are genuine.[35] However, this assumes that genes conferring susceptibility to multiple sclerosis are shared between populations especially if data sets are combined from ethnically diverse groups. In reality, it is probable that ubiquitous genes do exist which increase susceptibility to core aspects of the pathological process in multiple sclerosis—and perhaps also other autoimmune diseases—whereas others are restricted to particular populations. These considerations are clearly important when looking at meta-analyses, but the exercise has proved useful in selecting regions for the further study of positional candidates and establishing the probability that, in addition to the major histocompatibility complex, certain regions may encode genes which confer susceptibility across a range of autoimmune diseases.[36] This interpretation is consistent with the results of population-based studies demonstrating an increased recurrence risk for a variety of autoimmune diseases in the relatives of patients with multiple sclerosis—implicating, in particular, autoimmune thyroid disease.[37]

The lessons learned thus far from the analysis of complex traits, especially multiple sclerosis, are that no one gene makes a dominant contribution to susceptibility, although collectively their attributable risk determines a relative risk for siblings of around ×20. Knowing that multiple sclerosis is both linked and associated with the HLA-DR locus allows re-evaluation of the contribution made by other genomic regions on the basis of a stratified analysis. In the UK affected sibling pair survey, regions of interest clustered in those families which showed linkage to DR15 (1p, 5q, 17p, 17q and x), whereas others grouped with the non-DR15-sharing families (1 cen, 5 cen, 7p, 14q and 22q).[38] A further potential dividend from conditioning analyses is that regions which do not show any evidence for linkage using all families emerge as linked to the disease in one or other of the stratified groups. For example, there is evidence for linkage on 5q and 13p in DR15-sharing families and linkage to 16p and 20p in non-DR15-sharing families. These are not regions previously implicated as potential susceptibility loci in multiple sclerosis. Furthermore, conditioning for DR15 resolves broad sections of apparent linkage into discrete regions of interest, and this is especially evident on chromosomes 1 and 5. Thus, as knowledge accumulates, conditioned analyses may be essential in order to suggest or exclude new regions of interest or positional candidate susceptibility genes.

The presence of phenocopies is a major concern in the analysis of complex traits, where diagnosis depends on pattern recognition of symptoms, signs and laboratory investigations occurring in the absence of a test for the disease. Reassuringly, the cohort of cases included in the UK linkage genome screen was not contaminated by examples of cerebral autosomal-dominant arteriopathy with subcortical infarcts and leukoencephalopathy (CADASIL), spinocerebellar degenerations or adrenoleukodystrophy (in male–male pairs). However, this search did identify a potentially important aspect of genetic heterogeneity which may have implications for selective tissue vulnerability. Although there were no individuals having an excess of triplet repeats for SCA2, the 22-kb allele occurred at a higher frequency in cases than controls reported in the literature. This result prompted an assessment of transmission disequilibrium in family trios (see below) which supported an association between multiple sclerosis and the 22-kb allele.[39] A second data set showed similar findings, although the evidence for association weakened (S. Sawcer, unpublished observations). If confirmed, one interpretation of this finding would be that, in individuals who have a tendency

for autoimmunity as a result of the interplay between genetic susceptibility and environmental factors, the inflammatory process may be focused onto a particular system or pathway within the brain and spinal cord in those who have genetic polymorphisms exposing that pathway to tissue injury. In the case of SCA2, individuals with the normal 22-kb allele polymorphism may have disproportionate inflammatory demyelination of the spinocerebellar pathways—similar by analogy to involvement of the anterior visual pathway in Harding's disease.

Strategies for genetic analysis: family-based association

An alternative approach has been the use of family-based association methods in which the test is to show that a particular allele of a candidate gene, or a polymorphic marker in linkage disequilibrium with that gene, is transmitted to affected individuals more often than expected by chance. Transmission disequilibrium testing (TDT) uses trios consisting of single affecteds with both parents who are usually (but neeed not be) unaffected. Each parental allele has a 1:2 chance of being transmitted. The test provides evidence for an allelic association by demonstrating excess transmission, and identifies that allele which is responsible for disequilibrium in the sample. Although not every family will be informative, it follows that those markers which are in linkage disequilibrium with susceptibility genes for multiple sclerosis will be adequately represented. One further factor limiting the extent to which the sample of family trios may not prove fully informative for a particular polymorphic locus is the presence of homozygote parents. These are rejected in the analysis because the transmitted allele cannot be identified. Segregation distortion arises when a particular allele confers a survival advantage and therefore appears to be disproportionately transmitted. This allele will be preferentially transmitted to all surviving offspring, whether or not they have the disease trait in question. The issue can be resolved by studying affected and unaffected children in family quartets. But a new problem then arises which is offset by the affected family member approach, and that is the difficulty in assigning unaffected status to a young adult in a disease which may not manifest clinically until late in life—if at all, given the prevalence of pathologically verified but clinically silent disease in autopsy series. Because it is very unlikely that an investigator will choose to test for transmission disequilibrium at exactly the locus which encodes a disease susceptibility gene contributing to a complex trait, the dividend from family-based association methods depends crucially on the existence of linkage disequilibrium, and this is not resolved.[40] In this respect, TDT is no more or less constrained than case–control studies—TDT offering a more robust method but with lower statistical power than population associations detected in unrelated individuals. Conversely, TDT is statistically more powerful than family linkage for genes of small effect.

Linkage and association therefore provide different types of information. Each has its limitations and advantages. Assuming a reasonable sample size, any marker which is well distant from the true susceptibility locus will be linked but not associated. A marker which is close to the susceptibility locus will not be linked in sibling pairs if the sample size is inadequate (as are most currently available sibling pair studies) but it may nevertheless be associated. Only the combination of a close marker and an adequate sample will demonstrate both linkage and association.

Based on current strategies for complex traits and the available results, it might seem logical to focus entirely on family-based association studies. Here, the problem is that, for a systematic search, the extent of linkage disequilibrium in outbred populations demands a very dense set of microsatellite markers or SNPs and therefore a prodigious amount of genotyping. This can be reduced during the screening phase through the use of samples in which equal amounts of DNA from a large number of cases, controls or parents are pooled into a single sample and screened against a panel of microsatellites. Pooling can detect allelic frequency differences of about 5%. Thus one strategy is first to screen the genome with linkage to establish regions of interest and then to refine the map with TDT. However, whole genome linkage disequilibrium screening is now feasible. Power calculations indicate that the resource needed reliably to demonstrate transmission disequilibrium is much more attainable than that required for linkage. The density of markers must be sufficient to cover regions which are not in linkage disequilibrium (probably extending to no more than 0.25 cM), whereas linkage provides much greater topographical information for a given genotyping effort. Thus, a trade-off exists between the ease of collecting a definitive clinical resource and the laboratory work needed to screen the genome using family linkage and association methods. In addition to their disappointing initial showing in linkage screens in multiple sclerosis, genetic isolates having a high disease prevalence may also not confer an advantage through retaining

much more extensive linkage disequilibrium than outbred populations.[41,42]

The Genetic Analysis of Multiple sclerosis in EuropeanS (GAMES)

The burden of multiple sclerosis is not evenly distributed but is concentrated in northern Europe and in those regions where northern Europeans have migrated.[43] Although this distribution may in part relate to varying environmental risk-factor exposure, it also suggests a contribution from susceptibility genes which are presumed to have been distributed with the migration of northern Europeans. A European origin for genetic susceptibility in multiple sclerosis underlines the logic of studying susceptibility among the present populations of Europe and neighbouring regions. The varying frequency of multiple sclerosis in Europe is consistent with a dilution effect of genetic susceptibility factors originating in the north. This distribution has important consequences, since the power of genetic analysis is influenced by the regional frequency of each susceptibility allele. Paradoxically, the probability of detection is reduced where susceptibility factors are over-represented in the at-risk population or, conversely, very infrequent, since, although these fluctuations determine disease frequency, they also act to minimize the difference between cases and controls. Thus, the power to identify any susceptibility factor varies across the continent. It follows that some factors will be more easily detected in one place and others in another. Since it is not possible to anticipate in advance which regions will offer the greatest power to identify each susceptibility factor, a pan-European collaboration is necessary and can be expected to be highly informative.

Based on existing results, linkage disequilibrium mapping will be needed in order to advance knowledge on genetic susceptibility in multiple sclerosis. GAMES is predicated on the hypothesis that susceptibility factors in different parts of Europe will be identical by descent. If so, map resolution will be significantly improved by comparing different regions. Common ancestors for the various European populations are relatively ancient, and thus the identification of the same susceptibility haplotypes in different populations which are shown to be identical by descent will provide tighter resolution for the location of each susceptibility locus than can be achieved by studying these populations in isolation. The available linkage data in multiple sclerosis indicate that the genetic effect attributable to each susceptibility locus is modest and therefore the number of families required for a definitive study correspondingly large and almost certainly beyond the scope of any one investigator.

GAMES is planned to take forward the existing evidence from linkage to full linkage disequilibrium genome screens in the interval before new technologies for high-resolution mapping of susceptibility genes using SNPs become available.[28] GAMES assumes that several genes which vary in their frequency among at-risk populations contribute to susceptibility in multiple sclerosis and recognizes that the opportunity for identifying each will vary between populations. Factors which are universally present or absent in a given area will be very hard to identify, since they will invariably be either present or absent from cases and controls whereas the best opportunity may arise from the study of risk factors which have a moderate population frequency. GAMES acknowledges that the number of families needed to demonstrate linkage of genes conferring an excess risk of less than 1.5 may be several thousand and will therefore focus on linkage disequilibrium screening in case–control and family-based association methods. GAMES assumes that the extent of linkage disequilibrium in the outbred European population averages around 0.25 cM, making it necessary to screen the genome with more than 20 times as many markers as have been used collectively in linkage genome screens.

Therefore, GAMES will: (1) Use 6000 microsatellite markers to screen the genome; (2) compare cases and controls ($n = > 200$ of each) using pooled DNA to identify regions of interest; (3) confirm their status in pooled DNA from > 200 additional cases and their parents; (4) type these (or ideally a third set of 200) families individually across all emerging regions of interest; (5) preserve investigator independence but commit to a meta-analysis, posted at http://www.mrc-bsu.cam.ac.uk/MSgenetics; (6) create separate pools for primary progressive and relapsing secondary progressive forms of multiple sclerosis; (7) use strict diagnostic criteria and follow-up of individual cases in order later to stratify the analysis for genotypic and phenotypic subgroups reclassified using revised criteria;[44] (8) where more than 100 affected sibling pairs are available, carry out a conventional linkage genome screen in order to identify provisional regions of interest, since cumulative experience of linkage analysis in Europe should eventually cross the threshold for reliably identifying regions of interest; and (9) reduce the number of families required for linkage analysis in genetic isolates to 40.

GAMES predicts that: (1) some regions of interest will disappear—the *false positives*; (2) other regions of interest will be shared, to a varying extent, between players—the *ubiquitous* genes; and (3) some regions of interest will be confined to selected players—the *domestic genes*—providing evidence both for the effects of single quantitative traits and true heterogeneity which may be expressed as distinct clinical or laboratory phenotypes.

GAMES players are defined as: type 1—those performing the experiment in their own laboratory on receipt of the shared set of markers; type 2—those preferring to send an investigator with pooled DNA to one of two typing centres; type 3—those electing to collect DNA, create a pool and send this to one of the typing centres for local staff to complete the experiment; and type 4—those identifying cases but requiring an investigator from the coordinating centre to create the pool and type this at one of the central facilities. GAMES brings together collaborative European and Middle East ethnic groups representing regions of high, intermediate and low disease frequency. These are: Australia, Belgium, Cyprus, Denmark, Finland, France, Germany, Greece, Hungary, Iceland, Italy, The Netherlands, Norway, Poland, Portugal, Spain and the Canaries, Sweden, Turkey, and the UK.

CONCLUSIONS

Resolving the issues of complexity and heterogeneity in multiple sclerosis, and other complex traits, has practical dividends. Without knowledge linking aetiology to pathogenesis and phenotype, putative new treatments—selected on the basis of an imperfect understanding of the pathogenesis—will continue to be screened in cohorts who may or may not have an appropriate pathological substrate for that particular intervention.

REFERENCES

1. Spillantini MG, Goedert M. Tau protein pathology in neurodegenerative diseases. *Trends Neurosci* 1998; **21**: 428–433.
2. Hardy J, Gwinn-Hardy K. Genetic classification of primary neurodegenerative disease. *Science* 1998; **282**: 1075–1078.
3. Bird TD. Genotypes, phenotypes, and frontotemporal dementia. *Neurology* 1998; **50**: 1526–1527.
4. Spillantini MG, Van Swieten JC, Goedert M. Tau gene mutations in frontotemporal dementia and parkinsonism linked to chromosome 17 (FTDP-17). *Neurogenetics* 2000; **2**: 193–205.
5. Van Swieten JC, Stevens M, Rosso SM et al. Phenotypic variation in hereditary frontotemporal dementia with tau mutations. *Ann Neurol* 1999; **46**: 617–626.
6. Spillantini MG, Bird TD, Ghetti B et al. Frontotemporal dementia and parkinsonism linked to chromosome 17: a new group of tauopathies. *Brain Pathol* 1998; **8**: 387–403.

7. Spillantini MG, Crowther RA, Jakes R et al. α-Synuclein in filamentous inclusions of Lewy bodies from Parkinson's disease and dementia with Lewy bodies. *Proc Natl Acad Sci USA* 1998; **95**: 6469–6473.

8. Thompson AJ, Polman CH, Miller DH et al. Primary progressive multiple sclerosis (review). *Brain* 1997; **120**: 1085–1096.

9. Harding AE, Sweeney MG, Brockington M et al. Occurrence of a multiple sclerosis-like illness in women who have a Leber's hereditary optic neuropathy mitochondrial DNA mutation. *Brain* 1992; **115**: 979–989.

10. Yamasaki K, Horiuchi I, Minohara M et al. HLA-DPB1*0501-associated opticospinal multiple sclerosis: clinical, neuroimaging and immunogenetic studies. *Brain* 1999; **122**: 1689–1696.

11. Dean G, Bhighee AIG, Bill PLA et al. Multiple sclerosis in black South Africans and Zimbabweans. *J Neurol Neurosurg Psychiatry* 1994; **57**: 1064–1069.

12. Ferguson B, Matyszak MK, Esiri MM, Perry VH. Axonal damage in acute multiple sclerosis lesions. *Brain* 1997; **120**: 393–399.

13. Bitsch A, Schuchardt S, Bunkowski S, Kuhlmann T, Bruck W. Acute axonal injury in multiple sclerosis: correlation with demyelination and inflammation. *Brain* 2000; **123**: 1174–1183.

14. Trapp BD, Peterson J, Ransohoff RM et al. Axonal transection in the lesions of multiple sclerosis. *N Engl J Med* 1998; **338**: 278–285.

15. Luchinetti C, Bruck W, Parisi J et al. A quantitative analysis of oligodendrocytes multiple sclerosis lesions: a study of 117 cases. *Brain* 1999; **122**: 2279–2295.

16. Jeffery ND, Blakemore WF. Locomotor deficits induced by experimental spinal cord demyelination are abolished by spontaneous remyelination. *Brain* 1997; **120**: 27–37.

17. Scolding N, Franklin R, Stevens S et al. Oligodendrocyte progenitors are present in the normal adult human CNS and in the lesions of multiple sclerosis. *Brain* 1998; **121**: 2221–2228.

18. Wolswijk G. Chronic stage multiple sclerosis lesions contain a relatively quiescent population of oligodendrocyte precursor cells. *J Neurosci* 1998; **18**: 601–609.

19. Coles AJ, Paolili A, Molyneux P et al. Monoclonal antibody treatment exposes three mechanisms underlying the clinical course in multiple sclerosis. *Ann Neurol* 1999; **46**: 296–304.

20. Lee MA, Smith S, Palace J et al. Spatial mapping of T_2 and gadolinium-enhancing T_1 lesion volumes in multiple sclerosis: evidence for distinct mechanisms of lesion genesis. *Brain* 1999; **122**: 1261–1270.

21. Lucchinetti C, Bruck W, Parisi J et al. Heterogeneity for multiple sclerosis lesions: implications for the pathogenesis of demyelination. *Ann Neurol* 2000; **47**: 707–717.

22. Compston DAS. The genetic epidemiology of multiple sclerosis. *Phil Trans R Soc Lond B* 1999; **354**: 1623–1634.

23. Olerup O, Hillert J. HLA class II-associated genetic susceptibility in multiple sclerosis: a critical evaluation. *Tissue Antigens* 1991; **38**: 1–15.

24. Marrosu MG, Muntoni F, Murru MR et al. HLA-DQB1 genotype in Sardinian multiple sclerosis: evidence for a key role of DQB1.0201 and DQB1.0302 alleles. *Neurology* 1992; **42**: 883–886.

25. Hillert J, Gronning M, Hyland H, Link H, Olerup O. Immunogenetic heterogeneity in multiple sclerosis. *J Neurol Neurosurg Psychiatry* 1992; **55**: 887–890.

26. de la Concha EG, Arroyo R, Crusius JB et al. Combined effect of HLA-DRB1*1501 and interleukin-1 receptor antagonist gene allele 2 in susceptibility to relapsing/remitting multiple sclerosis. *J Neuroimmunol* 1997; **80**: 172–178.

27. Ma JJ, Nishimura M, Mine H et al. HLA-DRB1 and tumor necrosis factor gene polymorphisms in Japanese patients with multiple sclerosis. *J Neuroimmunol* 1998; **92**: 109–112.

28. Risch NJ. Searching for genetic determinants in the new millennium. *Nature* 2000; **405**: 847–856.

29. Sawcer S, Jones HB, Feakes R et al. A genome screen in multiple sclerosis reveals susceptibility loci on chromosome 6p21 and 17q22. *Nature Genet* 1996; **13**: 464–468.

30. Ebers GC, Kukay K, Bulman D et al. A full genome search in multiple sclerosis. *Nature Genet* 1996; **13**: 472–476.

31. Haines JL, Ter-Minassian M, Bazyk A et al. A complete genomic screen for multiple sclerosis underscores a role for the major histocompatibility complex. *Nature Genet* 1996; **13**: 469–471.

32. Kuokkanen S, Sundvall M, Terwilliger JD et al. A putative vulnerability locus to multiple sclerosis maps to 5p14–p12 in a region syntenic to the murine locus Eae2. *Nature Genet* 1996; **13**: 477–480.

33. Coraddu F, Sawcer S, D'Alfonso S et al. A genome screen for multiple sclerosis in Sardinian multiplex families. *Am J Human Genet* (in press).

34. Broadley S, Sawcer S, D'Alfonso et al. A genome screen for multiple sclerosis in Italian families. *Genes and Immunity* (in press).

35. The Transatlantic Multiple Sclerosis Genetics Cooperative. A meta-analysis of genome screens in multiple sclerosis. *Mult Scler* 2001; **7**: 3–11.

36. Becker KG, Simon RM, Bailey-Wilson JE. Clustering of non-major histocompatibility complex susceptibility candidate loci in human autoimune disease. *Proc Natl Acad Sci USA* 1998; **95**: 9979–9984.

37. Broadley S, Deans J, Sawcer SJ, Clayton D, Compston DAS. Autoimmune disease in first degree relatives of patients with multiple sclerosis in the United Kingdom. *Brain* 2000; **123**: 1102–1111.

38. Coraddu F, Sawcer S, Feakes R et al. HLA typing in the United Kingdom multiple sclerosis genome screen. *Neurogenetics* 1999; **2**: 24–33.

39. Chataway J, Sawcer S, Coraddu F et al. Allelic variants of the spinocerebellar ataxia genes contribute to multiple sclerosis susceptibility. *Neurogenetics* 1999; **2**: 91–96.

40. Kruglyak L. Prospects for whole-genome linkage disequilibrium mapping of common disease genes. *Nature Genet* 1999; **22**: 139–144.

41. Eaves IA, Merriman TR, Barber RA et al. The genetically isolated populations of Finland and Sardinia may not be a panacea for linkage disequilibrium mapping of common disease genes. *Nature Genet* 2000; **25**: 320–323.

42. Taillon-Miller P, Bauer-Sardina I, Saccone NL et al. Juxtaposed regions of extensive and minimal linkage disequilibrium in human Xq25 and Xq28. *Nature Genet* 2000; **25**: 324–328.

43. Compston DAS. Distribution of multiple sclerosis. In: Compston DAS, Ebers GC, Lassmann H, McDonald I, Matthews WB, Wekerle H, eds. *McAlpine's Multiple Sclerosis*, 3rd edn. London: Churchill Livingstone 1998, 63–100.

44. McDonald WI, Compston DAS, Edan G et al. International panel on the diagnosis of MS: new diagnostic criteria for MS. *Am Neurol* 2001 (in press).

3

Microglia and brain macrophages

Jack P Antel and Rosanne Seguin

INTRODUCTION

The immune system can be divided into two functionally distinct arms: the innate and the adaptive immune responses. As the name suggests, adaptive immune responses change and become enhanced following encounters with foreign material, resulting in amplified and specific immune responses against foreign targets. In contrast, the innate immune arm lacks this specificity, as it fails to discriminate among most foreign substances, and is not enhanced with each subsequent exposure. Both T- and B-lymphocytes are members of the adaptive immune response, while phagocytic cells such as neutrophils and macrophages, and circulating components of complement, are members of the innate immune response. It is important, however, as discussed later, to consider innate and adaptive immune arms as being integrated rather than separate and independent.[1]

We will consider the role of microglia and macrophages in the central nervous system (CNS) in the context of their physiological role in the systemic compartment. Stem cells in the bone marrow differentiate into monocytes which exit from the bone marrow to circulate throughout the body. Following entry into tissue, monocytes may differentiate fully into macrophages. Macrophages, as the name suggests, are 'big eaters', in that they engulf foreign targets and even self-tissues that have been injured or have died. Following internalization of the material, macrophages destroy the material by lysosomal enzymes. In addition to phagocytosis, macrophages secrete mediators that kill microbes and control the spread of infection. These toxins, however, may also injure normal cells in the immediate vicinity. Besides the production of chemokines and cytokines, macrophages secrete growth factors which may be used in repair of tissues.[2] These functions may be categorized as innate immune responses. Nevertheless, macrophages also provide an important link between innate and adaptive immune functions. Lymphocytes, the cells that specifically recognize and respond to foreign antigens, rely on the release of chemokines and cytokines by the innate immune cells for attraction to the site of infection. T-helper lymphocytes depend on non-lymphoid cells, called accessory cells, which include monocytes, macrophages and dendritic cells, for the presentation of molecules from foreign targets in a context that can be recognized by the T-helper lymphocytes.[2] These antigen-presenting cells (APCs) are required for maturation and activation of T-helper cells. However, along with the influence of macrophages on lymphocyte functions, there is also a bidirectional response whereby antigen-stimulated T-cells secrete cytokines, which in turn activate macrophages for phagocytosis and secretion of toxic molecules. Similarly, B-lymphocytes and, more specifically, their antibody products interact with macrophages such that once foreign material is coated by antibodies it can then readily be phagocytosed by macrophages, a process referred to as antibody-dependent cell cytotoxicity (ADCC). Therefore, in the periphery, macrophages not only act within the innate immune response to remove foreign material but also interact with adaptive immune responses, with the end-result of enhanced functions for both immune arms.

As regards the CNS, residing within the perivascular spaces surrounding cerebral and meningeal blood vessels are the perivascular macrophages. These cells are slowly but continuously replaced by blood-derived cells of the monocyte/macrophage lineage.[3] Distributed in the CNS parenchyma are the resident microglia, which are derived from bone marrow precursors that enter the CNS during early fetal development.[4–7] In contrast to astrocytes, which appear to play a role in the homeostatic control of the normal neuronal extracellular environment,[8] parenchymal microglia appear to mediate important functions when the brain has been damaged.[9] In normal conditions, microglia appear as ramified cells, characteristic of resting tissue macrophages, but progressively acquire a clear-cut activated macrophage phenotype in response to CNS inflammation and neuronal or myelin damage.[3] As both perivascular macrophages and microglia are derived from the same parental cell source, and there is currently a lack of truly microglia-specific antibodies, these cells may be considered collectively as 'brain macrophages'.

The brain has been considered to be an 'immunologically privileged' organ, in part due to the blood–brain barrier (BBB), which restricts immune cell entry into the CNS, and the lack of lymphatics, which limits egress of antigen from the CNS.[10] CNS-derived antigens are therefore not easily accessible to immune cells, so it was believed that the immune and nervous systems were separate. However, recent evidence suggests that resident immune cells of the CNS actively participate in communicating with the immune cells of the periphery, such that both innate and adaptive immune responses occur in the CNS. As demonstrated by neuroinflammatory disorders, large numbers of leukocytes can be recruited following chemokine release to the CNS from the periphery. The disruptive inflammation associated with the disease multiple sclerosis (MS) is believed to be initiated and perpetuated by T-cells infiltrating into the CNS. This response can be mimicked in the animal model of MS, experimental autoimmune encephalitis (EAE). Initiation of these T-cell responses against neurotrophic pathogens or CNS autoantigens occurs in peripheral lymphoid organs, after which the activated T-cells readily cross the blood–brain barrier (BBB) and enter the CNS.[11] Once in the CNS, the infiltrating T-cells need to re-encounter their specific antigen presented by local APCs at the target site.[3,10] The local APCs in the CNS are the perivascular macrophages. microglia and, to a lesser extent, astrocytes. We shall consider functions of brain macrophages, with regard to both innate immunity and their roles as APCs in inducing and promoting inflammation within the CNS.

One of the characteristic features of microglia in vivo is their rapid activation in response to infection, inflammation, and neural injury,[12] with a subsequent deactivation. As described for peripheral macrophages, various effector functions of brain macrophages may, in fact, result in damage to other tissues within the CNS. Therefore, the downregulation of these effector functions of activated brain macrophages could resolve the inflammation and destruction observed in neuroinflammatory disorders.

ROLE OF BRAIN MACROPHAGES IN INNATE IMMUNITY

Phagocytosis

Macrophages in the CNS have similar functions to those in the periphery. Perivascular macrophages and microglia phagocytose foreign material to limit inflammation and the spread of infection within the brain.[4] Microglia also have receptors for apoptotic cells and for an array of proteins such as β-amyloid that accumulate in specific neurodegenerative disease states. As mentioned earlier, ADCC is a process whereby immunoglobulin receptor-bearing microglia/macrophages are brought into proximity with antibody-coated target. Microglia become activated as a result of binding the Fc portion of antibody, as shown by increased NADPH oxidase activity.[13] With regard to autoimmune injury, microglia/macrophage attachment to myelin/oligodendrocytes with subsequent phagocytosis could be triggered by antibodies directed to antigens expressed on the surface of myelin.[14] In MS lesions, expression of all three Fcγ receptor classes is upregulated on microglia cells and macrophages.[13] Increased expression of the Fcγ receptors on brain-resident macrophages may be induced by cytokines, particular interleukin-1 (IL-1), IL-6 or tumour necrosis factor alpha (TNF-α). Cytokines also enhance myelin uptake and subsequent breakdown by macrophages and microglia.[15] Astrocyte-conditioned medium increases the phagocytosis of myelin by both microglia and macrophages three-fold, suggesting that, in the CNS environment, phagocytosis is a natural occurrence.[16] Therefore, it is possible that a typically protective immune response, such as phagocytosis, once misdirected can result in harm to the host.

Secretion of inflammatory molecules

TNF-α is a proinflammatory cytokine produced in large quantities by activated macrophages and microglia in response to various stimuli such as bacterial lipopolysaccharide products. However, members of the adaptive immune response, specifically activated human T-cells, have also been shown to induce microglia production of TNF-α.[17,18] TNF-α has been identified in MS plaques,[19] and elevated levels of TNF have been found in serum and cerebrospinal fluid (CSF) of MS patients. In addition to its immunoregulatory properties, such as enhancing cytokine secretion (IL-12) and activation of other cell types (natural killer (NK) cells), TNF-α can influence lymphocyte trafficking across endothelium by upregulating the expression of various adhesion molecules.[20] Thus the activation of microglia in response to an infectious stimulus may initiate a cascade of events which lead to the recruitment of T-cells into the CNS. These activated T-cells further enhance the activation of microglia. The activated microglia are then able to secrete a variety of mediators, some of which may be neurotoxins that damage oligodendrocytes and myelin, and eventually result in altered neuronal function by either axonal degeneration or other indirect effects as described in the following section.

TNF-α itself may act as a neurotoxin. Intravitreal injection of TNF-α has been shown to induce demyelination of mouse optic nerve axons.[21] Similarly, injection into mouse spinal cord causes an EAE-like response.[22] In passive transfer EAE, TNF antagonists inhibit the development or severity of disease.[23] These observations may be the result of either direct or indirect functions of TNF. In vitro, TNF-α causes demyelination and death of oligodendrocytes.[24] TNF-α does not cause lysis of the cells, but rather induces apoptosis of the oligodendrocytes. Human oligodendrocytes demonstrate TNF receptor 1 (TNFR1) expression in vitro.[25] TNFR1 has a death domain that is responsible for the induction of apoptosis.[26] Human oligodendrocytes in vitro are susceptible to high doses of TNF-α over long periods of time (5–7 days).[27,28] The concentrations of TNF-α required to mediate neurodegeneration are higher than one would expect to be present in brain, except perhaps in microenvironments immediately surrounding microglia. Cell-bound TNF may be more efficient than soluble TNF-α in mediating oligodendrocyte killing.[29] The mechanism by which TNF signals for apoptosis has not been delineated. It is known that TNF-α signals for increased levels of p53,[30] a well-characterized inducer of apoptosis. Besides p53 induction, TNF-α increases the expression of CD95 (fas) on the surface of oligodendrocytes as well as the ligand (CD95L) on the surface of effector cells. Oligodendrocytes are sensitive to CD95-mediated apoptosis.[31]

TNF-α can also contribute to neurotoxicity by increasing the activity of phospholipase A_2, which in turn cleaves phosphoglycerocholine to release platelet activating factor (PAF) and arachidonic acid.[32] Arachidonic acid may activate NMDA receptors in neurons, which leads to calcium influx and neuronal death.[33] Arachidonic acid metabolites may also impair the transport of glutamate in astrocytes, which is an important mechanism for the preservation of neuronal function.[34] Neurotoxicity has been attributed to increased extracellular glutamate.

Oligodendrocytes have only the AMPA/kainate type of excitatory glutamate receptor and are highly sensitive to glutamate excitotoxicity.[35] In passive transfer EAE, the addition of an AMPA/kainate antagonist reduced the neurological impairment of the recipient mice. Oligodendrocyte loss was reduced in the treated animals, but there was no observed effect on the inflammatory response associated with EAE. These observations would suggest that glutamate excitotoxicity mediated by AMPA/kainate receptors is important in CNS damage in EAE and possibly MS.

Quinolinic acid, which is a metabolite of tryptophan, may act as a NMDA receptor agonist to induce cell death.[36] Quinolinic acid is known to be produced by macrophages and may be one of the more important neurotoxins. Its neurotoxicity can be demonstrated not only under acute conditions, but also with chronic exposure at relatively low concentrations, which may be more relevant for a chronic disease.

Activated macrophages and microglia generate reactive oxygen species (ROS) that may also induce injury of myelin, oligodendrocytes and neurons. Contact between neurons and brain macrophages triggers production of superoxide anion and hydrogen peroxide by macrophages, which leads to neuronal death.[37] Nitric oxide (NO) has been implicated in neurotoxicity in many neurological diseases. Many studies using the murine system have implicated NO as key injury mediator in microglia-induced cytotoxicity to oligodendrocytes. However, unlike production by murine macrophages, which are known to produce large amounts of NO, the production of NO by human macrophages or microglia is controversial. Astrocytes, neurons and endothelial cells appear to be the major source of NO within the human CNS.[7]

INTERACTIONS OF BRAIN MACROPHAGES WITH ADAPTIVE IMMUNE RESPONSES

Brain macrophages as APCs

As described in the Introduction, infiltrating CD4+ T-helper cells in the CNS recognize antigenic peptides that have been processed and presented in the context of major histocompatibility complex (MHC) II molecules on the cell surface of the local APC. This antigen recognition is considered to be the first signal necessary for peripheral T-cell activation. A second signal is required, this time antigen-independent, which is provided by the interaction of costimulatory molecules (CD40, CD80, CD86) expressed by APCs with receptors/ligands on the T-cells (CD154,

CD28, CTLA-4). In addition to MHC II and costimu-latory molecule expression, several other features allow APCs to function efficiently.[2] Phagocytosis of particulate antigens is a prerequisite for competent antigen processing. Macrophages and microglia sample their mileau by endocytosis, and process and present these various ingested antigens on their surface. Receptors that mediate active endocytosis, include Fcγ and mannose receptors. Perivascular macrophages have been demonstrated to be compe-tent APCs both in vitro and in vivo. These cells not only exhibit constitutive expression of MHC II and costimulatory molecules, but also upregulate these molecules following exposure to inflammatory stimuli.[38,39] Similarly, resting parenchymal human microglia constitutively express MHC II, costimula-tory molecules (B7.2, CD40) and the Fcγ receptor class of immunoglobulin.[38,39] Parenchymal microglia activated following exposure to interferon gamma (IFN-γ) demonstrate enhanced expression of these molecules.[40] Macrophages and microglia in MS lesions express MHC class II antigens and costimu-latory molecules such as CD40, CD86 (B7.2) and CD80 (B7.1), indicating that these microglia are 'activated' and can perform immune functions such as antigen presentation and phagocytosis.[40] In the periphery, the most professional APCs are the dendritic cells (DCs). DCs acquire antigen in the periphery and then migrate to T-cell-rich areas of lymph nodes and spleen, where they are proficient at presenting protein antigens to naive T-helper cells. To date, DCs have not been described as residing in the CNS; however, IFN-γ-treated microglia have been shown to be capable of stimulating naive T-cells, and activated microglia induce secretion of Th1-type cytokines (IL-2, IFN-γ, TNF-α), albeit with a lower efficiency than DCs.[42] Furthermore, activated microglia are equally as capable as DCs in stimulat-ing polarized Th1 and Th2 cell lines to proliferate. Together, these observations suggest that microglia may play the role of DCs in the brain.

Encounter of peripheral T-cells with antigen presented by APCs in the absence of a co-stimulat-ing signal renders the T-cells anergic. Classical anergy is described as the inability to proliferate or produce cytokines upon challenge with antigen.[43,44] Subsequent exposure of the T-cells to IL-12, however, is sufficient to convert the T-cells into potent effectors.[45] Therapeutic treatments that would decrease APC functions, such as the inhibition of MHC II expression, or costimulatory molecules could possibly relieve the inflammation induced by the infiltrating T-cells by rendering these T-cells anergic.

Importance of IL-12 cytokine secretion by brain macrophages

Activated T-helper cells can be separated into at least two distinct phenotypes on the basis of their cytokine production profiles: IFN-γ, IL-2 and TNF-α are considered to be hallmarks of a Th1-type response, while IL-4, IL-5, IL-l0 and IL-13 represent a Th2–type response. Proinflammatory Th1 T-cells are considered central to the development of MS and its animal model (EAE).[46,47] In most experimental systems, IL-12 plays a critical role in the differentia-tion of naive T-cells into Th1 cells.[48] IL-12 also induces IFN-γ production by NK cells and T-cells, macrophage activation, and B-cell production of complement-fixing antibodies.[49] In adoptive transfer models of EAE, the inclusion of recombinant IL-12 during in vitro priming of the reactive T-cells resulted in increased severity and duration of the disease, and accelerated onset of the disease.[49] Neutralization of IL-12 following adoptive transfer of T-cells attenuated the incidence and severity of disease.[50] In the active immunization model of EAE, IL-12-knockout mice are completely resistant, suggesting that IL-12 is essential for pathogenesis.[51] In humans, increased expression of mRNA encoding IL-12p40 has been found in acute MS plaques but not in inflammatory cerebral infarcts or disease-free brain.[52]

Ligation of the costimulatory molecule CD40 on monocyte/macrophages with its ligand CD154 on T-cells is a potent stimulus for IL-12 secretion by monocytes. Immunohistochemical studies have colocalized Th cells expressing the CD40 ligand (CD154) and monocytic cells expressing CD40 in active MS and EAE lesions.[53] Murine microglia secrete IL-12 upon antigen-specific interactions with Th1 cells, CD40 ligation and TNF receptor ligation.[54] Similar increased T-cell-driven IL-12 secretion has been observed in peripheral blood mono-nuclear cells (PBMCs) from patients with progressive MS.[55] Culture of human microglia in vitro demonstrated that IL-12 secretion was triggered by microglia contact with T-cells that express CD40, with ligation playing an important role as a triggering signal. Addition of antagonists for IFN-γ and TNF-α reduced cytokine production, demonstrating that IL-12 was subject to both autocrine and paracrine regulation.[56,57]

In EAE, treatment of animals with a monoclonal antibody to CD154 inhibited IL-12 secretion and completely prevented disease.[53] Interference with CD154:CD40 ligation reduced the cytokine secretion by human microglia observed in culture.[58] The APC role of microglia and the subsequent production of

IL-12 following T-cell contact would suggest a mechanism whereby interactions between T-cells and microglial cells contribute to the persistent or recurrent proinflammatory Th1 immune response within human CNS. This initial inflammatory response facilitates the recuitment and activation of additional T-cells thereby perpetuating this cascade event.

Myelin membranes and oligodendrocytes do not express MHC class II molecules, suggesting that they are unlikely to be direct targets of T-cells. Although myelin-specific T-cells are clearly needed for triggering EAE, macrophages and microglia are integral to the tissue destruction that is associated with the disease.[49] As described previously, activated brain macrophages and microglia secrete a variety of inflammatory mediators, some of which may be neurotoxic and damage oligodendrocytes and myelin, and alter neuronal function. Potential therapeutics for MS would downregulate not only microglial APC functions for T-cell responses, but also inhibit many of the innate immune functions of microglia that may be causing oligodendrocyte damage.

POTENTIAL MECHANISMS OF SUPPRESSING BRAIN MACROPHAGE FUNCTIONS

Type I interferons

The previous discussion focused on activation of microglia. Now to be considered is whether active mechanisms are responsible for suppressing or terminating this activation state.

Deactivation of previously activated microglia is well recognized to occur in vivo.[12] Cytokines and molecules exist that reduce the proinflammatory effects of activated microglia and brain macrophages. Type 1 interferons, alpha and beta, are such candidate molecules and are produced by many cell types (macrophages, T-cells, Langerhans cells) in response to viral infection. IFN-β is currently used as therapy in MS, but its actual mechanism of action is unclear. IFN-β prevents differentiation of human Th1 cells in vitro by a mechanism that reduces IL-12 secretion by dendritic cells.[59] IFN-β specifically inhibits CD40-induced IL-12 production and not lipopolysaccharide (LPS)-induced IL-12 secretion, or CD40-induced IL-6 production.[60] IFN-β has been shown to inhibit TNF-α production by human microglia.[17]

Transforming growth factor-beta

Astrocyte-derived factors have been observed to downregulate MHC class II molecules on macrophages.[3] This may be a mechanism to inhibit the APC function of microglia. Neutralization of TGF-β eliminates the downregulatory effect, suggesting that TGF-β immunosuppresses activated microglia.[61] Both TGF-β_1 and TGF-β_2 inhibit endotoxin-induced NO production by rat microglia.[62] Antibodies against TGF-β enhance the clinical severity of EAE.[63] It is proposed that TGF-β is induced during the reactive inflammatory phase of disease and then exerts anti-inflammatory effects in the brain. TGF-β_1 has been shown to suppress the release of oxygen free radicals by cultured macrophages[64] and to selectively induce microglial apoptosis.[65] TGF-β is therefore a powerful candidate suppressor molecule, as it appears to mediate its inhibitory effects on a spectrum of microglial functions.

Interleukin-10

IL-10 is another anti-inflammatory cytokine. Elevated expression of IL-10 has been observed in brains of mice during the recovery phase of EAE, and IL-10-deficient mice develop accelerated and more severe disease than wild-type animals, suggesting that IL-10 plays a role in suppressing the inflammatory response seen in EAE.[66,67] IL-10 has an inhibitory effect on the process of antigen presentation, as it downregulates MHC II, B7.1 and B7.2 molecules expressed by microglia.[68] IL-10 has been shown to inhibit TNF-α and IL-12 production by monocytes, macrophages and microglia.[69,70] IL-10 plays a role in causing T-cells to undergo anergy.[71] Inhibition of APC functions and cytokine release of TNF-α and IL-12 may be a mechanism by which IL-10 reduces the aggravating effects of the activated microglia/macrophages.

SUMMARY

Brain macrophages appear to play a dual role, both as mediators of innate immunity to remove harmful material from the CNS, and acting as APCs to promote adaptive immune responses within the CNS. However, unchecked microglial function results in amplifying the effects of inflammation and mediating cellular degeneration. The balance between Th1-promoting and Th1-inhibiting influences within the CNS parenchyma appears to be a key factor in determining the magnitude and duration of CNS inflammation. Considering the ability of perivascular macrophages and microglia to act as efficient APCs, the intracerebral delivery of anti-inflammatory cytokines or molecules that block key costimulatory pathways might target important local loops for the amplification of T-cell response and provide an effective therapy for treating chronic inflammatory CNS disease. Microglia are also capable of effecting injury of oligodendrocytes and neurons by secreting a number of potential neurotoxins. Microglia also play a role in the process of remodeling and regeneration of the CNS. Understanding the nature of microglial activation is likely to offer therapeutic insights that strike a balance between the protective and destructive roles of these cells in the CNS.

REFERENCES

1. Medzhitov R, Janeway CAJ. Innate immunity impact on the adaptive immune response. *Curr Opin Immunol* 1997; **9**: 4–9.
2. Abbas AK, Lichtman AH, Pober JS. *Cellular and Molecular Immunology*. Philadelphia: WB Saunders, 1994.
3. Aloisi F, Ria F, Adorini L. Regulation of T cell responses by CNS-antigen presenting cell: different roles for microglia and astrocytes. *Immunol Today* 2000; **21**: 141–147.
4. Ling EA, Wong WC. The origin and nature of ramified and amoeboid microglia: a historical review and current concepts. *Glia* 1993; **7**: 9–18.
5. Streit WJ, Graeber MB. Heterogeneity of microglial and perivascular cell populations: insights gained from the facial nucleus paradigm. *Glia* 1993; **7**: 68–74.
6. Schmidtmayer J, Jacobsen C, Miksch G, Sievers J. Blood monocytes and spleen macrophage differentiate into microglia-like cells on monolayers of astrocytes: membrane currents. *Glia* 1994; **12**: 259–267.
7. Gonzalez-Scarano F, Baltuch G. Microglia as mediators of inflammatory and degenerative diseases. *Ann Rev Neurosci* 1999; **22**: 219–240.
8. Wilkin GP, Knott C. Glia: a curtain raiser in Parkinson's disease. *Adv Neurol* 1991; **80**: 3–7.
9. Gehrmann J, Matsumoto Y, Kreutzberg W. Microglia: intrinsic immunoeffector cell of the brain. *Brain Res Rev* 1995; **20**: 269–287.
10. Becher B, Prat A, Antel JP. Brain–immune connection: immuno-regulatory properties of CNS-resident cells. *Glia* 2000; **29**: 293–304.
11. Wekerle H, Sun D, Oropeza-Wekerle RL, Meyermann R. Immune reactivity in the nervous system: modulation of T-lymphocyte activation by glial cells. *J Exp Biol* 1987; **132**: 43–57.
12. Xiao BG, Link H. Is there a balance between microglia and astrocytes in regulating Th1/Th2-cell responses and neuropathologies? *Immunol Today* 1999; **20**: 477–479.
13. Ulvestad E, Williams K, Matre R, Nyland H, Olivier A, Antel JP. Fc receptors for IgG on cultured human microglia mediate cytotoxicity and phagocytosis of antibody-coated targets. *J Neuropathol Exp Neurol* 1994; **53**: 27–36.
14. Scolding NJ, Compston DA. Oligodendrocyte–macrophage interactions in vitro triggered by specific antibodies. *Immunology* 1991; **72**: 127–132.
15. Smith ME, van der Maesen K, Somera FP. Macrophage and microglial responses to cytokines in vitro: phagocytic activity, proteolytic enzyme release and free radical production. *J Neurosci Res* 1998; **54**: 68–78.
16. Smith ME, Hoerner MT. Astrocytes modulate macrophage phagocytosis of myelin in vitro. *J Neuroimmunol* 2000; **102**: 154–162.
17. Chabot S, Williams G, Yong VW. Microglia production of TNFalpha is induced by activated lymphocytes. Involvement of VLA-4 and inhibition by interferon-1B. *J Clin Invest* 1997; **100**: 604–612.
18. Becher B, Antel JP. Comparison of phenotypic and functional properties of immediately ex vivo and cultured human adult microglia. *Glia* 1996; **18**: 1–10.
19. Hofman FM, Hinton DR, Johnson K, Merrill JE. Tumor necrosis factor identified in multiple sclerosis brain. *J Exp Med* 1989; **170**: 607–612.
20. Springer TA. Adhesion receptors of the immune system. *Nature* 1990; **346**: 425–434.
21. Jenkins HG, Ikeda H. Tumor necrosis factor causes an increase in axonal transport of protein and demyelination in the mouse optic nerve. *J Neurol Sci* 1992; **108**: 99–104.
22. Simmons RD, Willenborg DO. Direct injection of cytokines into the spinal cord causes autoimmune encephalomyelitis-like inflammation. *J Neurol Sci* 1990; **100**: 37–42.
23. Ruddle NH, Bergman CM, McGrath KM et al. An antibody to lymphotoxin and tumor necrosis factor prevents transfer of experimental allergic encephalomyelitis. *J Exp Med* 1990; **172**: 1193–1200.
24. Selmaj K, Raine CS. Tumor necrosis factor mediates myelin and oligodendrocyte damage in organotypic culture of nervous tissue. *Ann NY Acad Sci* 1988; **540**: 568–570.
25. Wilt SC, Milward E, Zhou JM et al. In vitro evidence for a dual role of tumor necrosis factor alpha in human immunodeficiency virus type 1 encephalopathy. *Ann Neurol* 1995; **37**: 381–394.
26. Declercq W, Denecker G, Fiers W, Vandenabeele P. Cooperation of both TNF receptors in inducing apoptosis: involvement of the TNF receptor-associated factor binding domain of the TNF receptor 75. *J Immunol* 1998; **161**: 390–399.
27. D'Souza S, Alinauskas K, McCrea E, Goodyer C, Antel JP. Differential susceptibility of human CNS-derived cell populations to TNF-dependent and independent immune-mediated injury. *J Neurosci* 1995; **15**: 7293–7300.
28. Ladiwala U, Lachance C, Simoneau SJ, Khakar A, Barker PA, Antel JP. P75 neurotrophin receptor expression on adult human oligodendrocytes: signaling without cell death in response to NGF. *J Neurosci* 1998; **18**: 1297–1304.
29. Zajicek JP, Wing M, Scolding NJ, Compston DA. Interactions between oligodendrocytes and microglia. A major role for complement and tumor necrosis factor in oligodendrocyte adherence and killing. *Brain* 1992; **115**: 1611–1631.
30. Ladiwala U, Li H, Antel JP, Nalbantoglu J. p53 induction by tumor necrosis factor alpha and involvement of p53 in cell death of human oligodendrocytes. *J Neurochem* 1999; **73**: 605–611.

31. Pouly S, Becher B, Blain M, Antel JP. Interferon gamma modulates human oligodendrocyte susceptibility to Fas-mediated apoptosis. *J Neuropathol Exp Neurol* 2000; **59**: 280–286.

32. Bachwich PR, Censue SW, Larrick JW, Kunkel SL. Tumor necrosis factor stimulates interleukin-1 and prostaglandin E2 production in resting macrophages. *Biochem Biophys Res Commun* 1986; **136**: 94–101.

33. Lipton SA. Similarity of neuronal cell injury and death in AIDS dementia and focal cerebral ischemia: potential treatment with NMDA open-channel blockers and nitric oxide related species. *Brain Pathol* 1996; **6**: 507–517.

34. Chaudhry FA, Lehre KP, van Lookeren Campagne M et al. Glutamate transporters in glial plasma membranes: highly differentiated localizations revealed by quantitative ultrastructural immunocytochemistry. *Neuron* 1995; **15**: 711–720.

35. Pitt D, Werner P, Raine CS. Glutamate excitotoxicity in a model of multiple sclerosis. *Nature Med* 2000; **6**: 67–70.

36. Brew BJ, Rosenblum M, Cronin K, Price RW. AIDS dementia complex and HIV-1 brain infection: clinical–virological correlations. *Ann Neurol* 1995; **38**: 563–570.

37. Thery C, Stanley ER, Mallat M. Interleukin 1 and tumor necrosis factor alpha stimulate the production of colony-stimulating factor 1 by murine astrocytes. *J Neurochem* 1992; **59**: 1183–1186.

38. Bo L, Mork S, Kong PA, Nyland H, Pardo CA, Trapp BD. Detection of MHC class II-antigens on macrophages and microglia but not on astrocytes and endothelia in active multiple sclerosis lesions. *J Neuroimmunol* 1994; **51**: 135–146.

39. Ulvestad E, Willian K, Bo L, Trapp B, Antel J, Mork S. HLA class II molecules (HLA-DR, -DP, -DQ) on cells in the human CNS studied in situ and in vitro. *Immunology* 1994; **82**: 535–541.

40. Peress NS, Fleit HB, Perillo E, Kuljis R, Pezzullo C. Identification of Fc gamma RI, II and III on normal human brain ramified microglia and on microglia in senile plaques in Alzheimer's disease. *J Neuroimmunol* 1993; **48**: 71–79.

41. Ulvestad E, Williams K, Bjerkvig R, Tiekotter K, Antel J, Matre R. Human microglia cells have phenotypic and functional characteristics in common with both macrophages and dendritic antigen presenting cells. *J Leukocyte Biol* 1994; **56**: 732–740.

42. Aloisi F, Ria G, Columba-Cabezas S, Hess H, Penna G, Adorini L. Relative efficiency of microglia, astrocytes, dendritic cells and B cells in naive CD4+ T cell priming and Thl/Th2 stimulation. *Eur J Immunol* 1999; **29**: 2705–2714.

43. Jenkins MK. The ups and downs of T cell costimulation. *Immunity* 1994; **1**: 443–446.

44. Jenkins MK, Schwartz RH. Antigen presentation by chemically modified splenocytes induces antigen-specific T cell unresponsiveness in vitro and in vivo. *J Exp Med* 1987; **165**: 302–319.

45. Chang JT, Segal BM, Shevach EM. Role of costimulation in the induction of the IL-12/IL-12 receptor pathway and the development of autoimmunity. *J Immunol* 2000; **164**: 100–106.

46. Olsson T. Cytokine-producing cells in experimental autoimmune encephalomyelitis and multiple sclerosis. *Neurology* 1995; **45**: S11–S15.

47. Schulze-Koops H, Lipsky PE, Kavanaugh AF, Davis LS. Elevated Th1 or Th0 like cytokine mRNA in peripheral circulation of patients with rheumatoid arthritis.

Modulation by treatment with anti-ICAM-1 correlates with clinical benefit. *J Immunol* 1995; **155**: 5029–5037.

48. Gately MK, Renzetti LM, Magram J et al. The interleukin-12/interleukin-12-receptor system: role in normal and pathologic immune responses. *Annu Rev Immunol* 1998; **16**: 495–521.

49. Karp CL, Biron CA, Iranik DN. Interferon beta in multiple sclerosis: is IL-12 suppression the key? *Immunol Today* 2000; **121**: 24–28.

50. Leonard JP, Waldburger KE, Goldman SJ. Prevention of experimental autoimmune encephalomyelitis by antibodies against interleukin 12. *J Exp Med* 1995; **181**: 381–386.

51. Segal BM, Shevach EM. IL-12 unmasks latent autoimmune disease in resistant mice. *J Exp Med* 1996; **184**: 771–775.

52. Windhagen A, Newcombe J, Dangond F et al. Expression of costimulatory molecules B7-1 (CD80), B7-2 (CD86) and interleukin 12 cytokine in multiple sclerosis. *J Exp Med* 1995; **182**: 1985–1996.

53. Gerritse K, Laman JD, Noelle RJ et al. CD40–CD40 ligand interactions in experimental allergic encephalomyelitis and multiple sclerosis. *Proc Natl Acad Sci USA* 1996; **93**: 2499–2504.

54. Aloisi F, Penna G, Polazzi E, Minghetti L, Adorini L. CD40–CD154 interaction and IFN-gamma are required for IL-12 but not prostaglandin E2 secretion by microglia during antigen presentation to Th1 cells. *J Immunol* 1999; **162**: 1384–1391.

55. Balashov KE, Smith DR, Khoury SJ, Hafler DA, Weinder HL. Increased interleukin-12 production in progressive multiple sclerosis: induction of activated CD4+ T cells via CD40 ligand. *Proc Natl Acad Sci USA* 1997; **94**: 599–603.

56. Becher B, Dodelet V, Fedorowicz V, Antel JP. Soluble tumor necrosis factor receptor inhibits interleukin 12 production by stimulated human adult microglial cells in vitro. *J Clin Invest* 1996; **98**: 1539–1543.

57. Becher B, Blain M, Giacomini PS, Antel JP. Inhibition of Th1 polarization by soluble TNF receptor is dependent on antigen presenting cell derived IL-12. *J Immunol* 1999; **162**: 684–688.

58. Becher B, Blain M, Antel JP. CD40 engagement stimulates IL-12p70 production by human microglia cells. *J Neuroimmunol* 2000; **102**: 44–50.

59. McRae BL, Semnani RT, Hages MP, van Seventer GA. Type I interferons inhibit human dendritic cell IL-12 production and Th1 cell development. *J Immunol* 1998; **160**: 4298–4304.

60. McRae BL, Beilfuss BA, van Seventer GA. IFN-beta differentially regulates CD40-induced cytokine secretion by human dendritic cells. *J Immunol* 2000; **164**: 23–28.

61. Hailer NP, Heppner FL, Haas D, Nitsch R. Astrocytic factors deactivate antigen presenting cells that invade the central nervous system. *Brain Pathol* 1998; **8**: 459–474.

62. Vincent VA, Tilders FJ, van Dam AM. Inhibition of endotoxin-induced nitric oxide synthase production in microglial cells by the presence of astroglial cell: role for transforming growth factor beta. *Glia* 1997; **19**: 190–198.

63. Johns LD, Sriram S. Experimental allergic encephalomyelitis: neutralizing antibody to TGF beta 1 enhances the clinical severity of the disease. *J Neuroimmunol* 1993; **47**: 1–7.

64. Wing EJ, Ampel NM, Waheed A, Shadduk RK. Macrophage colony-stimulating factor (M-CSF)

enhances the capacity of murine macrophages to secrete oxygen reduction products. *J Immunol* 1985; **135**: 2052–2056.

65. Von Zahn J, Moller T, Kettenmann H, Nolte C. Microglial phagocytosis is modulated by pro- and anti-inflammatory cytokines. *Neuroreport* 1997; **8**: 3851–3856.

66. Kennedy MK, Torance DS, Picha KS, Mohler KM. Analysis of cytokine mRNA expression in the central nervous system of mice with experimental autoimmune encephalomyelitis reveals that IL-10 mRNA expression correlates with recovery. *J Immunol* 1992; **149**: 2496–2505.

67. Bettelli, E, Mercy PD, Howard ED, Weiner HL, Sobel RA, Kuchroo VK. IL-10 is critical in the regulation of autoimmune encephalomyelitis as demonstrated by studies of IL-10 and IL-4-deficient and transgenic mice. *J Immunol* 1998; **161**: 3229–3306.

68. De Waal Malefyt R, Abrams J, Bennett B, Figdor CG, de Vries JE. Interleukin 10 (IL-10) inhibits cytokine synthesis by human monocytes: an autoregulatory role of IL-10 produced monocytes. *J Exp Med* 1991; **174**: 1209–1220.

69. Bogdan C, Vodovotz Y, Nathan C. Macrophage deactivation by interleukin 10. *J Exp Med* 1991; **174**: 1549–1555.

70. Koch F, Stanzl U, Jennewein P et al. High levels of IL-12 production by murine dendritic cells: upregulation via MHC II and CD40 molecules and downregulation by IL-4 and IL-10. *J Exp Med* 1996; **184**: 741–746.

71. Akdis CA, Blesken T, Akdis M, Wuthrich B, Blaser K. Role of interleukin 10 in specific immunotherapy. *J Clin Invest* 1998; **102**: 98–106.

4

Humoral immune response and antibody-mediated brain injury

Nicole Kerlero de Rosbo and Avraham Ben-Nun

Multiple sclerosis (MS), characterized by neurological impairment of varying severity, is a human disease prototypic of immune-mediated brain tissue damage which presents as demyelinating lesions or 'plaques'. Autoimmune T-cells specific for myelin antigens are present at higher frequency in the immune repertoire of MS patients and are believed to be the basis for the immune-mediated pathogenesis of the disease. However, circumstantial, as well as experimental, evidence suggests that cellular immune effector mechanisms cannot solely account for the extensive destruction of myelin typical of MS, and it is likely that humoral immune effector mechanisms are also involved in disease pathogenesis. A biochemical marker for MS is an elevated level of immunoglobulins (Igs) in brain tissue and cerebrospinal fluid (CSF), which results mostly from intrathecal synthesis.[1] Myelinotoxicity of MS CSF and brain extract has been demonstrated,[1] and Igs isolated from MS, but not control brain tissue, were shown to stimulate the degradation of myelin basic protein (MBP) in human myelin.[2] That IgG possibly directed against some component of myelin participates locally in myelin breakdown in MS was suggested by the study of Prineas and Graham,[3] where capping of surface IgG was observed only on macrophages involved in myelin breakdown at plaque margins. Despite intensive work carried out to determine the specificity of Igs present in MS central nervous system (CNS), the target antigens are known for only a small proportion of the intrathecally synthesized Igs. Among these, myelin and viral components, particularly those cross-reacting with myelin antigens, would be of particular importance in antibody-mediated demyelination.

EXPERIMENTALLY INDUCED ANTIBODY-MEDIATED DEMYELINATION

Because of the difficulties in defining the specificities of demyelinating Igs in MS, antibodies experimentally raised to specific myelin components have been investigated for their demyelinating activity in vitro and in vivo.

In vitro demyelination

Experimental demyelination related to the humoral response was first demonstrated in vitro with sera from animals which, upon immunization with brain tissue homogenate, had developed experimental autoimmune encephalomyelitis (EAE), the purported experimental model for MS.[4–6] As demyelinating EAE sera show reactivity against total myelin, identification of the myelin antigens with the potential to induce antibodies with demyelinating activity has been attempted by assessing the effect on CNS cultures of antibodies experimentally raised to specific myelin components. Although antibodies against the major myelin proteins, MBP and proteolipid protein (PLP), can be present in EAE sera with demyelinating activity,[7–12] polyclonal antibodies raised against these proteins do not cause demyelination in cultured CNS tissue.[7,13–15] In contrast, antibodies directed against galactocerebroside (GalC), one of the main glycolipids of myelin, do initiate CNS myelin degradation in vitro.[8,16–21] However, the presence of detectable anti-glycolipid antibodies in EAE sera is not a prerequisite for demyelination in vitro,[11,13,18] and sera raised against the chloroform/methanol-insoluble fraction of myelin, which lacks MBP, PLP and lipids, demyelinated CNS explant cultures.[22] In this context, it is noteworthy that EAE sera devoid of reactivity against MBP, PLP and cerebrosides, but containing antibodies against the CNS-specific myelin glycoprotein M2, subsequently identified as myelin oligodendrocyte glycoprotein (MOG),[23] have been shown to demyelinate CNS tissue cultures.[13,24] That in vitro demyelination by EAE sera may indeed be attributed mainly to anti-MOG antibody activity is strongly supported by the specific dose-related demyelinating effect of purified monoclonal anti-MOG antibody in fetal rat brain aggregating cultures.[14]

In vivo demyelination

The demyelinating effect of antibodies to specific myelin components demonstrated in vitro has been extrapolated in vivo. The presence of anti-GalC antibody or anti-MOG antibody, but not anti-MBP antibody, within CNS tissue of laboratory animals results in extensive demyelination in vivo. Such experimentally induced in vivo antibody-mediated demyelination has been demonstrated using various routes for introducing the relevant antibody within CNS tissue. Intravenous administration of demyelinating sera from EAE animals into naive recipients does not cause CNS demyelination;[25,26] however, if the sera are injected intrathecally, demyelination does ensue.[27] The specificities of the in vivo demyelinating antibodies in EAE sera have not been defined as such; however, the specificities of in vitro demyelinating antibodies appear to be as relevant to in vivo demyelination. Thus, direct injection into the CNS of anti-GalC antibody,[28–30] or of monoclonal anti-MOG antibody,[31] resulted in CNS demyelination; such an effect was not observed with anti-MBP antibody.[28] In situ production of the putative demyelinating antibody specifically within the CNS in vivo has also demonstrated the demyelinating effect of anti-GalC antibodies: focal demyelinating lesions were induced in the spinal cord of rats following implantation of IgM anti-GalC-secreting hybridoma cells in the spinal cord.[32] A different approach, albeit based on a similar postulate, was taken by Litzenburger et al,[33] who generated transgenic mice engineered to produce high titers of monoclonal anti-MOG antibody shown to be pathogenic in vitro and in vivo. Although high-titer anti-MOG antibodies are detected in the serum of these mice, they do not result in clinical signs and demyelination. However, upon disturbance of the blood–brain barrier via induction of CNS inflammation following immunization with PLP, the transgene mice presented with accelerated development of EAE of increased severity and associated with

widespread CNS demyelination, at a time when the non-transgenic littermate showed no CNS lesions.[33] These studies support the repeated in vivo demonstrations that anti-MOG antibodies introduced into the circulation will cause CNS demyelination if they can reach the brain through a breached blood–brain barrier. These observations were first made in Lewis rats by Schluesener et al:[34] in the acute EAE produced in Lewis rats by injection of purified MBP or by passive transfer of monospecific MBP-reactive T-lymphocytes, there is little or no demyelination despite widespread inflammation.[35] Extensive demyelination could, however, be induced in these animals by intravenous injection of purified monoclonal anti-MOG antibody, at the time when the blood–brain barrier is breached, 7 days after immunization with MBP[34] or 3 days after adoptive transfer of the MBP-specific T-cells.[36,37] Similar observations were made with monoclonal anti-GalC antibody,[38] as well as with a monoclonal antibody raised against Theiler's murine encephalomyelitis virus and cross-reacting with a determinant on myelin and oligodendrocyte.[39] In contrast, injection of a monoclonal antibody directed against myelin-associated glycoprotein (MAG) under the same paradigm did not cause demyelination,[40] corroborating the in vitro findings that anti-MAG antibodies do not demyelinate CNS culture.[41] The demyelinating effect of the antibodies was independent of the antigen specificity of the T-cell line used to induce CNS inflammation and could be observed not only with encephalitogenic MBP- or MOG-specific T-cell lines,[36,37,42] but also with T-cell lines reactive with MAG or with the non-myelin brain antigens S100β or glial fibrillary acidic protein, which do not induce clinical EAE but cause CNS inflammation.[40,43,44]

EXPRESSION OF DEMYELINATION IN EAE IN THE CONTEXT OF ANTIBODIES

Increasing evidence correlates the presence and levels of anti-MOG antibodies with demyelination in EAE. This was first suggested by the demonstration that the demyelinating activity of chronic EAE sera assayed in vivo by intrathecal injection of normal rats is proportional to the anti-MOG antibody titer of the serum.[45] In guinea pigs with chronic EAE, antibodies against MOG are not always detected in sera but are always present in acid extract of CNS tissue, with levels correlating with severity of clinical signs and the intensity of demyelinating lesions; most importantly, in animals which did not develop chronic EAE, anti-MOG antibodies could not be detected and demyelination was absent.[11] The relationship between anti-MOG antibodies and demyelination has been shown best in the marmoset model of EAE. In these non-human primates, immunization with CNS white matter homogenate produces a demyelinating form of EAE, while adoptive transfer of MBP-reactive T-cell clones or active immunization with MBP produces only modest inflammation unaccompanied by demyelination,[46] unless anti-MOG antibody is administered sytemically.[47] Immunization of marmosets with MOG induces demyelinating EAE identical to that induced by immunization with CNS white matter homogenate,[47] and which can be exacerbated if the production of the pathogenic anti-MOG antibodies is enhanced.[48] Further convincing evidence linking demyelination with anti-MOG antibodies in marmoset EAE was obtained in marmosets immunized with MP4, a chimeric molecule composed of the human 21.5-kDa isoform of MBP and ΔPLP4, a recombinant form of human PLP lacking the hydrophobic domains. Severe symptomatic EAE developed in these animals and histopathological analysis revealed that lesions induced by MP4 could be either demyelinating or purely inflammatory, and that, while all animals developed significant titers of anti-MBP antibodies, a determinant spreading of the humoral response to MOG had occurred in all animals which exhibited demyelinating lesions, while animals with non-demyelinating disease did not develop antibodies against MOG.[49] That anti-MOG antibodies in MOG-induced EAE in marmosets are likely to be directly involved in myelin damage was recently suggested by in situ demonstration of MOG-specific auto-antibodies using gold-conjugated MOG peptides comprising epitopes located within amino acids 1–20, 21–40 and 61–80.[50] It is interesting to note that in severe demyelinating EAE induced by MOG in rhesus monkeys, non-human primates closely related to humans immunologically, anti-MOG antibodies, which appear early after immunization, also recognize epitopes within these MOG regions.[51]

Altogether, these data strongly implicate a role for anti-MOG antibodies as mediators of demyelination in EAE. It should, however, be noted that antibody-independent mechanisms of autoimmune demyelination exist, as demonstrated by recent studies with B-cell-deficient mice in which neither B-cells nor antibodies can be detected, and which developed EAE with primary demyelination upon immunization with the encephalitogenic MOG 35–55 peptide.[52,53] Of interest, and not fully understood, was the finding in one of these studies that while B-cell-deficient mice are susceptible to EAE induced by

MOG 35–55, they neither develop clinical disease nor show significant CNS pathology when immunized with the 120-amino acid-long recombinant MOG.[53]

ANTI-MYELIN ANTIBODY SPECIFICITIES IN MS AND THEIR IMPLICATIONS

The question as to whether cellular or humoral factors are primary participants in the myelin destruction characteristic of MS has not yet been resolved. The common theme of most early reports on myelin damage in MS was the involvement of antibodies, as in vitro demyelination by MS serum,[54] and later by MS CSF and brain extract,[1] was demonstrated. The direct participation of MS Igs in myelin breakdown[2,3] and the in vitro and in vivo EAE data strongly suggest that, also in MS, the deleterious autoantibody(ies) must be directed against a myelin component(s). Unfortunately, there is a paucity of data on myelin-specific Igs in MS lesions, and anti-myelin antibody specificity in MS has mostly been studied using serum and CSF samples. Through a variety of assays, antibodies to the most relevant myelin components, i.e. components present in relatively high amounts in CNS myelin, encephalitogenic components, as well as components shown to induce antibodies which mediate demyelination in vitro and/or in vivo, have all been demonstrated in MS CSF and/or serum. It can be expected that, depending on disease and blood–brain barrier status, relevant antibodies could be present in both serum and CSF concomitantly; however, CSF antibodies likely to represent intrathecal synthesis by plasma cells within demyelinating plaques[55] should be of greater relevance to antibody-mediated demyelination. Antibodies to MBP have been extensively studied. MBP-specific B-cells have been immunolocalized in MS lesions,[56] and were detected in CSF, and more rarely in blood, of most MS patients tested.[57] The MBP epitope most frequently recognized by MS CSF or Igs isolated from CNS tissue appears to be located within amino acids 83–97.[58,59] Although anti-MAG antibodies are more likely to be related to demyelination of the peripheral nervous sytem, cells secreting anti-MAG antibodies are present in CSF of MS patients,[60] and increased levels of anti-MAG antibodies could be detected in MS CSF.[61,62] Because of the highly hydrophobic nature of PLP, anti-PLP antibodies have been poorly studied. Nevertheless, anti-PLP antibody-secreting cells were detected in blood and more frequently in CSF from most MS patients.[63]

One would expect that the presence in MS of antibodies to components which induce antibodies shown to be non-demyelinating in vitro and/or in vivo, such as MBP, MAG and PLP, may be the result of a humoral response directed to myelin degradation products as disease progresses. In this context, studies have been conducted in patients with optic neuritis likely to develop into MS, to try and demarcate specificities more relevant to primary demyelination. So far, anti-MBP and anti-PLP antibody responses have mostly been analyzed, and the studies generally indicate a preponderance of such reactivities in optic neuritis patients as compared to controls.[64–66] The implications of these findings for demyelination in MS need to be evaluated further.

The presence in MS of B-cells and antibodies directed to the myelin components which can induce antibodies shown to be demyelinating in vitro and in vivo, GalC and MOG, may be more relevant to the initiation of demyelinating plaques. Anti-glycolipid antibodies, in particular anti-GalC antibodies, have been demonstrated in MS blood and CSF, and are apparently not present in significant amounts in healthy control individuals;[67–69] the demonstration that a significant amount of anti-GalC antibodies exist in MS CSF as immune complexes with GalC[67] may indicate their active involvement in demyelination. Original studies of the humoral response to MOG had indicated a preponderance of reactivity to MOG in MS patients as compared to controls. Thus, Sun et al[70] detected anti-MOG antibody-secreting cells in CSF of most of the patients they tested, but rarely so in their control individuals, while anti-MOG Igs were found in the CSF of a significantly greater proportion of MS patients than control individuals, and at higher levels, by Xiao et al.[71] Similar increased frequencies of antibody reactivity to MOG in MS as compared to healthy individuals were recently reported, albeit in analysis of serum antibody responses only, as CSF responses were not determined.[72] Interestingly, when responses to MOG were examined in the group of MS patients in the context of clinical course of the disease, the highest proportion of anti-MOG antibody-positives was found in the group of five patients who presented with a first manifestation of MS: all of these five newly diagnosed patients were seropositive for anti-MOG antibodies.[72] In another recent study, however, the proportion of MOG-reactive MS patients did not differ with clinical course; instead, anti-MOG antibodies demonstrated at first attack of MS persisted as disease progressed.[73] In this latter study, where MS patients were not compared with healthy controls, but with patients suffering from other neurological diseases, inflammatory (OIND) or non-inflammatory (ONND), the frequencies of serum antibody response to MOG were greater in MS patients than in ONND patients, who rarely responded, but not significantly different between MS and OIND patients; longitudinal analyses, however, revealed a transient response to MOG in ONID patients, while such a response persisted in MS patients.[73] Similar anti-MOG antibody frequencies were also observed in CSF of MS and OIND patients; however, comparison of anti-MOG antibody-specific IgG indices, total IgG indices, CSF cell counts and albumin quotient for CSF of anti-MOG antibody-positive MS and OIND patients indicated an intrathecal origin for anti-MOG antibody in MS, whereas in OIND the CSF anti-MOG antibodies were associated with pathological CSF mononuclear cell numbers and albumin quotient, indicating extensive blood–brain barrier damage and leakage from the peripheral blood.[73] Of particular interest were the findings that, while anti-MBP antibody responses were enhanced in advanced MS, as well as in OIND and ONND, indicating that an anti-MBP antibody response is a relatively common sequel to CNS injury in general, the frequency of anti-MBP antibody-positive patients presenting with a first attack of MS was significantly lower, suggesting that the anti-MBP antibody response accumulates over time as disease progresses[73] and may not be directly involved in the demyelinating process. In contrast, a recent immunocytochemical study suggests that anti-MOG antibodies may be directly associated with myelin damage in MS: in acute demyelinating lesions of recent origin in the brain of three MS cases, ongoing demyelination characterized by the transformation of normal lamellar myelin sheaths into vesiculated membranous networks around demyelinated axons was observed; such networks of vesiculated myelin showed positive immunoreactivity for IgG, apparently directed against specific regions of MOG, as indicated by colocalization with gold-labeled MOG peptides.[50,74] Moreover, the gold-labeled MOG peptides also reacted with droplets of myelin debris to which anti-MOG antibody was bound within surrounding macrophages.[50,74]

CONCLUDING REMARKS

Thus far, data obtained from experimentally induced demyelination in vitro and/or in vivo have clearly indicated that not all anti-myelin antibodies are demyelinating, but rather that antibodies directed against myelin components accessible to the immune system, i.e. located at the surface of the myelin sheath, are more likely to exhibit strong demyelinating activity. In this context, GalC and MOG are the best contenders as targets for antigen-specific antibody mediation of demyelination. It should, however, be noted that not all myelin components have been tested for their ability to elicit demyelinating antibodies. In particular, two recently uncovered myelin proteins, myelin-associated oligodendrocytic basic protein (MOBP) and oligodendrocyte-specific protein (OSP), have been shown to induce demyelinating EAE in mice,[75–78] and antibodies against these proteins should be tested for their demyelinating potential, particularly in view of the demonstration of elevated anti-OSP antibody levels in MS.[79] In MS, not all patients show humoral responses to known myelin components, which may indicate that, in these patients, antibody-mediated demyelination may be associated with myelin components other than those already tested; it is likely that MOG and GalC are not the only surface components of myelin which can be targeted by a pathogenic antibody response. It should also be considered that, particularly as indicated by experimental animal studies, CNS demyelination may occur in the absence of a humoral response,[52,53] and it has been suggested that B-cell-dependent demyelination may possibly be restricted to a minor subset of MS cases.[80]

ACKNOWLEDGEMENTS

We gratefully acknowledge the financial support of the Multiple Sclerosis Society of New York. Avraham Ben-Nun is the incumbent of the Eugene and Marcia Appelbaum Professorial Chair.

REFERENCES

1. Walsh MJ, Tourtellotte WW. The cerebrospinal fluid in multiple sclerosis. In: Hallpike JF, Adams CW, Tourtellotte WW, eds. *Multiple Sclerosis.* London: Chapman and Hall, 1983: 275–358.
2. Kerlero de Rosbo N, Bernard C. Multiple sclerosis brain immunoglobulins stimulate myelin basic protein degradation in human myelin: a new cause for demyelination. *J Neurochem* 1989; **53**: 513–518.
3. Prineas JW, Graham JS. Multiple sclerosis: capping of surface immunoglobulin G on macrophages engaged in myelin breakdown. *Ann Neurol* 1981; **10**: 149–158.
4. Bornstein MB, Appel SH. The application of tissue culture to the study of experimental 'allergic' encephalomyelitis: I. Patterns of demyelination. *J Neuropathol Exp Neurol* 1961; **20**: 141–157.
5. Appel SH, Bornstein MB. The application of tissue culture to the study of experimental 'allergic' encephalomyelitis: II. Serum factors responsible for demyelination. *J Exp Med* 1964; **119**: 303–312.
6. Grundke Iqbal I, Raine CS, Johnson AB, Brosnan CF, Bornstein MB. Experimental allergic encephalomyelitis:

characterization of serum factors causing demyelination and swelling of myelin. *J Neurol Sci* 1981; **50**: 63–79.
7. Seil FJ, Falk GA, Kies MW, Alvord EC. The in vitro demyelinating activity of sera from guinea pigs sensitized with whole CNS and purified encephalitogen. *Exp Neurol* 1968; **22**: 545–555.
8. Raine CS, Johnson AB, Marcus DM, Suzuki A, Bornstein MB. Demyelination in vitro. Absorption studies demonstrate that galactocerebroside is a major target. *J Neurol Sci* 1981; **52**: 117–131.
9. Lassmann H, Suchanek G, Kitz K, Stemberger H, Schwerer B, Bernheimer H. Antibodies in the pathogenesis of demyelination in chronic relapsing EAE (cr-EAE). In: Alvord EC, Kies MW, Suckling AJ, eds. *Experimental Allergic Encephalomyelitis: A Useful Model for Multiple Sclerosis.* New York: Alan Liss, 1983: 165–170.
10. Olsson T, Henriksson A, Link H, Kristensson K. IgM and IgG responses during chronic relapsing experimental allergic encephalomyelitis (r-EAE). *J Neuroimmunol* 1984; **6**: 265–281.
11. Lebar R, Baudrimont M, Vincent C. Chronic experimental autoimmune encephalomyelitis in the guinea pig. Presence of anti-M2 antibodies in central nervous system tissue and the possible role of M2 autoantigen in the induction of the disease. *J Autoimmun* 1989; **2**: 115–132.
12. Endoh M, Tabira T, Kunishita T. Antibodies to proteolipid apoprotein in chronic relapsing experimental allergic encephalomyelitis. *J Neurol Sci* 1986; **73**: 1–38.
13. Lebar R, Boutry J-M, Vincent C, Robinaux R, Voisin GA. Studies on autoimmune encephalomyelitis in the guinea pig. II. An in vitro investigation on the nature, properties, and specificities of the serum-demyelinating factor. *J Immunol* 1976; **116**: 1439–1446.
14. Kerlero de Rosbo N, Honegger P, Lassmann H, Matthieu J-M. Demyelination induced in aggregating brain cell cultures by a monoclonal antibody against myelin/oligodendrocyte glycoprotein. *J Neurochem* 1990; **55**: 583–587.
15. Seil FJ, Agrawal HC. Myelin proteolipid protein does not induce demyelinating or myelination inhibiting antibodies. *Brain Res* 1980; **194**: 273–277.
16. Dubois-Dalcq M, Niedieck B, Buyse M. Action of anticerebroside sera on myelinated nervous tissue culture. *Pathol Eur* 1970; **5**: 331–347.
17. Fry JM, Weissbarth S, Lehrer GM, Bornstein MB. Cerebroside antibody inhibits sulfatide synthesis and myelination and demyelinates in cord tissue cultures. *Science* 1974; **183**: 540–542.
18. Schwerer B, Kitz K, Lassmann H, Bernheimer H. Serum antibodies against glycosphingolipids in chronic relapsing experimental allergic encephalomyelitis. Demonstration by ELISA and relation to serum in vivo demyelinating activity. *J Neuroimmunol* 1984; **7**: 107–119.
19. Roth GA, Roytta M, Yu RK, Raine CS, Bornstein MB. Antisera to different glycolipids induce myelin alterations in mouse spinal cord tissue culture. *Brain Res* 1985; **339**: 9–18.
20. Kerlero de Rosbo N, Menon KK. Antibody-mediated demyelinating pathway: stimulation of the myelin protease is associated with specific recognition of externally located antigens of myelin. *J Neurochem* 1994; **63**(suppl 1): S42.
21. Menon KK, Piddlesden SJ, Bernard C. Demyelinating antibodies to myelin oligodendrocyte glycoprotein and galactocerebroside induce degradation of myelin basic

protein in isolated human myelin. *J Neurochem* 1997; **69**: 214–222.

22. Seil FJ, Garwood MM, Clark HB, Agrawal HC. Demyelinating and myelination inhibiting factors induced by chloroform–methanol insoluble proteins of myelin. *Brain Res* 1983; **288**: 384–388.

23. Lebar R, Lubetzki C, Vincent C, Lombrail P, Boutry J-M. The M2 autoantigen of central nervous system myelin, a glycoprotein present in oligodendrocyte membrane. *Clin Exp Immunol* 1986; **66**: 423–443.

24. Lebar R, Vincent C, Fisher-Le Boubenec F. Studies on autoimmune encephalomyelitis in the guinea pig. III. A comparative study of two autoantigens of central nervous myelin. *J Neurochem* 1979; **32**: 1451–1460.

25. Paterson PY. Multiple sclerosis—an immunologic reassessment. *J Chron Dis* 1973; **26**: 119–126.

26. Raine CS. The etiology and pathogenesis of multiple sclerosis—recent developments. *Pathobiol Ann* 1977; **7**: 347–384.

27. Lassmann H, Stemberger H, Kitz K, Wisniewski HM. In vivo demyelinating activity of sera from animals with chronic experimental allergic encephalomyelitis. Antibody nature of the demyelinating factor and the role of complement. *J Neurol Sci* 1983; **59**: 123–137.

28. Ozawa K, Saida T, Saida K, Nishitani H, Kameyama M. In vivo CNS demyelination mediated by anti-galactocerebroside antibody. *Acta Neuropathol (Berl)* 1989; **77**: 621–628.

29. Mastaglia FL, Carroll WM, Jennings AR. Spinal cord lesions induced by antigalactocerebroside serum. *Clin Exp Neurol* 1989; **26**: 33–44.

30. Woodruff RH, Franklin RJ. Demyelination and remyelination of the caudal cerebellar peduncle of adult rats following stereotaxic injections of lysolecithin, ethidium bromide, and complement/anti-galactocerebroside: a comparative study. *Glia* 1999; **25**: 216–228.

31. Lassmann H, Linington C. The role of antibodies against myelin surface antigens in demyelination in chronic EAE. In: Crescenzi GS, ed. *A Multidisciplinary Approach to Myelin Diseases*. New York: Plenum Press, 1987: 219–225.

32. Rosenbluth J, Schiff R, Liang WL, Dou WK, Moon D. Antibody-mediated CNS demyelination: focal spinal cord lesions induced by implantation of an IgM anti-galactocerebroside-secreting hybridoma. *J Neurocytol* 1999; **28**: 397–416.

33. Litzenburger T, Fassler R, Bauer J et al. B lymphocytes producing demyelinating autoantibodies: development and function in gene-targeted transgenic mice. *J Exp Med* 1998; **188**: 169–180.

34. Schluesener HJ, Sobel RA, Linington C, Weiner HL. A monoclonal antibody against a myelin oligodendrocyte glycoprotein induces relapses and demyelination in central nervous system autoimmune disease. *J Immunol* 1987; **139**: 4016–4021.

35. Raine C. Biology of disease. The analysis of autoimmune demyelination: its impact upon multiple sclerosis. *Lab Invest* 1984; **50**: 608–635.

36. Lassmann H, Brunner C, Bradi M, Linington C. Experimental allergic encephalomyelitis: the balance between encephalitogenic T lymphocytes and demyelinating antibodies determines size and structure of demyelinated lesions. *Acta Neuropathol (Berl)* 1988; **75**: 566–576.

37. Linington C, Bradl M, Lassmann H, Brunner C, Vass K. Augmentation of demyelination in rat acute allergic encephalomyelitis by circulating mouse monoclonal antibodies directed against a myelin/oligodendrocyte glycoprotein. *Am J Pathol* 1988; **130**: 443–454.

38. Fierz W, Heininger K, Schaefer B, Toyka KV, Linington CH, Lassmann H. Synergism in the pathogenesis of EAE induced by an MBP-specific T cell line and monoclonal antibodies to galactocerebroside or to a myelin oligodendroglial glycoprotein. *J Neuroimmunol* 1987; **16**: 55 (abstr).

39. Yamada M, Zurbriggen A, Fujinami RS. Monoclonal antibody to Theiler's murine encephalomyelitis virus defines a determinant on myelin and oligodendrocytes, and augments demyelination in experimental allergic encephalomyelitis. *J Exp Med* 1990; **171**: 1893–1907.

40. Weerth S, Berger T, Lassmann H, Linington C. Encephalitogenic and neuritogenic T cell responses to the myelin-associated glycoprotein (MAG) in the Lewis rat. *J Neuroimmunol* 1999; **95**: 157–164.

41. Seil FJ, Quarles RH, Johnson D, Brady RO. Immunization with purified myelin-associated glycoprotein does not evoke myelination-inhibiting or demyelinating antibodies. *Brain Res* 1981; **209**: 470–475.

42. Linington C, Berger T, Perry L et al. T cells specific for the myelin oligodendrocyte glycoprotein mediate an unusual autoimmune inflammatory response in the central nervous system. *Eur J Immunol* 1993; **23**: 1364–1372.

43. Kojima K, Berger T, Lassmann H et al. Experimental autoimmune panencephalitis and uveoretinitis transferred to the Lewis rat by T lymphocytes specific for the S100β molecule, a calcium binding protein of astroglia. *J Exp Med* 1994; **180**: 817–829.

44. Berger T, Weerth S, Kojima K, Linington C, Wekerle H, Lassmann H. Experimental autoimmune encephalomyelitis: the antigen specificity of T lymphocytes determines the topography of lesions in the central and peripheral nervous system. *Lab Invest* 1997; **76**: 355–364.

45. Linington C, Lassmann H. Antibody responses in chronic relapsing experimental allergic encephalomyelitis: correlation of serum demyelinating activity with antibody titre to the myelin/oligodendrocyte glycoprotein (MOG). *J Neuroimmunol* 1987; **17**: 61–69.

46. Genain C, Hauser SL. Allergic encephalomyelitis in common marmosets: pathogenesis of a multiple sclerosis-like lesion. *Methods* 1996; **10**: 420–434.

47. Genain C, Nguyen M-H, Letvin NL et al. Antibody facilitation of multiple sclerosis-like lesions in a nonhuman primate. *J Clin Invest* 1995; **96**: 2966–2974.

48. Genain C, Abel K, Belmar N et al. Late complications of immune deviation therapy in a nonhuman primate. *Science* 1996; **274**: 2054–2057.

49. McFarland HI, Lobito AA, Johnson MM et al. Determinant spreading associated with demyelination in a nonhuman primate model of multiple sclerosis. *J Immunol* 1999; **162**: 2384–2390.

50. Genain C, Cannella B, Hauser SL, Raine CS. Identification of autoantibodies associated with myelin damage in multiple sclerosis. *Nature Med* 1999; **5**: 170–175.

51. Kerlero de Rosbo N, Brok HP, Bauer J, Kaye JF, 't Hart BA, Ben-Nun A. Rhesus monkeys are highly susceptible to experimental autoimmune encephalomyelitis induced by myelin oligodendrocyte glycoprotein. Characterization of immunodominant cell epitope. *J Neuroimmunol* 2000; **110**: 83–96.

52. Hjelmstrom P, Juedes AE, Fjell J, Ruddle NH. B cell-deficient mice develop experimental allergic

encephalomyelitis with demyelination after myelin oligodendrocyte glycoprotein sensitization. *J Immunol* 1998; **161**: 4480–4483.

53. Lyons J-A, San M, Happ P, Cross AH. B cells are critical to induction of experimental allergic encephalomyelitis by protein but not by a short encephalitogenic peptide. *Eur J Immunol* 1999; **29**: 3432–3439.

54. Raine CS, Hummelgard A, Swanson E, Bornstein MB. Multiple sclerosis: serum-induced demyelination in vitro. A light and electron microscope study. *J Neurol Sci* 1973; **20**: 127–148.

55. Esiri MM. Multiple sclerosis: a quantitative and qualitative study of immunoglobulin containing cells in the central nervous system. *J Neuropathol Appl Neurobiol* 1980; **6**: 9–21.

56. Gerritse K, Deen C, Fasbender M, Ravid R, Boersma W, Claasen E. The involvement of specific anti-myelin basic protein antibody-forming cells in multiple sclerosis immunopathology. *J Neuroimmunol* 1994; **49**: 153–159.

57. Olsson T, Baig S, Hojeberg B, Link H. Antimyelin basic protein and antimyelin antibody-producing cells in multiple sclerosis. *Ann Neurol* 1990; **27**: 132–136.

58. Warren KG, Catz I, Steinman L. Fine specificity of the antibody response to myelin basic protein in the central nervous system in multiple sclerosis: the minimal B-cell epitope and a model of its features. *Proc Natl Acad Sci USA* 1995; **92**: 11061–11065.

59. Wucherpfennig KW, Catz I, Hausmann S, Strominger JL, Steinman L, Warren KG. Recognition of the immunodominant myelin basic protein peptide by autoantibodies and HLA-DR2-restricted T cell clones from multiple sclerosis patient. *J Clin Invest* 1997; **100**: 1114–1122.

60. Baig S, Olsson T, Yu-Ping J, Hojeberg B, Cruz M, Link H. Multiple sclerosis: cells secreting antibodies against myelin-associated glycoprotein are present in cerebrospinal fluid. *Scand J Immunol* 1991; **33**: 73–79.

61. Wajgt A, Gorny M. CSF antibodies to myelin basic protein and to myelin-associated glycoprotein in multiple sclerosis. Evidence of the intrathecal production of antibodies. *Acta Neurol Scand* 1983; **68**: 337–343.

62. Moller JR, Johnson D, Brady RO, Tourtellotte WW, Quarles RH. Antibodies to myelin-associated glycoprotein (MAG) in the cerebrospinal fluid of multiple sclerosis patients. *J Neuroimmunol* 1989; **22**: 55–61.

63. Sun JB, Olsson T, Wang WZ et al. Autoreactive T and B cells responding to myelin proteolipid protein in multiple sclerosis and control. *Eur J Immunol* 1991; **21**: 1461–1468.

64. Soderstrom M, Link H, Xu Z, Fredrikson S. Optic neuritis and multiple sclerosis: anti-MBP and anti-MBP peptide antibody-secreting cells are accumulated in CSF. *Neurology* 1993; **43**: 1215–1222.

65. Sellebjerg FT, Frederiksen JL, Olsson T. Anti-myelin basic protein and anti-proteolipid antibody-secreting cells in the cerebrospinal fluid of patients with acute optic neuritis. *Arch Neurol* 1994; **51**: 1032–1036.

66. Sellebjerg F, Madsen HO, Frederiksen JL, Ryder LP, Svejgaard A. Optic neuritis: myelin basic protein and proteolipid protein antibodies, affinity, and the HLA system. *Ann Neurol* 1995; **38**: 943–950.

67. Kasai N, Pachner AR, Yu RK. Anti-glycolipid antibodies and their immune complexes in multiple sclerosis. *J Neurol Sci* 1986; **75**: 33–42.

68. Ichioka T, Uobe K-I, Stoskopf M, Kishimoto Y, Tennekoon G, Tourtellotte WW. Anti-galactocerebroside antibodies in human cerebrospinal fluids determined by enzyme linked immunosorbent assay (ELISA). *Neurochem Res* 1988; **13**: 203–207.

69. Uhlig H, Dernick R. Monoclonal autoantibodies derived from multiple sclerosis patients and control persons and their reactivities with antigens of the central nervous system. *Autoimmunity* 1989; **5**: 87–99.

70. Sun J, Link H, Olsson T et al. T and B cell responses to myelin oligodendrocyte glycoprotein in multiple sclerosis. *J Immunol* 1991; **146**: 1490–1495.

71. Xiao B-G, Linington C, Link H. Antibodies to myelin–oligodendrocyte glycoprotein in cerebrospinal fluid from patients with multiple sclerosis and control. *J Neuroimmunol* 1991; **31**: 91–96.

72. Lindert R-B, Haase CG, Linington C, Wekerle H, Hohlfeld R. Multiple sclerosis: B- and T-cell responses to the extracellular domain of the myelin oligodendrocyte glycoprotein. *Brain* 1999; **122**: 2089–2099.

73. Reindl M, Linington C, Brehm U et al. Antibodies against the myelin oligodendrocyte glycoprotein and the myelin basic protein in multiple sclerosis and other neurological diseases: a comparative study. *Brain* 1999; **122**: 2047–2056.

74. Raine CS, Cannella B, Hauser SL, Genain CP. Demyelination in primate autoimmune encephalomyelitis and acute multiple sclerosis lesions: a case for antigen-specific antibody mediation. *Ann Neurol* 1999; **46**: 144–160.

75. Kaye JF, Kerlero de Rosbo N, Mendel I et al. The central nervous system-specific myelin oligodendrocytic basic protein (MOBP) is encephalitogenic and a potential target antigen in multiple sclerosis. *J Neuroimmunol* 2000; **102**: 189–198.

76. Holz A, Bielekova B, Martin R, Oldstone MBA. Myelin-associated oligodendrocytic basic protein: identification of an encephalitogenic epitope and association with multiple sclerosis. *J Immunol* 2000; **164**: 1103–1109.

77. Stevens DB, Chen K, Seitz RS, Sercarz EE, Bronstein JM. Oligodendrocyte-specific protein peptides induce experimental autoimmune encephalomyelitis in SJL/J mice. *J Immunol* 1999; **162**: 7501–7509.

78. Zhong M, Cohen L, Meshorer A, Kerlero de Rosbo N, Ben-Nun A. T-cells specific for soluble recombinant oligodendrocyte-specific protein induce severe clinical experimental autoimmune encephalomyelitis in H-2^b and H-2^s mice. *J Neuroimmunol* 2000; **105**: 39–45.

79. Bronstein JM, Lallone RL, Seitz RS, Ellison GW, Myers LW. A humoral response to oligodendrocyte-specific protein in MS. A potential molecular mimic. *Neurology* 1999; **53**: 154–161.

80. Lassmann H, Raine CS, Antel J, Prineas JW. Immunopathology of multiple sclerosis: report on an international meeting held at the Institute of Neurology, University of Vienna. *J Neuroimmunol* 1998; **86**: 213–217.

5

Antibody-mediated remyelination

Allan J Bieber, Arthur E Warrington, Virginia Van Keulen, Bogoljub Ciric, Larry R Pease and Moses Rodriguez

Multiple sclerosis (MS), an inflammatory demyelinating disease of the human central nervous system (CNS), is the most common cause of acquired non-traumatic neurologic disability in young adults. The pathologic hallmarks of the disease include damage to oligodendrocytes and CNS myelin, with subsequent demyelination, axonal loss and glial scarring. Active areas of disease display a prominent inflammatory response with tissue infiltration by mononuclear cells, primarily T-cells and macrophages. Although the exact causes of tissue damage in MS are largely unknown, the accumulation of demyelinated lesions probably accounts, at least in part, for the development of the neurologic deficits that are observed in patients with MS. Therapeutic strategies designed to promote remyelination may therefore hold promise for the treatment of this disease.

REMYELINATION IN MULTIPLE SCLEROSIS

Histologic studies indicating that remyelination can occur in MS lesions were first reported over 30 years ago.[1-3] Prineas and co-workers confirmed these initial reports when they described remyelination in several patients with chronic MS lesions.[4] Nerve fibers with abnormally thin sheaths and shorter than normal myelin internodes were observed at the margins of many of the chronic plaques that were examined. The extent of the observed remyelination was extremely limited.

In contrast, remyelination in acute lesions was much more substantial. Remyelination exceeding 10% of total lesion area was found in over 20% of the lesions that were examined from 15 patients with early-stage MS.[5] Numerous 'shadow plaques' were also observed which contained large numbers of thinly myelinated nerve fibers, suggesting that entire lesions had been remyelinated.

The strong remyelination response in acute MS lesions is reminiscent of remyelination following toxin-induced demyelination in animals.[6-8] Demyelination resulting from the injection of lysolecithin into the CNS is rapidly and completely reversed, with myelin sheaths that are uniformly thinner than normal and with characteristically shorter myelin internodes. The significant remyelination that is observed in MS lesions during the early stages of the disease, and the robust remyelination observed in non-inflammatory animal models of demyelination, suggest that complete myelin repair is possible and that stimulation of the endogenous repair process may be a potential therapeutic target.

THE ROLE OF ANTIBODIES IN MULTIPLE SCLEROSIS

Oligoclonal immunoglobulin bands in the cerebrospinal fluid (CSF) serve as an additional pathologic hallmark of MS.[9] The appearance of these immunoglobulin bands in the majority of patients with MS was initially interpreted as evidence for involvement of the humoral immune response in the pathogenesis of the disease. This notion has been supported by observations in rodents with experimental autoimmune encephalitis (EAE), using antibodies directed against the myelin oligodendrocyte glycoprotein (MOG). In these animals, intravenous injection of monoclonal antibodies (mAbs) against MOG has been shown to increase the severity of the disease, inducing relapses and enhancing demyelination.[10,11] In further support of the idea that antibodies might play a pathogenic role in demyelinating disease is the potential involvement of pathogenic autoantibodies in peripheral neurologic disorders, especially Guillain–Barré syndrome, an inflammatory demyelinating disease of peripheral nerves which is strongly associated with the presence of anti-GM1 and anti-GQ1b ganglioside antibodies.[12,13] However, there is currently little direct evidence to support a role for the humoral immune system in demyelinating diseases of the CNS, and there is no correlation between increased immunoglobulin levels in the CSF of MS patients and progression of the disease.

These observations leave open the possibility that elevated CSF immunoglobulin may represent a beneficial and potentially reparative physiologic response to myelin injury. Given the potential for complete CNS remyelination mentioned above, and the possibility that antibodies might play a beneficial role in the remyelination process, this laboratory has begun to explore the potential of antibody-based therapies for the enhancement of endogenous remyelination.

AUTOANTIBODIES PROMOTE REMYELINATION IN ANIMAL MODELS OF DEMYELINATING DISEASE

One of the first indications that autoreactive antibodies might actually enhance endogenous myelin repair came from studies in which EAE was induced in guinea pigs by immunization with homogenized spinal cord. After the disease was fully established, the animals were injected with myelin basic protein and galactocerebroside in incomplete Freund's adjuvant. Treatment with these myelin components was able to ameliorate the disease, resulting in significant clinical improvement and significantly fewer disease relapses.[14] Upon histologic examination, extensive remyelination of CNS lesions was observed. Based on these observations, this laboratory conducted similar experiments in a mouse model of demyelinating disease, the Theiler's murine encephalomyelitis virus (TMEV) model.

Persistent infection of susceptible mouse strains with TMEV results in chronic demyelination and is an excellent model for progressive MS.[15,16] Demyelination is characterized by viral persistence in oligodendrocytes and macrophages, with chronic demyelination and progressive loss of motor function. The pathology is immune-mediated, with animals demonstrating a wide range of disease phenotypes depending on their specific genetic background.[17] In the SJL strain, demyelination is evident within 30 days after infection. By 1–3 months, the animals begin to develop spasticity and gait abnormalities, weakness of the lower extremities and bladder incontinence, with paralysis eventually occurring by 6–9 months.[18] Spontaneous remyelination is minimal in the SJL strain, making this an excellent model for the study of strategies to promote endogenous remyelination.

To explore the possibility of a beneficial humoral immune response, chronic TMEV-infected mice were treated over a 5-week period with spinal cord homogenate (SCH) in incomplete Freund's adjuvant. Upon histologic examination of spinal cord lesions, immunized animals were found to have substantial CNS remyelination compared to control animals treated with adjuvant alone. Passive transfer of either antiserum[19] or purified immunoglobulin[20] from uninfected animals immunized with SCH was also found to promote remyelination, thus demonstrating a beneficial role for the humoral immune response in promoting myelin repair.

Based on these observations, spleens from SJL mice that had been immunized with SCH were used for the production of hybridomas in an attempt to identify mAbs which promote remyelination. A mouse mAb which enhances remyelination in the TMEV model was subsequently identified and designated SCH94.03.[21] SCH94.03 is a polyreactive IgM isotype antibody which is encoded by genes that are close to the germline immunoglobulin sequence.[22] Intriguingly, SCH94.03 binds to the surface of oligodendrocytes, suggesting that the remyelination-promoting activity of the antibody may involve direct stimulation of myelin-producing cells.[23] In subsequent studies, additional oligodendrocyte-specific mouse IgM mAbs were shown to promote CNS remyelination, further suggesting a direct relationship between oligodendrocyte binding and the remyelination-enhancing activity of the antibodies.[24,25]

HUMAN ANTIBODIES PROMOTE REMYELINATION IN TMEV-INFECTED MICE

Antibody treatment is currently being explored as a therapy for human demyelinating disease. Intravenous immunoglobulin (IVIg) has been used successfully to treat a variety of autoimmune neurologic diseases, including Guillain–Barré syndrome, chronic inflammatory demyelinating polyneuropathy, multifocal motor neuropathy, polymyositis, and myasthenia gravis.[26] Clinical studies in MS indicate that IVIg may be effective in stabilizing the course of the disease.[27] Given the demonstrated ability of a subset of mouse antibodies to promote CNS remyelination, and the potential efficacy of IVIg as therapy for MS in humans, we tested pooled human immunoglobulin for its ability to promote remyelination in the mouse TMEV model.

To determine if polyclonal human Ig (IVIg) could promote remyelination in the TMEV model of MS, chronically infected mice were treated with a single intraperitoneal injection of 1 mg of polyclonal human IgG, or approximately 0.05 g/kg body weight, which corresponds to one-eighth the dose frequently used for human IVIg treatment. Since all of the mouse mAbs that have promoted remyelination were of the IgM isotype, an additional group of mice were treated with a single 1 mg injection of polyclonal human IgM. Upon histologic examination of spinal cord sections 5 weeks after treatment, the area of oligodendrocyte remyelination in mice receiving either polyclonal human IgG or polyclonal human IgM was significantly greater than that observed in a saline-treated group (14.2% for IgG and 23.2% for IgM, compared to 6.74% for saline-treated; expressed as percentage of the total area of myelin pathology).[28] Treatment with polyclonal human IgM resulted in significantly more remyelination than was observed in mice treated with polyclonal human IgG.[28]

In general, individual lesions were either completely repaired or mostly unremyelinated. Few inflammatory cells or macrophages were present in the lesions of antibody-treated mice. In contrast, areas of myelin pathology in the mice treated with saline showed signs of active myelin destruction, with the presence of many inflammatory cells and macrophages, but contained few remyelinated axons. From these results, we conclude that polyclonal human antibodies, especially IgM antibodies, are able to promote significant myelin repair in a mouse model of demyelinating disease. These studies suggest that it may be possible to generate human mAbs which promote remyelination, analogous to those from mice which were initially characterized.

The previously identified mouse mAbs that promote CNS remyelination all bind to oligodendrocytes.[23,25] As a first step in the identification of candidate human mAbs for testing in the TMEV model, we assayed human mAbs for the ability to bind to the surface of rat oligodendrocytes presented in mixed primary culture. Our sources of human mAbs were serum-derived human monoclonal IgMs (sHIgM) and serum-derived human monoclonal IgGs (sHIgG) isolated from patients with monoclonal gammopathy, a condition characterized by high concentrations of monoclonal serum antibody. None of 50 sHIgGs bound to oligodendrocytes, but 6 of 52 sHIgMs bound to the surface of morphologically mature rat oligodendrocytes.[28] The oligodendrocyte-binding sHIgMs were then tested in vivo to determine whether they had remyelination-promoting activity. Among the sHIgMs tested, treatment with sHIgM22 resulted in the highest percentage area of oligodendrocyte remyelination, whereas sHIgM14 yielded no greater remyelination than the saline-treated group (17.1%, 8.4% and 6.7%

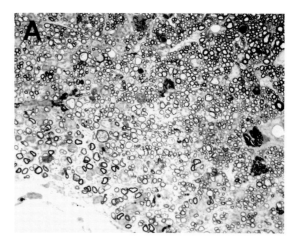

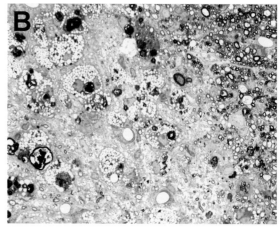

Figure 5.1 Remyelination with sHIgM22. sHIgM22, administered in a single 1 mg intraperitoneal injection, promoted significant remyelination in TMEV-infected SJL mice (A). Darkly staining normal myelin sheaths are apparent in the upper right corner of the panel. Thinner, lightly stained remyelination is evident throughout the rest of the tissue. In contrast, mice receiving saline exhibited many active regions of pathology, with little evidence of remyelination (B). Large numbers of macrophages, filled with vacuoles containing lipid and myelin debris, are evident in the lesions. Magnification ×600.

respectively).[28] The extent of remyelination promoted by sHIgM22 was significant in comparison to the spontaneous remyelination observed in the saline-treated group ($P < 0.05$). Fig. 5.1 shows a well-remyelinated lesion from a sHIgM22-treated animal and, for comparison, an unremyelinated lesion from the saline treatment group. In all treatment groups, the areas of white matter, areas of white matter pathology and percentage areas of remyelination were not statistically different.

sHIgM22 RECOGNIZES HUMAN OLIGODENDROCYTES

If the human mAbs are to be potentially successful in promoting remyelination in human demyelinating disease, their reactivity to surface antigens on human oligodendrocytes may be important in targeting the antibodies to areas of CNS pathology. The sHIgM22 antibody recognizes adult human oligodendrocytes in cultures established from adult human temporal lobe biopsies.[28] Unfixed human glial cells were immunolabeled at 4 days in culture, and oligodendrocytes were identified by labeling with mAb O4, an oligodendrocyte-specific antibody marker which recognizes sulfatide.[29] Most O4-positive cells also label with sHIgM22 (Fig. 5.2A). At later times in culture, human oligodendrocytes did not bind sHIgM22. This observation of transient antigen expression on the surface of oligodendrocytes has also been observed with the mouse mAbs that promote remyelination. Therefore, a direct effect on oligodendrocytes by the human and mouse mAbs that promote remyelination may be at a stage prior to complete oligodendrocyte differentiation, potentially a stage of partial dedifferentiation induced by damage. The sHIgM14 antibody also binds to human oligodendrocytes (Fig. 5.2B), but this antibody does not promote remyelination in vivo, indicating that simple binding to the oligodendrocyte cell surface is not sufficient to stimulate repair and that some form of antibody specificity is involved.

POTENTIAL MECHANISMS FOR THE ACTION OF REMYELINATION-PROMOTING ANTIBODIES

Little is known about the molecular biology of remyelination and even less about the role of antibodies in promoting this process. We propose two general hypotheses by which antibodies might promote remyelination. The antibodies may act by binding to unique receptors on the surface of oligodendrocytes or progenitor glial cells to induce remyelination, the direct hypothesis. Alternatively, the antibodies may work by binding to damaged oligodendrocytes or myelin, which then triggers a cascade of events by other resident CNS cells (astrocytes, microglia or neurons) or hematogenous cells (macrophages or immune T-cells), which in turn enhances myelin repair, the indirect hypothesis.

Since many of the mouse and human remyelination-promoting antibodies bind to oligodendrocytes and/or myelin, it is reasonable to hypothesize a direct effect on the cells being recognized. Work by

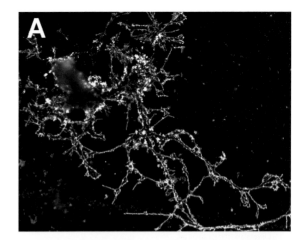

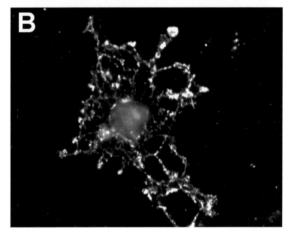

Figure 5.2 Human monoclonal antibody sHIgM22 binds to oligodendrocytes in culture. Cultured human oligodendrocytes were maintained in serum-free media for 3 weeks prior to immunolabeling. Human oligodendrocytes were identified by their labeling with O4 mAb, which binds to sulfatide on the cell surface (not shown). Cells which were positive for sulfatide also bound sHIgM22 (A) and sHIgM14 (B). Although both antibodies bind to the surface of oligodendrocytes, the sHIgM22 antibody actively promotes remyelination, while the sHIgM14 antibody does not. Magnification ×400.

other groups has demonstrated the principle that oligodendrocyte-specific antibodies can cause biochemical and morphologic changes in these cells. Dyer and co-workers have reported that several different antibodies directed against oligodendrocyte surface epitopes, including antibodies to galactocerebroside (GalC), sulfatide and myelin/oligodendrocyte-specific protein (MOSP), can induce changes in the organization of oligodendroglial membrane sheets and in the structure of the oligodendrocyte cytoskeleton.[30–32] These changes in cellular structure were preceded, and probably triggered, by antibody-induced calcium influx.[33–35] Antibody-mediated calcium influx may therefore play an important role in the regulation of oligodendrocyte function and could conceivably play a role in antibody-induced remyelination as well. In addition, Bansal and co-workers have reported that antibodies directed against oligodendrocyte surface antigens can either enhance the rate and extent of oligodendrocyte differentiation,[36] or can inhibit the differentiation of oligodendrocyte progenitors,[37,38] depending upon the specificity of the antibody.

Antibodies might also work to enhance myelin repair through more indirect mechanisms. An attractive hypothesis is that by binding to damaged oligodendrocytes and myelin, there may be opsonization and clearing of CNS debris by macrophages, thus allowing for the normal process of remyelination to ensue. The remyelination-promoting antibodies are all of the IgM isotype, and one of the properties of IgM antibodies is their efficient activation of complement. DeJong and Smith recently demonstrated that complement is a necessary factor for maximal efficiency of myelin phagocytosis by cultured macrophages and have proposed that one important effect of complement is to fragment myelin debris, making phagocytosis more efficient.[39] Large numbers of macrophages are often observed in demyelinated lesions, and phagocytosis of myelin debris may be an important prerequisite for efficient remyelination. Enhanced complement fixation following the binding of myelin debris by remyelination-promoting IgM antibodies may play a role in this process. Recent studies in culture have also demonstrated that treatment with polyclonal human immunoglobulins (IVIg) can act to stimulate the invasion of macrophages into injured nervous tissue and can enhance the phagocytosis and clearance of damaged myelin.[40]

Finally, remyelination-promoting antibodies have been shown to have immunomodulatory effects. A T-cell-mediated immune response has been shown to prevent spontaneous remyelination in chronic TMEV-infected SJL mice, and enhanced remyelination due to antibody-mediated suppression of an inhibitory immune response is another potential mechanism of action of remyelination-promoting antibodies. We have previously demonstrated that in chronic TMEV-infected mice, SCH94.03 treatment results in a 2–3-fold reduction in the number of CD4+ and CD8+ T-cells infiltrating the CNS, and also inhibits humoral antibody responses directed against several different immunizing antigens.[41] The observation that SCH94.03 has immunomodulatory activity is supported by its strong reactivity to dendritic cells of peripheral lymphoid organs, which may be involved in lymphocyte activation.[41]

We have also demonstrated an effect of SCH94.03 treatment on established relapsing EAE in SJL mice. EAE was induced by the adoptive transfer of myelin basic protein peptide-specific T-cells, and antibody treatment was initiated after recovery from the initial episode of clinical disease. Treatment with SCH94.03 reduced by half the percentage of mice that suffered clinical relapse, and prolonged relapse onset by an average of 6 days in those mice that did relapse.[42] The observation that SCH94.03 suppresses CNS inflammation in both the TMEV and EAE models argues strongly for a role for these antibodies as immunomodulatory agents.

SUMMARY

Promotion of CNS remyelination remains an important goal for the treatment of multiple sclerosis. Our laboratory has proposed the use of immunoglobulins directed at CNS antigens as an approach to enhance myelin repair. We have identified a panel of monoclonal antibodies which promote remyelination in a virus-induced model of demyelination in mice. These antibodies are primarily of the IgM isotype and react to surface antigens on oligodendrocytes. We are testing two major hypotheses to explain the mechanism of antibody-mediated myelin repair. The direct hypothesis proposes that antibodies react to surface antigens on oligodendrocytes to induce differentiation and/or proliferation of these cells. The indirect hypothesis proposes that antibodies bind to injured myelin and/or oligodendrocytes, resulting in more efficient scavenging by macrophages, thus allowing endogenous repair to take place. Alternatively, the antibodies may function as immunomodulatory agents and enhance remyelination indirectly through their effects on immune function. This approach to enhance repair is readily applicable to clinical trials in patients with CNS demyelination or injury.

ACKNOWLEDGEMENTS

We thank Mr and Mrs Eugene Applebaum and Acorda Therapeutics for their generous support. This work was also supported by grants from the NIH (NS24180) and the National Multiple Sclerosis Society (RG 3172-A-6).

REFERENCES

1. Perier O, Greqoire A. Electron microscopic features of multiple sclerosis lesions. *Brain* 1965; **88**: 937–952.
2. Feigin I, Popoff N. Regeneration of myelin in multiple sclerosis. *Neurology* 1966; **16**: 364–372.
3. Suzuki O, Andrews JM, Waltz JM, Terry RD. Ultrastructural studies in multiple sclerosis. *Lab Invest* 1969; **20**: 444–454.
4. Prineas JW, Connell F. Remyelination in multiple sclerosis. *Ann Neurol* 1979; **5**: 22–31.
5. Prineas JW, Barnard RO, Kwon EE, Sharer LR, Cho E-S. Multiple sclerosis: remyelination of nascent lesions. *Ann Neurol* 1993; **33**: 137–151.
6. Jeffery ND, Blakemore WF. Remyelination of mouse spinal cord axons demyelinated by local injection of lysolecithin. *J Neurocytol* 1995; **24**: 775–781.
7. Blakemore WF, Eames RA, Smith KJ, McDonald WI. Remyelination in the spinal cord of the cat following intraspinal injections of lysolecithin. *J Neurol Sci* 1977; **33**: 31–43.
8. Pavelko KD, van Engelen BG, Rodriguez M. Acceleration in the rate of CNS remyelination in lysolecithininduced demyelination. *J Neurosci* 1998; **18**: 2498–2505.
9. Mehta PD, Miller JA, Tourtellotte WW. Oligoclonal IgG bands in plaques from multiple sclerosis brains. *Neurology* 1982; **32**: 372–376.
10. Linington C, Engelhardt B, Kapocs G, Lassman H. Induction of persistently demyelinating lesions in the rat following the repeated adoptive transfer of encephalitic T-cells and demyelinating antibody. *J Neuroimmunol* 1992; **40**: 219–224.
11. Schluesener HJ, Sobel RA, Linington C, Weiner HL. A monoclonal antibody against a myelin oligodendrocyte glycoprotein induces relapses and demyelination in central nervous system autoimmune disease. *J Immunol* 1987; **139**: 4016–4021.
12. Willison HJ, Kennedy PGE. Gangliosides and bacterial toxins in Guillain–Barré syndrome. *J Neuroimmunol* 1993; **46**: 105–112.
13. Willison HJ, O'Hanlon G, Paterson G et al. Mechanisms of action of anti-GM1 and anti-GQ1b ganglioside antibodies in Guillain–Barré syndrome. *J Infect Dis* 1997; **176**(suppl 2): S144–S149.
14. Traugott U, Stone SH, Raine CS. Chronic relapsing experimental autoimmune encephalomyelitis: treatment with combinations of myelin components promotes clinical and structural recovery. *J Neurol Sci* 1982; **56**: 65–73.
15. Dal Canto MC, Lipton HL. A new model of persistent viral infection with primary demyelination. *Neurol Neurocir Psiquiatr* 1977; **18**: 455–467.
16. Rodriguez M, Oleszak E, Leibowitz J. Theiler's murine encephalomyelitis: a model of demyelination and persistence of virus. *Crit Rev Immunol* 1987; **7**: 325–365.
17. Lipton HL, Dal Canto MC. Susceptibility of inbred mice to chronic central nervous system infection by Theiler's murine encephalomyelitis virus. *Infect Immun* 1979; **26**: 369–374.
18. Lipton HL, Dal Canto MC. Chronic neurologic disease in Theiler's virus infection of SJL/J mice. *J Neurol Sci* 1976; **30**: 201–207.
19. Rodriguez M, Lennon VA, Benveniste EN, Merrill JE. Remyelination by oligodendrocytes stimulated by antiserum to spinal cord. *J Neuropathol Exp Neurol* 1987; **46**: 84–95.
20. Rodriguez M, Lennon VA. Immunoglobulins promote remyelination in the central nervous system. *Ann Neurol* 1990; **27**: 12–17.
21. Miller DJ, Sanborn KS, Katzmann JA, Rodriguez M. Monoclonal autoantibodies promote central nervous system repair in an animal model of multiple sclerosis. *J Neurosci* 1994; **14**: 6230–6238.
22. Miller DJ, Rodriguez M. A monoclonal autoantibody that promotes central nervous system remyelination in a model of multiple sclerosis is a natural autoantibody encoded by germline immunoglobulin genes. *J Immunol* 1995; **154**: 2460–2469.
23. Asakura K, Miller DJ, Murray K, Bansal R, Pfeiffer SE, Rodriguez M. Monoclonal autoantibody SCH94.03, which promotes central nervous system remyelination, recognizes an antigen on the surface of oligodendrocytes. *J Neurosci Res* 1996; **43**: 273–281.
24. Asakura K, Miller DJ, Pogulis RJ, Pease LR, Rodriguez M. Oligodendrocyte-reactive O1, O4, and HNK1 monoclonal antibodies are encoded by germline immunoglobulin genes. *Mol Brain Res* 1996; **34**: 282–293.
25. Asakura K, Miller DJ, Pease LR, Rodriguez M. Targeting of IgMkappa antibodies to oligodendrocytes promotes CNS remyelination. *J Neurosci* 1998; **18**: 7700–7708.
26. Dalakas MC. Intravenous immune globulin therapy for neurologic diseases. *Ann Intern Med* 1997; **126**: 721–730.
27. Frazekas F, Strasser-Fuchs S, Sorensen PS. Intravenous immunoglobulin trials in multiple sclerosis. *Int MSJ* 1999; **6**: 15–21.
28. Warrington AE, Asakura K, Bieber AJ et al. Human monoclonal antibodies reactive to oligodendrocytes promote remyelination in a model of multiple sclerosis. *Proc Natl Acad Sci USA* 2000; **97**: 6820–6825.
29. Sommer I, Schachner M. Monoclonal antibodies (O1 to O4) to oligodendrocyte cell surfaces: an immunocytological study in the central nervous system. *Dev Biol* 1981; **83**: 311–327.
30. Dyer CA, Matthieu JM. Antibodies to myelin/oligodendrocyte-specific protein and myelin/oligodendrocyte-specific glycoprotein signal distinct changes in the organization of cultured oligodendroglial membranes. *J Neurochem* 1994; **62**: 777–787.
31. Dyer CA, Benjamins JA. Antibody to galactocerebroside alters organization of oligodendroglial membrane sheets. *J Neurosci* 1988; **8**: 4307–4318.
32. Dyer CA, Benjamins JA. Organization of oligodendroglial membrane sheets: II. Galactocerebroside: antibody interactions signal changes in cytoskeleton and myelin basic protein. *J Neurosci Res* 1989; **24**: 212–221.
33. Dyer CA. Novel oligodendrocyte transmembrane signaling systems: investigations utilizing antibodies as ligands. *Mol Neurobiol* 1993; **7**: 1–22.
34. Dyer CA, Benjamins JA. Galactocerebroside and sulfatide independently mediate Ca^{2+} responses in oligodendrocytes. *J Neurosci Res* 1991; **30**: 699–711.
35. Dyer CA, Benjamins JA. Glycolipids and transmembrane signaling: antibodies to galactocerebroside cause an influx of calcium in oligodendrocytes. *J Cell Biol* 1990; **111**: 625–633.
36. Bansal R, Gard AL, Pfeiffer SE. Stimulation of oligodendrocyte differentiation in culture by growth in the presence of a monoclonal antibody to sulfated glycolipid. *J Neurosci Res* 1988; **21**: 260–267.

37. Bansal R, Pfeiffer SE. Reversible inhibition of oligodendrocyte progenitor differentiation by a monoclonal antibody against surface galactolipids. *Proc Natl Acad Sci USA* 1989; **86**: 6181–6185.

38. Bansal R, Pfeiffer SE. Regulation of gene expression in mature oligodendrocytes by the specialized myelin-like membrane environment: antibody perturbation in culture with the monoclonal antibody R-mAb. *Glia* 1994; **12**: 173–179.

39. DeJong BA, Smith ME. A role for complement in phagocytosis of myelin. *Neurochem Res* 1997; **22**: 491–498.

40. Kuhlman T, Bruck W. Immunoglobulins induce increased myelin debris clearance by mouse macrophages. *Neurosci Lett* 1999; **275**: 191–194.

41. Rodriguez M, Lindsley MD. Immunosuppression promotes CNS remyelination in chronic virus-induced demyelinating disease. *Neurology* 1992; **42**: 348–357.

42. Miller DJ, Bright JJ, Sriram S, Rodriguez M. Successful treatment of established relapsing experimental autoimmune encephalitis in mice with a monoclonal natural autoantibody. *J Neuroimmunol* 1997; **75**: 204–209.

6

Apoptosis in multiple sclerosis and experimental autoimmune encephalomyelitis

Daniel Offen, Ronit Mosberg-Galili and Eldad Melamed

INTRODUCTION

It is traditionally believed that the major pathogenetic substrate in multiple sclerosis (MS) is demyelination. However, accumulating evidence suggests that the disability in MS is due to progressive axonal damage and possibly neuronal loss rather than to the demyelination process. Various cell types are considered to be involved in the pathogenesis of MS: oligodendrocytes, microglia, macrophages, lymphocytes and neurons. The natural history of the disease and its severity are associated with the death of some cell types and the birth and proliferation of others. Cells die in various ways, mainly classified into either necrosis or apoptosis. These pathways differ in several parameters, including their morphology, physiology and biochemistry. In contrast to necrosis, which is a sporadic event, most commonly a result of a physiological insult, apoptosis is an active genetically controlled suicide. The apoptotic process is highly regulated by signals or proteins that control it at several crucial points. Cumulative evidence indicates that apoptosis plays a major dual role in the regulation of the inflammation and the progression of the autoimmune reaction in MS and in its animal model experimental autoimmune encephalomyelitis (EAE). Recently, it has been also demonstrated that axonal damage and neuronal loss are associated with the disease progression, possibly independent of inflammation or demyelinization. Here, we review recent studies demonstrating the role of apoptosis in immune cells and neurons in the pathogenesis of MS. The first line of evidence is based on the detection of the differential expression of 'apoptotic genes' such as the bcl-2 family, p53, Fas etc. The second is based on the detection of biochemical factors associated with apoptotic cell death and includes DNA degradation and activation of apoptotic proteins, such as the caspase family. The third line of evidence is derived from experimental animal models that are deficient in or overexpress certain apoptotic genes.

DETECTION OF APOPTOTIC CELL DEATH IN EAE AND MS

Evidence of involvement of the apoptotic process in immune cell death was first shown in EAE. During relapse, myelin-specific T-lymphocytes attack the myelinated tissue of the CNS. The severity of the disease is well correlated with the incidence of those T-cells in the infiltrate. Ultrastructural studies indicate that as much as 49% of the T-cells in EAE lesions at the time of recovery from a relapse show signs of apoptosis.[1] Apoptosis was confirmed in EAE brain macrophages and T-cells by the terminal deoxynucleotidyl transferase-mediated dUTP nick end-labeling (TUNEL) method, which demonstrated the typical DNA fragmentation in situ.[2] Using combined TUNEL and double immunofluorescent labeling, Ray et al[3] found apoptotic mononuclear phagocytes in spinal cord sections of rats with EAE. White et al[4] demonstrated that, in EAE, B-cells are eliminated from the CNS via the apoptotic pathway during spontaneous recovery. These apoptotic B-cells were identified by flow cytometry and electron microscopy in cells extracted from the spinal cord. Furthermore, they showed that B-cells expressing the apoptotic inducers Fas or Fas ligand were highly vulnerable, whereas those B-cells expressing high levels of the anti-apoptotic protein bcl-2 were relatively protected.

It has been shown in several studies that human autoreactive T-cells specific for CNS antigens are increased and activated in MS patients.[5,6] In vitro experiments have also demonstrated that cells from MS patients grown in the presence of apoptosis-blocking antibodies against the CD95 ligand show high numbers of myelin-specific T-cells.[7] The T-cells' CD95 system was also shown to be associated with apoptosis induced by interferon beta (IFN-β), which is widely used in MS therapy. Moreover, when IFN-β treatment failed, deterioration of the disease was associated with the increase in neutralized INF-β antibodies and soluble CD95.[8] Apoptotic T-cells were observed in the CNS in chronic-progressive EAE during recovery, while the antibodies prevented the generation and penetration of new inflammatory cells.[9] Nguyen et al[10] also reported that the beneficial clinical effect of glucocorticoid therapy in myelin basic protein (MBP)-induced EAE in rats is associated with the induction of apoptosis. A single subcutaneous injection of dexamethasone markedly augmented T- and B-cell (CD5), macrophage and microglial (CD11b) apoptosis in the CNS and peripheral nervous system (PNS).

Elimination of autoreactive T-cells by apoptosis has already been used as treatment in EAE models. Zhou et al[11] showed that bisindolylmaleimide VIII facilitates Fas-mediated apoptosis and inhibits the T-cell-mediated autoreaction. Although the early stages of MS are characterized by inflammation and demyelinization with relative preservation of the axons, axonal injury in advanced stages of the disease was demonstrated for the first time by Charcot in 1886.[12] Recent support for Charcot's autopsy findings has been provided by sophisticated diagnostic and imaging tools, which have confirmed the presence of axonal injury and neuronal loss in MS lesions and even in normal-appearing white matter. Ferguson et al[13] followed the accumulation of amyloid precursor protein, found only in axons near the lesions. They showed that the axonal transport is attenuated in the balb area, and this membrane blebbing was positively correlated with the concentration of the activated macrophages near the lesions. Moreover, using unique antibodies against the non-phosphorylated neurofilament typical of demyelinated axons, Trapp et al[14] demonstrated terminal axonal ovoids that indicate axonal transection. Furthermore, magnetic resonance spectroscopy (MRS) using the marker N-Acetyl-Aspartate (NAA) clearly showed axonal damage and brain atrophy in MS patients. Although axonal damage and neuronal loss have been observed, there is no direct evidence that neuronal apoptosis is involved in the progression of MS or EAE.

THE ROLE OF APOPTOTIC GENES IN MS AND EAE

Apoptosis is associated with activation or deactivation of proteolytic enzymes, such as caspases, that execute the death process by cutting the DNA into distinct fragments and deaggregating the DNA and proteins.[15] Studying the oligodendrocytes in the lesioned brain and spinal cord, Kuhlmann et al[16] demonstrated a strong association between the presence of bcl-2-positive oligodendrocytes and the presence of remyelination. Moreover, they found that the highest proportion of bcl-2-positive oligodendrocytes was observed in a subgroup of patients with a relapsing–remitting disease course, indicating that Bcl-2 increases the viability of the oligodendrocytes in MS. In EAE, it was also shown that expression of another anti-apoptotic protein, oligodendrocyte baculovirus p35 caspase inhibitor, protected mice from EAE.[17] Double staining of the EAE brains by the TUNEL method and immunocytochemistry revealed that astrocytes were more likely to be eliminated by apoptotic cell death than microglia.[3]

Extracts of EAE spinal cord showed that significantly increased expression of the two pro-apoptotic regulators, p53 and Bax, correlated with disease severity. This elevated expression could be seen in inflammatory cells but not in neurons or glia.[18] White et al[19] measured the expression of the apoptotic inducer proteins, Fas and Fas-ligand, and the Bcl-2 family of proteins in rat EAE induced by MBP. They found that cells over-expressing Fas and Fas-ligand were represented in the apoptotic population, in contrast to the cells expressing Bcl-2, which were protected from apoptotic cell death. Alcazar et al[20] found that cerebrospinal fluid (CSF) from patients with aggressive MS contains soluble mediators that induce axonal damage and apoptosis of neurons in culture. Furthermore, intraperitoneal or intracisternal administration of the apoptotic inhibitors Ac-YVAD-cmk and zVAD-fmk impaired the recovery or the earlier relapse.[21] The histological examination revealed that zVAD-fmk suppressed apoptotic cell death of inflammatory cells in the CNS of mice with EAE. This indicates that apoptosis of the infiltrated cells might be one of the recovery mechanisms in EAE.

EAE IN MUTANT AND TRANSGENIC ANIMALS

Mutant or transgenic animals provide a powerful tool for studying the physiological function of genes, whether they are overexpressed or absent. These methods enable us to target the genes studied into the relevant organs. One example of such manipulation is the transgenic mice that overexpress in the anti-apoptotic gene *bcl-xl* in their T-cells. These mice demonstrate an earlier onset and a chronic form of EAE.[22] Another study with mice deficient in *Fas*, the pro-apoptotic gene, shows a more severe clinical course of the disease.[23] In our study, we investigated the possible role of axonal damage and the role of anti-apoptotic regulation of neurons in the pathogenesis of MS. We used transgenic mice that overexpress the human *bcl-2* gene exclusively in their neurons, under the control of neuron-specific enolase (NSE) promoter. In previous studies, Bernard et al[24] have demonstrated that these mice contain increased numbers of neurons, due to greater resistance to neuronal death during development. Other studies have shown that these mice have a better performance in several behavioral assays.[25] The NSE–*bcl-2* mice are resistant to induced ischemia and to cell death induced by glutamate and free radicals.[26] The most important characteristic in the present context is their axonal resistance to crash and axotomy.[27] To study the effects of Bcl-2 overexpression in neurons on the pathogenesis of EAE, we compared the clinical manifestations of the disease in WT (C57BL/6) and transgenic NSE–*bcl-2* mice,[28] following disease induction with pMOG$_{35-55}$. We found that, 2 weeks after encephalitogenic challenge, WT mice developed severe EAE, characterized by complete hind limb paralysis (mean maximal score of 2.61 ± 0.18). In contrast, the NSE–*bcl-2* mice were significantly resistant to MOG-induced EAE. Half of the immunized transgenic mice remained disease-free, while the other half demonstrated mild clinical signs characterized by loss of tail tonicity and some weakness of the hind limbs, compared to WT mice (mean maximal score of 1.56 ± 0.39, $P = 0.017$). Thus, the disease induced in NSE–*bcl-2* mice was markedly reduced both in incidence and clinical severity.

Further characterization of spinal cords and brains of the WT animals revealed a widespread perivascular lymphohistiocytic inflammatory infiltrate with scattered neutrophils accompanied by severe demyelination and axonal damage. In contrast, sections of healthy NSE–*bcl-2* mice showed only focal perivascular lymphohistiocytic inflammation. Bielshowsky staining of spinal cord sections from immunized WT mice showed severe axonal damage. Only minimal axonal damage in regions surrounding inflammation was found in healthy immunized NSE–*bcl-2* mice.

To rule out the possibility that the differences in clinical manifestations of the disease in the NSE–*bcl-2* mice were due to generalized immune dysfunction associated with Bcl-2 overexpression in their neurons, the ability of the NSE–*bcl-2* mice to mount a T-cell response was compared to that of WT mice. NSE–*bcl-2* and WT mice were immunized with pMOG$_{35-55}$ and their recall T-cell proliferative response was compared. The immune potency of T-cells in developing a delayed-type hypersensitivity (DTH) response was assayed in both groups. We found that the DTH response against pMOG$_{35-55}$ or against pertussis protein derivative (PPD) was similar in both WT and NSE–*bcl-2* mice. These two experiments indicate that there are no differences between these groups in their capacity to elicit functional encephalitogenic T-cells specific for pMOG$_{35-55}$. We then compared free radical production in brain synaptosomes of WT and NSE–*bcl-2* mice following an oxidative burst by dechlorofluorocin (DCFH), and found that overexpression of Bcl-2 is associated with an increased free radical scavenger capacity of the synaptosomes.

In both EAE and MS, the inflammatory process in the CNS plays an important role in demyelination and axonal damage, consequently contributing to the disease progression. Such inflammatory changes are associated with the local production of highly destructive agents, including nitric oxide (NO) and reactive oxygen species (ROS), that may contribute to axonal damage.[29,30] It has been shown that in rodents with EAE, non-specific inhibitors of NO synthetase (NOS) partially ameliorate the disease.[31] It was suggested that the mechanism by which NO kills cells is not yet understood. However, it appears that NO, together with superoxide, forms highly toxic peroxynitrate, which, in turn, may generate additional free radicals with harmful effects, including lipid and protein oxidation.[32] Our study demonstrated that purified synaptosomes from CNS tissues of NSE–*bcl-2* mice produced significantly fewer free radicals than those of WT mice when challenged with H_2O_2 and NO.[28] Indeed, it has already been shown that oxidative stress is important in the pathogenesis of MBP-induced EAE, and treatment with free radical scavengers such as *N*-acetylcysteine inhibits disease development.[33]

Although the exact mechanism by which Bcl-2 protects cells from apoptotic death is not yet fully understood, it has been suggested that its anti-apoptotic effects are exerted by promoting the function of antioxidants via unknown mechanisms.[34,35] Several in vitro and in vivo studies have demonstrated that Bcl-2 protects cells from apoptosis induced by endogenous or exogenous oxidants and reduces ROS-induced damage.[36,37]

CONCLUSIONS

The mechanisms of progression, disease relapses and recovery from relapses in MS are unknown. However, there are indications that apoptotic death of the oligodendrocytes is a critical event in the pathogenesis of MS. It has also been sugessted that the axonal damage and the brain atrophy are results of apoptotic processes. Moreover, deletion of myelin-specific lymphocytes by apoptosis plays a role in termination of the inflammatory reactions. Cumulative evidence demonstrates that apoptosis plays a major dual role in the regulation of the inflammation and the progression of the autoimmune reaction in MS. Recent findings indicate that pro- and/or anti-apoptotic agents, targeted to the CNS or to the immune cells, might prove to be an important treatment modality for attenuating and delaying inflammation, axonal damage and disease progression in MS.

REFERENCES

1. Schmied M, Breitschopf H, Gold R et al. Apoptosis of T lymphocytes in EAE: evidence for programmed cell death as a mechanism to control inflammation in the brain. *Am J Pathol* 1993; **143**: 446–452.
2. Moon C, Kim S, Wie M et al. Increased expression of p53 and bax in the spinal cords of rats with EAE. *Neurosci Lett* 2000; **289**: 41–44.
3. Ray SK, Schaecher KE, Shields DC, Hogan EL, Banik NL. Combined TUNEL and double immunofluorescent labeling for detection of apoptotic mononuclear phagocytes in autoimmune demyelinating disease. *Brain Res Protoc* 2000; **5**: 305–311.
4. White CA, Nguyen KB, Pender MP. B cell apoptosis in the central nervous system in EAE: roles of B cell CD95, CD95L and Bcl-2 expression. *J Autoimmun* 2000; **14**: 195–204.
5. Zhang J, Markovic-Plese S, Lacet B, Raus J, Weiler HL, Hafler DA. Increased frequency of interleukin-2 responsive T-cells specific for myelin basic protein in peripheral and CSF of patients with multiple sclerosis. *J Exp Med* 1994; **179**: 973–984.
6. Zang YCQ, Kozovska MM, Hong J et al. Impaired apoptotic deletion of myelin basic protein reactive T cells in patients with multiple sclerosis. *Eur J Immuonol* 1999; **29**: 1692–1700
7. Zipp F, Martin R, Lichtenfels R et al. Human autoreactive and foreign antigen specific T cells resist apoptosis induced by recombinant CD95 ligand. *J Immunol* 1997; **159**: 2108–2115.

8. Zipp F, Weller M, Calabresi PA et al. Increased serum levels of soluble CD95 (APO1/Fas) in relapsing remitting multiple sclerosis. *Ann Neurol* 1998; **43**: 116–210.
9. Hyduk SJ, Karlik SJ. Apoptotic cells are present in the CNS throughout acute and chronic-progressive EAE in the absence of clinical recovery. *J Neuropathol Exp Neurol* 1998; **57**: 602–614.
10. Nguyen KB, McCombe PA, Pender MP. Increased apoptosis of T lymphocytes and macrophages in the central and peripheral nervous systems of Lewis rats with experimental autoimmune encephalomyelitis treated with dexamethasone. *J Neuropathol Exp Neurol* 1997; **56**: 58–69.
11. Zhou T, Song L, Yang P, Wong Z, Lui D, Jope RS. Bisindolylmaleimide-8 facilitates Fas mediated apoptosis and inhibits T cell mediated autoimmune diseases. *Nature Med* 1999; **5**: 42–48.
12. Charcot M. Histologie de la sclerose en plaques. *Gaz Hosp* 1868; **41**: 555–558
13. Ferguson B, Matyszak MK, Esivi MM et al. Axonal damage in acute multiple sclerosis lesions. *Brain* 1997; **120**: 292–399.
14. Trapp BD, Peterson J, Ransohoff RM et al. Axonal transection in the lesions of multiple sclerosis. *N Engl J Med* 1998; **338**: 278–285.
15. Earnshaw WC, Martins LM, Kaufmann SH. Mammalian caspases: structure, activation, substrates, and functions during apoptosis. *Annu Rev Biochem* 1999; **68**: 383–424.
16. Kuhlmann T, Lucchinetti CF, Zettl U, Bruck W. Bcl-2 expressing oligodendrocytes in multiple sclerosis lesions. *Glia* 1999; **28**: 34–39.
17. Hisahara S, Araki T, Sugiyama F et al. Targeted expression of baculovirus p35 caspase inhibitor in oligodendrocytes protects mice against autoimmune-mediated demyelination. *EMBO J* 2000; **9**: 341–348.
18. Moon C, Kim S, Wie M et al. Increased expression of p53 and bax in the spinal cords of rats with EAE. *Neurosci Lett* 2000; **289**: 41–44.
19. White CA, McCombe PA, Pender MP. The roles of Fas, Fas ligand and Bcl-2 in T cell apoptosis in the central nervous system in EAE. *J Neuroimmunol* 1998; **82**: 47–55.
20. Regidor I, Masjuan J, Salinas M, Alvarez-Cermeno JC. Axonal damage induced by cerebrospinal fluid from patients with relapsing–remitting multiple sclerosis. *J Neuroimmunol* 2000; **3**(104): 58–67.
21. Okuda Y, Sakoda S, Fujimura H, Yanagihara T. The effect of apoptosis inhibitors on experimental autoimmune encephalomyelitis: apoptosis as a regulatory factor. *Biochem Biophys Res Commun* 2000; **267**: 826–830.
22. Issazadeh S, Abdallah K, Chitnis T et al. Role of passive T-cell death in chronic experimental autoimmune encephalomyelitis. *J Clin Invest* 2000; **105**: 1109–1116.
23. Malipiero U, Frei K, Spanaus KS et al. Myelin oligodendrocyte glycoprotein-induced autoimmune encephalomyelitis is chronic/relapsing in perforin knockout mice, but monophasic in Fas- and Fas-ligand-deficient lpr and gld mice. *Eur J Immunol* 1997; **27**: 3151–3160.
24. Bernard R, Farlie P, Bernard O. NSE–bcl-2 transgenic mice, a model system for studying neuronal death and survival. *Dev Neurosci* 1997; **19**: 79–85.
25. Coleman GHJ, Bernard CC, Bernard O. Bcl-2 transgenic mice with increased number of neurons have a greater learning capacity. *Brain Res* 1999; **832**: 188–194.
26. Martinou JC, Dubois-Dauphin M, Staple JK et al. Overexpression of BCL-2 in transgenic mice protects neurons from naturally occurring cell death and experimental ischemia. *Nature* 1994; **13**: 1017–1030.

27. Chierzi S, Strettoi E, Cenni MC, Maffei L. Optic nerve crush: axonal responses in wild-type and bcl-2 transgenic mice. *J Neurosci* 1999; **19**: 8367–8376.

28. Offen D, Kaye JF, Merims D et al. MOG-induced EAE is attenuated in mice overexpressing bcl-2 in their neurons. *J Mol Neurosci* (in press).

29. Xiao BG, Zhang GX, Ma CG et al. The cerebrospinal fluid from patients with multiple sclerosis promotes neuronal and oligodendrocytes damage by delayed production of nitric oxide in vitro. *J Neurol Sci* 1996; **142**: 114–120.

30. Silber E, Sharief MK. Axonal degeneration in the pathogenesis of multiple sclerosis. *J Neurol Sci* 1999; **170**: 11–18.

31. Hooper DC, Bagasra O, Marini JC et al. Prevention of experimental allergic encephalomyelitis by targeting nitric oxide and peroxynitrite: implications for the treatment of multiple sclerosis. *Proc Natl Acad Sci USA* 1997; **94**: 2528–2533.

32. Lipton SA, Choi YB, Pan ZH et al. A redox-based mechanism for the neuroprotective and neurodestructive effects of nitric oxide and related nitroso-compounds. *Nature* 1993; **364**: 6438–6441.

33. Lehmann D, Karussis D, Misrachi-Koll R, Shezen E, Ovadia H, Abramsky O. Oral administration of the oxidant-scavenger N-acetyl-L-cysteine inhibits acute experimental autoimmune encephalomyelitis. *J Neuroimmunol* 1994; **50**: 35–42.

34. Hockenbery DM, Oltvai ZN, Yin XM, Milliman CL, Korsmeyer SJ. Bcl-2 functions in an antioxidant pathway to prevent apoptosis. *Cell* 1993; **75**: 241–251.

35. Offen D, Beart P, Choung S et al. Transgenic mice expressing human bcl-2 in their neurons are resistant to 6-OH-dopamine and MPTP neurotoxicity. *Proc Natl Acad Sci USA* 1998; **95**: 5789–5794.

36. Offen D, Ziv I, Panet H et al. Dopamine-induced apoptosis is inhibited in PC12 cells expressing Bcl-2. *Mol Cell Neurobiol* 1997; **17**: 289-304.

37. Hochman A, Sternin H, Gorodin S et al. Enhanced oxidative stress and altered antioxidants in brains of Bcl-2 deficient mice. *J Neurochem* 1998; **71**: 741–748.

7

Cell migration and adhesion molecules at the blood–brain barrier in experimental autoimmune encephalomyelitis and multiple sclerosis

Juan J Archelos, Bernd C Kieseier and Hans-Peter Hartung

INTRODUCTION

Although the blood–brain barrier (BBB) constitutes one of the tightest blood–organ barriers known in the human body,[1] a variety of immune cells are found in lesions of the central nervous system (CNS) in inflammatory demyelination. Only activated T-cells and presumably other activated immune cell types can pass the intact BBB.[2] The degree of accessibility of a pathologically open BBB for non-activated leukocytes is less well characterized. From numerous in vitro and in vivo experiments, it has emerged that adhesion molecules, matrix metalloproteinases, chemokines and their regulators such as cytokines are crucial molecules to direct the migration of T-cells into the CNS during inflammation. Here we review the evidence to implicate these molecules in T-cell migration at the BBB in multiple sclerosis (MS), the prototype chronic inflammatory disease of the CNS, and in its animal model, experimental autoimmune encephalomyelitis (EAE).

ADHESION MOLECULES

Structural and functional features

On a molecular level, adhesion molecules (AMs) are critically involved in all steps of the immune response.[3–5] Based on their structure, three main classes of AM can be distinguished: (1) members of the immunoglobulin superfamily; (2) integrins; and (3) selectins[5] (Table 7.1).

Upregulation of adhesion molecules in inflammation of the CNS

Experimental autoimmune encephalomyelitis
In the acute phase of EAE, both ICAM-1 and VCAM-1 are upregulated on lesion- and non-lesion-associated blood vessels. PECAM-1 seems to be redistributed and enriched at the endothelial tight junctions without an increase of expression, while MAdCAM-1, P-selectin and E-selectin are not found at any stage of the disease.[6–9] Endothelial integrins are modulated in EAE and exhibit a defined spatiotemporal expression pattern at the BBB[10,11] (Fig. 7.1). Clinical relapses, BBB breakdown and parenchymal infiltration are preceded by an upregulation of certain AMs on blood vessels.[12]

Multiple sclerosis
Similar to the situation in EAE, in the acute and chronic active MS lesion ICAM-1, VCAM-1 and E-selectin are upregulated on endothelial cells[11,13,14] and integrins are modulated on endothelial cells at the BBB.[15] In situ, the immune molecule expression patterns of infiltrating T-cells and resident neural cells have been described in the MS lesion[11,16,17] (Fig. 7.2). It is noteworthy that ICAM-1/LFA-1 expression is present at relatively high levels in plaques of all ages. In contrast, VCAM-1/VLA-4 is lowest in acute lesions and increased in chronic lesions. Certain integrin subunits have been associated with a chronic breakdown of the BBB in MS.[15] The presence of a variety of AMs on mononuclear cells in EAE and MS and their upregulation on endothelial cells at the

Table 7.1 Adhesion molecules (AMs) putatively involved in transendothelial migration of T-cells at the blood–brain barrier in EAE and MS

AM	Expression	Ligands
ICAM-1	E, T, B, Ma, Mi, A	$\alpha_L\beta_2$ (LFA-1), Mac-1, CD43
VCAM-1	E, Ma, Pe	$\alpha_4\beta_1$ (VLA-4), $\alpha_4\beta_7$
PECAM-1	E, T, Ma, NK	PECAM-1, $\alpha_v\beta_3$
$\alpha_4\beta_1$ (VLA-4)	T, B, Ma	VCAM-1, FN, VLA-4, $\alpha_4\beta_7$
$\alpha_L\beta_2$ (LFA-1)	T, Ma, Mi	ICAM-1, -2, -3
$\alpha_4\beta_7$ (LPAM-1)	T	VCAM-1, FN, MAdCAM-1
$\alpha_M\beta_2$ (Mac-1)	Ma, Mi, NK	ICAM-1, FN, C3bi
E-selectin	E	sLewis^x, ESL-1
L-selectin	T, B, Ma	sLewis^x, mucins
P-selectin	E	sLewis^x, PSGL-1
CD44	T, B, Ma, A, O	ECM

Only cellular distributions and functions of AMs with potential relevance for the pathogenesis of MS are given. Cellular distribution: A, astrocytes; B, B-cells; E, endothelial cells; Ma, macrophages, monocytes; Mi, microglia; NK, natural killer cells; Pe, pericytes; O, oligodendrocytes; T, T-cells. Abbreviations: C3bi, complement factor 3bi; ECM, hyaluronate, collagen, fibrinectin, laminin; ESL-1, E-selectin ligand-1; FN, fibronectin; ICAM-1, intercellular cell adhesion molecule-1; LFA-1, lymphocyte function-associated molecule-1; LPAM-1, lymphocyte Peyer´s patch adhesion molecule-1; Mac-1, macrophage glycoprotein associated with complement receptor function; MAdCAM-1, mucosal addressin cell adhesion molecule-1; PECAM-1, platelet/endothelial cell adhesion molecule-1; PSGL-1, P-selectin glycoprotein ligand-1; VCAM-1, vascular cell adhesion molecule-1; VLA-4, very late antigen-4. Mucins: CD34, GlyCAM, MAdCAM, PSGL-1.

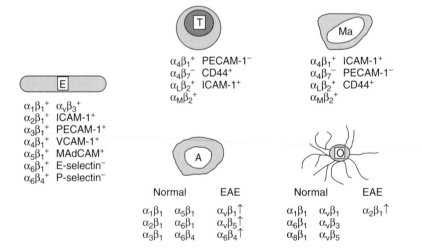

Figure 7.1 Expression of adhesion molecules and integrins on CNS endothelium and infiltrating immune cells in experimental autoimmune encephalomyelitis (EAE), and on glia in EAE. In rodent EAE, endothelial cells (E) of the CNS, infiltrating T-cells (T) and macrophages (Ma) have an adhesion molecule phenotype characteristic of a T-helper-1-mediated disease. Astrocytes (A) and oligodendrocytes (O) express a variety of integrins in normal rats. In acute EAE, there is an upregulation of the vitronectin and laminin receptors on astrocytes and neo-expression of $\alpha_2\beta_1$ on oligodendrocytes, both mediated in vitro by tumor necrosis factor alpha (TNF-α), a central proinflammatory cytokine in EAE.

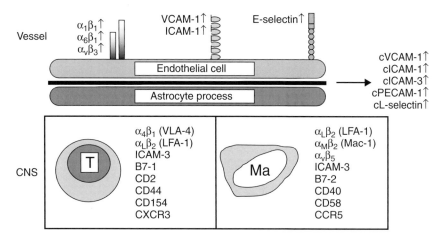

Figure 7.2 Expression of integrins and immune molecules in the active MS lesion. Integrins are expressed and regulated on endothelial, neural and infiltrating mononuclear cells in MS. Together with other immunomodulating molecules present on the surface of these cells, they contribute to the development and maintenance of the inflammatory process. cICAM-1 and cVCAM-1, circulating integrin ligands, are elevated in remitting–relapsing MS and correlate with disease activity on cranial MRI. Only the expression patterns described in MS lesions are listed. Data from EAE, although they may apply to MS, are not included. B7, B-cell activation antigen B7; CD40L (CD154), ligand of CD40; CXR, chemokine receptors; ICAM-3 (CD50), intercellular cell adhesion molecule-3; LFA-1 (CD58), lymphocyte function-associated molecule-3; VCAM-1 (CD106), vascular cell adhesion molecule-1.

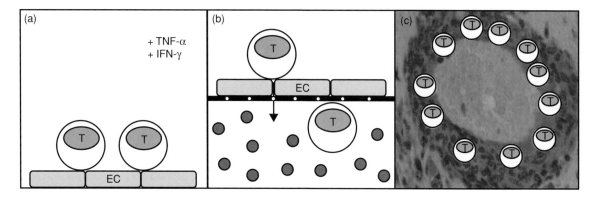

Figure 7.3 Commonly used in vitro assays to elucidate the functional role of AMs. Essentially, three types of in vitro adhesion assay have been used to study T-cell adhesion and migration at the BBB. (a) Brain endothelial cells (ECs) are cultured as a monolayer and incubated with T-cells, which adhere to a variable degree to ECs depending on the activation status of both cell types (e.g. resting versus activated by cytokines such as TNF-α or interferon gamma (IFN-γ)), the incubation temperature, the cell types used (e.g. primary cells versus cell lines), and the duration of interaction. The role of AMs in this initial T-cell adhesion is evaluated by incubation of the cells with monoclonal antibodies (mAbs) to a defined AM. Significant inhibition of cell adhesion by a defined antibody suggests an important role of the corresponding AM in this initial adhesion step. (b) The transmigration of T-cells across an endothelial cell layer is studied in Boyden chambers. This two-chamber model allows us to introduce chemoattractants in the lower chamber and to examine their role in transmigration. More complex models use an extracellular matrix coated membrane on which the ECs are grown. (c) A more direct approach involves the adhesion of resting or activated T-cells to inflamed vessels on tissue sections obtained from the CNS of EAE animals and the blockade of adhesion by incubation with mAb to AM.

BBB during active disease suggests a pathophysiological role of AMs in the initiation of CNS inflammation. The role of AMs in the transmigration of T-cells across the BBB has been studied in a variety of in vitro assays and in animal models.

Function of adhesion molecules

In vitro assays

Despite large variations in experimental setting, three basic assay types have been used (Fig. 7.3). Recent observations suggest that the initial adhesion of T-cells to cytokine-stimulated endothelial cells (ECs) is mediated by ICAM-1 and VCAM-1 and the following transmigration by ICAM-1, PECAM-1 and E-selectin.[18–20] Laschinger and Engelhardt[21] studied an encephalitogenic T-cell line and found that α_L, α_4, α_7, β_1, ICAM-1 and VCAM-1 mediate the initial adhesion, and α_L and ICAM-1 the transmigration, of these EAE-inducing cells. In elegant adhesion assays utilizing inflamed vessels isolated from EAE animals, adhesion of T-cells to inflamed endothelium has been shown to depend on α_4, $\times_1$, ICAM-1, LFA-1 and VCAM-1.[22,23] The differing findings obtained with these in vitro assays reflect the high variability that results from a critical role of several other parameters (Fig. 7.3). In MS, in vitro assays showed that T-cells adhere more avidly to ECs during exacerbation[24–26] and engage in transendothelial migration ex vivo.[27,28]

In vivo studies

To obtain more conclusive evidence for a pathogenic role of AMs in EAE, several groups studied the effects of therapeutic manipulation with monoclonal antibodies (mAbs). Antibodies to AMs putatively involved in transendothelial migration at the BBB did indeed prevent the development of clinical disease and reduced mononuclear infiltration and demyelination[5,16,29–32] (Table 7.2). The mechanisms underlying suppression of EAE achieved with such intervention vary considerably, depending on which AM is targeted. In rodent models of EAE, not all antibodies masking a specific AM are equipotent: some prevent clinical signs completely, while others only retard disease. Even worsening of EAE with antiadhesion monoclonal antibody treatment was observed.[29] In addition, severe side-effects such as focal spleen and liver necrosis, generalized immunosuppression,[33] cerebral bleeding,[34] and severe lymphopenia have been described in the Lewis rat EAE model.[35] Potentially opposing actions and even severe adverse effects noted with these antibodies underscore the complexity of the biological role of cell adhesion molecules and emphasize the need for

Table 7.2 Treatment efficacy of monoclonal antibodies to adhesion molecules (AMs) in EAE

AM	EAE	Efficacy	No. of studies
$\alpha_4\beta_1$	Active	++	> 4
	AT	++	> 5
VCAM-1	Active	ND	0
	AT	+	1
$\alpha_4\beta_7$	Active	0	1
	AT	0/+	1/1
ICAM-1	Active	+	3
	AT	0/+	1/3
LFA-1	Active	+	1
	AT	–/+	2/1
PECAM-1	Active	ND	0
	AT	0	1
L-selectin	Active	0/+	1/1
	AT	0	2
E-selectin	Active	0	1
	AT	0	1
P-selectin	Active	0	1
	AT	0	1
CD44	Active	0	1
	AT	++	2

Active, EAE induction with an encephalitogenic protein or peptide; AT, adoptive transfer of encephalitogenic T-cells to induce EAE; 0, no significant effect; +, moderately effective suppression; ++, very effective suppression; –, worsening of disease; ND, not done.

careful experimentation in appropriate animal models. To understand the multitude of individual functions and to be able to target the most appropriate ones with high specificity, further studies are needed using antibodies with well-characterized specificity or those engineered to react with defined epitopes/domains.

In addition to studies of the role of AMs in the acute transendothelial migratory process, attempts to link specific AMs to different stages in the generation of the chronic inflammatory lesion have been reported[22,23,30–33,36–38] (Fig. 7.4).

Summarizing in vitro and in vivo experimentation, a cascade of sequentially interacting pairs of AMs seems to be responsible for the crucial transendothelial migration of T-cells into the target organ.[3–5] Integrins and members of the immunoglobulin superfamily are essentially involved in the

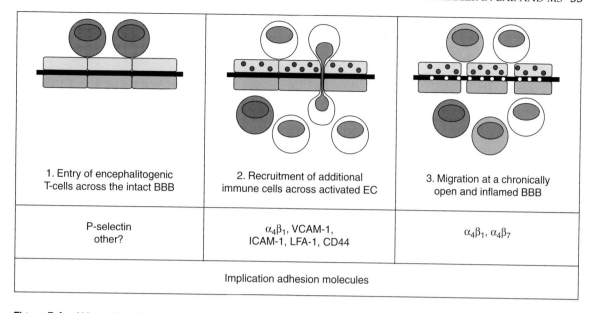

1. Entry of encephalitogenic T-cells across the intact BBB	2. Recruitment of additional immune cells across activated EC	3. Migration at a chronically open and inflamed BBB
P-selectin other?	$\alpha_4\beta_1$, VCAM-1, ICAM-1, LFA-1, CD44	$\alpha_4\beta_1$, $\alpha_4\beta_7$
Implication adhesion molecules		

Figure 7.4 AMs mediate T-cell recruitment in different stages of EAE. Summary of the currently available in vivo evidence for a crucial role of AMs at different stages of lesion development in EAE.

trafficking of T-cells and monocytes/macrophages across vessel walls. Selectins are necessary for T-cell recirculation and for transendothelial migration. Based on the studies published to date, the α_4 chains of VLA-4, CTLA-4 and ICAM-1 appear to be the most promising targets for intervention. The validity of this concept of AM-dependent T-cell migration at the BBB in inflammation was examined recently in a first phase II clinical trial with a humanized mAb against α_4 in MS.[39] Two single antibody injections reduced the number of new active lesions to 50% in the first 3 months. However, the complexity of anti-AM-treatment was underscored by the observation of increased relapse rates in the treatment group after discontinuation of antibody administration. Interestingly, approved immune-modulating therapies for MS modify T-cell migration and downregulate expression of putatively important AM and matrix metalloproteinases by T-cells and brain endothelium[27,28,40–47] (Table 7.3).

Circulating adhesion molecules in MS

Not only are AMs present at the BBB as anchored transmembrane molecules, but some, after interaction with the corresponding ligand, are cleaved or shed and circulate as soluble forms in body fluids.[48]

Table 7.3 Effect of immunomodulatory treatment on T-cell migration and AM expression

Treatment	T-cell adhesion/migration	Possible mechanisms	AM on ECs/T-cells
MP	Adhesion ↓	MMP-2/-9 ↓	E-selectin, ICAM-1, VLA-4, LFA-1 ↓
IFN-β_1	Migration ↓	MMP-9 ↓	VLA-4 ↓
	Adhesion ↓		
GA	Migration ↓	Not defined	No effect
	No effect		

EC, endothelial cell at the BBB; GA, glatiramer acetate; MMP, matrix metalloproteinases; MP, methylprednisolone; IFN-β_1, interferon-β_1.

Table 7.4   Circulating AM levels in MS

cAM	Serum levels	Correlation with clinical DA	Correlation with MRI DA	Studies +/−
cICAM-1	↑	+	+	> 9/5
cVCAM-1	↑	+	+	> 6/3
cPECAM-1	↑	ND	+	1
cL-selectin	↑	+	+	2/2
cE-selectin	↑[a]	+	−	4/1

[a]Primary progressive form of MS. DA, disease activity; ND, not done; studies +/−, number of studies which support (+) or do not support (−) the presence of elevated levels of cAMs in MS.

Areas of interest are the cellular origin of the circulating forms, the molecules inducing cleavage and shedding, and the physiological function of circulating adhesion molecules (cAMs). In addition, in MS an easy-to-measure disease activity marker is much needed. cAMs could be promising candidates.

In MS, circulating forms of ICAM-1, ICAM-3, VCAM-1, PECAM-1, E-selectin and L-selectin have been associated with clinical and MRI disease activity[16] (Table 7.4).

CHEMOKINES

The burgeoning family of chemoattractant cytokines, so-called chemokines, comprises a large and diverse group of 8–10-kDa proteins that display between two and four N-terminal cystein amino acid residues. Based on the relative positions of these cystein residues in the mature protein, chemokines are divided into the CXC (or α), CC (or β), C (or γ), and CX$_3$C (or δ) subfamilies. To date, over 50 different chemokines have been recognized.

Secreted by a variety of leukocytes and other cell types, chemokines are functionally characterized by their capacity to induce the directional migration and activation of leukocytes. Furthermore, they promote humoral and cell-mediated immune reactions, and regulate cell adhesion, leukocyte trafficking, and homing.[49–51]

Chemokines exert their effects by binding to homologous transmembrane G protein-coupled receptors on target cells. To date, four human CXC chemokine receptors, eight human CC chemokine receptors and one human CX$_3$C chemokine receptor have been identified. All receptors are expressed on various types of leukocytes—some appear to be restricted to certain cell types, whereas others are more widely displayed. Furthermore, in some cell types, chemokine receptors are found to be constitutively expressed, whereas they are inducible in others.[2] This diversity is also reflected in the expression pattern noted on T-helper cells: Th1 cells preferentially express CXCR3 and CCR5, whereas Th2 cells preferentially express CCR4 and CCR3. The migratory responsiveness is mirrored by the chemokine receptor expression pattern identifiable on these cell subtypes.[52]

Several studies have revealed a strong and consistent relationship between chemokine expression in the CNS and clinical symptoms of EAE, and a good correlation of the chemokine expression pattern and morphological changes due to inflammation. Glabinski and colleagues demonstrated that chemokine expression immediately followed the earliest entry of leukocytes into the CNS,[52,53] thus potentially mediating an amplification of the inflammatory reaction. Astrocytes in particular were detected as primary sources of various chemokines, such as monocyte chemotactic proteins 1 (MCP-1), 2 (MCP-2), and 3 (MCP-3), as well as interferon (IFN) inducible protein 10 (IP-10), and growth-regulated oncogene α (GRO-α).[53,54] In chronic EAE models, a dramatic increase of MCP-1, IP-10, GRO-α, RANTES (Regulated on Activation, Normal T-cells, Expressed and Secreted) and macrophage inflammatory protein 1α (MIP-1α) was detectable during relapses; the first three were observed in astrocytes surrounding inflammatory foci, whereas the latter two were displayed by invading mononuclear cells within inflammatory lesion.[55]

The clinical course of EAE could be modulated by antibodies blocking chemokine function,[56] underscoring the important role of chemokines in the pathogenesis of inflammatory demyelination. Studies performed on brain tissue confirmed findings obtained in the animal model, and revealed the expression of MCP-1, MCP-2 and MCP-3 by reactive astrocytes in active and chronic–active MS lesions. Furthermore, inflammatory cells within the lesion expressed these proteins, as well as ECs, which were positive for MCP-3[58–59] Activated perivascular T-cells were demonstrated to express RANTES in active MS plaques[60] as well as surrounding astrocytes.[58] Moreover, MIP-1α was recognized on astrocytes and macrophages within the plaque, whereas MIP-1β was expressed by macrophages and microglia within the lesion and microglia in surrounding white matter.[58] In the cerebrospinal fluid (CSF) of MS patients, increased levels of MIP-1α,[61] IP-10, RANTES and monokine induced by IFN-γ-(Mig) could be detected. In vitro studies revealed that MIP-1α, MIP-1β, and IP-10 are secreted from myelin proteolipid protein-specific CD8+ T-cell lines derived from MS patients.[62]

Recently, Ransohoff and co-workers were able to demonstrate a distinct pattern of chemokine receptor expression in MS lesions:[63] CXCR3 was found to be expressed by mononuclear cells, whereas CCR5 could be localized to lymphocytic cells, macrophages, and microglia cells. Strikingly, increased numbers of CD4+ cells displaying CXCR3 and CD4+CD8+ cells carrying CCR5 were detected in the CSF compared to the peripheral venous blood of MS patients. Similar observations were reported by an independent group, demonstrating increased numbers of CXCR3+ and CCR5+ peripheral blood T-cells in MS patients.[64] These findings emphasize the need to further elucidate the complex interaction of chemokines and their receptors in the initiation, perpetuation and resolution of inflammatory demyelination.

MATRIX METALLOPROTEINASES

The matrix metalloproteinases (MMPs) comprise a large group of endoproteinases that share some structural features in the N-terminal catalytic domains. At least 23 members are known, and these can be categorized into the subfamilies of the collagenases, gelatinases, stromelysins, matrilysin, and membrane-type metalloproteinases. With the exception of the membrane type MMPs, which are bound to the cellular surface, all other MMPs are secreted into the extracellular space by a wide range of cell types as latent pro-enzymes requiring activation by proteolytic cleavage of an N-terminal domain to expose the active catalytic site. Since MMPs can catalyze the degradation of all protein components of the extracellular matrix, their finely tuned regulation is of critical importance to prevent tissue destruction.[65,66]

In recent in vitro studies, the spectrum of MMP substrates was extended to pro-forms of MMPs, enzyme inhibitors, cell membrane-bound adhesion molecules, cytokine precursors, and cytokine receptors. The shedding of the pro-form of the pro-inflammatory cytokine tumor necrosis factor alpha (TNF-α) was, in particular, attributed to MMPs.[67,68] However, recent work suggests that the TNF-α-converting enzyme (TACE) is not an MMP; indeed, TACE has been cloned independently by two groups and identified as a unique disintegrin metalloproteinase with notable sequence identity to the adamalysin family of metalloproteinases.[69]

A growing body of evidence indicates that the contribution of MMPs to the pathogenesis of EAE might be manifold. This evidence is based in part on the observation that all important effector cells potentially involved in the pathogenesis of EAE, such as T-lymphocytes, macrophages, astrocytes, and microglial cells, apparently express different MMPs. Increased levels of MMP-9 were detected in the CSF of rodents with EAE. On the mRNA level, a differential regulation of MMPs during the clinical course of EAE has been found. MMP-7 and -9 were dramatically upregulated at the peak of clinical disease.[70,71] We were able to localize MMP-9 to infiltrating mononuclear cells and to the perivascular area.[71] The injection or induction of MMP-9 and MMP-2 resulted in breakdown of the extracellular matrix and opening of the BBB in rats.[72,73] These studies suggested that MMPs might be critically involved in BBB damage. In fact, recent evidence has confirmed this notion. When MMP-7, -8 and -9 were injected into the brain parenchyma of rats in a delayed-type hypersensitivity model of MS, leukocyte recruitment and BBB breakdown were observed.[74] Earlier in vitro studies had already indicated that MMPs, in particular MMP-9, apparently promote trans-basement membrane migration of T-lymphocytes.[75] Given the essential role of T-cell migration from blood into brain to the genesis of organ-specific autoaggression, MMPs are in all likelihood strategic effector mediators in the evolution of autoimmune CNS demyelination.

The myelin sheath is another potential target for proteolytic MMPs, since these proteases are known to degrade myelin basic protein (MBP) in vitro.[76] Thus, MMPs would act as immediate effector molecules in the process of demyelination and could perpetuate the immunoinflammatory response by generating additional immunogenic peptides.

The application of broad-spectrum MMP inhibitors has been shown to suppress the development of and to reverse established EAE in a dose-dependent way.

This was paralleled by restoration of the damaged BBB in the inflammatory phase of the disease, and a significant reduction in MMP-9 activity within the CSF. However, no change in the degree of inflammation and demyelination was noted.[77,78] In a delayed-type hypersensitivity, non-CNS antigen, rodent model of MS that causes focal demyelinating lesions morphologically similar to MS plaques, MMP inhibition was able to prevent both inflammation and demyelination.[79] In chronic relapsing EAE, a synthetic MMP inhibitor was shown to completely block acute and to reverse established severe disease. In this study, mRNAs for TNF-α and the cell death signaling molecule FasL were found to be downregulated, whereas mRNA for the anti-inflammatory Th2 cytokine IL-4 was upregulated.[80]

Several studies have attempted to elucidate the expression pattern of MMPs in the human brain. In autopsied brain samples from patients without any demyelinating disease of the CNS, MMP-1, -2, -3 and -9 could be localized to microglia and astrocytes. An increase in the expression of these MMPs was noticeable in samples from MS patients. In addition, perivascular macrophages were found to stain positive for MMP-9. The cytokines known to induce MMP-9 expression are also detectable within active MS lesions, both in perivascular cells and in activated microglia.[81,82]

Further evidence is available to suggest that MMPs are important mediators in BBB breakdown in MS. In the CSF of MS patients, raised levels of MMP-9 are associated with a leaky BBB as demonstrated by enhanced gadolinium passage into the brain parenchyma on magnetic resonance imaging. In addition, treatment with high-dose methylprednisolone, a drug known to negatively influence the transcription of MMPs, reduced both gadolinium enhancement and CSF levels of MMP-9.[83] Other investigators have noted an increase of MMP-9 during clinical relapses in the CSF[84] and in serum. High mean serum MMP-9 levels were associated with significantly more gadolinium-enhancing T1 MRI lesions.[85]

In summary, several lines of evidence suggest that the aberrant expression of MMPs may be of critical importance to the demyelinative process in the inflamed CNS. Damage to the BBB, leukocyte migration, myelin damage, and, potentially, TNF-α activation are crucial effector mechanisms in inflammatory demyelination, all of which seem to be mediated through the proteolytic activity of MMPs. Further research should shed light on the precise pathogenetic role of different MMPs, and allow the development of specific MMP inhibitors that may be applied therapeutically in MS.

CONCLUSION

The BBB as a defined anatomical structure is essential for the maintenance of tissue integrity, and its dysfunction is a crucial early step in the pathogenesis of immune-mediated diseases of the CNS. AMs, chemokines and MMPs expressed at the BBB and their corresponding ligands present on immune cells are of major importance for the transendothelial migration of T-cells and monocytes across the BBB. This step initiates the local immune response in the target tissue and leads to mononuclear infiltration, demyelination and eventually axonal loss with the associated neurological symptoms. The molecular mechanisms operating at the BBB during migration of T-cells into the CNS have been widely explored in EAE. These findings may have considerable therapeutic implications in the near future. A better understanding of the BBB in physiology and pathology will in all likelihood enlarge the therapeutic options in immune-mediated diseases of the CNS.

SUMMARY

MS is an immune-mediated disease of the CNS and constitutes a major cause of transient and permanent neurological disability, particularly in young adults. The etiology and pathogenesis of MS are only partially understood. On a cellular level, focal mononuclear cell infiltration with demyelination and eventual axonal loss are crucial pathogenetic events. In this chapter we have reviewed the evidence that AMs, chemokines and MMPs expressed at the BBB and by T-cells play a central role in immune cell recruitment to the CNS and hence in the development of organ-specific autoaggression. Therapeutic targeting of these molecules has been very successful in the corresponding animal model of experimental autoimmune encephalomyelitis, and holds promise as a novel treatment strategy to combat human immune-mediated disorders of the CNS.

REFERENCES

1. Pardridge WM. Drug delivery to the brain. *J Cereb Blood Flow Metab* 1997; **17**: 713–731.
2. Hickey WF, Hsu BL, Kimura H. T-lymphocyte entry into the central nervous system. *J Neurosci Res* 1991; **28**: 254–260.
3. Springer TA. Traffic signals for lymphocyte recirculation and leukocyte emigration: the multistep paradigm. *Cell* 1994; **76**: 301–314.
4. Butcher E, Picker LJ. Lymphocyte homing and homeostasis. *Science* 1996; **272**: 60–66.
5. Archelos JJ, Hartung H-P. The role of adhesion molecules in multiple sclerosis: biology, pathogenesis

and therapeutic implications. *Mol Med Today* 1997; **3**: 310–321.

6. Engelhardt B, Vestweber D, Hallmann R, Schulz M. E- and P-selectin are not involved in the recruitment of inflammatory cells across the blood–brain barrier in experimental autoimmune encephalomyelitis. *Blood* 1997; **90**: 4459–4472.

7. Williams KC, Zhao RW, Ueno K, Hickey WF. PECAM-1 (CD31) expression in the central nervous system and its role in experimental allergic encephalomyelitis in the rat. *J Neurosci Res* 1996; **45**: 747–757.

8. Dopp JM, Brenemann SM, Olschowka JA. Expression of ICAM-1, VCAM-1, L-selectin, and leukosialin in the mouse central nervous system during the induction and remission stages of experimental allergic encephalomyelitis. *J Neuroimmunol* 1994; **54**: 129–144.

9. Lindsey JW, Steinman L. Competitive PCR quantification of CD4, CD8, ICAM-1, VCAM-1, and MHC class II mRNA in the central nervous system during development and resolution of experimental allergic encephalomyelitis. *J Neuroimmunol* 1993; **48**: 227–234.

10. Previtali S, Archelos JJ, Hartung H-P. Modulation of the expression of integrins on glial cells during experimental autoimmune encephalomyelitis. A central role for TNF-α. *Am J Pathol* 1997; **151**: 1425–1435.

11. Archelos JJ, Previtali SC, Hartung H-P. The role of integrins in immune-mediated diseases of the nervous system. *Trends Neurosci* 1999; **22**: 30–38.

12. Cannella B, Cross AH, Raine CS. Upregulation and coexpression of adhesion molecules correlate with relapsing autoimmune demyelination in the central nervous system. *J Exp Med* 1990; **172**: 1521–1524.

13. Raine CS. Multiple sclerosis: immune system molecule expression in the central nervous system. *J Neuropathol Exp Neurol* 1994; **53**: 328–337.

14. Cannella B, Raine CS. The adhesion molecule and cytokine profile of multiple sclerosis lesions. *Ann Neurol* 1995; **37**: 424–435.

15. Sobel RA, Hinojoza JR, Maeda A, Chen M. Endothelial cell integrin laminin receptor expression in multiple sclerosis lesions. *Am J Pathol* 1998; **153**: 405–415.

16. Archelos JJ, Hartung H-P. Adhesion molecules in multiple sclerosis: a review. In: Siva A, Thompson A, Kesselring J, eds. *Frontiers in Multiple Sclerosis*, Vol. 2. London: Martin Dunitz, 1999: 85–116.

17. Lee SJ, Benveniste EN. Adhesion molecule expression and regulation on cells of the central nervous system. *J Neuroimmunol* 1999; **98**: 77–88.

18. Pryce G, Male D, Campbell I, Greenwood J. Factors contolling T-cell migration across rat cerebral endothelium in vitro. *J Neuroimmunol* 1997; **75**: 84–94.

19. Reiss Y, Hoch G, Deutsch U, Engelhardt B. T-cell interaction with ICAM-1 deficient endothelium in vitro: essential role for ICAM-1 and ICAM-2 in transendothelial migration of T-cells. *Eur J Immunol* 1998; **28**: 3086–3099.

20. Wong D, Prameya R, Dorovini-Zis K. In vitro adhesion and migration of T lymphocytes across monolayers of human brain microvessel endothelial cells: regulation by ICAM-1, VCAM-1, E-selectin and PECAM-1. *J Neuropathol Exp Neurol* 1999; **58**: 138–152.

21. Laschinger M, Engelhardt B. Interaction of alpha4-integrin with VCAM-1 is involved in adhesion of encephalitogenic T-cell blasts to brain endothelium but not in their transendothelial migration in vitro. *J Neuroimmunol* 2000; **102**: 32–43.

22. Yednock TA, Cannon C, Fritz LC et al. Prevention of experimental autoimmune encephalomyelitis by antibodies against α4β1 integrin. *Nature* 1992; **356**: 63–66.

23. Steffen BJ, Butcher EC, Engelhardt B. Evidence for involvement of ICAM-1 and VCAM-1 in lymphocyte interaction with endothelium in experimental autoimmune encephalomyelitis in the central nervous system in the SJL/J mouse. *Am J Pathol* 1994; **145**: 189–201.

24. Tsukada N, Matsuda M, Miyagi K, Yanagisawa N. Adhesion of cerebral endothelial cells to lymphocytes from patients with multiple sclerosis. *Autoimmunity* 1993; **4**: 329–333.

25. Vora AJ, Perkin GD, McCoy T, Dumonde DC, Brown KA. Enhanced binding of lymphocytes from patients with multiple sclerosis to tumour necrosis factor-alpha (TNF-alpha)-treated endothelial monolayers: associations with clinical relapse and adhesion molecule expression. *Clin Exp Immunol* 1996; **105**: 155–162.

26. Lou J, Chofflon M, Juillard C et al. Brain microvascular endothelial cells and leukocytes derived from patients with multiple sclerosis exhibit increased adhesion capacity. *Neuroreport* 1997; **8**: 629–633.

27. Prat A, Al-Asmi A, Duquette P, Antel JP. Lymphocyte migration and multiple sclerosis: relation with disease course and therapy. *Ann Neurol* 1999; **46**: 253–256.

28. Uhm JH, Doley NP, Stüve O et al. Migratory behavior of lymphocytes isolated from multiple sclerosis patients: effects of interferon β-1b therapy. *Ann Neurol* 1999; **46**: 319–324.

29. Cannella B, Cross AH, Raine CS. Anti-adhesion molecule therapy in experimental autoimmune encephalomyelitis. *J Neuroimmunol* 1993; **46**: 43–56.

30. Gordon EJ, Myers KJ, Dougherty JP, Rosen H, Ron Y. Both anti-CD11a (LFA-1), and anti-CD11b (MAC-1) therapy delay the onset and diminish the severity of experimental autoimmune encephalomyelitis. *J Neuroimmunol* 1995; **62**: 153–160.

31. Brennan FR, O'Neill JK, Allen SJ, Butter C, Nuki G, Baker D. CD44 is involved in selective leucocyte extravasation during inflammatory central nervous system disease. *Immunology* 1999; **98**: 427–435.

32. Brocke S, Piercy C, Steinman L, Weissman IL, Veromaa T. Antibodies to CD44 and integrin alpha4, but not L-selectin, prevent central nervous system inflammation and experimental encephalomyelitis by blocking secondary leukocyte recruitment. *Proc Natl Acad Sci USA* 1999; **96**: 6896–6901.

33. Archelos JJ, Jung S, Mäurer M et al. Inhibition of experimental autoimmune encephalomyelitis by an antibody to the intercellular adhesion molecule ICAM-1. *Ann Neurol* 1993; **34**: 145–154.

34. Soilu-Hänninen M, Roytta M, Salmi A, Salonen R. Therapy with antibody against leukocyte integrin VLA-4 (CD49d) is effective and safe in virus-facilitated experimental allergic encephalomyelitis. *J Neuroimmunol* 1997; **72**: 95–105.

35. Archelos JJ, Jung S, Rinner W, Lassmann H, Miyasaka M, Hartung H-P. Role of leukocyte adhesion molecule L-selectin in experimental autoimmune encephalomyelitis. *J Neurol Sci* 1998; **159**: 127–134.

36. Keszthelyi E, Karlik S, Hyduk S et al. Evidence for a prolonged role of α4 integrin throughout active experimental allergic encephalomyelitis. *Neurology* 1996; **47**: 1053–1059.

37. Carrithers MD, Visintin I, Kang SJ, Janeway CA. Differential adhesion molecule requirements for immune

surveillance and inflammatory recruitment. *Brain* 2000; **123**: 1092–1101.

38. Kanwar JR, Harrison JEB, Wang D et al. β7 integrins contribute to demyelinating disease of the central nervous system. *J Neuroimmunol* 2000; **103**: 146–152.

39. Tubridy N, Behan PO, Capildeo R et al. The effect of anti-alpha4 integrin antibody on brain lesion activity in MS. The UK Antegren Study Group. *Neurology* 1999; **53**: 466–472.

40. Cronstein BN, Kimmel SC, Levin RI, Martiniuk F, Weissmann G. A mechanism for the antiinflammatory effects of corticosteroids: the glucocorticoid receptor regulates leukocyte adhesion to endothelial cells and expression of endothelial-leukocyte adhesion molecule-1 and intercellular adhesion molecule-1. *Proc Natl Acad Sci USA* 1992; **89**: 9991–9995.

41. Leppert D, Waubant E, Burk MR, Oksenberg JR, Hauser SL. Interferon beta-1b inhibits gelatinase secretion and in vitro migration of human T-cells: a possible mechanism for treatment efficacy in multiple sclerosis. *Ann Neurol* 1996; **40**: 846–852.

42. Soilu-Hänninen M, Salmi A, Salonen R. Interferon-beta downregulates expression of VLA-4 antigen and antagonizes interferon-gamma-induced expression of HLA-DQ on peripheral blood monocytes. *J Neuroimmunol* 1996; **60**: 99–106.

43. Stüve O, Dooley NP, Uhm JH et al. Interferon β-1b decreases the migration of T lymphocytes in vitro: effects on matrix metalloproteinase-9. *Ann Neurol* 1996; **40**: 853–863.

44. Corsini E, Gelati M, Dufour A et al. Effects of beta-IFN-1b treatment in MS patients on adhesion between PBMNCs, HUVECs and MS-HBECs: an in vivo and in vitro study. *J Neuroimmunol* 1997; **79**: 76–83.

45. Pitzalis C, Sharrack B, Gray IA, Lee A, Hughes RA. Comparison of the effects of oral versus intravenous methylprednisolone regimens on peripheral blood T lymphocyte adhesion molecule expression, T-cell subsets distribution and TNF alpha concentrations in multiple sclerosis. *J Neuroimmunol* 1997; **74**: 62–68.

46. Elovaara I, Lalla M, Spare E, Lehtimaki T, Dastidar P. Methylprednisolone reduces adhesion molecules in blood and cerebrospinal fluid in patients with MS. *Neurology* 1998; **51**: 1703–1708.

47. Dufour A, Corsini E, Gelati M, Massa G, Tarcic N, Salmaggi A. In vitro glatiramer acetate treatment of brain endothelium does not reduce adhesion phenomena. *Ann Neurol* 1900; **47**: 680–681.

48. Hartung HP, Archelos JJ, Zielasek J et al. Circulating adhesion molecules and inflammatory mediators in demyelination. *Neurology* 1995; **45**(suppl 6): S22–S32.

49. Taub DD, Oppenheim JJ. Chemokines, inflammation and the immune system. *Ther Immunol* 1994; **1**: 229–246.

50. Luster AD. Chemokines—chemotactic cytokines that mediate inflammation. *N Engl J Med* 1998; **338**: 436–445.

51. Ward SG, Bacon K, Westwick J. Chemokines and T lymphocytes: more than an attraction. *Immunity* 1998; **9**: 1–11.

52. Bonecchi R, Bianchi G, Bordignon PP et al. Differential expression of chemokine receptors and chemotactic responsiveness of type 1 T helper cells (Th1s) and Th2s. *J Exp Med* 1998; **187**: 129–134.

53. Glabinski AR, Balasingam V, Tani M et al. Chemokine monocyte chemoattractant protein-1 is expressed by astrocytes after mechanical injury to the brain. *J Immunol* 1996; **156**: 4363–4368.

54. Tani M, Glabinski AR, Tuohy VK, Stoler MH, Estes ML, Ransohoff RM. In situ hybridization analysis of glial fibrillary acidic protein mRNA reveals evidence of biphasic astrocyte activation during acute experimental autoimmune encephalomyelitis. *Am J Pathol* 1996; **148**: 889–896.

55. Glabinski AR, Tani M, Strieter RM, Tuohy VK, Ransohoff RM. Synchronous synthesis of alpha- and beta-chemokines by cells of diverse lineage in the central nervous system of mice with relapses of chronic experimental autoimmune encephalomyelitis. *Am J Pathol* 1997; **150**: 617–630.

56. Karpus WJ, Lukacs NW, McRae BL, Strieter RM, Kunkel SL, Mille SD, An important role for the chemokine macrophage inflammatory protein-1a in the pathogenesis of the T cell-mediated autoimmune disease experimental autoimmune encephalomyelitis. *J Immunol* 1995; **155**: 5003–5010.

57. McManus C, Berman JW, Brett FM, Staunton H, Farrell M, Brosnan CF. MCP-1, MCP-2 and MCP-3 expression in multiple sclerosis lesions: an immunohistochemical and in situ study. *J Neuroimmunol* 1998; **86**: 20–29.

58. Simpson JE, Newcombe J, Cuzner ML, Woodroofe MN. Expression of monocyte chemoattractant protein-1 and other beta-chemokines by resident glia and inflammatory cells in multiple sclerosis lesions. *J Neuroimmunol* 1998; **84**: 238–249.

59. van der Voorn P, Tekstra J, Beelen RHJ, Tensen CP, van der Valk P, de Groot CJA. Expression of MCP-1 by reactive astrocytes in demyelinating multiple sclerosis lesions. *Am J Pathol* 1999; **154**: 45–51.

60. Hvas J, McLean C, Justesen J et al. Perivascular T cells express the pro-inflammatory chemokine RANTES mRNA in multiple sclerosis lesions. *Scand J Immunol* 1997; **46**: 195–203.

61. Mijagishi R, Kikuchi S, Fukazawa T, Tashiro K. Macrophage inflammatory protein-1 alpha in the cerebrospinal fluid of patients with multiple sclerosis and other inflammatory neurological diseases. *J Neurol Sci* 1995; **129**: 223–227.

62. Biddison WE, Taub DD, Cruikshank WW, Center DM, Connor EW, Honma K. Chemokine and matrix metalloproteinase secretion by myelin proteolipid protein-specific CD8+ T cells: potential roles in inflammation. *J Immunol* 1997; **158**: 3046–3053.

63. Sorensen TL, Tani M, Jensen J et al. Expression of specific chemokines and chemokine receptors in the central nervous system of multiple sclerosis patients. *J Clin Invest* 1999; **103**: 807–815.

64. Balashov KE, Rottman JB, Weiner HL, Hancock WW. CCR5+ and CXCR3+ T-cells are increased in multiple sclerosis and their ligands MIP-1α and IP-10 are expressed in demyelinating brain lesions. *Proc Natl Acad Sci USA* 1999; **96**: 6873–6878.

65. Woessner JF Jr. The family of matrix metalloproteinases. *Ann NY Acad Sci* 1994; **732**: 11–21.

66. Yong VW, Krekoski CA, Forsyth PA, Bell R, Edwards DR. Matrix metalloproteinases and diseases of the CNS. *Trends Neurosci* 1998; **21**: 75–80.

67. Gearing AJH, Beckett P, Christodoulou M et al. Processing of tumor necrosis factor-α precursor by metalloproteinases. *Nature* 1994; **370**: 555–557.

68. Mohler KM, Sleath PR, Fitzner JN et al. Protection against lethal dose of endotoxin by an inhibitor of tumor necrosis factor processing. *Nature* 1994; **370**: 218–220.

69. Moss ML, Jin S-LC, Milla ME. Cloning of a disintegrin metalloproteinase that processes precursor tumor necrosis factor-α. *Nature* 1997; **385**: 733–736.

70. Clements JM, Cossins JA, Wells GMA et al. Matrix metalloproteinase expression during experimental autoimmune encephalomyelitis and effects of a combined matrix metalloproteinase and tumor necrosis factor-α inhibitor. *J Neuroimmunol* 1997; **74**: 85–94.

71. Kieseier BC, Kiefer R, Clements JM et al. Matrix metalloproteinase-9 and -7 are regulated in experimental autoimmune encephalomyelitis. *Brain* 1998; **121**: 159–166.

72. Rosenberg GA, Kornfeld M, Estrada E, Kelley RO, Liotta LA, Stetler-Stevenson WG. TIMP-2 reduces proteolytic opening of blood–brain barrier by type IV collagenase. *Brain Res* 1992; **576**: 203–207.

73. Rosenberg GA, Dencoff JE, McGuire PG, Liotta LA, Stetler-Stevenson WA. Injury-induced 92-kilodalton gelatinase and urokinase expression in rat brain. *Lab Invest* 1994; **71**: 417–422.

74. Anthony DC, Miller KM, Fearn S et al. Matrix metalloproteinase expression in an experimentally-induced DTH model of multiple sclerosis in the rat CNS. *J Neuroimmunol* 1998; **87**: 62–72.

75. Leppert D, Waubant E, Galardy R, Bunnett NW, Hauser SL. T cell gelatinases mediate basement membrane transmigration in vitro. *J Immunol* 1995; **154**: 4379–4389.

76. Chandler S, Coates R, Gearing A, Lury J, Wells G, Bone E. Matrix metalloproteinases degrade myelin basic protein. *Neurosci Lett* 1995; **201**: 223–226.

77. Gijbels K, Galardy RE, Steinman L. Reversal of experimental autoimmune encephalomyelitis with a hydroxamate inhibitor of matrix metalloproteinases. *J Clin Invest* 1994; **94**: 2177–2182.

78. Hewson AK, Smith T, Leonard JP, Cuzner ML. Suppression of experimental allergic encephalomyelitis in the Lewis rat by the matrix metalloproteinase inhibitor Ro31-9790. *Inflamm Res* 1995; **44**: 345–349.

79. Matyszak MK, Perry VH. Delayed-type hypersensitivity lesions in the central nervous system are prevented by inhibitors of matrix metalloproteinases. *J Neuroimmunol* 1996; **69**: 141–149.

80. Liedtke W, Cannella B, Mazzaccaro RJ et al. Effective treatment of models of multiple sclerosis by matrix metalloproteinase inhibitors. *Ann Neurol* 1998; **44**: 35–46.

81. Cuzner ML, Gveric D, Strand C et al. The expression of tissue-type plasminogen activator, matrix metalloproteases and endogenous inhibitors in the central nervous system in multiple sclerosis: comparison of stages in lesion evolution. *J Neuropathol Exp Neurol* 1996; **55**: 1194–1204.

82. Maeda A, Sobel RA. Matrix metalloproteinases in the normal human central nervous system, microglial nodules, and multiple sclerosis lesions. *J Neuropathol Exp Neurol* 1996; **55**: 300–309.

83. Rosenberg GA, Dencoff JE, Correa N, Reiners M, Ford CC. Effect of steroids on CSF matrix metalloproteinases in multiple sclerosis: relation to blood–brain barrier injury. *Neurology* 1996; **46**: 1626–1632.

84. Leppert D, Ford J, Stabler G et al. Matrix metalloproteinase-9 (gelatinase B) is electively elevated in CSF during relapses and stable phases of multiple sclerosis. *Brain* 1998; **121**: 2327–2334.

85. Lee MA, Palace J, Stabler G, Ford J, Gearing A, Miller K. Serum gelatinase B, TIMP-1 and TIMP-2 levels in multiple sclerosis: a longitudinal clinical and MRI study. *Brain* 1999; **122**: 191–197.

8

Matrix metalloproteinases and their inhibitors in brain injury and repair

Ariel Miller, Sarah Shapiro, Nitza Lahat and Yanina Galboiz

Matrix metalloproteinases (MMPs), a family of zinc-dependent proteolytic enzymes, together with their endogenous tissue inhibitors, TIMPs, are involved in remodeling of the extracellular matrix (ECM) under a variety of physiological conditions. Recent studies, however, have implicated MMPs in various pathological conditions such as tumor invasion and metastasis, arteriosclerosis, and inflammatory and autoimmune diseases.

MMPs appear to play a key role in the pathogenesis of central nervous system (CNS) disorders, contributing to blood–brain barrier (BBB) eruption, brain edema, immune cell infiltration, myelin degradation and glial-scar formation. Increased activity of MMPs has recently been reported in experimental animal models of demyelinating diseases as well as in multiple sclerosis (MS) patients. Similarly, increased levels of MMPs, and in particular MMP-2 and -9, have been detected in experimental cerebral ischemia as well as in stroke patients. Modulation of MMP/TIMP profiles seems to be associated also with bacterial and viral meningoencephalitis. Additionally, though results are still controversial, MMPs seem to be involved in the deposition of β-amyloid protein in Alzheimer's diseases (AD).

The association of MMPs with CNS disorders has raised considerable interest, as they may represent potential biomarkers for disease activity as well as attractive targets for novel therapeutic strategies, aimed at inhibiting MMP activity. Thus, understanding the structure and function of these key enzymes may have significant implications for arresting evolving brain injury and promoting CNS repair.

THE EXTRACELLULAR MATRIX

The extracellular matrix (ECM), in addition to maintaining the structural integrity of different tissues, is involved in determining the uniqueness and characteristics of the distinct tissues and in providing functional signals that dictate a wide range of cellular behavior, including growth, differentiation, proliferation and cell death. ECM-mediated signals and remodeling are also essential for migration of immune cells into inflammatory sites and the initiation or aggravation of tissue injury.[1] The ECM consists mainly of collagen, fibronectin, laminin and various proteoglycans. Breakdown and remodeling of the ECM, by enzymes of the matrix MMP family, are essential in a variety of physiological conditions, such as ovulation and implantation, growth, wound-healing and angiogenesis. On the other hand, excessive breakdown of the ECM is a key process in numerous pathological conditions, e.g. tumor growth and metastasis, atherosclerosis, periodontal diseases and autoimmune diseases such as rheumatoid arthritis.[2,3] Several lines of evidence also implicate MMPs in the pathogenesis of diverse CNS diseases.[4]

MATRIX METALLOPROTEINASES

The MMPs are a family of structurally and functionally related ECM-degrading endopeptidases with the potential to affect a wide variety of physiological and pathological processes. These enzymes are distinguished from other metalloproteinases by a unique, highly conserved motif in the propeptide domain and a zinc-binding motif in the catalytic domain[5] (Fig. 8.1). The MMP family currently consists of 20 enzymes divided into subgroups according to their structure and substrate specificity (Table 8.1). The subgroups include: collagenases (MMP-1, MMP-8, and MMP-13), capable of degrading fibrillar collagen; gelatinases (MMP-2 and MMP-9), capable of degrading collagen types IV and V, gelatin and laminin; stromelysins (MMP-3, MMP-7,

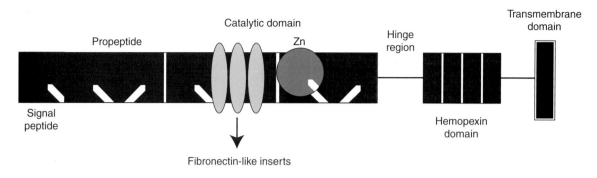

Figure 8.1 Structure of human matrix metalloproteinase.

Table 8.1 The MMP family			
Main substrate	**MMP**		**Subgroup**
Fibrillar collagen	Fibroblast collagenase	MMP-1	Collagenase
	Neutrophil collagenase	MMP-8	
	Collagenase 3	MMP-13	
Collagen type IV and V, gelatin and fibronectin	Gelatinase A	MMP-2	Gelatinases
	Gelatinase B	MMP-9	
Laminin, fibronectin and elastin	Stromelysin 1	MMP-3	Stromelysins
	Stromelysin 2	MMP-10	
	Stromelysin 3	MMP-11	
	Metalloelastase	MMP-12	
	Matrilysin	MMP-7	
Collagen, gelatin and Pro-MMP-2	MT1–MMP	MMP-14	Membrane-type (MT) MMPs
	MT2-MMP	MMP-15	
	MT3-MMP	MMP-16	
	MT4-MMP	MMP-17	
Unknown	Enamelysin	MMP-19	Others
		MMP-20	

MMP-1O, and MMP-12), capable of degrading a wide spectrum of proteoglycans, laminin, fibronectin, and elastin; and membrane-type (MT) MMPs (MMP-14, MMP-15, MMP-16, and MMP-17), capable of degrading a wide spectrum of matrix components and also involved in MMP-2 activation.[4,6] The majority of MMPs are secreted as inactive zymogen forms whose activation occurs outside the cell in a stepwise manner.[5] As of today, four TIMPs have been identified. TIMPs suppress MMP activity by binding to the highly conserved zinc catalytic domain of MMPs;

they are also known to bind to other domains of MMP-2 and MMP-9.[7] Owing to their potentially deleterious nature, expression and activation of MMPs are tightly controlled at different levels. Regulation takes place at the level of transcription, the level of pro-enzyme activation such as binding with MT-MMPs, integrins and plasmin, or inhibition through interactions with TIMPs and other serum proteins.[4,7,8] Cytokines are also involved in the regulation of MMP expression and activity. The net balance between MMP and TIMP expression appears to determine the outcome of ECM degradation, whether beneficial or destructive.

MMPs IN MULTIPLE SCLEROSIS

MS, the most common disabling neurological disorder among young adults, is pathologically characterized by T-cell and macrophage infiltration into the CNS, demyelination and secondary axonal injury.[9,10] Pro-inflammatory cytokines, such as interferon gamma (IFN-γ) and tumor necrosis factor alpha (TNF-α) are also increased and contribute to MS pathology. Several lines of evidence suggest that MMPs are involved in the pathogenesis of MS. Elevated levels of both MMP-2 and MMP-9 were demonstrated in the cerebrospinal fluid (CSF) of MS patients and experimental autoimmune encephalomyelitis (EAE) mice, an MS animal model.[11,12] Increased levels of MMP-9 and MMP-7 mRNA were detected in brain tissue from EAE animals.[13,14] MMP-2, MMP-7 and MMP-9 expression was also found to be upregulated in MS lesions.[15–17] The MMP-9 level in serum of relapsing–remitting (RR) MS patients was found to be elevated, and an additional elevation was observed during relapse.[18,19] We have recently demonstrated elevated levels of MMP-7 and MT1-MMP mRNA expressed by peripheral blood leukocytes from RR and secondary progressive (SP) MS patients.[20] Moreover, we found that IFN-γ treatment was associated with distinct modulation of the MMP/TIMP profile in RR MS though not in SP MS patients.[21] Additionally, steroids, which serve as a treatment for acute relapses, were found to decrease MMP-9 levels in CSF of MS patients,[22] while administration of synthetic MMP inhibitors led to the suppression of disease activity in EAE.[23–25]

The involvement of MMPs in the pathogenesis of MS appears to include a number of mechanisms, among which are degradation of cerebral vascular basement membrane leading to disruption of the BBB integrity, brain edema and immune cell infiltration into the CNS.[26] An increase in cerebral vascular permeability, demonstrated following MMP-2 injection into rats, and a decrease of this phenomenon following co-injection of both MMP-2 and its inhibitor, TIMP-2, supports a direct role of MMPs in BBB damage.[27] MMPs may also be involved in the demyelination process owing to their ability to degrade myelin basic protein, a major component of central myelin.[28] This process of demyelination is followed by release of new immunogenic peptides which may lead to spreading autoimmunity.[29] Additionally, MMPs are also involved in the conversion of TNF-α, a potent pro-inflammatory cytokine implicated in the pathogenesis of MS, to its active form.[18]

MMPs IN ALZHEIMER'S DISEASE

AD, the most common cause of dementia in the elderly, is predominantly a degenerative disease of the CNS gray matter. The pathological and diagnostic hallmarks of the disease are the presence of extracellular deposits of β-amyloid protein and intracellular aggregation of neurofibrillary tangles. Although the disease is degenerative in nature, recent evidence implicates inflammatory mechanisms. Activated microglial cells, which are capable of secreting pro-inflammatory cytokines, especially interleukin (IL)-1, have been demonstrated in the periphery of the β-amyloid plaques. Furthermore, elevated levels of IL-1 have been detected in brain tissue, CSF and serum from AD patients.[30,31] In addition, β-amyloid has been shown to stimulate the production of TNF-α in cultured astrocyte.[31] The β-amyloid protein arises from the proteolytic cleavage of a larger membrane protein, β-amyloid precursor protein (APP). APP can be cleaved by the action of proteases, leading to the secretion of β-amyloid.[4] Reports on MMP involvement in AD are at present preliminary and controversial. It has been reported that MMP-2 can cleave β-amyloid and that APP has a domain that inhibits MMP-2 activity.[32] Independently, it has been shown that MMP-2 can cleave APP in a manner preventing β-amyloid accumulation.[33] In contrast, others have shown that MMP-2 might be amyloidogenic.[34] Moreover, β-amyloid has been shown to be a potent stimulator of MMP-2, MMP-9, and MMP-3 in mixed hippocampal and astrocyte cultures, findings that support a role for MMPs in the development or progression of neuritic plaques.[35] In glioblastoma cells as well, β-amyloid was found to increase MT-MMP expression, leading to increased MMP-2 activity.[36] Increased amounts of latent MMP-9 have been reported in hippocampal specimens from AD patients, suggesting that lack of activation of this enzyme may contribute to β-amyloid deposition.[37] TIMP immunoreactivity has also been demonstrated in β-amyloid plaques and neurofibrillary tangles co-distributed with APP, further supporting a possible role for MMPs and TIMPs in the evolution of these lesions.[38] In summary, MMPs seem to be involved in the deposition of β-amyloid protein in AD, and their role will be further clarified by additional research in the field.

MMPs IN INFECTIOUS MENINGITIS

The breakdown of the BBB is a typical histopathological feature of meningitis, leading to development of brain edema and CNS infiltration by immune cells. An emerging body of evidence points to MMPs as important contributors to the pathogenesis of meningitis. A dramatic increase in MMP-9 levels was observed in the CSF of animals infected with *Streptococcus pneumoniae*. The increase in MMP-9 correlated with both an increase in CSF cell number and an increase in total protein concentration.[39] A similar increase in MMP-9 levels and activity was also observed in brain tissue from a rat model of meningococcal meningitis. Elevated expression of MMP-3 and MMP-13, capable of activating MMP-9, was also observed in those animal models.[40] In accordance with the findings reported in experimental models of bacterial meningitis, augmented MMP-9 activity was recorded in CSF samples taken from patients with bacterial meningitis. In patients, increased expression of TIMP-1 was also observed.[41] Similar findings were observed in patients with viral meningitis.[42] In a recent study conducted in our laboratory, elevated levels of MMP-2 and MMP-9 as well as elevated levels of IL-8 were observed in CSF of patients with either bacterial or viral meningitis.[43] The source of these enzymes may be either the invading pathogen(s), the inflammatory cells or resident CNS cells. The use of synthetic MMPs inhibitors in the rat model of meningococcal meningitis, with significantly reduced BBB disruption,[41] emphasizes the role of MMPs in meningitis.

MMPs IN CEREBRAL ISCHEMIA

Cerebral ischemia (stroke) is the leading cause of death resulting from neurological injury. Ischemic injury to the CNS leads to damage of cerebral vascular endothelium, disruption of the BBB, brain edema, extensive leukocyte recruitment and neuronal injury.[17] In the brain of a primate model of cerebral ischemia, a significant elevation in MMP-2 levels can be detected as early as 1 h after middle cerebral artery occlusion (MCAO).[44] MMP-2 expression was highly correlated with the extent of neuronal injury. Increases in MMP-9 levels were observed only in cases of hemorrhagic transformation. These findings point to a potential role for MMP-2 in the primary events leading to neuronal injury, and to the potential association of MMP-9 with hemorrhagic transformation after focal cerebral ischemia.[44] In the rat model of cerebral ischemia following MCAO, MMP-2 activity was significantly increased by 24 h and peaked after 5 days, while a significant increase in MMP-9 activity was observed after 12 h, peaking by 24 h.[45,46] In these studies, unlike MMP-2 and MMP-9, TIMP-1 was identified at comparable levels in both control and ischemic tissue. Rats injected with MMP-9 neutralizing monoclonal antibody exhibited significantly reduced infarct size,[45] implicating the potential therapeutic significance of MMP inhibitors in reducing brain injury after stroke.[45] In brain autopsies of patients who died between less than 2 h and several years after a stroke, MMP-9 activity was markedly elevated in the infarcted tissue at 2 days post-infarction and remained elevated in tissues from patients who died months after the event. A significant increase in MMP-2 activity was observed only in patients who died 4 months or later after the event.[47] Studies conducted in our laboratory have demonstrated a positive correlation between MMP-2 and MMP-9 levels in the CSF of patients following stroke, and the size of the peri-infarct edema.[48,49]

MMPs IN BRAIN REPAIR

The upregulation of distinct MMPs identified as part of the cascade of events following various CNS injuries discussed above, as well as following traumatic brain insult, supports their potential involvement both in the pathogenesis of CNS disorders and in promoting CNS repair. Degradation of the ECM, occurring following tissue injury and cell death, enables remodeling of the damaged area. Tissue recovery also requires formation of new blood vessels (angiogenesis), which is a MMP-dependent process. MMPs seem to contribute also to the migration of phagocytes into the injured tissue in the process of debris engulfing and wound-healing. Additionally, preliminary data suggest that MMPs play an essential role in neuronal and oligodendrocyte precursor cells' migration to the injured tissue in the process of remyelination[50,51] as well as axonal growth and synaptic reconnections.[52]

Continuing research is required in order to elucidate the role of the distinct members of the MMP/TIMP family in the pathogenesis as well as repair of the various CNS disorders. These studies may be implemented in the development of selective MMP inhibitors or enhancers as part of the therapeutic strategies for neurological diseases.

ACKNOWLEDGEMENT

This work was supported by funds provided by the Rappaport Institute for Research in the Medical Sciences, Chutick Fund for Brain Research, Technion-Israel Institute of Technology, Haifa, Israel and a grant of the Israeli Ministry of Health, Jerusalem, Israel.

REFERENCES

1. Sobel RA. The extracellular matrix in multiple sclerosis lesions. *J Neuropathol Exp Neurol* 1998; **57**: 205–217.
2. Nagase H. Matrix metalloproteinases. In: Hooper NM, ed. *Zinc Metalloproteinases in Health and Disease.* 1996: Taylor & Francis, London, 153–204.
3. Cawston T. Matrix metalloproteinases and TIMPs: properties and implications for the rheumatic disease. *Mol Med Today* 1998; **3**: 130–137.
4. Yong VW, Krekoski CA, Forsyth PA et al. Matrix metalloproteinases and diseases of the CNS. *Trends Neurosci* 1998; **21**: 75–80.
5. Nagase W. Activation mechanisms of matrix metalloproteinases. *Bio Chem* 1997; **378**: 151–160.
6. Westermarck J, Veli-Matti K. Regulation of matrix metalloproteinase expression in tumor invasion. *FASEB J* 1999; **13**: 781–792.
7. Gomez DE, Alonso DF, Yoshiji H, Thorgeirsson UP. Tissue inhibitors of metalloproteinases: structure, regulation and biological functions. *Eur J Cell Biol* 1997; **74**: 111–122.
8. Borden P, Heller RA. Transcriptional control of matrix metalloproteinases and the tissue inhibitors of matrix metalloproteinases. *Crit Rev Eukaryotic Gene Expression* 1997; **7**: 159–178.
9. Amor S, Baker D, Layward L et al. Multiple sclerosis: variations on a theme. *Immunol Today* 1997; **18**: 368–371.
10. Trapp BD, Peterson J, Ransohoff RM et al. Axonal transection in the lesion of multiple sclerosis. *N Engl J Med* 1998; **338**: 278–285.
11. Gijbels K, Masure S, Carton H, Opdenakker G. Gelatinase in the cerebrospinal fluid of patients with multiple sclerosis and other inflammatory neurological diseases. *J Neuroimmunol* 1992; **41**: 29–34.
12. Gijbels K, Proost P, Masure S et al. Gelatinase B is present in the cerebrospinal fluid during experimental autoimmune encephalomyelitis and cleaves myelin basic protein. *J Neurosci Res* 1993; **36**: 432–440.
13. Clements JM, Cossins JA, Wells GMA et al. Matrix metalloproteinase expression during experimental autoimmune encephalomyelitis and effects of combined matrix metalloproteinase and tumour necrosis factor alpha inhibitor. *J Neuroimmunol* 1997; **74**: 85–94.
14. Kieseier B, Kiefer R, Clements JM et al. Matrix metalloproteinase-9 and -7 are regulated in experimental autoimmune encephalomyelitis. *Brain* 1998; **121**: 159–166.
15. Cuzner ML, Gveric D, Strand C et al. The expression of tissue type plasminogen activator, matrix metalloproteinases and endogenous inhibitors in the central nervous system in multiple sclerosis: comparison of stages in lesion evolution. *J Neuropathol Exp Neurol* 1996; **55**: 1194–1204.
16. Maeda A, Sobel RA. Matrix metalloproteinases in the normal human central nervous system, microglial nodules and multiple sclerosis lesions. *J Neuropathol Exp Neurol* 1996; **55**: 300–309.
17. Anthony DC, Ferguson B, Matyzak MK et al. Differential matrix metalloproteinase expression in cases of multiple sclerosis and stroke. *Neuropathol Appl Neurobiol* 1997; **23**: 406–415.
18. Chandler S, Miller KM, Clements JM et al. Matrix metalloproteinases, tumor necrosis factor and multiple sclerosis: an overview. *J Neuroimmunol* 1997; **72**: 155–161.
19. Lee MA, Palace J, Stabler G et al. Serum gelatinase B, TIMP-1 and TIMP-2 levels in multiple sclerosis. *Brain* 1999; **122**: 191–197.
20. Galboiz Y, Shapiro S, Lahat N, Miller A. The profile of matrix metalloproteinases (MMPs) and tissue inhibitors of metalloproteinases (TIMPs) in multiple sclerosis. *J Neurol* 1999; **24**(Suppl 1): 89–90.
21. Galboiz Y, Shapiro S, Lahat N et al. Matrix metalloproteinases (MMPs) and their tissue inhibitors (TIMPs) as markers of disease subtype and response to interferon-β therapy in relapsing and secondary progressive multiple sclerosis patients. *Ann Neurol*, in press.
22. Rosenberg GA, Dencoff JE, Corea N et al. Effect of steroids on CSF matrix metalloproteinases in multiple sclerosis: relation to blood–brain barrier injury. *Neurology* 1996; **46**: 1626–1632.
23. Liedtke W, Cannella B, Mazzaccaro RJ et al. Effective treatment of models of multiple sclerosis by matrix metalloproteinase inhibitors. *Ann Neurol* 1998; **44**: 35–46.
24. Hewson AK, Smith T, Leonard JP, Cuzner ML. Suppression of experimental allergic encephalomyelitis in the Lewis rat by the matrix metalloproteinase inhibitor Ro31-9790. *Inflamm Res* 1995; **44**: 345–349.
25. Gijbels K, Galardy RE, Steinman L. Reversal of experimental autoimmune encephalomyelitis with hydroxamate inhibitor of matrix metalloproteases. *J Clin Invest* 1994; **94**: 2177–2182.
26. Leppert D, Waubant E, Galardy R et al. T cell gelatinases mediate basement membrane transmigration in vitro. *J Immunol* 1995; **154**: 4379–4389.
27. Rosenberg GA, Kornfeld M, Estrada E et al. TIMP-2 reduces proteolytic opening of blood–brain barrier by type IV collagenase. *Brain Res* 1992; **576**: 203–207.
28. Chandler S, Coates R, Gearing AJ et al. Matrix metalloproteinases degrade myelin basic protein. *Neurosci Lett* 1995; **201**: 223–226.
29. Opdenakker G, Van Damme J. Cytokine-regulated proteases in autoimmune diseases. *Immunol Today* 1994; **15**: 103–107.
30. Yates SL, Burgess LH, Kocsis-Angle J et al. Amyloid beta and amylin fibrils induce increases in proinflammatory cytokine and chemokine production by THP-1 and murine microglia. *J Neurochem* 2000; **74**: 1017–1025.
31. Sutton ET, Thomas T, Bryant MW et al. Amyloid beta peptide induced inflammatory reaction is mediated by the cytokines tumor necrosis factor and interleukin-1. *J Submicrosc Cytol Pathol* 1999; **31**: 313–323.
32. Miyazaki K, Hasegawa M, Funahashi K, Umeda M. A metalloproteinase inhibitor domain in Alzheimer amyloid protein precursor. *Nature* 1993; **362**: 839–841.
33. Roher AE, Kasunic TC, Woods AS et al. Proteolysis of A beta peptide from Alzheimer disease brain by gelatinase A. *Biochem Biophys Res Commun* 1994; **205**: 1755–1761.
34. LePage RN, Fosang AJ, Fuller SJ et al. Gelatinase A possesses a beta-secretase-like activity in cleaving the amyloid protein precursor of Alzheimer's disease. *FEBS Lett* 1995; **377**: 267–270.
35. Deb S, Gottschall PE. Increased production of matrix metalloproteinases in enriched astrocyte and mixed hippocampal cultures treated with beta-amyloid peptides. *J Neurochem* 1996; **66**: 1641–1647.
36. Deb S, Zhang JW, Gottschall PE. Activated isoforms of MMP-2 are induced in U87 human glioma cells in response to beta-amyloid peptide. *J Neurosci Res* 1999; **55**: 44–53.

37. Lim PG, Russell MJ, Cullen MJ, Tokes ZA. Matrix metalloproteinases in dog brains exhibiting Alzheimer-like characteristics. *J Neurochem* 1997; **68**: 1606–1611.

38. Peress N, Perillo E, Zucker S. Localization of tissue inhibitor of matrix metalloproteinases in Alzheimer's disease and normal brain. *J Neuropathol Exp Neurol* 1995; **54**: 16–22.

39. Azeh I, Mader M, Smirnov A et al. Experimental pneumococcal meningitis in rabbits: the increase of matrix metalloproteinase-9 in cerebrospinal fluid correlates with leukocyte invasion. *Neurosci Lett* 1998; **256**: 127–130.

40. Kieseier B, Paul R, Koedel U et al. Differential expression of matrix metalloproteinases in bacterial meningitis. *Brain* 1999; **122**: 1579–1587.

41. Paul R, Lorenzl S, Koedel U et al. Matrix metalloproteinases contribute to the blood brain barrier disruption during bacterial meningitis. *Ann Neurol* 1998; **44**: 592–600.

42. Kolb SA, Lahrtz F, Paul R et al. Matrix metalloproteinases and tissue inhibitors of metalloproteinases in viral meningitis: upregulation of MMP-9 and TIMP-1 in cerebrospinal fluid. *J Neuroimmunol* 1998; **84**: 143–150.

43. Shapiro S, Lerner A, Lahat N, Sobel E, Miller A. Matrix metalloproteinases (MMPs), IL-8 and sICAM-1 in bacterial and viral meningitis. *J Neurol* 1999; **246**(suppl 1): 13.

44. Heo JH, Lucero J, Abumiya T et al. Matrix metalloproteinases increase very early during experimental focal cerebral ischemia. *J Cereb Blood Flow Metab* 1999; **19**: 624–633.

45. Romanic AM, White RF, Arleth AJ et al. Matrix metalloproteinase expression increases after cerebral focal ischemia in rats: inhibition of matrix metalloproteinase-9 reduces infarct size. *Stroke* 1998; **29**: 1020–1030.

46. Rosenberg GA, Navratil M, Barone F, Feuerstein G. Proteolytic cascade enzymes increase in focal cerebral ischemia in rat. *J Cereb Blood Flow Metab* 1996; **16**: 360–366.

47. Clarck AW, Krekoski CA, Bou SS et al. Increased gelatinase A (MMP-2) and gelatinase B (MMP-9) activities in human brain after focal ischemia. *Neurosci Lett* 1997; **238**: 53–56.

48. Braker C, Shapiro S, Lahat N, Honigman S, Miller A. Matrix metalloproteinases (MMPs) and IL-8 CSF levels are correlated with brain edema following cerebral infarction. In: List, Muller, John, eds. *Advances in Critical Care Testing 1999*. Springer, Berlin,1999: 103–104.

49. Shapiro S, Lahat N, Finkelstein, Bitterman H, Miller A. Effects of hypoxia, reoxygenation and tumor necrosis factor (TNF)-α on the secretion of MMP-2 by human endothelial cells. *J Neurol* 1999; **246**(suppl 1): 76.

50. Amberger VR, Avellana-Adalid V, Hensel T et al. Oligodendrocyte-type 2 astrocyte progenitors use metalloendoprotease to spread and migrate on CNS myelin. *Eur J Neurosci* 1997; **9**: 151–162.

51. Uhm JH, Dooley NP, Oh LY, Yong VW. Oligodendrocytes utilize a matrix metalloproteinase, MMP-9, to extend processes along an astrocyte extracellular matrix. *Glia* 1998; **22**: 53–63.

52. Nordstrom LA, Lochner J, Yeung W, Ciment G. The metalloproteinase stromelysin-1 (transin) mediates PC12 cell growth cone invasiveness through basal laminae. *Mol Cell Neurosci* 995; **6**: 56–68.

9

Monitoring progression of multiple sclerosis: *p*-cresol sulfate is the dominant component of urine myelin basic protein-like material

John Whitaker, Lori Coward, Marion Kirk, Patricia Jackson and Ligong Cao

INTRODUCTION

Multiple sclerosis (MS) is a heterogeneous disorder with varied clinical presentations and features,[1] a range or subsets of histopathological abnormalities in the central nervous system (CNS),[2] and diverse and often asymptomatic alterations on craniospinal MRI or spectroscopy.[3] This situation has led to the recognition of different subtypes of MS[4] defined by profiles of the clinical events of relapses, remissions, and progression. Patients with progressive MS, whether preceded by or mixed with relapses and remissions, i.e. secondary progressive (SP) MS, or devoid of clinically manifested relapses and remissions, i.e. primary progressive (PP) MS, comprise the most disabling and difficult-to-treat population of MS patients. Effective treatment of relapsing–remitting (RR) MS with interferon beta-1b,[5] interferon beta-1a[6] or glatiramer acetate[7] has not yet been translated into consistently effective treatment of SP or PP MS.[8,9]

For the treatment and management of MS to advance, clinical trials must be well designed with feasible and objective outcomes to identify effective agents.[10] The most critical need in seeking to therapeutically alter the basic disease process in MS is an objective and feasible test(s) which marks or parallels the clinical events of relapses, remissions, and progression. Such a test could serve as a surrogate marker to determine as soon as possible the eventual clinical success or failure of treatments used for this chronic disease. Associated with the breakdown of the CNS myelin sheath in MS, material immunoreactive with antibodies to myelin basic protein (MBP) can be detected in cerebrospinal fluid (CSF).[11,12] Since immunoreactivity may occur through molecular or structural mimicry, the designation of immunoreactive material detected in CSF, and subsequently in urine,[13] with antibodies to MBP acknowledged the lack of a validation by bioassay or delineation of chemical features. The limited amounts of CSF MBP-like material (MBPLM) restricted its characterization, and the difficulty of obtaining multiple CSF specimens from the same patient led to the investigation of blood and urine to improve the clinical feasibility of the approach. An acceptable assay for blood MBPLM is unavailable, but MBPLM can be detected in urine.[13]

CSF and urine MBPLM are quite different in immunochemical characteristics and disease relationships.[13–15] Thus, CSF MBPLM is large, suggesting that it is bound to another molecule, appears to be an epitope in MBP peptide 80–89 that is present in the intact MBP molecule, and is found or increased during periods of acute CNS myelin damage, irrespective of cause. In contrast, urinary MBPLM is small, estimated to be less than 1000 Da, has the immunoreactivity of a cryptic epitope in MBP peptide 83–89 not present in MBP, is found in normals, does not rise in relapses of MS, but increases in progressive MS, both SP and PP disease.[13,16–19]

SELECTED FEATURES OF MBP

MBP accounts for 30% of CNS myelin proteins,[20] is encoded by a single gene of seven exons located on chromosome 18,[21] and is normally expressed only by oligodendrocytes and Schwann cells. Alternate splicing of the MBP transcript gives rise to at least four isoforms of human MBP, with the major ones having molecular masses of 21.5 kDa (encoded by all seven exons) and 18.5 kDa (encoded by exons 1 and 3–7).[22] The 18.5 kDa isoform containing 170 amino acid residues dominates in adult human CNS myelin. In addition to multiple isoforms, MBP may have a number of post-translational modifications, such as N-terminal acylation, selected phosphorylation of serine and threonine, deamidation of glutamine, loss of C-terminal arginine, methylation of the arginine at residue 107, and citrullination of arginines that may result in charged isomers.[23]

MBP has multiple independent epitopes throughout its 170 residues, and a multideterminant model is likely.[24,25] Certain regions of MBP appear to have special relevance to MS. One of these comprises residues 80–100. There is evidence for intramolecular folding and β-sheet structure in this region.[26] Antibodies to MBP in CSF and brain extracts[27,28] frequently react with this MBP region. Moreover, MBP peptide 87–99 contains the encephalitogenic epitopes for the SJL mice[29] and a minor I-E restricted encephalitogenic epitope in the Lewis rat.[30] This is also a prominent region recognized by MBP-sensitive T-cells derived from MS patients[31] and similar to the B-cell epitope commonly recognized by CSF antibody to MBP.[28] The fine specificities of epitopes bound by polyclonal and monoclonal antibodies to MBP implicate three or more epitopes, two of which are cryptic, in MBP peptide 80–89.[32,33]

MBPLM IN URINE

The detection of MBPLM in urine required the recognition of a cryptic epitope in MBP peptide 80–89,[13,32] the corrected primary sequence at positions 83 and 84 of MBP,[34] and a suitable and selective polyclonal antiserum.[13] The immunochemical behavior of MBP peptide 80–89 reveals two cryptic, or unexposed, epitopes, one in residues 83–89 recognized by polyclonal antibody R110,[13] and a second in residues 80–85 recognized by monoclonal antibody (mAb) F41.[33] Although mAb F41 detects MBPLM in urine, MBPLM measurements with mAb F41 do not correlate well with clinical events of disease progression.[17]

Available information on the characteristics and correlates of urinary MBPLM indicates that it: (1) cross-reacts with a cryptic epitope in MBP peptide 83–89;[13] (2) is normally present but low in neonates and rises above adult levels in childhood;[35] (3) is normal in RR MS but elevated in SP MS and, to a lesser degree, in PP MS;[17,19] (4) does not correlate

with disease activity in MS;[16] (5) when elevated correlates with a transition to the SP phase of MS from RR MS;[17,18] (6) when elevated, correlates with lesion number and volume of T2-weighted CNS lesions manually identified and quantitated on 0.15T cranial MRI;[17] and (7) is significantly correlated with black hole volume on T1-weighted post-gadolinium cranial MRI, especially in SP MS without relapse which is moderately advanced with an Expanded Disability Status Scale score of ≥ 5.5.[36]

p-CRESOL SULFATE IS THE MAJOR COMPONENT OF URINARY MBPLM

In its original description, urinary MBPLM was estimated to have a molecular size of less than 1000 Da.[13] Using a combination of isolation methods, especially high-performance liquid chromatography (HPLC), followed by mass spectrometry and NMR, it has been demonstrated that p-cresol sulfate is the dominant chemical moiety in urinary MBPLM.[37] This conclusion was based on the following observations. First, purified MBPLM shows a peak of 187 on negative electrospray mass spectrometry which has the same spectral features as any of the three isomers of cresol sulfate. Second, MBPLM and p-cresol sulfate have the same properties by multiple reaction monitoring. Third, and most conclusively, both the ^{1}H and ^{13}C NMR spectra of urinary MBPLM and p-cresol sulfate are identical but different from the spectra for m-cresol sulfate and o-cresol sulfate. Fourth, p-cresol sulfate has immunoreactivity in parallel with MBPLM in the radioimmunoassay (RIA) used for its detection. Based on fractionation by HPLC and monitoring with RIA, p-cresol sulfate is the dominant but not the only component of urinary MBPLM. m-Cresol sulfate and o-cresol sulfate react similarly to each other but considerably less than p-cresol sulfate. Fifth, p-cresol sulfate has the same properties in the separation systems, including HPLC, applied for the purification of MBPLM.

The immunochemical cross-reactivity of p-cresol sulfate and the cryptic epitope in MBP peptide 83–89 could not have been anticipated. Small peptides from MBP peptide 80–89 have a surprising conformational increase in structure by removal of residues from the N-terminus of this decapeptide.[38] There is a growing appreciation of the extent of molecular mimicry of antigenic material which shares immunochemical reactivity. This includes immunoglobulin peptides and small organic molecules,[39] DNA and peptides,[40] and cryptococcal polysaccharides and peptides.[41] The shared molecular structure between MBP peptide 83–89 and a small molecule whose dominant component is p-cresol sulfate can be added to this list.

MEASUREMENT OF *p*-CRESOL SULFATE IN URINE AND SERUM

With the determination that *p*-cresol sulfate was the dominant component of urinary MBPLM, studies were then undertaken to measure *p*-cresol sulfate in urine by MRM and to correlate it with the level of MBPLM quantitated in urine by RIA. *p*-Cresol sulfate and urinary MBPLM values were highly correlated ($r = 0.780$), and in a small series values for all MS patients, especially those with SP and PP MS, were higher than those for normal controls.[42] With the RIA for urinary MBPLM, an assay on serum could not be validated due to the interference by serum proteins. Using MRM, *p*-cresol sulfate has been detected in serum at a level of about 2–5% that of urine. Serum *p*-cresol sulfate correlates well ($r = 0.822$) with urine *p*-cresol sulfate values, adjusted to reflect renal function and urine dilution, for creatinine content.

CONCLUSIONS

The identification of *p*-cresol sulfate as the dominant component of urinary MBPLM and the detection of it in serum will provide a more direct means to delineate further the relationship of *p*-cresol sulfate to progressive MS. Characterization of the other portion(s) of the material linked with *p*-cresol sulfate and definition of the metabolic origin and fate of *p*-cresol sulfate should make it possible to understand the role of *p*-cresol sulfate in the pathobiological events of MS and possibly to use it as a marker for determining disease progression and the effects of agents used to treat it.

ACKNOWLEDGEMENTS

The research described in this report was supported by the Research Program of the Veterans Administration, the National Multiple Sclerosis Society Grant #RG 2667-A-7, and the National Institutes of Health (PO1 NS29719). Mrs Jeanine Goodwin furnished excellent technical assistance, and Ms. Linda Brent provided excellent assistance in the preparation of the manuscript.

REFERENCES

1. Whitaker JN, Mitchell GW. Clinical features of multiple sclerosis. In: Raine CS, McFarland HF, Tourtellotte WW, eds. *Multiple Sclerosis, Clinical and Pathogenic Basis.* London: Chapman & Hall, 1997: 3–19.
2. Lucchinetti CF, Bruck W, Rodriguez M, Lassmann H. Distinct patterns of multiple sclerosis pathology indicates heterogeneity in pathogenesis. *Brain Pathol* 1996; **6**: 259–274.
3. Arnold DL. Magnetic resonance spectroscopy: imaging axonal damage in MS. *J Neuroimmunol* 1999; **98**: 2–6.
4. Lublin FD, Reingold SC. Defining the clinical course of multiple sclerosis: results of an international survey. *Neurology* 1996; **46**: 907–911.
5. The IFNB Multiple Sclerosis Study Group. Interferon beta-1b is effective in relapsing-remitting multiple sclerosis. I. Clinical results of a multicenter, randomized, double-blind, placebo-controlled trial. *Neurology* 1993; **43**: 655–661.
6. Jacobs LD, Cookfair DL, Rudick RA et al. Intramuscular interferon beta-1a for disease progression in relapsing multiple sclerosis. *Ann Neurol* 1996; **39**: 285–294.
7. Johnson KP, Brooks BR, Cohen JA et al. Copolymer 1 reduces relapse rate and improves disability in relapsing-remitting multiple sclerosis: results of a phase III multicenter, double-blind, placebo-controlled trial. *Neurology* 1995; **45**: 1268–1276.
8. Bornstein MB, Miller A, Slagle S et al. A placebo-controlled, double-blind, randomized, two-center, pilot trial of Cop 1 in chronic progressive multiple sclerosis. *Neurology* 1991; **41**: 533–539.
9. Kappos L, Moeri D, Radue EW et al. Predictive value of gadolinium-enhanced magnetic resonance imaging for relapse rate and changes in disability or impairment in multiple sclerosis: a meta-analysis. *Lancet* 1999; **353**: 964–969.
10. Whitaker JN, McFarland HF, Rudge P, Reingold SC. Outcomes assessment in multiple sclerosis clinical trials: a critical analysis. *Mult Scler* 1995; **1**: 37–47.
11. Cohen SR, Herndon RM, McKhann GM. Radioimmunoassay of myelin basic protein in spinal fluid: an index of active demyelination. *N Engl J Med* 1976; **295**: 1455–1457.
12. Whitaker JN. Myelin encephalitogenic protein fragments in cerebrospinal fluid of persons with multiple sclerosis. *Neurology* 1977; **27**: 911–920.
13. Whitaker JN. The presence of immunoreactive myelin basic protein peptide in urine of persons with multiple sclerosis. *Ann Neurol* 1987; **22**: 648–655.
14. Whitaker JN. Myelin basic protein in cerebrospinal fluid and other body fluids. *Mult Scler* 1998; **4**: 16–21.
15. Whitaker JN, Kachelhofer RD, Mitchell GW et al. Urine myelin basic protein-like material in multiple sclerosis during treatment with interferon beta-1b. *Neurology* 1998; **50**: A343.
16. Whitaker JN, Williams PH, Layton BA et al. Correlation of clinical features and findings on cranial magnetic resonance imaging with urinary myelin basic protein-like material in patients with multiple sclerosis. *Ann Neurol* 1994; **35**: 577–585.
17. Whitaker JN, Kachelhofer RD, Bradley EL et al. Urinary myelin basic protein-like material as a correlate of the progression of multiple sclerosis. *Ann Neurol* 1995; **38**: 625–632.
18. Whitaker JN, Layton BA, Bartolucci AA et al. Urinary myelin basic protein-like material in patients with multiple sclerosis during interferon beta-1b treatment. *Arch Neurol* 1999; **56**: 687–691.
19. Bashir K, Whitaker JN. Clinical and laboratory features of primary progressive and secondary progressive multiple sclerosis. *Neurology* 1999; **53**: 765–771.
20. Morell P, Quarles RH, Norton WT. Formation, structure and biochemistry of myelin. In: Siegel G, Agranoff B, Albers RW, Molinoff P, eds. *Basic Neurochemistry.* New York: Raven Press, 1989: 109–136.

21. Roach A, Boylan K, Harvath S, Prusiner SB, Hood L. Characterization of cloned cDNA representing rat myelin basic protein: absence of expression in brain in shiverer mutant mice. *Cell* 1983; **42**: 799–806.

22. Kamholz J, Toffenetti J, Lazzarini RA. Organization and expression of the human myelin basic protein gene. *J Neurosci Res* 1988; **21**: 62–70.

23. Moscarello MA. Myelin basic protein: a dynamically changing structure. In: Hashim GA, Moscarello M, eds. *Dynamic Interactions of Myelin Proteins*. New York: John Wiley & Sons, 1990: 25–48.

24. Whitaker JN, Chou CHJ, Chou FCH, Kibler RF. Antigenic regions for the humoral response to myelin basic protein. *Mol Immunol* 1979; **16**: 495–501.

25. Day ED, Potter NT. Monoclonal and polyclonal antibodies to myelin basic protein determinants. *J Neuroimmunol* 1986; **10**: 289–312.

26. Stoner GL. Predicted folding of β-structure in myelin basic protein. *J Neurochem* 1984; **43**: 433–447.

27. Warren KG, Catz I. Increased synthetic peptide specificity of tissue-CSF bound anti-MBP in multiple sclerosis. *J Neuroimmunol* 1993; **43**: 87–96.

28. Warren KG, Catz I, Steinman L. Fine specificity of the antibody response to myelin basic protein in the central nervous system in multiple sclerosis: the minimal B-cell epitope and a model of its features. *Proc Natl Acad Sci USA* 1995; **92**: 11061–11065.

29. Kono DH, Urban JL, Horvath SJ et al. Two minor determinants of myelin basic protein induce experimental allergic encephalomyelitis in SJL/J mice. *J Exp Med* 1988; **168**: 213–227.

30. Offner H, Hashim GA, Celnik B et al. T cell determinants of myelin basic protein include a unique encephalitogenic I-E-restricted epitope for Lewis rats. *J Exp Med* 1989; **170**: 355–367.

31. Ota K, Matsui M, Milford EL, et al. T-cell recognition of an immunodominant myelin basic protein epitope in multiple sclerosis. *Nature* 1990; **346**: 183–187.

32. Whitaker JN, Chou CHJ, Chou FCH, Kibler RF. Molecular internalization of a region of myelin basic protein. *J Exp Med* 1977; **146**: 317–331.

33. Whitaker JN, McKeehan A, Freeman DW. Monoclonal and polyclonal antibody responses to the myelin basic protein epitope present in human urine. *J Neuroimmunol* 1994; **52**: 53–60.

34. Gibson BW, Gilliom RD, Whitaker JN, Biemann K. Amino acid sequence of human myelin basic protein peptide 45–89 as determined by mass spectrometry. *J Biol Chem* 1984; **259**: 5028–5031.

35. Percy AK, Lane JB, Goodwin J, Kachelhofer RD, Whitaker JN. Age-related changes in the level of urinary myelin basic protein-like material during childhood. *Neurology* 1998; **51**: 1339–1341.

36. Whitaker JN, Wolinsky JS, Narayana PA et al. Urinary myelin basic protein-like material correlates with black hole volume on T1-weighted cranial MRI in advanced multiple sclerosis. *Arch Neurol* 2001; **58**: 49–54.

37. Cao LG, Kirk MC, Coward LU, Jackson P, Whitaker JN. p-Cresol sulfate is the dominant component of urinary myelin basic protein like material. *Arch Biochem Biophys* 2000; **377**: 9–21.

38. Whitaker JN, Moscarello MA, Herman PK, Epand RM, Surewicz WK. Conformational correlates of the epitopes of human myelin basic protein peptide 80–89. *J Neurochem* 1990; **55**: 568–576.

39. Kang C-Y, Brunck TK, Kieber-Emmons T, Blalock JE, Kohler H. Inhibition of self-binding antibodies (autobodies) by a V_H-derived peptide. *Science* 1988; **240**: 1034–1036.

40. Putterman C, Deocharan B, Diamond B. Molecular analysis of the autoantibody response in peptide-induced autoimmunity. *J Immunol* 2000; **164**: 2542–2549.

41. Valadon P, Nussbaum G, Oh J, Scharff MD. Aspects of antigen mimicry revealed by immunization with a peptide mimetic of *Cryptococcus neoformans* polysaccharide. *J Immunol* 1998; **161**: 1829–1836.

42. Whitaker JN, Coward L, Kirk M et al. A urinary p-cresol sulfate in multiple sclerosis. *Ann Neurol* 1999; **46**: 935 (abstr).

10

Immunomodulation and therapy in multiple sclerosis

Arnon Karni, Karim Makhlouf, Samia J Khoury and Howard L Weiner

INTRODUCTION

Although the etiology and pathogenesis of multiple sclerosis (MS) may still be considered by many to be 'unknown', the working hypothesis of most investigators is that MS is a cell-mediated autoimmune disease directed against central nervous system (CNS) myelin and is related in some way to a viral infection.[1] Furthermore, with recent advances in our understanding of the immune system and the demonstration that certain treatments can affect the clinical course of MS, it is now possible to approach the disease in more positive terms.

The pathologic picture of MS is one consistent with cell-mediated immune damage to the myelin sheath.[2-4] Inflammation is associated with increased expression of IFN-γ, endothelial cell activation with expression of class II and adhesion molecules, and macrophage-mediated destruction of myelin via receptor-mediated endocytosis. IL-12 expression and B7.1 upregulation in the active lesions are consistent with a Th1-type or cell-mediated autoimmune process.[5] The picture is consistent with a delayed-type hypersensitivity (DTH) response in the CNS. In support of this, reactivity of cells against several myelin antigens (MBP, PLP, myelin oligodendrocyte glycoprotein (MOG)) has been demonstrated in the peripheral blood and cerebrospinal fluid (CSF) of MS patients.[6-8] These are identical to cells that cause an MS-like disease in the animal model of MS, experimental allergic encephalomyelitis (EAE), and since they have been found in MS patients, they can be considered pathogenic cells capable of cell-mediated CNS inflammation. In some instances there may be a large number of myelin autoreactive cells.[9] Autoantibodies to myelin antigens have also been demonstrated in MS,[10] and although they do not appear to be important in initiating the disease, they could

play an important secondary role in the disease process by causing demyelination. For example, in animals, antibody against MOG has been shown to enhance demyelination when inflammation is present,[11,12] although alone these antibodies have minimal pathologic effects. To date, anti-MOG antibodies have not been consistently demonstrated in patients with MS, though there may be other antibodies that play a role in the process. Thus, the primary immunologic and pathologic event that causes MS is the generation of Th1-type CD4[+] cells that become activated, secrete IFN-γ and other proinflammatory cytokines, and are specific for antigens in the myelin sheath. Although CD8[+] cells could also theoretically participate in CNS inflammation, this has not been demonstrated, and defects in CD8[+] cells may be related to altered immunoregulation in the disease.

For many years it was felt that identification of 'the' autoantigen in MS would be the key to understanding and treating the disease. This theory was analogous to the demonstration that the acetylcholine receptor was the primary autoantigen in

---

Table 10.1   Multiple sclerosis as a Th1–type cell-mediated autoimmune disease

Exacerbation of MS induced by administration of IFN-γ

Elevated production of IFN-γ and tumor necrosis factor in blood and CNS

Increased production of IL-12 in progressive MS

Presence of IL-12 and B7.1 in MS lesions

Similarities of MS to EAE, which is a Th1 cell-mediated autoimmune disease

myasthenia gravis. This is no longer a valid assumption, as it has now been demonstrated that even though CNS inflammation may be initiated by a cell-meditated attack against a specific myelin antigen such as MBP, there is spreading of immune reactivity to other antigens in the target organ. This has been shown in animal models of EAE[13-15] and in another prototypic organ-specific autoimmune disease, diabetes in the NOD mouse.[16,17] Indeed, in MS, reactivity to multiple myelin autoantigens has been demonstrated,[6-8,18] and in the NOD mouse model of diabetes, similar spreading of autoreactivity has been demonstrated with reactivity to insulin, GAD, heat shock proteins and other islet antigens.[19] In MS, it is possible that spreading of reactivity among antigens and their epitopes may be responsible for causing different attacks of the disease. Furthermore, other cells such as γ–δ cells may be recruited to the CNS once inflammation has been initiated and also participate in the pathologic inflammatory process.[20,21] Thus, there is no single autoantigen that is the target of an autoimmune attack, but reactivity to multiple myelin antigens. This makes therapy directed at eliminating specific cells that react to only one myelin antigen or that have a unique T-cell receptor problematic.

There must be a triggering event or a series of triggering events that initiate the disease. The immune system has evolved to protect the host against environmental pathogens, and in MS the immune system is misdirected in an organ-specific fashion and attacks myelin components in the CNS. Thus, the initiation of the disease involves sensitization initiated by an infectious process that also confers specificity for myelin components, and this occurs via infectious agents that have components that cross-react with myelin antigens or by a self-limited infection of the brain that releases myelin antigens and results in sensitization.

A major advance in our understanding of the function and regulation of the immune response is an understanding of the type or 'class' of immune response that is induced (Table 10.2). Th1-type responses are characterized by IFN-γ secretion, and are important in the generation of DTH responses and in immune responses against viruses. Th1-type responses also induce cell-mediated autoimmune diseases such as EAE in animals, and by inference Th1-type responses against myelin antigens would induce MS in humans. Administration of IFN-γ to MS patients caused worsening of disease.[22] Th1 responses, however, are important in protection against certain parasitic infections (e.g. leishmaniasis).[23] Th2-type responses are characterized by IL-4

Table 10.2 Class of immune response

	Th1	Th2	Th3
Cytokine[a]	IFN-γ	IL-4	TGF-β
Help	DTH/IgG$_{2a}$	IgG$_1$/IgE	IgA
Suppression	Th2	Th1	Th1/2
Immunity[b]	Cell-mediated	Humoral	Mucosal

[a]The primary cytokine associated with each class of immune response is presented. In vivo, there can also be mixed cytokine patterns.
[b]Different types of immunity are favored by each type of T-cell, but are not exclusive. Thus, although secretion of TGF-β is favored in mucosal immunity, it is seen as part of systemic immunity as well, and Th3 responses involve cells that may secrete IL-4 and IL-10. TR1 cells are a recently described class of regulatory cells that primarily secrete IL-10.[25]

secretion, and regulate Th1-type responses, and IL-4 administration is protective in EAE.[24] CD4+ regulatory T-cells that suppress Th1 responses and primarily secrete IL-10 have also recently been described.[25] Th3-type responses are characterized by TGF-β secretion and are preferentially induced following mucosal presentation of antigen.[26] Furthermore, natural recovery from EAE is associated with the appearance of cells that secrete TGF-β[27,28] According to this paradigm, the response of a non-susceptible individual exposed to a myelin antigen is either not to respond or to generate a Th2 or Th3 response which is non-pathogenic and protective, whereas in patients with MS, a pathogenic Th1-type response is generated. Thus, the central concept that underlies whether MS is initiated and perpetuated and that forms the basis for treatment is the class of immune response (Table 10.3).

Major histocompatibility complex (MHC) linkage to MS is well known, with DR2 being the most closely linked factor associated with MS.[29] MHC may

Table 10.3 Factors which influence the class of immune responses

Route of antigen exposure
Type of antigen
Genetics of the host
Environmental exposure
Adjuvant
Local milieu

be linked to disease in several ways: (1) it could determine the ability of a person to generate pathogenic autoreactive T-cells by determining which myelin peptides are presented to T-cells; (2) it could determine the shape of the T-cell repertoire at the time of T-cell development during thymic ontogeny and during peripheral deletion; and (3) it could determine the class of immune response based on the binding affinity of peptides in the MHC groove. Of note is the fact that HLA-DR2 is linked to increased production of lymphotoxin and TNF-α (Th1-type cytokines) by T-cells.[30] However, it is also clear that non-MHC genes are important in determining the class of immune response to myelin antigens. For example, in animal models there are non-MHC-linked genes that determine whether an animal is susceptible or not to EAE. B10.S and SJL mice are both H-2[s], yet only SJL animals are susceptible to EAE.[31] It appears that susceptibility is determined by the class of immune response generated, as when SJL animals are immunized with MOG or MBP in complete Freund's adjuvant, Th1-type T-cells are induced, whereas when B10.S animals are immunized in an identical fashion, Th2 and Th3 cells are induced.[32] The importance of non-MHC genes in determining the class of immune response and susceptibility or resistance to autoimmunity has also been observed in the collagen arthritis model.[33] Another non-MHC-linked immune factor that can influence the class of immune response is the type of costimulation that occurs when antigen is presented by an antigen-presenting cell to a T-cell.[34] A recent study supports the hypothesis that MS patients may be genetically predisposed to Th1 responses, as they have less IgE-mediated allergic diseases which represent a Th2-mediated disease.[35]

Other factors besides genetics must play a role in MS, as it is known that identical twins are not 100% concordant for MS.[36] Even though identical twins raised in the same house are exposed to a similar environment, their exposure to infectious agents is not identical, and this differential environmental exposure accounts for the non-concordance rate. Differential environmental exposure impacts on the development of MS by creating an immune milieu that leads to a Th1 versus a Th2 or Th3 response against myelin antigens. As discussed above, environmental antigens may also lead to the generation of myelin cross-reactive populations of memory cells. In addition, the age at which an individual is exposed to environmental agents may also play an important role in generating different classes of immune responses against myelin antigens. In this regard, there is some evidence that MS may be related to a viral infection that occurs at a certain time in childhood.[37] Also, it is known that there are seasonal variations in MS attacks,[38] and we have recently found that progressive MS patients, but not controls, have increased anti-CD3-induced IFN-γ secretion in the winter months.[39]

Defects in immune regulation have been described in MS but have never been completely understood, in part because of our incomplete understanding of immune regulation and tolerance maintenance (Table 10.4). These defects include a number of defects in antigen-non-specific suppressor mechanisms.[40,41] However, a generalized defect of immune regulation or tolerance in MS does not explain the specificity of the autoimmune responses against myelin antigens, or the lack of generalized autoimmunity in MS. It may be, however, that defects in regulation or tolerance are simply related to regulation of the class of immune response generated (Th1 versus Th2/Th3) or the state of immune activation of T-cells in MS patients. There theoretically could also be defects related to innate immune responses which could also determine class of immune response or affect mechanisms associated with deletion.

MS is not a localized disease of the CNS, but one that is driven by the movement of cells from the peripheral immune system into the CNS.[42] Thus, immune abnormalities related to the disease process can be identified and monitored in the peripheral blood of MS patients. Activated T-cells are present in both the peripheral blood and the CNS of MS patients.[43–45] However, local immune responses may subsequently be established in the CNS, one of the best characterized being the local production of immunoglobulin. In addition, there may be local activation of microglia. Nonetheless, migration of cells into the nervous system plays a crucial role in initiating and perpetuating the disease, especially in the earlier stages.

MS is not a uniform disease, but one with different subtypes. For example, subtypes of MS may be related to immune reactivity against different myelin antigens, e.g. MBP versus PLP versus MOG. Studies in the EAE model suggest that differences in lesion

Table 10.4	Mechanisms of immune tolerance
Deletion:	Death of cell
Anergy:	'Paralyzed' cell, lack of costimulation
Regulation:	Active suppression by regulatory T-cells

distribution in MS may reflect differences in the myelin specificity of autoreactive T-cells.[46] In addition, there may be different disease subtypes related to immune response genes, and subtypes related to an individual's unique environmental exposure. Also, spinal MS and primary progressive MS may represent a specifically unique subtype.[47] The existence of different subtypes complicates the investigation and treatment of the disease.

One of the clinical features of relapsing–remitting MS is that patients generally recover from an attack. This implies that there are natural regulatory mechanisms that are affecting the immune process to the benefit of the host. In the EAE model, immune mechanisms associated with recovery include apoptosis of pathogenic T-cells[48] and a class switch from Th1 to Th2/Th3 responses.[27,49,50] Evidence for a class switch during recovery from attacks is beginning to accumulate in MS as well. For example, patients who are in a recovery stage from an acute attack appear to have an increase in IL-10-secreting PLP-reactive cells.[51] Understanding these natural regulatory mechanisms and determining ways to augment them is likely to help us deal with the disease process.

It is the chronic progressive form of MS that usually leads to disability. There is recent evidence that changes in the immune system occur when patients change from the relapsing–remitting to the chronic progressive form of the disease. These changes involve the emergence of activated T-cells which drive the immune system towards a Th1 bias. Specifically, T-cells from patients with progressive forms of MS differentiate into cells that drive non-T-cells to produce IL-12, a powerful inducer of Th1-type responses.[52] and may be independent of costimulation requirements. We have also found an increase in IL-12-secreting monocytes in progressive MS and of Th1-type chemokine receptor expression.[53,54]

We have also recently investigated the regulation of IFN-γ by IL-18 in patients with MS. Peripheral blood mononuclear cells from 33 MS patients (19 relapsing–remitting (RR) and 14 secondary progressive (SP)) and 14 healthy controls were stimulated with anti-CD3 plus anti-CD28. IFN-γ and IL-18 were measured in the presence or absence of neutralizing anti-IL-18, anti-IL-12 or isotype control antibody. IFN-γ production in SP-MS was $22\,201 \pm 14\,615$ pg/ml versus 3142 ± 402 pg/ml in RR-MS ($P = 0.04$). IL-18 was higher in SP-MS (72.4 ± 21.4 pg/ml) versus RR-MS (22.2 ± 9.1 pg/ml) ($P = 0.04$). There were no significant differences in the expression of the receptor for IL-18 on T-cells in SP-MS patients versus RR-MS

patients and controls. IFN-γ levels were reduced by neutralizing anti-IL-18 in healthy controls ($P = 0.05$), RR-MS patients ($P = 0.006$) and SP-MS patients ($P = 0.04$). IFN-γ was also reduced by neutralizing anti-IL-12 ($P = 0.04$, $P = 0.05$ and $P = 0.0001$, respectively) and by a combination of neutralizing anti-IL-18 and anti-IL-12 ($P = 0.03$, $P = 0.003$ and $P = 0.001$, respectively). These results demonstrate that IL-18 is a potent inducer of IFN-γ in SP-MS patients, is elevated in these patients, and, in conjunction with IL-12, drives the immune system towards a Th1-type bias in MS.[55]

These results are important, as they demonstrate that there is a basic difference in the peripheral immune system in progressive versus relapsing–remitting MS. By inference, there may be different responses to immunomodulatory therapy in relapsing–remitting versus chronic progressive patients. More important, these results imply that the study of MS should involve not only the investigation of what initiates the disease, but also what occurs when the disease switches from the relapsing–remitting to the progressive form. It is also likely that changes within the CNS itself occur in the progressive form, such as the development of axonal atrophy and localized CNS immune responses.

If one assumes that MS is a cell-mediated CNS autoimmune disease directed against myelin components, it is analogous to EAE.[56] EAE involves a well-defined series of immunologic events leading to myelin destruction and occurs in relapsing and progressive forms (Table 10.5). Interruption of this pathway at different stages in the cascade has an ameliorating effect on EAE. Although imperfect, EAE has served as an important working model for testing treatment approaches prior to clinical trials in MS. One of the major differences between treatment of MS and EAE is that many treatments tested in EAE are given at a restricted time during the course of EAE or prior to immunization. Also, EAE is

Table 10.5   EAE and immune therapy of MS
Activation of myelin-reactive T-cells in the peripheral immune system
Migration of cells into the CNS
Recruitment of additional cells
Release of inflammatory mediators
Sensitization to new antigens in the CNS
Suppression of autoimmune response
Tissue repair

studied in inbred strains of animals, whereas MS occurs in an outbred population. Furthermore, treatment of MS requires chronic therapy of an immune system that may already be activated or in a state of differentiation. One of the unexplained differences between EAE and MS is the protective role of IFN-γ in EAE under some circumstances,[57–59] although defects in IFN-γ suppression by CD8 cells have been observed in progressive MS.[60] Nonetheless, EAE remains an important model for the study of mechanisms by which cell-mediated immunity against myelin antigens causes myelin damage and can be regulated.

In the past it was argued that there were no effective treatments for MS. It has now become clear that there are numerous immune-modulating treatments that can affect the disease process, albeit imperfectly and not under all circumstances.[61] These are listed in Table 10.6. A treatment may have a positive effect on MS even though all trials may not have demonstrated a positive clinical effect. Differences may relate to dosage schedules and differential responses in patient subgroups. For example, we have found that patients with primary progressive MS do not respond as well to pulse cyclophosphamide.[62] Antibiotics would not benefit all patients with pneumonia in a trial that mixed both viral and bacterial pneumonia. MS is different from other CNS diseases such as amyotrophic lateral sclerosis, in which there are not many drugs that can impact on the disease process. Thus, it is important to consider MS as a disease in which immunomodulatory drugs

can affect the disease process, and to understand the manner in which these drugs positively impact on the disease. Furthermore, it is unlikely that each of these drugs is acting differently; it is more probable that they act through a limited number of pathways that ultimately impact on one final common pathway.

If MS is a Th1 cell-mediated disease, then an increase in Th1-type myelin-reactive cells would be associated with worsening of disease, and Th2- or Th3-type myelin-reactive cells would have an ameliorating effect on the disease process. This is the theoretical basis for treatment with oral tolerance,[63] which increases Th3-type myelin-reactive cells,[64] or altered peptide ligand, which increases Th2-type myelin-reactive cells.[65] Thus one could postulate that effective treatment of MS will relate to the balance of Th2 + Th3/Th1 myelin-reactive cells. Nonetheless, even if a treatment affects this balance, it must do so with a strong enough biological effect to impact on the disease process, something which argues for combination therapy.

Regulatory cells that are specific for an autoantigen secrete anti-inflammatory cytokines when they encounter the autoantigen in the target tissue and will thus suppress inflammation in the organ under attack, independent of the autoantigen. This has been termed bystander suppression,[66] and has been demonstrated in a number of animal models. Thus, in the EAE model one can suppress PLP-induced EAE by feeding MBP.[67] Also, in the LCMV viral model of diabetes, the LCMV protein is expressed in the pancreatic islets on the insulin promoter. When animals are infected with the virus, viral-specific immune responses result in diabetes. Feeding insulin generates insulin-specific regulatory cells that suppress the viral-induced diabetes by migrating to the islets, reacting with insulin and secreting anti-inflammatory cytokines.[68] Oral MBP can decrease stroke size in rat models by increasing TGF-β levels in the brain and suppressing inflammation associated with stroke.[69] Although bystander suppression was initially described in association with mucosally induced regulatory cells, any immune manipulation that induces a class switch and Th2 or Th3 regulatory cells would have the same effect. It has been argued that this is one of the mechanisms by which copolymer 1 is effective; copolymer 1 induces Th2-type cells that cross-react with myelin basic protein.[70] Also, altered peptide ligands that induce IL-4 and T-cell receptor vaccination may also act via this mechanism.[65] Bystander suppression solves the conundrum of having to know what the autoantigen is for antigen-specific therapy.

Table 10.6 Immune therapy which helps MS
Azathioprine[79]
Interferon-α[80]
Interferon-β$_{1a}$[81]
Interferon-β$_{1b}$[82]
Cladribine[83]
Copolymer 1[84]
Corticosteroids[85]
Cyclophosphamide[86,87]
Cyclosporin[88]
IVIg[89]
Linomide[90,91]
Methotrexate[92]
Mitoxanthrone[93]
Plasma exchange[94,95]
Total lymphoid irradiation[96]

It may be that most treatments that affect the disease process ultimately impact on antigen-specific myelin-reactive cells either by decreasing IFN-γ-secreting or increasing Th2 of Th3 myelin-reactive cells. Thus, even 'antigen-non-specific' immuno-modulatory treatments have their effect by affecting the balance of Th1 versus Th2/3 myelin-reactive cells in the nervous system. For example, we have found that IFN-β causes a class switch by decreasing anti-CD3 induced IFN-γ secretion and increasing IL-4 secretion,[71] and IFN-β has also been shown to increase IL-10.[72] Unexpectedly, we have also found that cyclophosphamide, thought to be a general immunosuppressant, induces a marked immune deviation, with an increase in IL-4 and TGF-β and a decrease in IFN-γ and IL-12.[54] In addition, there is an increase of IL-4-secreting MBP- and PLP-specific cells in cyclophosphamide-treated patients.[73] There are some exceptions to this rule, e.g. treatments aimed at affecting trafficking of cells into the CNS or decreasing antigen-non-specific inflammatory mediators such as TNF.

Until all the factors associated with the disease are known, it is unlikely that a single treatment given once will be effective or that a single treatment will be effective in all forms of MS. This is especially true if the disease process is being randomly and intermittently triggered by environmental factors. Also, it is clear that the disease is more active as viewed by MRI than can be observed clinically, so continuous or pulse therapy will be required. Furthermore, although there are now treatments that can ameliorate MS, they are only partially effective. Effective therapy will require combination therapy. Combination therapy has been the rule in medicine and one would expect the same to be true for MS. Furthermore, if the immune system is constantly being driven towards a Th1 response in MS patients, continuous or pulse therapy will be required to counterbalance this effect unless a more permanent change in the immune system can be induced.

If MS is truly an immune-mediated disease and immune therapy is effective, then the ultimate proof of this hypothesis will be the identification of immune measures that are linked both to clinical course and to response to therapy. A major effort in MS by investigators is being made to find immune surrogate markers that link to disease activity and/or response to therapy.[43,71,72,74] Such immune measures would also provide a rationale for which type of combination therapy to administer and when to initiate or stop a particular treatment. Towards this end, we recently investigated immunologic correlates of disease activity in MS as related to disease stage and MRI. We investigated IL-12, activation markers and serum ICAM and TNF-R.

We investigated IL-12 and the relationship between IL-12 and disease activity on MRI in a larger number of patients.[75] Blood was collected prospectively from MS patients: 277 samples were obtained from 196 patients. Disease type and activity, rating on the EDSS and AI scales and ongoing treatment were assessed at the time of blood sampling. MRI of the brain with and without gadolinium (Gd) was performed at the discretion of the treating physician. We measured the percentage of IL-12-expressing monocytes in the blood by flow cytometry. We obtained the following results.

(1) When compared to healthy controls ($n = 10$, mean IL-12 = 7.13%), all groups of MS patients had significantly higher IL-12 expression (unpaired t-test)

(2) Relapsing–remitting: $n = 90$, IL-12 = 16.97%, $P = 0.0004$

(3) Relapsing–remitting progressive: $n = 23$, IL-12 = 23.42%, $P = 0.0006$

(4) Primary progressive: $n = 17$, IL-12 = 20.73%, $P = 0.0194$

(5) Secondary progressive (SP): $n = 137$, IL-12 = 22.04%, $P < 0.0001$.

SP patients also had significantly higher IL-12 expression than RR patients ($P = 0.011$). The presence of GD-enhancing lesions on MRI was used as a measure of disease activity. There was significantly higher expression of IL-12 among patients with enhancing lesions on MRIs done within 30 (enhancing: $n = 17$, IL-12 = 29%; non-enhancing: $n = 38$, Il-12 = 14%; $P = 0.01$, Wilcoxon), 60 (enhancing: $n = 19$, IL-12 = 31%; non-enhancing: $n = 44$, IL-12 = 15%; $P = 0.006$) or 90 (enhancing: $n = 19$, IL-12 = 31%; non-enhancing: $n = 48$, IL-12 = 15%; $P = 0.005$) days from blood sampling.

We also investigated whether changes in activation markers on peripheral blood T-cells correlate with disease activity in patients with multiple sclerosis.[76] We found that: (1) a change in the percentage of cells expressing the activation markers IL-2 receptor (CD25), class II MHC (I3), or surface dipeptidyl peptidase (CD26) correlated significantly with a change in lesion volume on MRI or a change in number of Gd-enhancing lesions; and (2) changes in CD25+ cells and in CD4+ cells expressing class II MHC also correlated with changes in disability as measured by EDSS in patients with RR disease and changes in CD4+CD25+ cells correlated with the occurrence of attacks in patients with RR disease.

We found that in terms of serum ICAM and TNF-R, circulating forms of adhesion molecules or soluble receptors may be released from cells as a consequence of activation and may be useful markers for inflammation. Patients with relapsing–progressive disease had the highest levels of sICAM-1, whereas patients with progressive disease had the highest levels of sTNF-Rs. Fluctuations in sICAM-1 correlated with the occurrence of attacks in patients with relapsing and relapsing–progressive disease. In patients with relapsing–progressive MS, an increase in sICAM-1 level preceded the appearance of new Gd-enhancing lesions on MRI, whereas a decrease in sICAM-1 levels correlated with the appearance of new Gd-enhancing lesions.[77]

It has sometimes been assumed that if a treatment is found for MS, it should help all patients. However, a very important treatment concept in MS is that there will be responders and non-responders to each 'effective' therapy. Thus, because an individual patient does not respond to a particular treatment does not mean that the treatment is ineffective. Furthermore, since the disease is heterogeneous, one of the most important aims of clinical and immunologic research in MS is to understand why people are responders or non-responders. For example, in our studies of pulse cyclophosphamide we recently found that the length of time a person is chronic progressive correlates with whether they respond to therapy.[62] Furthermore, as with any disease process in medicine, it would be expected that the disease would be easiest to arrest at early stages and that later stages would be less responsive to therapy. Towards this end, we are beginning to test the use of 6 months of 'rescue therapy' with pulse cyclophosphamide in relapsing–remitting patients who are IFN-β non-responders. Clearly, one of the primary goals of therapy is to prevent the progressive forms of the disease. This is especially true for immune therapy as it would not be effective to treat axonal damage to the nervous system. Furthermore, if the immune system becomes differentially activated in the progressive forms of the illness,[52] treatment that is effective in the relapsing stage may not be effective in the progressive stages. Finally, MS may be a more irreversible disease than previously appreciated, since axonal transection occurs in MS lesions.[78]

ACKNOWLEDGEMENTS

Arnon Karni is the recipient of a fellowship from the national Multiple Sclerosis Society. Supported by NIH grants NS23132, a grant from the National Multiple Sclerosis Society, The Foundation for Neurological Diseases and The Nancy Davis Center Without Walls.

REFERENCES

1. Martin R, McFarland HF, McFarlin DE. Immunological aspects of demyelinating diseases. *Annu Rev Immunol* 1992; **10**: 153–187.
2. Raine CS. The Dale McFarlin memorial lecture. The immunology of the MS lesion. *Ann Neurol* 1994; **36**: S61–S72.
3. Prineas JW. Pathology of multiple sclerosis. In: Cook SD, ed. *Handbook of Multiple Sclerosis*, Vol. 10. Newark: Marcel Dekker, Inc., 1996: 223–.
4. Lassmann H. *Comparative Neuropathology of Chronic Experimental Allergic Encephalomyelitis and Multiple Sclerosis.* Berlin: Springer-Verlag, 1983.
5. Windhagen A, Newcombe J, Dangond F et al. Expression of costimulatory molecules B7–1 (CD80), B7–2 (CD86), and interleukin 12 cytokine in multiple sclerosis lesions. *J Exp Med* 1995; **182**: 1985–1996.
6. Olsson T, Wang W-Z, Höjeberg B et al. Autoreactive T-lymphocytes in multiple sclerosis determined by antigen-induced secretion of interferon-gamma. *J Clin Invest* 1990; **86**: 981–985.
7. Allegretta M, Nicklas J, Sriram S, Albertini R. T-cells responsive to myelin basic protein in patients with multiple sclerosis. *Science* 1990; **247**: 718.
8. Zhang J, Markovic S, Raus J, Lacet B, Weiner HL, Hafler DA. Increased frequency of IL-2 responsive T-cells specific for myelin basic protein and proteolipid protein in peripheral blood and cerebrospinal fluid of patients with multiple sclerosis. *J Exp Med* 1993; **179**: 973–984.
9. Bieganowska KD, Ausubel LJ, Modabber Y, Slovik E, Messersmith W, Hafler DA. Direct ex vivo analysis of activated, fas-sensitive autoreactive T-cells in human autoimmune disease. *J Exp Med* 1997; **185**: 1585–1594.
10. Warren KG, Catz I, Johnson E, Mielke B. Anti-myelin basic protein and anti-proteolipid protein specific forms of multiple sclerosis. *Ann Neurol* 1994; **35**: 280–289.
11. Linington C, Bradi M, Lassmann H, Brunner C, Vass K. Augmentation of demyelination in rat acute allergic encephalomyelitis by circulating mouse monoclonal antibodies directed against a myelin/oligodendrocyte glycoprotein. *Am J Pathol* 1988; **130**: 443.
12. Schluesener H, Sobel R, Linington C, Weiner HL. A monoclonal antibody against a myelin oligodendrocyte glycoprotein induces relapses and demyelination in CNS autoimmune disease. *J Immunol* 1987; **139**: 4016.
13. Lehmann P, Forsthuber T, Miller A, Sercarz E. Spreading of T-cell autoimmunity to cryptic determinants of an autoantigen. *Nature* 1992; **358**: 155.
14. McCarron R, Fallis R, McFarlin D. Alterations in T-cell antigen specificity and class II restriction during the course of chronic relapsing experimental allergic encephalomyelitis. *J Neuroimmunol* 1990; **29**: 73–79.
15. Cross AH, Tuohy VK, Raine CS. Development of reactivity to new myelin antigens during chronic relapsing autoimmune demyelination. *Cell Immunol* 1993; **146**: 261–270.
16. Kaufman DI, Clare-Salzler M, Tian J et al. Spontaneous loss of T-cell tolerance to glutamic acid decarboxylase in murine insulin-dependent diabetes. *Nature* 1993; **366**: 69–72.

17. Tisch R, Yang X-D, Singer SM, Liblau RS, Fugger L, McDevitt HO. Immune response to glutamic acid decarboxylase correlates with insulitis in non-obese diabetic mice. *Nature* 1993; **366**: 72–75.

18. Kerlero de Rosbo N, Milo R, Lees MB, Burger D, Bernard CCA, Ben-Nun A. Reactivity to myelin antigens in multiple sclerosis: peripheral blood lymphocytes respond predominantly to myelin oligodendrocyte glycoprotein. *J Clin Invest* 1993; **92**: 2602–2608.

19. Harrison LC. Islet cell antigens in insulin-dependent diabetes: Pandora's box revisited. *Immunol Today* 1992; **13**: 348–352.

20. Shimonkevitz R, Colburn C, Burnham J, Murray RS, Kotzin BL. Clonal expansion of activated gamma/delta T-cells in recent onset multiple sclerosis. *Proc Natl Acad Sci USA* 1993; **90**: 923–927.

21. Wucherpfennig KW, Newcombe J, Kebby C, Cuzner ML, Hafler DA. Gamma/delta T-cell receptor repertoire in acute demyelinating multiple sclerosis lesions. *Proc Natl Acad Sci USA* 1992; **89**: 4588–4592.

22. Panitch HS, Hirsch RL, Haley AS, Johnson KP. Exacerbations of multiple sclerosis in patients treated with gamma interferon. *Lancet* 1987; **1**: 893.

23. Seder RA, Paul WE. Lymphocyte responses and cytokines. *Cell* 1994; **76**: 241–251.

24. Racke MK, Bonomo A, Scott DE et al. Cytokine-induced immune deviation as a therapy for inflammatory autoimmune disease. *J Exp Med* 1994; **180**: 1961–1966.

25. Groux H, O'Garra A, Bigler M et al. A CD4+ T-cell subset inhibits antigen-specific T-cell responses and prevents colitis. *Nature* 1997; **389**: 737–742.

26. Chen Y, Kuchroo VK, Inobe J-I, Hafler DA, Weiner HL. Regulatory T-cell clones induced by oral tolerance: suppression of autoimmune encephalomyelitis. *Science* 1994; **265**: 1237–1240.

27. Khoury SJ, Hancock WW, Weiner HL. Oral tolerance to myelin basic protein and natural recovery from experimental autoimmune encephalomyelitis as associated with downregulation of inflammatory cytokines and differential upregulation of transforming growth factor b, interleukin 4, and prostaglandin E expression in the brain. *J Exp Med* 1992; **176**: 1355–1364.

28. Karpus W, Swanborg R. CD4+ suppressor cells inhibit the function of effector cells of experimental autoimmune encephalomyelitis through a mechanism involving transforming growth factor beta. *J Immunol* 1991; **146**: 1163–1168.

29. Steinman L. Multiple sclerosis and its animal models: the role of the major histocompatibility complex and the T-cell receptor repertoire. *Semin Immunopathol* 1992; **14**: 79–93.

30. Zipp F, Weber F, Huber S et al. Genetic control of multiple sclerosis: increased production of lymphotoxin and tumor necrosis factor-alpha by HLA-DR2+ T-cells. *Ann Neurol* 1995; **38**: 723–730.

31. Segal BM, Shevach EM. IL-12 unmasks latent autoimmune disease in resistant mice. *J Exp Med* 1996; **184**: 771–775.

32. Maron R, Hancock WW, Slavin A, Hattori M, Kuchroo V, Weiner HL. Genetic susceptibility or resistance to autoimmune encephalomyelitis in MHC congenic mice is associated with differential production of pro- and anti-inflammatory cytokines. *Int Immunol* 1999; **11**: 1573–1580.

33. Mussener A, Lorentzen JC, Kleinau S, Klareskog L. Altered Th1/Th2 balance associated with non-major histocompatibility complex genes in collagen-induced arthritis in resistant rat strains. *Eur J Immunol* 1997; **27**: 695–699.

34. Kuchroo V, Prabhu Das M, Brown JA et al. B7-1 and B7-2 costimulatory molecules differentially activate the Th1/Th2 developmental pathways: application to autoimmune disease therapy. *Cell* 1995; **80**: 707–718.

35. Oro AS, Guarino TJ, Driver R, Steinman L, Umetsu DT. Regulation of disease susceptibility: decreased prevalence of IgE-mediated allergic disease in patients with multiple sclerosis. *J Allergy Clin Immunol* 1996; **97**: 1402–1408.

36. Sadovnick AD, Rice GP, Armstrong H. A population-based study of multiple sclerosis in twins: update. *Ann Neurol* 1993; **33**: 281–285.

37. Kurtzke JF. Epidemiology of multiple sclerosis. In: Vinken PJ, Bruyn GW, Klawans HL et al, eds. *Handbook of Clinical Neurology*, Vol. 3. New York: Elsevier Science Publishers, 1985: 259–287.

38. Bamford CR, Sibley WA, Thies C. Seasonal variation of multiple sclerosis exacerbations in Arizona. *Neurology* 1983; **33**: 897–701.

39. Balashov KE, Olek MJ, Smith DR, Khoury SJ, Weiner HL. Seasonal variation of interferon-gamma production in progressive multiple sclerosis. *Ann Neurol* 1998; **44**: 824–828.

40. Antel J, Arnason B, Medof M. Suppressor cell function in multiple sclerosis: correlation with clinical disease activity. *Ann Neurol* 1978; **5**: 338.

41. Hafler DA, Weiner HL. Immunologic mechanisms and therapy in multiple sclerosis. *Immunol Rev* 1995; **144**: 75–107.

42. Hafler DA, Weiner HL. *In vivo* labeling of peripheral blood T-cells using monoclonal antibodies: rapid traffic into cerebrospinal fluid in multiple sclerosis. *Ann Neurol* 1987; **22**: 90–93.

43. Bongioanni P, Meucci G. T-cell tumor necrosis factor-alpha receptor binding in patients with multiple sclerosis. *Neurology* 1997; **48**: 826–831.

44. Noronha A, Toscas A, Jensen MA. Interferon beta augments suppressor cell function in multiple sclerosis. *Ann Neurol* 1990; **27**: 207–210.

45. Hafler D, Fox D, Manning M, Schlossman S, Reinherz E, Weiner H. *In vivo* activated T lymphocytes in the peripheral blood and cerebrospinal fluid of patients with multiple sclerosis. *N Engl J Med* 1985; **312**: 1405–1411.

46. Berger T, Weerth S, Kojima K, Linington C, Wekerle H, Lassmann H. Experimental autoimmune encephalomyelitis: the antigen specificity of T lymphocytes determines the topography of lesions in the central and peripheral nervous system. *Lab Invest* 1997; **76**: 355–364.

47. Revesz T, Kidd D, Thompson AJ et al. A comparison of the pathology of primary and secondary progressive multiple sclerosis. *Brain* 1994; **117**: 759–765.

48. Schmied M, Breitschopf H, Gold R et al. Apoptosis of T lymphocytes in experimental autoimmune encephalomyelitis. Evidence for programmed cell death as a mechanism to control inflammation in the brain. *Am J Pathol* 1993; **143**: 446–452.

49. Kennedy MK, Torrance DS, Picha KS, Mohler KM. Analysis of cytokine mRNA expression in the central nervous system of mice with experimental autoimmune encephalomyelitis reveals that IL-10 mRNA expression correlates with recovery. *J Immunol* 1992; **149**: 2496–2505.

50. Chen Y, Hancock WW, Marks R, Gonnella PA, Weiner HL. Mechanisms of recovery from experimental allergic encephalomyelitis: T-cell deletion and immune deviation in myelin basic protein T-cell receptor transgenic mice. *J Neuroimmunol* 1998; **82**: 149–159.

51. Correale J, Gilmore W, McMillan M et al. Patterns of cytokine secretion by autoreactive proteolipid protein-specific T-cell clones during the course of multiple sclerosis. *J Immunol* 1995; **154**: 2959–2968.

52. Balashov KE, Smith DR, Khoury SJ, Hafler DA, Weiner HL. Increased IL-12 production in progressive multiple sclerosis: induction by activated CD4+ T-cells via CD40 ligand. *Proc Natl Acad Sci USA* 1997; **94**: 599–603.

53. Balashov KE, Rottman JB, Weiner HL, Hancock WW. CCR5(+) and CXCR3(+) T cells are increased in multiple sclerosis and their ligands MIP-1alpha and IP-10 are expressed in demyelinating brain lesions. *Proc Natl Acad Sci USA* 1999; **96**: 6873–6878.

54. Comabella M, Balashov K, Issazadeh S, Smith D, Weiner HL, Khoury SJ. Elevated interleukin-12 in progressive multiple sclerosis correlates with disease activity and is normalized by pulse cyclophosphamide therapy. *J Clin Invest* 1998; **102**: 671–678.

55. Karni A, Koldzic G, Khoury SJ. Elevated interferon-gamma in secondary progressive multiple sclerosis is linked to both interleukin-18 and interferon-12. *Ann Neurol* 2000; **48**: 450.

56. Martin R, McFarland HF. Immunological aspects of experimental allergic encephalomyelitis and multiple sclerosis. *Crit Rev Clin Lab Sci* 1995; **32**: 121–182.

57. Lublin FD, Knobler RL, Kalman B et al. Monoclonal anti-gamma interferon antibodies enhance experimental allergic encephalomyelitis. *Autoimmunity* 1993; **16**: 267–274.

58. Ferber IA, Brocke S, Taylor-Edwards C et al. Mice with disrupted IFN-γ gene are susceptible to the induction of experimental autoimmune encephalomyelitis (EAE). *J Immunol* 1996; **156**: 15–7.

59. Billiau A, Heremans H, Vandekerckhove F et al. Enhancement of experimental allergic encephalomyelitis by antibodies against IFN-γ. *J Immunol* 1988; **140**: 1506–1510.

60. Balashov KE, Khoury SJ, Hafler DA, Weiner HL. Inhibition of T-cell responses by activated human CD8+ T-cells is mediated by interferon-γ and is defective in chronic progressive multiple sclerosis. *J Clin Invest* 1995; **95**: 2711–2719.

61. Weiner H, Hohol M, Khoury S, Dawson D, Hafler D. Therapy for MS. *Neurol Clin* 1995; **13**: 173–196.

62. Hohol MJ, Olek MJ, Orav EJ et al. Treatment of progressive multiple sclerosis with pulse cyclophosphamide/methylprednisolone: response to therapy is linked to the duration of progressive disease. *Mult Scler* 1999; **5**: 403–409.

63. Faria AMC, Weiner HL. Oral tolerance: mechanisms and therapeutic applications. *Adv Immunol* 1999; **73**: 153–264.

64. Fukaura H, Kent SC, Pietrusewicz MJ, Khoury SJ, Weiner HL, Hafler DA. Induction of circulating myelin basic protein and proteolipid protein-specific transforming growth factor-beta1–secreting Th3 T-cells by oral administration of myelin in multiple sclerosis patients. *J Clin Invest* 1996; **98**: 70–77.

65. Nicholson L, Greer J, Sobel R, Lees M, Kuchroo V. An altered peptide ligand mediates immune deviation and prevents EAE. *Immunity* 1995; **3**: 397–405.

66. Miller A, Lider O, Weiner HL. Antigen-driven bystander suppression following oral administration of antigens. *J Exp Med* 1991; **174**: 791–798.

67. Al-Sabbagh A, Miller A, Santos LMB, Weiner HL. Antigen-driven tissue-specific suppression following oral tolerance: orally administered myelin basic protein suppresses proteolipid induced experimental autoimmune encephalomyelitis in the SJL mouse. *Eur J Immunol* 1994; **24**: 2104–2109.

68. Von Herrath MG, Dyrberg T, Oldstone MBA. Oral insulin treatment suppresses virus-induced antigen-specific destruction of beta cells and prevents autoimmune diabetes in transgenic mice. *J Clin Invest* 1996; **98**: 1324–1331.

69. Becker KJ, McCarron RM, Ruetzler C et al. Immunologic tolerance to myelin basic protein decreases stroke size after transient focal cerebral ischemia. *Proc Natl Acad Sci USA* 1997; **94**: 10873–10878.

70. Aharoni R, Teitelbaum D, Sela M, Arnon R. Copolymer 1 induces T-cells of the T helper type 2 that crossreact with myelin basic protein and suppress experimental autoimmune encephalomyelitis. *Proc Natl Acad Sci USA* 1997; **94**: 10821–10826.

71. Smith DR, Balashov KE, Hafler DA, Khoury SJ, Weiner HL. Immune deviation following pulse cyclophosphamide/methylprednisolone treatment of multiple sclerosis: increased interleukin-4 production and associated eosinophilia. *Ann Neurol* 1997; **42**: 313–318.

72. Rudick R, Ransohoff R, Peppler R. Interferon beta induces IL-10 expression: relevance to multiple sclerosis. *Ann Neurol* 1996; **40**: 618–627.

73. Takashima H, Smith DR, Fukaura H, Khoury SJ, Hafler DA, Weiner HL. Pulse cyclophosphamide plus methylprednisolone induces myelin-antigen-specific IL-4-secreting T cells in multiple sclerosis patients. *Clin Immunol Immunopathol* 1998; **88**: 28–34.

74. Genc K, Dona D, Reder AT. Increased CD80+ B cells in active multiple sclerosis and reversal by interferon β-1b therapy. *J Clin Invest* 1997; **99**: 2664–2671.

75. Makhlouf K, Weiner HL, Khoury SJ. Correlation between increased interleukin-12 expression and the presence of active lesions on magnetic resonance imaging in multiple sclerosis patients. *Ann Neurol* 2000; **48**: 477.

76. Khoury SJ, Guttmann CR, Orav EJ, Kikinis R, Jolesz FA, Weiner HL. Changes in activated T cells in the blood correlate with disease activity in multiple sclerosis. *Arch Neurol* 2000; **57**: 1183–1189.

77. Khoury SJ, Orav EJ, Guttmann CRG, Kikinis R, Jolesz FA, Weiner HL. Changes in serum levels of ICAM and TNF-R correlate with disease activity in multiple sclerosis. *Neurology* 1999; **53**: 758–764.

78. Trapp BD, Peterson J, Ransohoff RM, Rudick R, Mork S, Bo L. Axonal transection in the lesions of multiple sclerosis. *N Engl J Med* 1998; **338**: 278–285.

79. Yudkin PL, Ellison GW, Ghezzi A et al. Overview of azathioprine treatment in multiple sclerosis. *Lancet* 1991; **338**: 1051–1055.

80. Durelli L, Bongioanni MR, Ferrero B et al. Interferon alpha-2a treatment of relapsing-remitting multiple sclerosis: disease activity resumes after stopping treatment. *Neurology* 1996; **47**: 123–129.

81. Jacobs L, Cookfair D, Rudick R et al Results of a phase III trial of intramuscular recombinant beta interferon as treatment for multiple sclerosis. *Ann Neurol* 1994; **36**: 259.

82. The IFNB Multiple Sclerosis Study Group and The University of British Columbia MS/MRI Analysis Group. Interferon beta-1b in the treatment of multiple sclerosis: final outcome of the randomized controlled trial. *Neurology* 1995; **45**: 1277–1285.

83. Beutler E, Sipe JC, Romine JS, Koziol JA, McMillan R, Zyroff J. The treatment of chronic progressive multiple sclerosis with cladribine. *Proc Natl Acad Sci USA* 1996; **93**: 1716–1720.

84. Johnson KP, Brooks BR, Cohen JA et al. Copolymer 1 reduces relapse rate and improves disability in relapsing-remitting multiple sclerosis: results of a phase III multicenter, double-blind placebo-controlled trial. The Copolymer 1 Multiple Sclerosis Study Group. *Neurology* 1995; **45**: 1268–1276.

85. Beck RW, Cleary PA, Trobe JD et al. The effect of corticosteroids for acute optic neuritis on the subsequent development of multiple sclerosis. *N Engl J Med* 1993; **239**: 1764–1769.

86. Weiner HL, Mackin GA, Orav EJ et al. Intermittent cyclophosphamide pulse therapy in progressive multiple sclerosis: final report of the Northeast Cooperative Multiple Sclerosis Treatment Group. *Neurology* 1993; **43**: 910–918.

87. Hommes OR, Lamers KJB, Reekers P. Effect of intensive immunosuppression on the course of chronic progressive multiple sclerosis. *J Neurol* 1980; **223**: 177–190.

88. Group TMSS. Efficacy and toxicity of cyclosporine in chronic progressive multiple sclerosis: a randomized, double-blinded, placebo-controlled clinical trial. *Ann Neurol* 1990; **27**: 591–605.

89. Fazekas F, Deisenhammer F, Strasser-Fuchs S, Nahler G, Mamoli B. Randomized placebo-controlled trial of monthly intravenous immunoglobulin therapy in relapsing-remitting multiple sclerosis. *Lancet* 1997; **349**: 589–593.

90. Anderson O, Lycke J, Tollesson PO et al. Linomide reduces the rate of active lesions in relapsing-remitting multiple sclerosis. *Neurology* 1996; **47**: 895–900.

91. Karussis DM, Meiner Z, Lehmann D et al. Treatment of secondary progressive multiple sclerosis with the immunomodulator linomide: a double blind, placebo-controlled pilot study with monthly magnetic resonance imaging evaluation. *Neurology* 1996; **47**: 341–346.

92. Goodkin DE, Rudick RA, VanderBrug Medendorp S. Low-dose (7.5 mg) oral methotrexate reduces the rate of progression in chronic progressive multiple sclerosis. *Ann Neurol* 1995; **37**: 30–40.

93. Edan G, Miller D, Clanet M et al. Therapeutic effect of mitoxantrone combined with methylprednisolone in multiple sclerosis: a randomised multicenter study of active disease using MRI and clinical criteria. *J Neurol, Neurosurg Psychiatry* 1997; **62**: 112–118.

94. Weiner HL, Dau PC, Khatri BO et al. Double-blind study of true vs. sham plasma exchange in patients treated with immunosuppression for acute attacks of multiple sclerosis. *Neurology* 1989; **39**: 1143–1149.

95. Rodriguez M, Karnes WE, Bartleson JD, Pineda AA. Plasmapheresis in acute episodes of fulminant CNS inflammatory demyelination. *Neurology* 1993; **43**: 1100–1104.

96. Cook SD, Devereux C, Troiano R et al. Total lymphoid irradiation in multiple sclerosis. In: Rudick RA, Goodkin DE, eds. *Treatment of Multiple Sclerosis: Trial Design, Results, and Future Perspectives*. New York: Springer-Verlag, 1992: 267–280.

11

Immunogene therapy for autoimmune demyelination

Roberto Furlan, Pietro L Poliani, Alessandra Bergami, Francesca Ruffini, Elena Brambilla,
Peggy C Marconi, Giancarlo Comi and Gianvito Martino

INTRODUCTION

The peripheral delivery of drugs in patients affected by central nervous system (CNS)-confined diseases is therapeutically ineffective because of the presence of the blood–brain barrier (BBB), which forms an inaccessible wall to the majority of CNS targeting molecules. When 'therapeutic' molecules have been systemically administered to patients affected by a chronic inflammatory demyelinating disease of the CNS, such as multiple sclerosis (MS), results have been disappointing. A successful therapeutic approach in MS should therefore consider the delivery of 'therapeutic' molecules directly into the CNS in order to inhibit blood-borne CNS-confined mononuclear cells acting as ultimate effector cells, to rescue surviving oligodendrocytes, or to induce oligodendrocyte progenitor migration and differentiation into demyelinating areas. Biological and physical vectors engineered with heterologous genes coding for anti-inflammatory cytokines and/or growth factors might represent the appropriate tool to deliver therapeutic genes into the CNS. Here we provide a brief review of the various gene therapy attempts made so far in experimental demyelination and a critical overview of the advantages and disadvantages of the different delivery techniques employed.

THE BLOOD–BRAIN BARRIER: AN INPENETRABLE WALL

Given the choice, most of the patients affected by CNS-confined disorders would prefer to receive drugs through a systemic injection over a hole drilled in the skull. Unfortunately, many of the new therapies developed for brain diseases are only partially effective when administered through the bloodstream, because they scarcely cross the BBB. This barrier is formed by close, interacting endothelial cells, glial cells (mainly astrocytes) and pericytes forming an almost inpenetrable wall preventing many 'detrimental' molecules, such as toxins, from getting into the brain from the bloodstream and thus tainting the brain's nerve cell habitat.[1] Under physiological conditions, molecules are able to cross the BBB either via lipid-mediated transport, restricted to small molecules with molecular masses lower than approximately 700 Da and usually proportional to the lipid solubility of the molecule, or catalyzed transport, including carrier-mediated or receptor-mediated mechanisms.[1] To allow access to the CNS of 'therapeutic' compounds, research is now developing novel technologies mainly based on an assault on the brain's gates (i.e. opening the BBB using the sugar mannitol) or on coupling the 'drugs' to molecules that already cross the BBB (i.e. nerve cell-protecting molecules).[1] In this chapter, we discuss another emerging technology for delivering therapeutic molecules into the CNS and which is mainly based on the use of gene therapy devices such as plasmids and/or biological vectors.

THERAPEUTIC TARGETS IN MS

MS is characterized by the presence, within the CNS, of inflammatory infiltrates containing a few autoreactive T-cells and a multitude of pathogenetic non-specific lymphocytes determining the typical patchy CNS demyelination, ranging from demyelination with preservation of oligodendrocytes to complete oligodendrocyte and axonal loss and severe glial scarring.[2,3] CNS antigen-specific T-cells are believed to provide the organ specificity of the pathogenic process and to regulate the recirculation within the CNS of non-antigen-specific lymphomononuclear cells that, by directly destroying oligodendrocytes and/or by releasing myelinotoxic substances, act as final effector cells.[2] In most instances, however, oligodendrocytes or their precursors are morphologically preserved in demyelinating plaques, remaining able to differentiate and remyelinate.[3] A successful therapeutic approach to MS should therefore include inhibition of antigen- and non-antigen-specific immune cells and/or the rescue of surviving oligodendrocytes within demyelinating plaques.

CYTOKINE-BASED THERAPIES IN HUMAN AND EXPERIMENTAL DEMYELINATION

Preliminary considerations

Among the putative mechanisms orchestrating the immunological network sustaining the activation of antigen- and non-antigen-specific immune cells in MS, those initiated and sustained by pro-inflammatory cytokines are considered essential. Pro-inflammatory cytokines (i.e. tumor necrosis factor (TNF)-α/β, interferon (IFN)-γ, interleukin (IL)-$1\alpha/\beta$) are mainly secreted by monocytes/macrophages and T-cells belonging to the Th1 subset (see ref. 4 for review). In the pathogenic mechanism underlying MS, these molecules can (1) sustain the primary CNS-confined inflammatory process leading to the development of myelin-specific T-cells, (2) activate myelin-specific T-cells and shape their repertoire (Th1 versus Th2 pattern), and (3) induce the CNS recruitment from the periphery of myelinotoxic effector cells, including non-antigen-specific T- and B-cells and monocyte/macrophages.[5] Finally, certain pro-inflammatory cytokines can determine direct oligodendrotoxicity (e.g. TNF-α).[6]

Although pro-inflammatory cytokines represent a suitable therapeutic target in MS, therapies based on the use of cytokines with an anti-inflammatory profile (IFN-β, IL-4, transforming growth factor (TGF)-β, IL-10) so far attempted in MS patients have been mostly disappointing. Subcutaneous as well as intramuscular administration of IFN-β in patients with relapsing–remitting MS is only partially effective[7,8] since it reduces by one-third the disease exacerbation rate and does not change substantially the progression of disability. Systemic administration of TGF-β does not induce any change in the disability status of patients or in the appearance of brain magnetic resonance imaging lesions.[9] Intravenous injection of the recombinant TNF receptor p55 immunoglobulin fusion protein Lenercept in MS patients induces an increase in the number of patients experiencing exacerbations.[10]

As previously mentioned, the administration route of cytokines in MS patients can partially explain the disappointing results obtained so far. Along with the scarce BBB crossing of systemically injected cytokines,[11] severe unpredictable and undesirable side-effects have been observed. TGF-β administration in MS patients determines reversible nephrotoxicity.[9] Moreover, systemic administration of IFN-β as well as of the Lenercept molecule causes the formation of anti-cytokine-binding as well as neutralizing antibodies,[10,12] thus further limiting the therapeutic effect, if present, of these molecules. The delivery of potentially therapeutic cytokines directly into the CNS may overcome some of the above-mentioned limitations, although practical considerations (e.g. injection schedule) as well as the potential toxicity of intrathecal treatments should be taken into consideration.

Anti-inflammatory cytokine-based gene therapy in experimental autoimmune encephalomyelitis

To date, gene therapy has never been attempted in MS patients. Some experiments, mainly based on anti-inflammatory cytokine gene delivery, have been performed in animals affected by experimental autoimmune encephalomyelitis (EAE), the animal model of MS. Gene therapy approaches so far attempted in EAE can be divided into two distinct categories: (1) cytokine genes incorporated into viral vectors or plasmids and injected into the bloodstream or into circulating encephalitogenic T-cells; and (2) cytokine genes transferred directly into the CNS using viral vectors, plasmids or engineered cell lines. Here is a brief summary of the results obtained.

Concerning peripheral approaches, EAE was ameliorated when IL-4[13] or IL-10[14] genes were transferred into autoreactive encephalitogenic T-cells. Murine latent TGF-β_A cDNA engineered into a myelin basic protein (MBP)-specific BALB/c T-helper 1 (Th1) clone injected into SJLxBALB/c F1 12–15 days after immunization also significantly delayed and ameliorated proteolipid protein (PLP)-induced EAE.[15] Intravenous injection of vaccinia virus (VV)-derived vectors showed that disease amelioration was obtained when IL-6, TNF-α, IL-1β, IL-2, IL-10 but not IL-4 or IFN-γ were administered.[16] Naked plasmid DNA expression vectors encoding either TGF-β (pVR-TGF-β_1) or an IL-4–IgG$_1$ chimeric protein (pVR-IL-4–IgG$_1$) injected intramuscularly into MBP-induced EAE mice[17] resulted in production of TGF-β_1 or IL-4-IgG$_1$, respectively, and protection from clinical and histopathological signs of EAE through a pronounced downregulatory effect on MBP-specific T-cells, as demonstrated by in vitro assays for antigen-specific proliferation and production of IFN-γ and TNF-α. In the CNS, treatment with either vector suppressed IL-12 and IFN-γ mRNA expression, while IL-4 and TGF-β_1 mRNA levels were increased compared to control mice.[17]

Concerning target organ-oriented gene therapy approaches, direct CNS injection using DNA–liposome constructs was therapeutically successful in EAE when IL-4, TGF-β, IFN-β, p75TNF receptor but not IL-10 were delivered.[18] Gene delivery of CTLA4-human Ig into mice CNS using a non-replicating adenoviral vector was more effective than a single injection of CTLA4-human Ig protein in ameliorating EAE induction and progression.[19] Finally, a conditionally immortalized syngeneic fibroblast line established using a temperature-sensitive SV40 large T Ag-expressing retrovirus, infected with a retrovirus expressing soluble dimeric p75 TNF receptor (dTNFR) construct and CNS-injected into EAE mice, significantly ameliorated both acute and relapsing EAE.[20]

Cytokine gene delivery using HSV-1-derived vectors

We have been working on a CNS delivery system for cytokine genes based on viral vectors. An ideal CNS delivery tool should be able to reach different CNS areas (MS is a multifocal disease with a preferential periventricular distribution), should persist long enough within the CNS, should be completely non-toxic for CNS resident cells and should be unable to induce peripheral side-effects. We developed a novel system to deliver cytokine genes into the CNS based on the use of non-replicative HSV type 1-derived vectors. These vectors are considered an alternative to classical retroviral and adenoviral vectors, mainly because HSV is able to accommodate multiple foreign genes and to infect postmitotic cells, such as neurons.[21–24] We used an HSV-1-derived vector named d120,[24,25] obtained from the HSV-1 Kos strain by deletion of both copies of the IE ICP4 gene. In this non-replicating mutant, we inserted the murine IL-4 gene, driven by the ICP4 promoter, into the thymidine kinase locus. In vivo preliminary experiments indicated that d120 is easily transferred within the CNS, diffuses consistently in all cerebrospinal fluid (CSF) spaces, and is able to efficiently infect the layer of ependymal cells surrounding the ventricles as well as choroidal and leptomeningeal cells. Within the CNS, the HSV-1 vector redirects the infected cell

machinery to produce discrete amounts of the cytokine in the CSF of mice up to 28 days post-injection.[26] We then used the IL-4-containing vector as a therapeutic tool in EAE mice. IL-4 was administered intracerebrally in Biozzi AB/H mice immunized with myelin oligodendrocyte glycoprotein (MOG)$_{40–55}$ before[27] and after[28] the appearance of EAE signs. No toxic reactions were observed. A significant amelioration of the clinical and pathological CNS features of EAE was observed with both therapeutic protocols. The protective effect of this therapy was mostly due to the ability of IL-4 to downregulate in situ production of pro-inflammatory chemokines (monocyte chemoattractant chemokines, and RANTES) and pro-inflammatory cytokines (i.e. IL-1β, TNF-α). Furthermore, we found that lymph node cells from IL-4-treated versus non-treated mice were able to process and proliferate in response, to the encephalitogenic antigen as well as to drive an appropriate Th1 response, thus indicating a lack of interference of the IL-4 gene therapy approach we used on the proper functioning of the immune system in the periphery.

We also used another non-replicative HSV-1-derived viral vector created in an HSV-1 triple deletion mutant backbone lacking the two copies of the ICP4 gene, the ICP27 gene, and the ICP22 gene and containing the mouse IL-1 receptor antagonist (IL-1ra) gene.[23] The deletion of the ICP4, ICP22 and ICP27 genes, which are essential for viral in vitro and in vivo replication and viral cytotoxicity, reduces considerably the intrinsic cytotoxicity of this HSV-1-derived mutant.[23] After assessing the proper in vivo distribution of the vector into naive mice, we intracerebrally injected the IL-1ra-containing HSV-1-derived vector into C57/BL6 mice immunized with MOG$_{35–55}$. The treatment was performed either before or after the onset of EAE. The results (R. Furlan, unpublished) indicate that the IL-1ra vector was able to significantly delay the onset and reduce the severity of EAE when preventively injected, but not when the vector was injected after EAE onset. No interference with the proper functioning of the peripheral immune system has been observed when using the IL-1ra-containing vector.

GENE THERAPY OF REMYELINATION: FUTURE APPLICATIONS

The two major target candidates for the immune-mediated pathogenic process in MS are oligodendrocytes and myelin components.[3] Conceivably, both are involved in the disease, which would explain the clinical heterogeneity of MS by virtue of target heterogeneity. In the chronic form of MS, oligodendrocytes seem to represent the primary target of the pathological process, and are almost completely lost in demyelinating areas, so that no spontaneous remyelination takes place. In contrast, in the acute relapsing–remitting form of the disease, the persistence of oligodendrocytes in demyelinating areas in which remyelination takes place suggests that the primary targets in this form are myelin components such as MBP, PLP, MOG or others. This latter disease form, which accounts for more than 80% of MS patients, might therefore benefit from therapies aimed at stimulating oligodendrocytes to remyelinate. For a long time it was believed that repair of myelin sheaths does not occur in MS. However, more recently, a detailed analysis of MS pathology provided evidence for extensive remyelination.[29,30] Remyelination is prominent during the early stage of disease evolution and apparently depends upon the availability of oligodendrocytes or their progenitor cells within the lesions.[31,32] In the late chronic stage of the disease, repair of myelin is sparse and, if present at all, restricted to a small rim at the plaque edge. It is as yet unclear which cells in the CNS accomplish remyelination. They could in part be recruited from oligodendrocytes that have survived the acute phase of demyelination.[33] However, recent experimental data suggest that mature, terminally differentiated oligodendrocytes are incapable of synthesizing new myelin.[34] In contrast, in most experimental situations, remyelinating cells are derived from the pool of undifferentiated glial precursor cells, which are present even in the adult CNS tissue and can also be found in low numbers in demyelinated MS plaques. Thus, it is suggested that the failure of myelin repair in late chronic MS lesions is due to a depletion of this progenitor cell pool, which is likely to occur in areas of repeated demyelinating episodes.[29,35] On the other hand, some oligodendrocyte progenitor cells can be found even in old demyelinated scars of MS patients.

All these findings suggest that myelin repair in MS lesions could be therapeutically approached by introducing into the pathological tissue growth factors which prevent destruction of oligodendrocytes and stimulate undifferentiated glial precursor cells to divide, differentiate and remyelinate axons. The use of growth factors in humans, however, is subject to the following considerations: (1) growth factors may drive terminally differentiated mature oligodendrocytes into apoptosis;[36] and (2) rescue of oligodendrocytes and/or their progenitor cells in demyelinating conditions depends upon the mechanisms of myelin injury. Nevertheless, a gene therapy

safety study using a growth factor named ciliary neurotrophic factor (CNTF) has been already performed in humans affected by amyotrophic lateral sclerosis (ALS), a neurodegenerative disease of the motor neurons.[37] This study showed that introduction of heterologous genes coding for CNTF into the CSF using encapsulated genetically modified CNTF-producing myoblasts is feasible and nontoxic. Moreover, experiments aimed at delivering genes coding for other neurotropic factors have also been performed in non-human primates affected by an experimental model of Parkinson's disease in which therapeutic effects have been observed without any side-effects related to the procedure or to the vector toxicity.

While no attempts have been made to transfer growth factor genes into MS patients in order to induce oligodendrocyte progenitor proliferation, some experimental evidence is available from EAE animals. It has been recently shown that autoreactive T-cells isolated from SWXJ mice immunized with $PLP_{139-151}$ and transfected with an antigen-inducible transgene coding for platelet-derived growth factor-α (PDGF), a growth factor important in regulating the development of oligodendrocytes, upon adoptive transfer, migrated to the CNS and ameliorated ongoing EAE.[38] Moreover, we found that the intrathecal injection into C57BL/6 mice of an HSV-1-derived vector engineered with the basic fibroblast growth factor (bFGF) gene, after the onset of MOG_{35-55}-induced EAE, is feasible and non-toxic and induces migration of oligodendrocyte progenitors into demyelinated areas, thus supporting remyelinating processes and prevention of axonal loss. In bFGF-treated EAE mice, but not in controls, PDGF-R^+ cells (surface marker of oligo precursors) have been found in demyelinating areas of the spinal cord where remyelination was ongoing (F. Ruffini, submitted). In conclusion, although preliminary, these studies indicate that delivery of neuroprotective agents such as growth factor genes into the CNS can be easily approached using gene therapy systems employing viral vectors without overt undesirable toxic effects.

CONCLUSIONS

The gene therapy results obtained so far, including our own, are encouraging due to the wide range of therapeutic flexibility that biological vectors possess (Fig. 11.1). However, gene therapy techniques used in EAE models might have major limitations when transferred to humans: (1) autoreactive T-cells can be easily isolated in the animal model of MS but not in

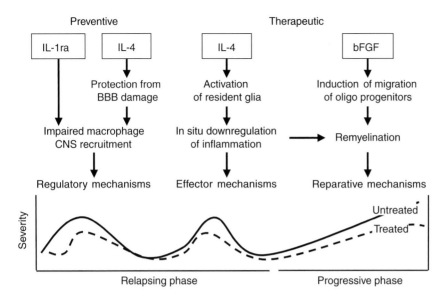

Figure 11.1 Summary of the results obtained using HSV-1-derived vectors in EAE. Both the preventive use of IL-4 and IL-1ra (intracerebral injection of the vector 10–15 days before EAE onset) and the therapeutic treatment (intracerebral injection of the vector after EAE onset) with IL-4 of bFGF-containing vectors ameliorated the clinicopathological signs of EAE in mice. Preventive treatment with IL-4- or IL-1ra-containing vectors led to downregulation of CNS recruitment of macrophages from the periphery. Therapeutic treatment with IL-4 induced in situ downregulation of inflammation via inhibition of pro-inflamamtory cytokine and chemokine production by CNS-resident cells as well as blood-borne immune cells. Treatment with bFGF led to the recruitment of oligodendrocyte precursors in areas of demyelination, thus protecting mice from demyelination as well axonal loss. HSV-1-derived vectors possess a wide range of therapeutic flexibility that can be of help in any of the phases of immunomediated demyelinating diseases.

humans, where the MS antigen is still unknown; (2) DNA liposomes as well as VVs have limited transfection efficiency when introduced into post-mitotic cells such as those resident in the CNS; (3) regulatory sequences used in plasmids for naked DNA vaccination can per se modulate cytokine production in vivo, thus suppressing EAE;[39] (4) VVs as well as adenoviral vectors still have residual toxicity and immunogenicity; and (5) CG repeated motifs contained in bacterial plasmids used to transfer heterologous genes into EAE animals might per se induce EAE.[40] Some of these limitations have been overcome by the use of HSV-1-derived vectors, which, in our hands, have been shown to be easily transferred within the CNS through the CSF circulation with no major reactions of the resident cells whose intracellular machinery was used to produce the heterologous gene (e.g. cytokine and growth factor genes). The main advantages of this system are: (1) the availability of high cytokine/growth factor levels in different areas of the CNS; (2) the persistent therapeutic effect (i.e. 4 weeks) after a single vector administration; and (3) the lack of interference of this procedure with the proper functioning of the peripheral immune system. Moreover, the possibility of accommodating multiple genes within the HSV-1-derived vectors suggests that this therapeutic device might be useful to take advantage of cytokines with synergistic activity in the near future. On the other hand, the short-lasting effect of these vectors (no more than 4 weeks after in vivo delivery) as well as the impossibility of regulating the gene transcription are the major limiting factors of HSV-1-based therapy developed for chronic diseases such as MS. Nevertheless, the new improvements in viral vector technology should overcome these constraints and soon lead to: (1) 'inducible' vectors in which the transcription of the heterologous gene contained in the vector could be exogenously induced or inhibited; (2) chimeric vectors able to integrate into host DNA of postmitotic cells (e.g.

retroviruses combined with herpesviruses); and (3) short versus long-term expressing vectors.

ACKNOWLEDGEMENTS

Our work is supported by MURST, the Minister of Health (Progetti Finalizzati) and the Italian National Multiple Sclerosis Society (AISM). We thank Joseph Glorioso for providing the vectors we used and encouraging our research.

REFERENCES

1. Saunders NR, Habgood MD, Dziegielewska KM. Barrier mechanisms in the brain, I. Adult brain. *Clin Exp Pharmacol Physiol* 1999; **26**: 11–19.

2. Martino G, Hartung HP. Immunopathogenesis of multiple sclerosis: the role of T-cells. *Curr Opin Neurol* 1999; **12**: 309–321.

3. Lucchinetti CF, Brück W, Rodriguez M, Lassmann H. Distinct patterns of multiple sclerosis pathology indicate heterogeneity on pathogenesis. *Brain Pathol* 1996; **6**: 269–274.

4. Abbas AK, Murphy KM, Sher A. Functional diversity of helper T lymphocytes. *Nature* 1996; **383**: 787–793.

5. Kieseier B, Storch MK, Archelos JJ, Martino G, Hartung HP. Effector pathways in immune mediated central nervous system demyelination. *Curr Opin Neurol* 1999; **12**: 323–336.

6. Selmaj KW, Raine CS. Tumor necrosis factor mediates myelin and oligodendrocyte damage in vitro. *Ann Neurol* 1988; **23**: 339–346.

7. The IFNB Multiple Sclerosis Study Group. Interferon beta-1b is effective in relapsing–remitting multiple sclerosis. I. Clinical results of a multicenter, randomized, double-blind, placebo-controlled trial. *Neurology* 1993; **43**: 655–661.

8. Weinstock-Guttman B, Ransohoff RM, Kinkel RP, Rudick RA. The interferons: biological effects, mechanisms of action, and use in multiple sclerosis. *Ann Neurol* 1995; **37**: 7–15.

9. Calabresi PA, Fields NS, Maloni HW et al. Phase 1 trial of transforming growth factor beta 2 in chronic progressive MS. *Neurology* 1998; **51**: 289–292.

10. The Lenercept Multiple Sclerosis Study Group and University of British Columbia MS/MRI Analysis Group. TNF neutralization in MS: results of a randomized, placebo-controlled multicenter study. *Neurology* 1999; **53**: 457–465.

11. Khan OA, Xia Q, Bever CT Jr, Johnson KP, Panitch HS, Dhib-Jalbut SS. Interferon beta-1b serum levels in multiple sclerosis patients following subcutaneous administration. *Neurology* 1996; **46**: 1639–1643.

12. The IFNB Multiple Sclerosis Study Group and the University of British Columbia MS/MRI Analysis Group. Neutralizing antibodies during treatment of multiple sclerosis with interferon beta-1b: experience during the first three years. *Neurology* 1996; **47**: 889–894.

13. Shaw MK, Lorens JB, Dhawan A et al. Local delivery of interleukin 4 by retrovirus-transduced T lymphocytes ameliorates experimental autoimmune encephalomyelitis. *J Exp Med* 1997; **185**: 1711–1714.

14. Mathisen PM, Yu M, Johnson JM, Drazba JA, Tuohy VK. Treatment of experimental autoimmune encephalomyelitis with genetically modified memory T-cells. *J Exp Med* 1997; **186**: 159–164.

15. Chen LZ, Hochwald GM, Huang C et al. Gene therapy in allergic encephalomyelitis using myelin basic protein-specific T-cells engineered to express latent transforming growth factor-beta1. *Proc Natl Acad Sci USA* 1998; **95**: 12516–12521.

16. Willenborg DO, Fordham SA, Cowden WB, Ramshaw IA. Cytokines and murine autoimmune encephalomyelitis: inhibition or enhancement of disease with antibodies to select cytokines, or by delivery of exogenous cytokines using a recombinant vaccinia virus system. *Scand J Immunol* 1995; **41**: 31–40.

17. Piccirillo CA, Prud'homme GJ. Prevention of experimental allergic encephalomyelitis by intramuscular gene transfer with cytokine-encoding plasmid vectors. *Hum Gene Ther* 1999; **10**: 1915–1922.

18. Croxford JL, Triantaphyllopoulos K, Podhajcer OL, Feldmann M, Baker D, Chernajovsky Y. Cytokine gene therapy in experimental allergic encephalomyelitis by injection of plasmid DNA–cationic liposome complex into the central nervous system. *J Immunol* 1997; **160**: 5181–5187.

19. Croxford JL, O'Neill JK, Ali RR et al. Local gene therapy with CTLA4–immunoglobulin fusion protein in experimental allergic encephalomyelitis. *Eur J Immunol* 1998; **28**: 3904–3916.

20. Croxford JL, Triantaphyllopoulos KA, Neve RM, Feldmann M, Chernajovsky Y, Baker D. Gene therapy for chronic relapsing experimental allergic encephalomyelitis using cells expressing a novel soluble p75 dimeric TNF receptor. *J Immunol* 2000; **164**: 52776–52781.

21. Glorioso JC, Goins WF, Meaney CA, Fink DJ, DeLuca NA. Gene transfer to brain using herpes simplex virus vectors. *Ann Neurol* 1994; **35**: S28–S34.

22. Martino G, Poliani PL, Marconi P, Comi G, Furlan R. Cytokine gene therapy of autoimmune demyelination revisited using herpes simplex virus type-1-derived vectors. *Gene Ther* 2000; **7**: 1087–1093.

23. Marconi P, Krisky D, Oligino T et al. Replication-defective herpes simplex virus vectors for gene transfer in vivo. *Proc Natl Acad Sci USA* 1996; **93**: 11319–11320.

24. DeLuca NA, McCarthy AM, Schaffer PA. Isolation and characterization of deletion mutants of herpes simplex virus type 1 in the gene encoding immediate-early regulatory protein ICP4. *J Virol* 1985; **56**: 558–570.

25. Kuklin NA, Daheshia M, Marconi PC et al. Modulation of mucosal and systemic immunity by enteric administration of non-replicating herpes simplex virus expressing cytokines. *Virology* 1998; **240**: 245–253.

26. Martino G, Furlan R, Galbiati F et al. A gene therapy approach to treat demyelinating diseases using non-replicative herpetic vectors engineered to produce cytokines. *Mult Scler* 1998; **4**: 222–227.

27. Furlan R, Poliani PL, Galbiati F et al. Central nervous system delivery of interleukin-4 by a non-replicative herpes simplex type 1 viral vector ameliorates autoimmune demyelination. *Hum Gene Ther* 1998; **9**: 2605–2617.

28. Furlan R, Poliani PL, Marconi PC et al. Interleukin-4 gene delivery in the central nervous system at the time of disease onset inhibits progression of autoimmune demyelination. *Gen Ther* 2001; **8**: 13–19.

29. Prineas JW, Barnard RO, Kwon EE, Sharer LR, Cho ES. Multiple sclerosis: remyelination of nascent lesions. *Ann Neurol* 1993; **33**: 137–151.

30. Rodriguez M. Central nervous system demyelination and remyelination in multiple sclerosis and viral models of disease. *J Neuroimmunol* 1992; **40**: 255–263.

31. Brück W, Schmied M, Suchanek G et al. Oligodendrocytes in the early course of multiple sclerosis. *Ann Neurol* 1994; **35**: 65–73.

32. Ozawa K, Suchanek G, Breitschopf H et al. Patterns of oligodendroglia pathology in multiple sclerosis. *Brain* 1994; **117**: 1311–1322.

33. Targett MP, Sussman J, Scolding N, O'Leary MT, Compston DA, Blakemore WF. Failure to achieve remyelination of demyelinated rat axons following transplantation of glial cells obtained from the adult human brain. *Neuropathol Appl Neurobiol* 1996; **22**: 199–206.

34. Ludwin SK. Central nervous system demyelination and remyelination in the mouse: an ultrastructural study of cuprizone toxicity. *Lab Invest* 1978; **39**: 597–612.

35. Linington C, Engelhardt B, Kapocs G, Lassmann H. Induction of persistently demyelinated lesions in the rat following the repeated adoptive transfer of encephalitogenic T-cells and demyelinating antibody. *J Neuroimmunol* 1992; **40**: 219–224.

36. Muir DA, Compston DA. Growth factor stimulation triggers apoptotic cell death in mature oligodendrocytes. *J Neurosci Res* 1996; **44**: 1–11.

37. Aebischer P, Schluep M, Déglon N et al. Intrathecal delivery of CNTF using encapsulated genetically modified xenogeneic cells in amyotrophic lateral sclerosis patients. *Nature Med* 1996; **2**: 696–699.

38. Mathisen PM, Yu M, Yin L et al. Th2 T-cells expressing transgene PDGF-A serve as vectors for gene therapy in autoimmune demyelinating disease. *J Autoimmun* 1999; **13**: 31–38.

39. Boccaccio GL, Mor F, Steinman L. Non-coding plasmid DNA induces IFN-gamma in vivo and suppresses autoimmune encephalomyelitis. *Int Immunol* 1999; **11**: 289–296.

40. Tsunoda I, Tolley ND, Theil DJ, Whitton JL, Kobayashi H, Fujinami RS. Exacerbation of viral and autoimmune animal models for multiple sclerosis by bacterial DNA. *Brain Pathol* 1999; **9**: 481–493.

12

DNA vaccination for central nervous system autoimmune diseases

Nathan Karin

Conceptually, gene therapy has been used as an efficient methodology to circumvent genetic deficiency by transfection of cDNA encoding the appropriate functional gene product. It is therefore conceivable that the best candidates for this form of therapy would be genetic diseases associated with a single gene mutation, such as X-linked agammaglobulinemia (XLA) or cystic fibrosis (CF). Paradoxically, it appears that gene therapy needs to confront similar levels of technological challenges when encountering genetic disorders, such as XLA or CF, to those a involved in a successful intervention in multifactorial diseases. Yet, while genetic disorders that involve a mutation in a single gene are rare, multifactorial diseases comprise a major cause of illness and death in the developed countries. This has motivated scientists to explore gene therapy strategies in multifactorial disorders. This chapter discusses the use of a modification of gene therapy named DNA vaccination to provide novel ways of interfering in the regulation of the inflammatory process in T-cell-mediated autoimmune diseases, such as mutiple sclerosis (MS), and thus provide protective immunity against these multifactorial diseases. One approach to applying gene therapy in T-cell-mediated autoimmunity involves in vitro transfection of antigen-specific autoimmune T-cells with a regulatory gene of interest, such as interleukin-4 (IL-4) or IL-10.[1,2] Upon injection of the manipulated T-cells into the circulation, the cells are expected to home to the target autoimmune organ and propagate the response to the specific autoimmune determinate.[1,2] While so doing, they produce and secrete the desired regulatory gene product at this site and restrain the relevant autoimmune disease.[1,2] My group has utilized another modification of gene therapy, by which the immune system could be 're-educated' to restrain its harmful activities.

Experimental autoimmune encephalomyelitis (EAE) is a paralytic autoimmune disease of the central nervous system that serves as an animal model for MS. In both diseases, circulating leukocytes enter the brain blood to interact with their target antigens, resulting in impaired nerve conduction and paralysis. The disease can be induced in various susceptible strains of animals, one of which is the Lewis strain of rats. Upon a single immunization with myelin basic protein (MBP) emulsified in an appropriate adjuvant, these rats develop active EAE.[3] MBP-specific CD4[+] T-cell clones and lines selected from EAE rats are capable of transferring the disease to naive recipients.[3] When being attenuated to become non-encephalitogenic, or if administered at a sub-pathogenic dose, these cells can endow recipients with a high state of resistance to any further attempt to induce the disease.[4–6] The suggested mechanism includes elicitation of a self-specific anti-idiotypic response, which includes CD4[+6] and CD8[+7,8] regulatory T-cells. These studies suggest that some cells of the specific arm of the immune system not only do not participate in the induction of antigen-specific effector function, but also regulate the harmful function of autoimmune effector T-cells. As discussed below, my group has recently defined another mechanism by which immune cells mount an immune response against self-antigens (pro-inflammatory cytokines and chemokines) to restrain the harmful activity of autoimmune T-cells.

The role of cytokines and chemokines in the regulation of T-cell-mediated autoimmunity has been extensively studied. Based on their cytokine profile, CD4[+] T-cells can be divided into: Th1 cells that produce large amounts of interferon gamma (IFN-γ) and tumor necrosis factor alpha (TNF-α), and, to a much lesser extent, IL-4 and IL-10; and Th2 cells that produce IL-4, IL-10, and IL-13, and, to a much lesser extent, IFN-γ and TNF-α.[9–18] More recently defined subsets comprise the Th3 cells that produce significant amounts of transforming growth factor beta (TGF-β) and have been associated with oral tolerance,[19] and the high-IL-10- low-IL-4-producing regulatory T-cells that have been implicated in colitis.[20] Th1 cells selected in response to various autoantigens transfer T-cell-mediated autoimmune diseases, whereas IL-4-secreting Th2 cells, selected in response to these same antigens, either inhibit or exert no profound effect on the inflammatory process.[13,21–33] High levels of IFN-γ and low levels of IL-4 positively select for Th1 cells, whereas low levels of IFN-γ together with high levels of IL-4 mediate Th2 selection.[9–14] In a recent study, Wildbaum and Youssef isolated mRNA encoding rat IFN-γ inducing factor (IGIF, IL-18) from the EAE brain, generated neutralizing antibodies against its gene product, and used them to explore the role of IGIF in T-cell deviation and function.[34] These antibodies significantly reduced the production of IFN-γ by primed T-cells proliferating in response to their target MBP epitope and by Con A-activated T-cells from naive donors. When administered to rats during the development of either active or transferred EAE, these antibodies significantly blocked the development of disease. Splenic T-cells from protected rats were cultured with the encephalitogenic MBP epitope and evaluated for production of IL-4 and IFN-γ. These cells, which proliferated, exhibited a profound increase in IL-4 production, accompanied by a significant decrease in IFN-γ and TNF-α production.[34] This study demonstrates, again, that by simple means one may interfere in a natural mechanism by which self-tolerance is maintained by the peripheral immune system to keep autoreactive lymphocytes under control.[34] As an alternative approach to treat T-cell-mediated autoimmune diseases, one may use antibodies to key adhesion molecules that mediate leukocyte migration to their target organ. Eight years ago, we defined the $\alpha_4 \beta_1$ integrin (VLA-4) as the key adhesion molecule that mediates T-cell and monocyte transmigration to the target autoimmune site in EAE, and demonstrated that VLA-4-specific antibodies can inhibit the development and progression of disease.[35] The underlying mechanism includes blockade of the secondary influx of leukocytes that is required for the development and progression of disease.[36] Once again, this form of therapy is not disease, or organ, specific and is dependent on continuing exposure to these antibodies.

In an attempt to develop a highly specific therapeutic strategy, we have explored the abilities of dominant epitopes of MBP, or even soluble altered analogs of these epitopes, to inhibit an ongoing disease.[37–39] In a recent study, we demonstrated that an engagement of the antigenic determinant to one major histocompatibility complex (MHC) anchor and to one TCR binding site of an MBP determinant could be sufficient for the generation of antigen-specific T-cell tolerances,[37] whereas five–seven simultaneous engagements of an MBP determinant to MHC and TCR are required for mounting an encephalitogenic response in self-reactive T-cells.[37] Perhaps during the evolution of self–non-self recognition, the immune system has evolved to induce self-specific unresponsiveness more readily than self-specific pro-inflammatory responses. The major advantage of using such a non-pathogenic altered antigen analog for therapy resides in its specificity. Yet, as with previous means of therapy discussed above, it requires continuing administration, which is impractical for the treatment of long-lasting chronic diseases.

In an attempt to overcome the above disadvantage, we have recently explored two ways by which the immune system could be 're-educated' to restrain the aggressiveness of autoimmune T-cells EAE is attenuated. The first approach interferes in the polarization of MBP-specific T-cells during the neonatal period of life. The other approach uses naked DNA vaccination to generate self-specific immunity cytokines/chemokines capable of neutralizing the harmful effect of autoimmune T-cells and macrophages. The autoimmune response of T-cells to components of the central nervous system (CNS) begins with recognition of a single or limited number of self-determinants, and then expands into a reaction to several self-determinants on the same molecule, termed intramolecular epitope spreading, or to other molecules within the nervous system, termed intermolecular epitope spreading.[40–43] The first approach explores determinate spread following neonatal exposure to encephalitogenic determinants. The embryonic and neonatal periods have been thought of as a window in ontogeny during which the developing immune system is particularly susceptible to tolerization. Thus, antigenic challenge in neonatal life may result in specific T-cell unresponsiveness in the adult.[44–48] Antigen-specific T-cell deletion was suggested to be a pivotal mechanism by which central tolerance, including tolerance to neonatally administered antigens, is induced and maintained.[49,50] Our observations clearly show that neonatal exposure to MBP epitopes results not only in antigen-specific T-cell deletion, but also in altered deviation of some of the escaping CD4+ antigen-specific T-cells. In adult life, these cells can endow disease resistance that spreads in an intramolecular manner.[51,52] As with soluble peptide therapy,[38] here again the tolerant state is IL-4 dependent.[51,52] Most importantly, our observations indirectly suggest that tolerizing T-cells selected during the neonatal period of life, to maintain central tolerance, become effective when they encounter their target antigen in the periphery during adult life.[51,52]

The second approach which we have recently proposed suggests that some of the autoreactive lymphocytes that escape central selection elicit the production of neutralizing antibodies to pro-inflammatory mediators of the immune system, such as TNF-α and pro-inflammatory chemokines.[53–55] As this response in not sufficient to prevent the development and progression of an autoimmune condition, we have looked for ways in which this response could be amplified in accordance with the development and progression of the autoimmune condition. For this purpose, we have selected a modification of gene therapy named naked DNA vaccination. A major current use of this technology is to increase the cell-mediated antigen-specific immune response against infectious agents such as tuberculosis and HIV, and allergens such as mite proteins.[56–62] The interesting work of Waisman et al paved the way for applying this powerful technology to elicit protective immunity to experimental autoimmune diseases.[63] In their study, Waisman et al inhibited EAE by immunizing mice with cDNA encoding the T-cell receptor V genes.[63] In our studies, we tried to use naked DNA vaccination to break down tolerance to pro-inflammatory mediators of the autoimmune process, thus generating immunological memory against these pro-inflammatory factors.[53,54] Thus each gene of interest was cloned into a mammalian vector with a strong viral promoter (cytomegalovirus (CMV)) and a repeated immunostimulatory sequence (ISS).[60,61] We have demonstrated that upon repeated administrations of each vaccine, tolerance to its gene product was broken and immunological memory was established.[53,54] In these experiments, rats were immunized with MBP/CFA to induce active EAE 2 months after the last administration of each vaccine. At this time, the self-specific antibody titer to each gene product regressed to background levels. Interestingly, immunization with MBP/CFA to induce active EAE, and not with the CFA alone, to elicit a local inflammatory process, elicited the rapid production of self-specific antibodies to the product of each given vaccine.[53,54] Thus, rats that were previously subjected to naked DNA vaccines encoding MIP-1α, MCP-1 or TNF-α were EAE resistant, and at that time exhibited a marked antibody titer against the gene product of each vaccine. Each titer

accelerated in accordance with the progression of disease in control EAE rats and regressed background levels upon recovery. MCP-1-, MIP-1α- and TNF-α-specific antibodies generated in EAE-resistant rats were neutralizing in vitro, and could transfer EAE resistance in adoptive transfer experiments.[53,54] Thus by applying pro-inflammatory cytokine/chemokine-based naked DNA vaccination, one may re-educate the immune system to use self-specific immunity to restrain its own harmful activities.[53,54]

The biological significance of the association between the elevated levels of TNF-α or C-C chemokine mRNA at a privileged autoimmune site (CNS) and the enhancement in anti-self-response against pro-inflammatory cytokines and chemokines is apparent. After all, an ideal immune system would be selected in evolution to centralize its destructive competence against invading microbes rather than against the self-tissues it was designed to protect.[64–66] The underlying mechanism by which the immune system distinguishes a gene product transcribed at a privileged autoimmune site from the same gene product transcribed at a local site of inflammation is, however, still elusive. A partial explanation for these intriguing observations was previously suggested by Cyster et al.[67] This group provided compelling evidence to suggest that peripheral clonal exclusion of self-reactive B-cells occurs in germinal centers of lymph nodes that drain tissues lacking immune surveillance (i.e. immune privileged areas), where competition for follicular niches does not exclude self-reactive cells from the recirculating B-cell repertoire.[67] This may suggest that the expression and production of pro-inflammatory cytokines/chemokines will lead to the exclusion of self-specific B-cells, capable of generating an immune response to these self-gene products, unless they are transcribed and produced at an autoimmune site, such as the CNS.[67] Pro-inflammatory chemokine/cytokine-based DNA vaccination probably amplifies this process of tolerance breakdown.

From the basic science perspective, the above observations may provide a new perspective for understanding the role of T-cell and B-cell selection in induction and maintenance of tolerance to self. In the process of negative selection, self-reactive T-cells die when they encounter self-antigen in the thymus.[49,50] Similarly, self-specific pre-B-cells either die or undergo receptor editing in the bone marrow.[68] It is believed that those cells escaping central tolerance are subjected to various mechanisms acting outside the thymus or the bone marrow to keep them under control. This type of control has been termed peripheral tolerance. T-cell anergy,[69] active suppression,[30,69–71] T-cell deletion[72,73] and generation of anti-idiotypic immunity[74] have been described as key mechanisms that contribute to the maintenance of peripheral tolerance. The current study suggests for the first time that self-specific T- and B-cells, capable of mounting self-specific immunity against pro-inflammatory mediators, escape central tolerance to provide the immune system with a powerful tool with which to keep its dangerous anti-self activity under control and thus maintain tolerance to self in the periphery. Moreover, as microbes and self-components are constructed from similar 'building blocks' and as central selection manifests its own limitations, anti-self immunity cannot be avoided, but rather has to be restrained by peripheral mechanisms. Moreover, it could well be that a substantial increase in the competence of the immune system to effectively limit its T- and B-cell repertoire would result in a constrained ability to effectively confront infectious diseases. The case of natural immunity to TNF-α, evoked during the course of a T-cell-mediated autoimmune disease, demonstrates how the immune system has evolved to benefit from its own limited competence to effectively select against self-reactivity.

From a clinical perspective, the advantage of interfering in the autoimmune process with cytokine and chemokine DNA vaccines is apparent. A major disadvantage in treating chronic diseases with xenogenic neutralizing antibodies lies in their immunogenicity. This has motivated investigators to develop chimeric humanized antibodies (review: Riethmuller et al[75]) and monoclonal antibodies engineered with human Ig heavy and light chain yeast artificial chromosome (YAC).[76] However, following repeated immunization, these engineered antibodies do trigger an apparently allotypic response. The therapeutic strategy suggested by our studies has an advantage over the above methods, since it resulted in the generation of immunity to autologous antigen only during the course of disease at the time when mRNA encoding the pro-inflammatory cytokine is profoundly evated at the site of inflammation. Yet another major disadvantage of applying anti-chemokine/cytokine immunotherapy in T-cell-mediated autoimmunity is that the treatment is not disease specific and may lead to suppression/alteration of other immunological functions. Ultimately, an ideal DNA vaccine would exert a maximal effect on the clinical manifestation of an autoimmune condition with a minimal effect on other immunological functions. We believe that the next breakthrough in the development of

genetic vaccines for T-cell-mediated autoimmunity will depend on defining disease-specific chemokine/cytokine encoding DNA vaccines. This goal is still dependent on future characterization of organ-specific/disease-specific pro-inflammatory factors.

REFERENCES

1. Shaw MX, Lorens JB, Dhawan A et al. Local delivery of interleukin 4 by retrovirus-transduced T lymphocytes ameliorates experimental autoimmune encephalomyelitis. *J Exp Med* 1997; **185**(9): 1711–1714.
2. Mathisen PM, Tuohy VK. Gene therapy in treatment of autoimmune diseases. *Immunol Today* 1998; **19**(3): 193–195.
3. Ben-Nun A, Wekerle H, Cohen IR. The rapid isolation of clonable antigen-specific T lymphocyte lines capable of mediating autoimmune encephalomyelitis. *Eur J Immunol* 1981; **11**(3): 195–199.
4. Ben-Nun A, Wekerle H, Cohen IR. Vaccination against autoimmune encephalomyelitis with T-lymphocyte line cells reactive against myelin basic protein. *Nature* 1981; **292**(5818): 60–61.
5. Beraud E, Lider O, Baharav E, Reshef T, Cohen IR. Vaccination against experimental autoimmune encephalomyelitis using a subencephalitogenic dose of autoimmune effector cells (1). Characteristics of vaccination. *J Autoimmun* 1989; **2**(1): 75–86.
6. Lider O, Beraud E, Reshef T, Friedman A, Cohen IR. Vaccination against experimental autoimmune encephalomyelitis using a subencephalitogenic dose of autoimmune effector T cells. (2). Induction of a protective anti-idiotypic response. *J Autoimmun* 1989; **2**(1): 87–99.
7. Sun D, Ben-Nun A, Wekerle H. Regulatory circuits in autoimmunity: recruitment of counter-regulatory CD8+ T cells by encephalitogenic CD4+ T line cells. *Eur J Immunol* 1984; **18**(12): 1993–1999.
8. Sun D, Qin Y, Chluba J, Epplen JT, Wekerle H. Suppression of experimentally induced autoimmune encephalomyelitis by cytolytic T–T cell interactions. *Nature* 1988; **332**(6167): 843–845.
9. O'Garra A, Murphy K. Role of cytokines in determining T-lymphocyte function. *Curr Opin Immunol* 1994; **6**(3): 458–466.
10. Abbas AK, Murphy KM, Sher A. Functional diversity of helper T lymphocytes. *Nature* 1996; **383**(6603): 787–793.
11. Swain SL, Weinberg AD, English M, Huston G. IL-4 directs the development of Th2-like helper effectors. *J Immunol* 1990; **145**: 3796–3806.
12. Lederer JA, Perez VL, DesRoches L, Kim SM, Abbas AK, Lichtman AH. Cytokine transcriptional events during helper T cell subset differentiation. *J Exp Med* 1996; **184**(2): 397–406.
13. Seder RA, Gazzinelli R, Sher A, Paul WE. IL-12 acts directly on CD4+ T cells to enhance priming for IFN-γ production and diminishes IL-4 inhibition of such priming. *Proc Natl Acad Sci USA* 1993; **90**: 10188–10192.
14. Seder RA, Paul WE, Davis MM, Fazekas de St Groth B. The presence of interleukin-4 during in vitro priming determines the cytokine-producing potential of CD4+ T cells from T cell receptor transgenic mice. *J Exp Med* 1992; **176**: 1091–1098.

15. Fiorentino DF, Zlotnik A, Vieira P et al. IL-10 acts on the antigen presenting cell to inhibit cytokine production by Th1 cells. *J Immunol* 1991; **146**(10): 3444–3451.

16. Mosmann TR, Coffman RL. Th1 and Th2 cells: different patterns of lymphokine secretion lead to different functional properties. *Annu Rev Immunol* 1989; **9**: 145–173.

17. Mosmann T, Moor K. The role of IL-10 in the cross-regulation of Th1 and Th2 responses. *Immunol Today* 1989; **12**(2): A49–A53.

18. Huang H, Hu-Li J, Chen H, Ben-Sasson SZ, Paul WE. IL-4 and IL-13 production in differentiated T helper type 2 cells is not IL-4 dependent. *J Immunol* 1997; **159**(8): 3731–3738.

19. Fukaura H, Kent SC, Pietrusewicz MJ, Khoury SJ, Weiner HL, Hafler DA. Induction of circulating myelin basic protein and proteolipid protein-specific transforming growth factor-beta1-secreting Th3 T cells by oral administration of myelin in multiple sclerosis patients. *J Clin Invest* 1996; **98**(1): 70–77.

20. Groux H, O'Garra A, Bigler M et al. A CD4+ T-cell subset inhibits antigen-specific T-cell responses and prevents colitis. *Nature* 1997; **389**(6652): 737–742.

21. Racke MK, Bonomo A, Scott DE et al. Cytokine-induced immune deviation as a therapy for inflammatory autoimmune disease. *J Exp Med* 1994; **180**(5): 1961–1966.

22. Cash E, Minty A, Ferrara P, Caput D, Fradelizi D, Rott O. Macrophage-inactivating IL-13 suppresses experimental autoimmune encephalomyelitis in rats. *J Immunol* 1994; **153**(9): 4258–4267.

23. Kuchroo VK, Das MP, Brown JA et al. B7-1 and B7-2 costimulatory molecules activate differentially the Th1/Th2 developmental pathways: application to autoimmune disease therapy. *Cell* 1999; **80**(5): 707–718.

24. Leonard JP, Waldburger KE, Goldman SJ. Prevention of experimental autoimmune encephalomyelitis by antibodies against interleukin 12. *J Exp Med* 1995; **181**(1): 381–386.

25. Healey D, Ozegbe P, Arden S, Chandler P, Hutton J, Cooke A. In vivo activity and in vitro specificity of CD4+ Th1 and Th2 cells derived from the spleens of diabetic NOD mice. *J Clin Invest* 1995; **95**(6): 2979–2985.

26. Khoruts A, Miller SD, Jenkins MK. Neuroantigen-specific Th2 cells are inefficient suppressors of experimental autoimmune encephalomyelitis induced by effector Th1 cells. *J Immunol* 1995; **155**(10): 5011–5017.

27. Ando DG, Clayton J, Kono D, Urban JL, Sercarz EE. Encephalitogenic T cells in the B10.PL model of experimental allergic encephalomyelitis (EAE) are of the Th-1 lymphokine subtype. *Cell Immunol* 1989; **124**(1): 132–143.

28. Katz JD, Benoist C, Mathis D. T helper subsets in insulin dependent diabetes. *Science* 1995; **268**: 1185–1188.

29. Liblau RS, Singer SM, McDevitt HO. Th1 and Th2 CD4+ T-cells in the pathogenesis of organ-specific autoimmune diseases. *Immunol Today* 1995; **16**: 34–38.

30. Saoudi A, Kuhn J, Huygen K et al. TH2 activated cells prevent experimental autoimmune uveoretinitis, a TH1-dependent autoimmune disease. *Eur J Immunol* 1993; **23**(12): 3096–3103.

31. Rapoport MJ, Jaramillo A, Zipris D et al. Interleukin-4 reverses T cell proliferative unresponsiveness and prevents the onset of diabetes in nonobese diabetic mice. *J Exp Med* 1993; **178**: 87–99.

32. Rott O, Fleischer B, Cash E. Interleukin-10 prevents experimental allergic encephalomyelitis in rats. *Eur J Immunol* 1994; **24**(6): 1434–1440.

33. Trinchieri G. Interleukin-12 and its role in the generation of Thi cells. *Immunol Today* 1993; **14**: 335–337.

34. Wildbaum G, Youssef S, Grabie N, Karin N. Prevention of experimental autoimmune encephalomyelitis by antibodies to interferon gamma inducing factor. *J Immunol* 1998; **161**(11): 6368–6374.

35. Yednock TA, Cannon C, Fritz LC, Sanchez MF, Steinman L, Karin N. Prevention of experimental autoimmune encephalomyelitis by antibodies against alpha 4 beta 1 integrin. *Nature* 1992; **356**(6364): 63–66.

36. Karin N, Szafer F, Mitchell D, Gold DP, Steinman L. Selective and nonselective stages in homing of T lymphocytes to the central nervous system during experimental allergic encephalomyelitis. *J Immunol* 1993; **150**(9): 4116–4124.

37. Karin N, Binah O, Grabie N et al. Short peptide based tolerogens without antigenic activity reverse autoimmunity. *J Immunol* 1998; **160**(10): 5188–5194.

38. Brocke S, Gijbels K, Allegretta M et al. Treatment of experimental encephalomyelitis with a peptide analogue of myelin basic protein. *Nature* 1996; **379**(6563): 343–346.

39. Karin N, Mitchell JD, Brocke S, Ling N, Steinman L. Reversal of experimental autoimmune encephalomyelitis by a soluble peptide variant of a myelin basic protein epitope: T cell receptor antagonism and reduction of IFN-γ and TNF-α production. *J Exp Med* 1994; **180**: 2227–2237.

40. Offner H, Hashim GA, Celnik B et al. T cell determinants of myelin basic protein include a unique encephalitogenic I-E-restricted epitope for Lewis rats. *J Exp Med* 1989; **170**(2): 355–367.

41. Offner H, Vainiene M, Gold DP et al. Characterization of the immune response to a secondary encephalitogenic epitope of basic protein in Lewis rats. I. T cell receptor peptide regulation of T cell clones expressing cross-reactive V beta genes. *J Immunol* 1992; **148**(6): 1706–1711.

42. Lehmann PV, Forsthuber T, Miller A, Sercarz EE. Spreading of T-cell autoimmunity to cryptic determinants of an autoantigen. *Nature* 1992; **358**(6382): 155–157.

43. Mor F, Cohen lR. Shifts in the epitopes of myelin basic protein recognized by Lewis rat T cells before, during, and after the induction of experimental autoimmune encephalomyelitis. *J Clin Invest* 1993; **92**(5): 2199–2206.

44. Qin YF, Sun DM, Goto M, Meyermann R, Wekerle H. Resistance to experimental autoimmune encephalomyelitis induced by neonatal tolerization to myelin basic protein: clonal elimination vs. regulation of autoaggressive lymphocytes. *Eur J Immunol* 1989; **19**(2): 373–380.

45. Clayton TP, Gammon GM, Ando DG, Kono DH, Hood L, Sercarz EE. Peptide-specific prevention of experimental allergic encephalomyelitis. Neonatal tolerance induced to the dominant T cell determinant of myelin basic protein. *J Exp Med* 1989; **169**(5): 1681–1691.

46. Vandenbark AA, Vainiene M, Celnik B, Hashim GA, Buenafe A, Offner H. Definition of encephalitogenic and immunodominant epitopes of guinea pig myelin basic protein (Gp-BP) in Lewis rats tolerized neonatally with Gp-BP or Gp-BP peptides. *J Immunol* 1994; **153**(2): 852–861.

47. Gammon GM, Oki A, Shastri N, Sercarz EE. Induction of tolerance to one determinant on a synthetic peptide does not affect the response to a second linked determinant. Implications for the mechanism of neonatal tolerance induction. *J Exp Med* 1986; **164**(2): 667–672.

48. Gammon G, Don K, Shastri N, Oki A, Wilbur S, Sercarz EE. Neonatal T-cell tolerance to minimal immunogenic peptides is caused by clonal inactivation. *Nature* 1986; **309**: 413–415.

49. Ramsdell F, Fowlkes BJ. Clonal deletion versus clonal anergy: the role of the thymus in inducing self tolerance. *Science* 1990; **248**(4961): 1342–1348.

50. Kappler J, Roehm N, Marrack P. T cell tolerance by clonal elimination in the thymus. *Cell* 1987; **49**: 273–280.

51. Grabie N, Karin N. Expansion of neonatal tolerance to self in adult life: II. Tolerance preferentially spreads in an intramolecular manner. *Int Immunol* 1999; **11**(6): 907–913.

52. Grabie N, Wohl I, Youssef S, Wildbaum G, Karin N. Expansion of neonatal tolerance to self in adult life: I. The role of a bacterial adjuvant in tolerance spread. *Int Immunol* 1999; **11**(6): 899–906.

53. Wildbaum G, Karin N. Augmentation of natural immunity to a pro-inflammatory cytokine (TNF-α) by targeted DNA vaccine confers long lasting resistance to experimental autoimmune encephalomyelitis. *Gene Therapy* 1999; **6**: 1128–1138.

54. Youssef S, Wildbaum G, Maor G et al. Long lasting protective immunity to experimental autoimmune encephalomyelitis following vaccination with naked DNA encoding C-C chemokines. *J Immunol* 1998; **161**(8): 3870–3879.

55. Youssef S, Wildbaum G, Karin N. Prevention of experimental autoimmune encephalomyelitis by MIP-1alpha and MCP-1 naked DNA vaccines. *J Autoimmun* 1999; **13**(1): 21–29.

56. Boyer JD, Ugen KE, Wang B et al. Protection of chimpanzees from high-dose heterologous HIV-1 challenge by DNA vaccination. *Nature Med* 1997; **3**(5): 526–532.

57. Kim JJ, Ayyavoo V, Bagarazzi MT et al. In vivo engineering of a cellular immune response by co-administration of IL-12 expression vector with a DNA immunogen. *J Immunol* 1997; **158**(2): 816–826.

58. Kim JJ, Bagarazzi ML, Trivedi N et al. Engineering of in vivo immune responses to DNA immunization via codelivery of costimulatory molecule genes. *Nature Biotechnol* 1997; **15**(7): 641–646.

59. Raz E, Watanabe A, Baird SM et al. Systemic immunological effects of cytokine genes injected into skeletal muscle. *Proc Natl Acad Sci USA* 1999; **90**(10): 4523–4527.

60. Raz E, Tighe H, Sato Y et al. Preferential induction of a Th1 immune response and inhibition of specific IgE antibody formation by plasmid DNA immunization. *Proc Natl Acad Sci USA* 1996; **93**(10): 5141–5145.

61. Sato Y, Roman M, Tighe H et al. Immunostimulatory DNA sequences necessary for effective intradermal gene immunization. *Science* 1996; **273**: 352–357.

62. Tascon RE, Colston MJ, Ragno S, Stavropoulos E, Gregory D, Lowrie DB. Vaccination against tuberculosis by DNA injection. *Nature Med* 1996; **2**(8): 888–892.

63. Waisman A, Ruiz PJ, Hirschberg DL et al. Suppressive vaccination with DNA encoding a variable region gene of the T-cell receptor prevents autoimmune encephalomyelitis and activates Th2 immunity. *Nature Med* 1996; **2**(8): 899–905.

64. Steinman L. Escape from 'horror autotoxicus': pathogenesis and treatment of autoimmune disease. *Cell* 1995: **80**(1): 7–10.

65. Matzinger P. Tolerance, danger, and the extended family. *Annu Rev Immunol* 1994; **12**: 991–1045.

66. Janeway CA, Jr. The immune system evolved to discriminate infectious nonself from noninfectious self. *Immunol Today* 1992; **13**(1): 11–16.

67. Cyster JG, Hartley SB, Goodnow CC. Competition for follicular niches excludes self-reactive cells from the recirculating B-cell repertoire. *Nature* 1994; **371**(6496): 389–395.

68. Melamed D, Benschop RJ, Cambier JC, Nemazee D. Developmental regulation of B lymphocyte immune tolerance compartmentalizes clonal selection from receptor selection. *Cell* 1998; **92**(2): 173–182.

69. Friedman A, Weiner HL. Induction of anergy or active suppression following oral tolerance is determined by antigen dosage. *Proc Natl Acad Sci USA* 1994; **91**(14): 6688–6692.

70. Chen Y, Kuchroo VK, Inobe J, Hafler D, Weiner HL. Regulatory T-cell clones induced by oral tolerance: suppression of autoimmune encephalomyelitis. *Science* 1994; **265**: 1237–1240.

71. Khoury SJ, Hancock WW, Weiner HL. Oral tolerance to myelin basic protein and natural recovery from experimental autoimmune encephalomyelitis are associated with downregulation of inflammatory cytokines and differential upregulation of transforming growth factor beta, interleukin 4, and prostaglandin E expression in the brain. *J Exp Med* 1992; **176**(5): 1355–1364.

72. Critchfield JM, Racke MK, Zuniga PJ et al. T cell deletion in high antigen dose therapy of autoimmune encephalomyelitis. *Science* 1994; **263**(5150): 1139–1143.

73. Critchfield JM, Lenardo MJ. Antigen-induced programmed T cell death as a new approach to immune therapy. *Clin Immunol Immunopathol* 1995; **75**(1): 13–19.

74. Lider O, Reshef T, Beraud E, Ben-Nun A, Cohen IR. Anti-idiotypic network induced by T cell vaccination against experimental autoimmune encephalomyelitis. *Science* 1988; **239**: 181–183.

75. Riethmuller G, Rieber EP, Kiefersauer S et al. From antilymphocyte serum to therapeutic monoclonal antibodies: first experiences with a chimeric CD4 antibody in the treatment of autoimmune disease. *Immunol Rev* 1992; **129**: 81–104.

76. Green LL, Hardy MC, Maynard-Currie CE et al. Antigen-specific human monoclonal antibodies from mice engineered with human Ig heavy and light chain YACs. *Nature Genet* 1994; **7**(1): 13–21.

13

Stem cell transplantation for neurological diseases: new hope for disorders of myelin?

Tamir Ben-Hur

Recent advances in stem cell biology have ignited enthusiastic expectations of healing central nervous system (CNS) diseases by transplantation of regenerating cells and genes. In this chapter I shall review briefly the potential application of stem cell transplantation in neurological patients, with special reference to demyelinating disorders, and mention some problematic issues that still face this therapeutic approach.

EXISTENCE OF NEURAL PRECURSOR CELLS IN THE ADULT MAMMALIAN BRAIN

Stem cells are defined as precursor cells that have the potential for continuous self-renewal and are pluripotent in their ability to generate progeny cells of different lineages.[1] Neural stem cells that proliferate in the ventricular zone and later in the subventricular zone of the developing brain give rise to the three neural lineages of the CNS, i.e. neurons, astrocytes and oligodendrocytes. The identification of neural stem cells as well as progenitor cells of specific lineages in the adult CNS[2,3] has changed considerably the past view of the adult brain as an organ without potential for cell renewal. Neural stem cells that were isolated from the adult rodent CNS showed similar characteristics to their embryonic counterparts in their response to mitogenic factors and their potential to generate the three neural lineages.[4] Precursor cells have been identified in several specific regions of the adult rodent CNS, where they continue to generate neural progeny. New neurons are continuously generated in the anterior subventricular zone, from which they migrate via the rostral migratory stream to the olfactory epithelium.[5] Also, precursor cells in the dentate gyrus generate hippocampal granular neurons throughout life.[6] One specific population of cells that

has been recently suggested to consist of neural stem cells is the ventricular and spinal ependymal cell layer, which may represent the residua of the embryonic ventricular zone.[7] Similar precursors may exist in the ventricular wall of the adult human brain[8] and there may be ongoing neuronogenesis in the adult human hippocampus as well.[9] Precursor cells of glial lineages exist in the adult brain too. Oligodendrocyte progenitor cells have been isolated from various adult rodent CNS regions.[10,11] Similar adult human oligodendrocyte progenitors were grown in vitro[12] and identified in the adult human brain[13] and spinal cord[14] in vivo.

PRECURSOR CELLS IN THE ADULT CNS ARE RESPONSIBLE FOR REGENERATION OF OLIGODENDROCYTES AND MYELIN

Several studies have investigated the nature of the cells that remyelinate the adult CNS after induction of lesions in the myelin sheaths. Although oligodendrocytes may survive within such lesions, they are unable to rebuild myelin sheaths.[15] The lack of spontaneous remyelination in experimentally demyelinated lesions that were X-irradiated to kill proliferating cells suggests that cell division is an absolute prerequisite for myelin regeneration.[15] While mature astrocytes retain the potential to react to injury and divide, there is no convincing evidence that fully differentiated oligodendrocytes are able to revert into a proliferating state. Therefore, it is thought that remyelination depends mainly on proliferating oligodendrocyte progenitors that react to injury.[16] Oligodendrocyte progenitors, identified by expression of NG2 on their cell surface, are probably the major cycling cell population that reacts to demyelination.[17–19] The adult subventricular zone (SVZ) contains neural precursor cells that express the embryonic, polysialylated form of the neural cell adhesion molecule (PSA-NCAM). Such SVZ PSA-NCAM+ cells also react to demyelination by proliferating and differentiating, generating astrocytes and remyelinating oligodendrocytes.[20] Stem cells of the spinal ependymal layer react to traumatic injury by increased proliferation and migration into the lesion and participate in formation of the glial scar.[7] It is not known whether these cells participate in myelin regeneration.

WHY DOES MYELIN REGENERATION FAIL IN MULTIPLE SCLEROSIS?

In different experimental models of focal demyelination, it has been shown that the adult rodent CNS has endogenous potential for regenerating oligodendrocytes and myelin. Attempts to regenerate myelin can also be recognized pathologically in brains of multiple sclerosis patients by the existence of shadow plaques, which are partially remyelinated lesions.[21–23] However, as disease advances, there is subsequent failure of remyelination. Data from experimental models of demyelination and from human brain tissue suggest that several factors may play a role in limiting myelin regeneration in the adult brain and its subsequent failure. In experimental focal demyelination it has been shown that only a subpopulation of local progenitor cells react to injury and generate new oligodendrocytes and myelin.[17] Although progenitor cells were demonstrable in acute and chronic multiple sclerosis (MS) lesions, they did not exhibit reactive increases in cell number as compared to normal white matter.[13,24,25] This suggests that the response of the progenitor cell population to the demyelinating process is deficient in the human brain as well. Analysis of brain tissue from MS patients suggested that there are several different pathological patterns of demyelination. In some patients, there was progressive loss of oligodendrocytes and myelin without reactive remyelination, whereas in others, who exhibited strong T-cell and macrophage activity, there was robust remyelination.[26]

Cell migration seems to be another limiting factor in myelin regeneration. It has been shown that only progenitor cells that reside at the margins of experimental lesions migrate into the lesion core and remyelinate it, whereas long-distance migration of progenitor cells does not occur in the brain parenchyma.[16,27] The limited recruitment of oligodendrocyte progenitor cells in the adult CNS may be related to their apparent dormant state. Adult oligodendrocyte progenitor cells have a consider-

ably slower cell cycle than progenitor cells of the developing brain, and they require prolonged exposure to multiple growth factors before they convert into rapidly proliferating cells.[28] It may be hypothesized that mobilization of the adult progenitor cells is limited by insufficient supply of environmental signals in the brain. It has also been suggested that repeated demyelinating episodes in chronic and relapsing multiple sclerosis cause a depletion in the endogenous pool of progenitor cells. Although progenitor cells decrease in number after experimental focal demyelination,[17] this was not observed in pathological specimens of chronic MS lesions.[13,24,25]

Bidirectional trophic interactions between oligodendrocytes and axons are necessary for their long-term survival. In fact, the chronic and supposedly irreversible neurological disability in MS patients is thought to correlate best with the degree of axonal loss in the CNS.[29,30] Moreover, there is recent evidence that axonal transection occurs already in acute multiple sclerosis lesions.[31] Therefore, achieving remyelination prior to development of axonal damage is crucial in any therapeutic strategy. It has been suggested that CNS regeneration, and specifically remyelination, are closely linked to the acute inflammatory phase of the disease, whereas in the chronic stage regeneration does not occur.[32]

In conclusion, both environmental factors and basic properties of endogenous adult progenitor cells limit the degree of spontaneous remyelination. The apparent linkage between the acute inflammatory phase and myelin regeneration, and the necessity to remyelinate before axonal damage occurs, may define a narrow time window when remyelination is feasible. While this time window may be too narrow for adequate endogenous progenitor cell mobilization, it also determines the window of opportunity for therapeutic cell transplantation.

RATIONALE FOR CELL TRANSPLANTATION INTO THE CNS TO REPAIR MYELIN

Cell transplantation into the CNS has been suggested for genetic dysmyelinating disorders as well as for acquired demyelinating diseases. In some leukodystrophies, endogenous oligodendrocyte lineage cells are unable to cover axons with stable myelin. Transplantation of myelin-forming cells rather than replacing the missing gene in such patients is a mode of delivering the entire 'cell factory' that manufactures myelin. This approach may be advantageous over other modes of gene therapy, where targeting the gene to specific cells and tissues, and controlling its degree of expression, may be problematic or even detrimental.[33–36] Various cell populations that were transplanted into embryonic and newborn brains of animals with genetic defects in myelin produced extensive, normal-appearing and compact myelin. Glial cell transplants myelinated the spinal cords of shaking (*sh*) pups, the canine X-linked model of human Pelizaeus–Merzbacher disease, in which there is a mutation in the proteolipid protein gene.[37] Similarly, cell transplants myelinated the CNS in other genetic models of dysmyelination, including the myelin-deficient (*md*) rat[38] and shiverer (*shi*) mouse.[39] In acquired demyelinating diseases, such as MS, growth factor therapy to enhance the endogenous brain's capacity for repair may serve as an alternative to transplantation strategies. In fact, both therapeutic approaches have shown promising results in experimental animals. Transplanted myelin-forming cells remyelinated focal lesions in the optic nerve and spinal cord and restored normal conduction properties, indicating fully functional regenerated myelin.[40,41] Insulin-like growth factor-1 (IGF-1) and glial growth factor-2 (GGF2) are neurotrophic factors that promote survival and proliferation in the oligodendrocyte lineage. Treatment with these factors was beneficial clinically and pathologically in animals with experimental autoimmune encephalomyelitis (EAE).[42–44]

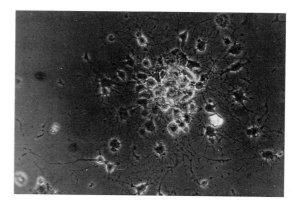

Figure 13.1 Differentiation of glial cells from a sphere. Newborn rat striatal stem cells were expanded as floating spheres in culture conditions that promote the adoption of a glial fate. After the spheres were attached to an adherent surface, many cells migrated out and differentiated into typical multipolar oligodendrocytes and process-bearing astrocytes. Such spheres can generate remyelinating cells in vivo after transplantation into a demyelinated lesion.

PROBLEMATIC ISSUES IN CELL TRANSPLANTATION FOR DEMYELINATING DISEASES

Several issues need to be considered in designing therapeutic cell transplantation for MS.

Which cell to use?

Various cell populations were shown to myelinate efficiently following their transplantation into experimental animals. In the oligodendrocyte lineage, progenitor cells had significantly better myelinating properties than mature cells.[45] Early glial precursor cells, which have similar growth properties to stem cells but are committed to a glial fate,[46] remyelinated 95–100% of the axons in the dorsal columns of rats,[47] as compared to only 70% remyelinated axons expected from oligodendrocyte progenitors. Multipotential neural stem cells may have good myelinating properties as well. Expansion of cells in the form of spheres may be a preferable method to obtain large volumes of cells that are needed for transplantation. This has been achieved

not only with stem cells (termed neurospheres) but also with glial precursors ('oligospheres', Fig. 13.1).[46,48,49] Also, it has recently been shown that embryonic stem cells, which are the totipotent stem cells that generate the entire repertoire of cells in the body, can be expanded in vitro and then generate myelin-forming cells upon transplantation into embryonic brains of rats with a genetic defect in myelin.[50] Moreover, recent discoveries have demonstrated a plasticity of stem cells to the degree of promiscuity, where stem cells of one tissue generated cells of other tissues.[51] These observations have expanded the potential options for using stem cells for transplantation. In particular, it may not be mandatory to introduce glial-committed cells for remyelination in vivo, as the developing and acutely demyelinated CNS may instruct other cells to differentiate into the required lineage. However, this may not be true in CNS tissue afflicted with a chronic degenerative disease. For example, in animal models of Parkinson's disease, there was limited survival and differentiation of transplanted stem cells and these became mostly astrocytes rather than tyrosine hydroxylase[+] neurons.[52–54]

Remyelination of the CNS is not dependent on oligodendrocytes alone and may be achieved by other myelin-forming cells as well. Table 1 lists some advantages and disadvantages of the major cell types that may be used in transplantation for myelination. Schwann cells, the peripheral myelin-forming cells,

Table 13.1 Potential use of different cell populations for transplantation		
Cell type	Advantages	Disadvantages
Embryonic stem cells	Totipotent, self-renewing	Teratoma formation, non-migrating, uncommitted
Neural stem cells	Multipotential, self-renewing	Non-migrating, uncommitted
Glial-committed precursor cells	Proven remyelinating capacity, migratory	Restricted to glia
Oligodendrocyte progenitors	Proven remyelinating capacity, migratory	Probably less efficient than earlier glial precursors, limited source
Schwann cells	Proven remyelinating capacity, migratory, autograft possible	Restricted to myelin-forming cells
Olfactory nerve-ensheathing cells	Proven remyelinating capacity, migratory, autograft possible	Restricted to myelin-forming cells

have excellent myelinating properties in the CNS. They produce thick and compact myelin after transplantation into the CNS,[55,56] and can restore normal conduction velocity in the dorsal columns of the spinal cord, indicating functional recovery.[57] Schwann cells can be isolated from a nerve biopsy of patients affected with a myelin disorder of the CNS. The ability to expand Schwann cells in vitro and then introduce them back into the CNS as an autograft is an important advantage in their potential use. Olfactory nerve-ensheathing cells are another cell population with a capacity to grow in vitro and to remyelinate and improve conduction properties after transplantation into the adult rat spinal cord.[58] These cells are unique in that they continue to develop throughout life in the olfactory epithelium, from which they migrate to the olfactory bulb and myelinate central olfactory neurons.[59,60] These cells seem also to promote axonal growth.[61,62] Thus, the relative availability of these cells and their apparent myelinating and axonal growth-promoting properties make them another candidate for therapeutic transplantation.

When to transplant?

The timing of transplantation is probably another important consideration. Human multipotential neural stem cells that were transplantated into embryonic rat brain generated mostly neurons,[63] whereas after transplantation into newborn brains (in which neuronogenesis was complete and gliogenesis was in action) the stem cells generated mostly glia.[64] This suggests that the developing brain directs the fate of transplanted uncommitted cells according to the

normal pattern of development at that stage. In the adult CNS, transplanted oligodendrocyte progenitors integrate well in acutely lesioned tissue, but they do not survive in normal tissue.[65] This may be because normal brain tissue expresses the minimal amount of trophic factors, enough to maintain the survival of resident cells but insufficient for supporting the survival of transplanted cells. When progenitor cells were transplanted into the spinal cord of animals with experimental autoimmune encephalomyelitis and an ongoing inflammatory process, they survived much better in vivo.[66] As MS is a chronic and relapsing disease, it would be necessary to maintain long-term survival of transplanted cells both through phases of inflammation and remissions. Moreover, as the time window for remyelination is considered to be narrow, it may be best to introduce remyelinating cells as early as possible, in a form that will keep their survival independent of tissue support so that they are ready for immediate mobilization upon tissue demand.

Where to transplant in multifocal and disseminated diseases?

Cell migration is a major limiting factor in remyelination. However, it is impossible to transplant cells into all foci of disease in MS. Recent studies have shown that intraventricular transplantation of oligodendrocyte progenitors or stem cells leads to widespread myelination in the genetic dysmyelinating models of the shiverer mouse[39] and myelin-deficient rat.[67] As mentioned above, the adult brain may prove much more problematic in supporting transplanted cell migration and integration. We have recently studied the response of glial precursor cell spheres to inflammation in EAE, the animal model of MS. We found that, following intraventricular transplantation of spheres, cells migrated into inflamed periventricular white matter tracts, but not into gray matter. There was a general correlation between the severity of the inflammatory response and the degree of transplanted cell migration into the brain. As most white matter tracts that are involved in MS are in close proximity to ventricular and spinal subarachnoid spaces, intraventricular and intrathecal transplantation may serve as an efficient route of delivering remyelinating cells.

EXPERIENCE WITH HUMAN STEM CELLS

Several lines of human neural stem cells have been established. These cells, like their rodent counterparts, proved to proliferate in vitro for a long time, without losing their multipotentiality. The possibility of expanding and freezing these non-transformed neural stem cell lines enabled their banking, thus establishing a source of potentially unlimited amount of transplantable cells.[68,69] In addition, several lines of human embryonic stem cells were developed,[70,71] from which neurons could be obtained.[71] One potential hazard in stem cell transplantation is the risk of tumor formation. To date, no laboratory has reported on tumors arising from transplanted neural stem cells. However, embryonic stem cells are defined, in part, by their ability to form teratomas after transplantation. These teratomas contain cells of the three embryonic layers, i.e. ectoderm, mesoderm and endoderm. Multiple in vitro passages of the embryonic stem cells and their exposure to various growth factors in order to generate neural precursors may eliminate this problem.[50]

Most studies in which xenotransplantation of human cells into rodents were performed reported that graft rejection did not pose a significant problem, raising hopes that transplanted stem cells will not be rejected as allografts by the patient's immune system. If graft rejection does prove to be a major obstacle, then in the future nuclear transfer from somatic cells to oocyte or stem cells may be attempted in order to generate the patient's own stem cell line for syngeneic transplantation.

ETHICAL CONSIDERATIONS

As the potential use of embryonic cells moves closer to clinical practice, there is increasing public dispute on the legitimacy of abortions and whether the utilization of material obtained from aborted embryos for medical purposes is ethical. Promising experience has been gained in the last decade with transplantation of fetal mesencephalic tissue into patients suffering from advanced Parkinson's disease.[72,73] The large amount of fetal tissue that is required for this technique poses a major obstacle to its widespread use. In addition to the basic ethical discussion on the use of abortion material for medical purposes, concerns were raised that the practice of embryonic tissue transplantation will increase the pressure to perform abortions and create a black market in which pregnancy and aborted tissues will be sold to the highest bidder. The development of stem cell lines that are expanded in vitro to create an almost unlimited source of cells for transplantation may solve some of the ethical issues at stake. As in other cases where medical and scientific advances have found society without the means to deal with their ethical, legal and social consequences, it is important to discuss these issues in public, with the active participation of the medical and scientific community.

REFERENCES

1. McKay R. Stem cells in the central nervous system. *Science* 1997; **276**: 66–71.
2. Reynolds BA, Weiss S. Generation of neurons and astrocytes from isolated cells of the adult mammalian central nervous system. *Science* 1992; **255**: 1707–1710.
3. Gritti A, Parati EA, Cova L et al. Multipotential stem cells from the adult mouse brain proliferate and self-renew in response to basic fibroblast growth factor. *J Neurosci* 1996; **16**: 1091–1100.
4. Johe KK, Hazel TG, Muller T, Dugich-Djordjevic MM, McKay RD. Single factors direct the differentiation of stem cells from the fetal and adult central nervous system. *Genes Dev* 1996; **10**: 3129–3140.
5. Lois C, Garcia-Verdugo JM, Alvarez-Buylla A. Chain migration of neuronal precursors. *Science* 1996; **271**: 978–981.
6. Kuhn HG, Dickinson-Anson H, Gage FH. Neurogenesis in the dentate gyrus of the adult rat: age-related decrease of neuronal progenitor proliferation. *J Neurosci* 1996; **16**: 2027–2033.
7. Johansson CB, Momma S, Clarke DL, Risling M, Lendahl U, Frisen J. Identification of a neural stem cell in the adult mammalian central nervous system. *Cell* 1999; **96**: 25–34.
8. Johansson CB, Svensson M, Wallstedt L, Janson AM, Frisen J. Neural stem cells in the adult human brain. *Exp Cell Res* 1999; **253**: 733–736.
9. Eriksson PS, Perfilieva E, Bjork-Eriksson T et al. Neurogenesis in the adult human hippocampus. *Nat Med* 1998; **4**: 1313–1317.
10. Wolswijk G, Noble M. Identification of an adult-specific glial progenitor cell. *Development* 1989; **105**: 387–400.
11. Reynolds R, Hardy R. Oligodendroglial progenitors labeled with the O4 antibody persist in the adult rat cerebral cortex in vivo. *J Neurosci Res* 1997; **47**: 455–470.

12. Scolding NJ, Rayner PJ, Sussman J, Shaw C, Compston DA. A proliferative adult human oligodendrocyte progenitor. *Neuroreport* 1995; **6**: 441–445.

13. Scolding N, Franklin R, Stevens S, Heldin CH, Compston A, Newcombe J. Oligodendrocyte progenitors are present in the normal adult human CNS and in the lesions of multiple sclerosis. *Brain* 1998; **121**: 2221–2228.

14. Horner PJ, Power AE, Kempermann G et al. Proliferation and differentiation of progenitor cells throughout the intact adult rat spinal cord. *J Neurosci* 2000; **20**: 2218–2228.

15. Keirstead HS, Blakemore WF. Identification of post-mitotic oligodendrocytes incapable of remyelination within the demyelinated adult spinal cord. *J Neuropathol Exp Neurol* 1997; **56**: 1191–1201.

16. Gensert JM, Goldman JE. Endogenous progenitors remyelinate demyelinated axons in the adult CNS. *Neuron* 1997; **19**: 197–203.

17. Keirstead HS, Levine JM, Blakemore WF. Response of the oligodendrocyte progenitor cell population (defined by NG2 labelling) to demyelination of the adult spinal cord. *Glia* 1998; **22**: 161–170.

18. Levine JM, Reynolds R. Activation and proliferation of endogenous oligodendrocyte precursor cells during ethidium bromide-induced demyelination. *Exp Neurol* 1999; **160**: 333–347.

19. Di Bello IC, Dawson MR, Levine JM, Reynolds R. Generation of oligodendroglial progenitors in acute inflammatory demyelinating lesions of the rat brain stem is associated with demyelination rather than inflammation. *J Neurocytol* 1999; **28**: 365–381.

20. Nait-Oumesmar B, Decker L, Lachapelle F, Avellana-Adalid V, Bachelin C, Van Evercooren AB. Progenitor cells of the adult mouse subventricular zone proliferate, migrate and differentiate into oligodendrocytes after demyelination. *Eur J Neurosci* 1999; **11**: 4357–4366.

21. Prineas JW, Barnard RO, Kwon EE, Sharer LR, Cho ES. Multiple sclerosis: remyelination of nascent lesions. *Ann Neurol* 1993; **33**: 137–151.

22. Raine CS, Wu E. Multiple sclerosis: remyelination in acute lesions. *J Neuropathol Exp Neurol* 1993; **52**: 199–204.

23. Compston A. Remyelination in multiple sclerosis: a challenge for therapy. The 1996 European Charcot Foundation Lecture. *Mult Scler* 1997; **3**: 51–70.

24. Wolswijk G. Chronic stage multiple sclerosis lesions contain a relatively quiescent population of oligodendrocyte precursor cells. *J Neurosci* 1998; **18**: 601–609.

25. Chang A, Nishiyama A, Peterson J, Prineas J, Trapp BD. NG2–positive oligodendrocyte progenitor cells in adult human brain and multiple sclerosis lesions. *J Neurosci* 2000; **20**: 6404–6412.

26. Lucchinetti C, Bruck W, Parisi J, Scheithauer B, Rodriguez M, Lassmann H. A quantitative analysis of oligodendrocytes in multiple sclerosis lesions. A study of 113 cases. *Brain* 1999; **122**: 2279–2295.

27. Franklin RJ, Gilson JM, Blakemore WF. Local recruitment of remyelinating cells in the repair of demyelination in the central nervous system. *J Neurosci Res* 1997; **50**: 337–344.

28. Wolswijk G, Noble M. Cooperation between PDGF and FGF converts slowly dividing O-2A adult progenitor cells to rapidly dividing cells with characteristics of O-2A perinatal progenitor cells. *J Cell Biol* 1992; **118**: 889–900.

29. De Stefano N, Matthews PM, Fu L et al. Axonal damage correlates with disability in patients with relapsing-remitting multiple sclerosis. Results of a longitudinal magnetic resonance spectroscopy study. *Brain* 1998; **121**: 1469–1477.

30. Trapp BD, Ransohoff R, Rudick R. Axonal pathology in multiple sclerosis: relationship to neurologic disability. *Curr Opin Neurol* 1999; **12**: 295–302.

31. Trapp BD, Peterson J, Ransohoff RM, Rudick R, Mork S, Bo L. Axonal transection in the lesions of multiple sclerosis. *N Engl J Med* 1998; **338**: 278–285.

32. Sharief MK. Cytokines in multiple sclerosis: pro-inflammation or pro-remyelination? *Mult Scler* 1998; **4**: 169–173.

33. Scherer SS, Chance PF. Myelin genes: getting the dosage right. *Nat Genet* 1995; **11**: 226–228.

34. Winter CG, Saotome Y, Saotome I, Hirsh D. CNTF overproduction hastens onset of symptoms in motor neuron degeneration (mnd) mice. *J Neurobiol* 1996; **31**: 370–378.

35. Rubio F, Kokaia Z, Arco A et al. BDNF gene transfer to the mammalian brain using CNS-derived neural precursors. *Gene Ther* 1999; **6**: 1851–1866.

36. Inoue K, Osaka H, Imaizumi K et al. Proteolipid protein gene duplications causing Pelizaeus–Merzbacher disease: molecular mechanism and phenotypic manifestations. *Ann Neurol* 1999; **45**: 624–632.

37. Archer DR, Cuddon PA, Lipsitz D, Duncan LD. Myelination of the canine central nervous system by glial cell transplantation: a model for repair of human myelin disease. *Nat Med* 1997; **3**: 54–59.

38. Hammang JP, Archer DR, Duncan ID. Myelination following transplantation of EGF-responsive neural stem cells into a myelin-deficient environment. *Exp Neurol* 1997; **147**: 84–95.

39. Yandava BD, Billinghurst LL, Snyder EY. 'Global' cell replacement is feasible via neural stem cell transplantation: evidence from the dysmyelinated shiverer mouse brain. *Proc Natl Acad Sci USA* 1999; **96**: 7029–7034.

40. Groves AK, Barnett SC, Franklin RJ et al. Repair of demyelinated lesions by transplantation of purified O-2A progenitor cells. *Nature* 1993; **362**: 453–455.

41. Kocsis JD. Restoration of function by glial cell transplantation into demyelinated spinal cord. *J Neurotrauma* 1999; **16**: 695–703.

42. Yao DL, Liu X, Hudson LD, Webster HD. Insulin-like growth factor I treatment reduces demyelination and up-regulates gene expression of myelin-related proteins in experimental autoimmune encephalomyelitis. *Proc Natl Acad Sci USA* 1995; **92**: 6190–6194.

43. Li W, Quigley L, Yao DL et al. Chronic relapsing experimental autoimmune encephalomyelitis: effects of insulin-like growth factor-I treatment on clinical deficits, lesion severity, glial responses, and blood brain barrier defects. *J Neuropathol Exp Neurol* 1998; **57**: 426–438.

44. Cannella B, Hoban CJ, Gao YL et al. The neuregulin, glial growth factor 2, diminishes autoimmune demyelination and enhances remyelination in a chronic relapsing model for multiple sclerosis. *Proc Natl Acad Sci USA* 1998; **95**: 10100–10105.

45. Warrington AE, Barbarese E, Pfeiffer SE. Differential myelinogenic capacity of specific developmental stages of the oligodendrocyte lineage upon transplantation into hypomyelinating hosts. *J Neurosci Res* 1993; **34**: 1–13.

46. Ben-Hur T, Rogister B, Murray K, Rougon G, Dubois-Dalcq M. Growth and fate of PSA-NCAM+ precursors of the postnatal brain. *J Neurosci* 1998; **18**: 5777–5788.

47. Keirstead HS, Ben-Hur T, Rogister B, O'Leary MT, Dubois-Dalcq M, Blakemore WF. Polysialylated neural cell adhesion molecule-positive CNS precursors generate both oligodendrocytes and Schwann cells to remyelinate the CNS after transplantation. *J Neurosci* 1999; **19**: 7529–7536.

48. Vitry S, Avellana-Adalid V, Hardy R, Lachapelle F, Baron-Van Evercooren A. Mouse oligospheres: from pre-progenitors to functional oligodendrocytes. *J Neurosci Res* 1999; **58**: 735–751.

49. Zhang SC, Lipsitz D, Duncan ID. Self-renewing canine oligodendroglial progenitor expanded as oligospheres. *J Neurosci Res* 1998; **54**: 181–190.

50. Brustle O, Jones KN, Learish RD et al. Embryonic stem cell-derived glial precursors: a source of myelinating transplants. *Science* 1999; **285**: 754–756.

51. Bjornson CR, Rietze RL, Reynolds BA, Magli MC, Vescovi AL. Turning brain into blood: a hematopoietic fate adopted by adult neural stem cells in vivo. *Science* 1999; **283**: 534–537.

52. Svendsen CN, Clarke DJ, Rosser AE, Dunnett SB. Survival and differentiation of rat and human epidermal growth factor-responsive precursor cells following grafting into the lesioned adult central nervous system. *Exp Neurol* 1996; **137**: 376–388.

53. Svendsen CN, Caldwell MA, Shen J et al. Long-term survival of human central nervous system progenitor cells transplanted into a rat model of Parkinson's disease. *Exp Neurol* 1997; **148**: 135–146.

54. Herrera DG, Garcia-Verdugo JM, Alvarez-Buylla A. Adult-derived neural precursors transplanted into multiple regions in the adult brain. *Ann Neurol* 1999; **46**: 867–877.

55. Baron-Van Evercooren A, Gansmuller A, Duhamel E, Pascal F, Gumpel M. Repair of a myelin lesion by Schwann cells transplanted in the adult mouse spinal cord. *J Neuroimmunol* 1992; **40**: 235–242.

56. Baron-Van Evercooren A, Avellana-Adalid V, Lachapelle F, Liblau R. Schwann cell transplantation and myelin repair of the CNS. *Mult Scler* 1997; **3**: 157–161.

57. Honmou O, Felts PA, Waxman SG, Kocsis JD. Restoration of normal conduction properties in demyelinated spinal cord axons in the adult rat by transplantation of exogenous Schwann cells. *J Neurosci* 1996; **16**: 3199–3208.

58. Imaizumi T, Lankford KL, Waxman SG, Greer CA, Kocsis JD. Transplanted olfactory ensheathing cells remyelinate and enhance axonal conduction in the demyelinated dorsal columns of the rat spinal cord. *J Neurosci* 1998; **18**: 6176–6185.

59. Barnett SC, Hutchins AM, Noble M. Purification of olfactory nerve ensheathing cells from the olfactory bulb. *Dev Biol* 1993; **155**: 337–350.

60. Barnett SC, Alexander CL, Iwashita Y et al. Identification of a human olfactory ensheathing cell that can effect transplant-mediated remyelination of demyelinated CNS axons. *Brain* 2000; **123**: 1581–1588.

61. Li Y, Field PM, Raisman G. Repair of adult rat corticospinal tract by transplants of olfactory ensheathing cells. *Science* 1997; **277**: 2000–2002.

62. Ramon-Cueto A, Cordero MI, Santos-Benito FF, Avila J. Functional recovery of paraplegic rats and motor axon regeneration in their spinal cords by olfactory ensheathing glia. *Neuron* 1900; **25**: 425–435.

63. Brustle O, Choudhary K, Karram K et al. Chimeric brains generated by intraventricular transplantation of fetal human brain cells into embryonic rats. *Nat Biotechnol* 1998; **16**: 1040–1044.

64. Flax JD, Aurora S, Yang C et al. Engraftable human neural stem cells respond to developmental cues, replace neurons, and express foreign genes. *Nat Biotechnol* 1998; **16**: 1033–1039.

65. O'Leary MT, Blakemore WF. Oligodendrocyte precursors survive poorly and do not migrate following transplantation into the normal adult central nervous system. *J Neurosci Res* 1997; **48**: 159–167.

66. Tourbah A, Linnington C, Bachelin C, Avellana-Adalid V, Wekerle H, Baron-Van Evercooren A. Inflammation promotes survival and migration of the CG4 oligodendrocyte progenitors transplanted in the spinal cord of both inflammatory and demyelinated EAE rats. *J Neurosci Res* 1997; **50**: 853–861.

67. Learish RD, Brustle O, Zhang SC, Duncan ID. Intraventricular transplantation of oligodendrocyte progenitors into a fetal myelin mutant results in widespread formation of myelin. *Ann Neurol* 1999; **46**: 716–722.

68. Vescovi AL, Parati EA, Gritti A et al. Isolation and cloning of multipotential stem cells from the embryonic human CNS and establishment of transplantable human neural stem cell lines by epigenetic stimulation. *Exp Neurol* 1999; **156**: 71–83.

69. Carpenter MK, Cui X, Hu ZY et al. In vitro expansion of a multipotent population of human neural progenitor cells. *Exp Neurol* 1999; **158**: 265–278.

70. Thomson JA, Itskovitz-Eldor J, Shapiro SS et al. Embryonic stem cell lines derived from human blastocysts [published erratum appears in *Science* 1998; **282**(5395): 1827]. *Science* 1998; **282**: 1145–1147.

71. Reubinoff BE, Pera MF, Fong CY, Trounson A, Bongso A. Embryonic stem cell lines from human blastocysts: somatic differentiation in vitro. *Nat Biotechnol* 2000; **18**: 399–404.

72. Tabbal S, Fahn S, Frucht S. Fetal tissue transplantation in Parkinson's disease. *Curr Opin Neurol* 1998; **11**: 341–349.

73. Brundin P, Pogarell O, Hagell P et al. Bilateral caudate and putamen grafts of embryonic mesencephalic tissue treated with lazaroids in Parkinson's disease. *Brain* 2000; **123**: 1380–1390.

Part 2

Infections and lymphoproliferative disorders

14

Viruses in neurological disease

Jill R Breen and Donald H Gilden

Neurotropic virus infection is a frequent cause of morbidity and mortality worldwide. This chapter reviews the most common viruses that infect the nervous system. It begins with the human herpesvirus family, not only because they are a common cause of serious disease involving the central and peripheral nervous systems, but also because some of the herpesviruses respond to antiviral treatment. The second section discusses the neurological complications of HIV, the most common viral cause of neurological disease worldwide. HTLV-1 myelopathy is discussed in the same section. Finally, the last section reviews the neurological complications produced by a wide spectrum of enteroviruses, myxoviruses, arthropod-borne viruses, adenoviruses, arenaviruses, papovaviruses, parvoviruses, filoviruses, rhabdoviruses and paramyxoviruses.

HUMAN HERPESVIRUSES

There are eight known human herpesviruses: herpes simplex virus (HSV)-1, HSV-2, varicella-zoster virus (VZV), cytomegalovirus (CMV), Epstein–Barr virus (EBV), and herpes 6, 7 and 8. Each of the human herpesviruses is a large double-stranded DNA virus that establishes latent infection in ganglia (HSV and VZV) or blood mononuclear cells (all other herpesviruses).

Herpes simplex virus type 1

Initial HSV-1 infection usually occurs before age 20 years. Virus becomes latent, primarily in trigeminal and other cranial nerve ganglia, and reactivates under stress or sunlight exposure to produce recurrent herpes labialis.

HSV encephalitis

The most serious complication of HSV-1 is acute encephalitis, which results from the combined effects of virus replication, cerebral inflammation and the predilection of HSV-1 to replicate in the medial temporal lobe and orbital surface of the frontal lobes. HSV-1 encephalitis occurs at any time of the year and is characterized by the acute onset of fever, headache, irritability, lethargy, confusion, seizures, aphasia and focal deficits.[1] Before acyclovir, the mortality, often due to uncal herniation, was 60–70%. Even with treatment, the mortality approaches 30%, and survivors often have permanent seizure disorders, memory loss, higher cognitive dysfunction, aphasia and focal neurological deficits.[2]

As early as 3 days into illness, a CT scan may reveal low-density temporal lobe lesions associated with a mild mass effect. MRI is more sensitive and demonstrates gyral edema on T1-weighted imaging in 80% of cases. Contrast enhancement is present in 50% of patients,[3] and high signal intensity may be evident in the temporal lobe or cingulate gyrus on T2-weighted scans.[4] The signal abnormalities may extend into the insula but spare the putamen. Cerebrospinal fluid (CSF) examination reveals normal or high opening pressure, a mononuclear pleocytosis, elevated protein and IgG index, and normal glucose; rarely, the CSF glucose is low. The CSF Gram stain is negative, and cultures are sterile. Red blood cells and xanthochromia may also be found in the CSF, reflecting hemorrhagic necrosis in the brain. During acute HSV-1 encephalitis, virus usually cannot be isolated from CSF, but PCR for HSV DNA in CSF confirms the diagnosis. In early HSV encephalitis, the EEG shows generalized slowing, sometimes predominating over the affected temporal lobe(s).[5] Within several days, periodic sharp-slow wave complexes every 2–3 s develop.[6] In the setting of fever and neurological deficits, this finding provides strong presumptive evidence of HSV encephalitis. Grossly, hemorrhagic necrosis and edema are found in the medial temporal and orbital frontal lobes. Microscopic examination of meninges and parenchyma reveals inflammatory infiltrates and Cowdry A intranuclear inclusions (eosinophilic inclusions that displace nuclear chromatin).

HSV encephalitis is treated with intravenous acyclovir, 15–30 mg/kg three times daily for 10 days. Because cerebral edema is a frequent cause of death, intubation and hyperventilation to bring the partial pressure of carbon dioxide to 25 mmol/l may be critical. Dexamethasone should also be given intravenously at an initial dose of 10 mg, followed by 4–8 mg every 4–5 h for the next 3 days. Total fluid intake should be reduced to one-half to two-thirds of maintenance, and the patient's head should be elevated to 30°. Mannitol can be given in repeated doses of 0.25–2 g/kg, and serum osmolality should be monitored and kept below 310 mOsm/l. The effectiveness of mannitol decreases with repeated use, and rebound increases in intracranial pressure may occur. Anticonvulsant medications are used if seizures develop; there are no data to support seizure prophylaxis in this situation.

Although HSV encephalitis is typically acute and non-recurrent, HSV was cultured from the brain of one patient and from CSF of another, both of whom displayed subacute symptoms.[7] A third subject developed recurrent HSV encephalitis confirmed by brain biopsy after treatment with intravenous adenine arabinoside (ara-A). After the second bout, the patient was treated successfully with a second course of ara-A followed by oral prednisone for life.[8] Ever since the advent of acyclovir, relapses after HSV encephalitis, often presenting with choreoathesosis, have been reported; however, virological documentation is lacking.[86]

Herpes simplex virus type 2

Just as HSV-1 causes recurrent herpes labialis, HSV-2 causes recurrent genital herpes (pelvic or genital pain with rash).

Clinical syndromes

ASEPTIC MENINGITIS

The most common central nervous system (CNS) complication of HSV-2 infection is aseptic meningitis (headache, fever, and stiff neck). Aseptic meningitis may follow recurrent genital infection. HSV-2 aseptic meningitis occurs any time of year and can recur.[9] The CSF contains a mononuclear pleocytosis. Unlike HSV-1 in encephalitis, HSV-2 can readily be isolated from CSF during aseptic meningitis.[10] Infection is

self-limited and not life-threatening, and treatment is supportive.

RADICULONEUROPATHY

Reactivation of HSV-2 along peripheral nerves is accompanied initially by neuralgia, malaise and fever followed by a painful vesicular rash on an erythematous base with pain and numbness along the affected dermatome. Although the first attack may be confused with VZV eruption, recurrent 'zoster' in an otherwise immunocompetent individual is due to HSV-2, not VZV. The 'below the waist' location of most recurrent neuropathy suggests that HSV-2 rather than HSV-1 is the causative agent. Although no trials have been performed to establish treatment protocols, oral acyclovir, 800 mg five times daily, or famciclovir, 500 mg three times daily for 7–10 days, are reasonable choices.

ENCEPHALITIS

HSV-2 encephalitis is rare and occurs primarily in newborns and immunocompromised adults, especially HIV-infected individuals with concurrent CMV infection. Neurological features include seizures, altered mental status and focal neurological deficits. Unlike the restriction of HSV-1 encephalitis to the temporal and frontal lobes, HSV-2 encephalitis is usually diffuse.[11] Even so, a few cases of HSV-2 encephalitis with primary temporal lobe involvement have been reported in adults.[12] Treatment of acute encephalitis is the same as for HSV-1 encephalitis (above). In AIDS patients, long-term treatment with oral acyclovir or famciclovir has been used; however, acyclovir-resistant strains of HSV have emerged.[13]

Varicella-zoster virus

VZV causes chickenpox (varicella), becomes latent in cranial and dorsal root ganglia, and may reactivate decades later to produce shingles (zoster). Reactivation occurs most commonly in elderly and immunocompromised individuals. Although zoster rash is usually temporally associated with neurological disease, all of the above conditions, most notably meningoencephalitis, cranial neuropathies and myelitis, may occur without antecedent rash.[14]

Clinical syndromes

ZOSTER

Herpes zoster consists of dermatomal distribution vesicular rash on an erythematous base associated with burning pain and mixed hypesthesia and hyperpathia. Elderly patients may develop a toxic encephalopathy during acute zoster. Zoster occurs at any time of year. Rash begins to resolve within a week, but pain usually lasts for 4–6 weeks. Nearly all zoster is due to viral reactivation, but clusters of zoster outbreaks have been reported.[15,16] Zoster is more common in immunocompromised hosts such as bone marrow transplant recipients and patients with cancer, lymphoma, leukemia and AIDS. Zoster may also occur at the site of X-irradiation. In immunocompetent individuals, zoster does not usually recur.[17]

Zoster most commonly involves thoracic or trigeminal dermatomes and frequently involves the ophthalmic division of the trigeminal nerve. Arm weakness and loss of reflexes may accompany cervical distribution zoster.[18] Lumbosacral zoster may produce leg weakness and loss of reflexes as well as bowel or bladder dysfunction. Cranial neuropathies also occur, including zoster oticus (rash in the ear) with ipsilateral facial paralysis (Ramsay–Hunt syndrome). Cranial neuropathies often develop weeks after zoster and may affect multiple nerves.[19] These features suggest that cranial neuropathies result from occlusion of vasa vasorum with resultant microinfarction of nerves, a process initiated by migration of VZV from afferent cranial nerve fibers to these small arteries. This is analogous to the migration of VZV from trigeminal afferents to the larger carotid arteries that produces granulomatous arteritis (described below).

Treatment of zoster pain includes extra-strength acetaminophen and 30–60 mg codeine every 6 h. Phenytoin (300–400 mg daily), carbamazepine (400–1200 mg daily)[14] and gabapentin (900 mg daily) are often useful. Oral acyclovir (800 mg five times daily) or famciclovir (500 mg three times daily) reduce the duration of rash but do not prevent postherpetic neuralgia (PHN).[20,21] All patients with ophthalmic distribution zoster should be treated with an antiviral agent. Steroids have not been shown to prevent PHN, but are often given for 3–5 days during acute zoster to reduce rash duration.[22,23]

PRE- AND POST-HERPETIC NEURALGIA

Although the rash of zoster and pain typically occur within days of each other, there are reports of dermatomal distribution pain that precedes rash by 7–100 days (pre-herpetic neuralgia).[24] PHN, pain that persists for more than 4–6 weeks after zoster, is common, and affects more than 40% of zoster patients over age 60.[25–27] Double-blinded placebo-controlled trials have shown that patients obtain relief with topical aspirin in chloroform,[28] gabapentin,[29] tricyclic antidepressants and anticonvulsants.[30] No single drug or treatment regimen has emerged as clearly superior.

GRANULOMATOUS ARTERITIS

From 2 weeks to 6 months after an attack of trigeminal distribution zoster, patients may develop contralateral neurological symptoms attributable to granulomatous arteritis. These symptoms include transient ischemic attacks (TIAs), mental status changes or hemiplegia. Ipsilateral central artery occlusion,[31] brainstem infarcts[32,33] and thalamic infarcts[34] have also been reported. These complications occur in persons over the age of 60 without any gender predilection, and mortality is 25%. The CSF contains a mononuclear pleocytosis with less than 100 cells/mm³, an increased IgG index and oligoclonal bands.[35] Focal and segmental stenosis of the middle cerebral, internal carotid and anterior cerebral arteries is often evident on angiography. Strokes, more often ischemic[36] than hemorrhagic,[37] are common in large-vessel territories. Based on the clinical, pathological and virological findings, intravenous acyclovir (10–15 mg/kg three times daily for 7–10 days) and a short course of oral steroids (60–80 mg prednisone for 3–5 days) are recommended.

SMALL-VESSEL ENCEPHALITIS

This condition is usually seen in immunocompromised patients. Initial symptoms include headache, fever, vomiting, mental status changes, focal deficits and seizures. Disease is often subacute or chronic.[38] The CSF contains a mononuclear pleocytosis and may also reveal red blood cells, mild protein elevation, and normal to low glucose. PCR may reveal VZV DNA in CSF. MRI reveals mixed ischemic or hemorrhagic infarcts, with deep-seated lesions that involve white more than gray matter. Pathological examination reveals perivenous encephalomalacia with focal hemorrhage and necrosis. Plaque-like demyelinating lesions situated at gray–white junctions are common.[39] Brain vessels and parenchyma contain inclusions and viral antigen and DNA. Aggressive treatment with intravenous acyclovir, 30 mg/kg three times daily, is recommended. Immunocompromised individuals who survive VZV small-vessel encephalitis may need to be maintained on oral acyclovir or famciclovir to prevent further virus reactivation.

VENTRICULITIS AND MENINGITIS

In AIDS patients, VZV may preferentially infect ependyma and meninges more than brain. Patients often present with a gait disorder and hydrocephalus. MRI shows enhancing ventricular lesions. In instances of meningoencephalitis, the CSF contains thousands of mononuclear cells, protein elevation to several grams and enhancing meningeal lesions on MRI. In fatal cases, histopathology demonstrates necrotizing vasculitis of the meninges.[40]

MYELITIS

VZV myelitis develops in both immunocompetent and immunocompromised individuals. Acute paraparesis, bowel and bladder incontinence and a sensory level usually develop 1–2 weeks after zoster.[14] MRI reveals T2 hyperintensity with or without spinal cord swelling. In immunocompromised patients, myelitis may be protracted, and MRI reveals more extensive longitudinal enhancing lesions. CSF shows a mild mononuclear pleocytosis and slight protein elevation. PCR usually reveals amplifiable VZV DNA.[41] Immunocompromised patients should be treated with intravenous acyclovir, 30 mg/kg three times daily,[42] with or without a short course of steroids. A standard treatment for immunocompetent individuals has not been established.

ZOSTER SINE HERPETE

Prolonged, burning radicular pain without rash can be caused by VZV. Proof was evident in two subjects with long-standing radicular pain without rash in which PCR demonstrated VZV DNA in the CSF. Both patients were successfully treated with intravenous acyclovir, 15 mg/kg three times daily for 14 days.[43]

VZV 'CEREBELLITIS'

Ataxia, nystagmus and nausea with movement may be associated with acute chickenpox and develop either before[44] or after[45] rash. In one subject,[44] the EEG showed bilateral slowing with sharp bursts of theta waves and lack of sleep spindles. Brain imaging does not usually reveal lesions in the cerebellum or brainstem, and the CSF is normal. Symptoms and signs usually resolve spontaneously. No antiviral treatment appears to be necessary.

Cytomegalovirus

Congenital CMV infection

Infants infected in utero with CMV may be born with microcephaly, spastic weakness and a seizure disorder.[46] CMV also produces a neonatal meningoencephalitis characterized by lethargy and coma. Although both ganciclovir and foscarnet kill CMV in vitro, no studies have been performed to establish dose or duration of treatment in patients.

Neurological disease in immunocompetent adults

Guillain–Barré syndrome (GBS) is characterized by a rapid onset of ascending paralysis and sensory deficit that may extend to respiratory muscles and cranial nerves. Neuropathy may be primarily demyelinating or axonal. A four-fold or greater rise in antibody titer to CMV has been associated with 40% of cases of acute demyelinating polyneuropathy,[47] in contrast to the axonal form of acute polyneuropathy that is often associated with *Campylobacter* infection.[48]

Neurological disease in immuncompromised adults

POLYRADICULITIS

The most common neurological disease produced by CMV in immunocompromised individuals is polyradiculitis. This condition is characterized by progressive distal weakness, paresthesias, incontinence and sensory loss that simulate a cauda equina syndrome. The CSF may contain either a polymorphonuclear or monocytic pleocytosis with increased protein and normal or low glucose. PCR will amplify CMV DNA present in CSF.

MONONEURITIS MULTIPLEX

In late HIV disease (CD4 count below 50 cells/mm^3), patients may develop extensive mononeuritis with rapid progression[49] and, without treatment, may die within 3 months.[50] EMG shows multiple axonal mononeuropathies beginning distally and spreading proximally. Biopsy may show necrotizing vasculitis, cryglobulinemia, axonal and demyelinating lesions, and CMV inclusions.[51] Gancyclovir may stabilize[50] or reverse[49] the deficits in CMV-induced mononeuropathy multiplex, and plasmapheresis provided improvement in one patient with HIV and cryoglobulinemia.[52]

ENCEPHALITIS–VENTRICULITIS

CMV encephalitis is usually subacute and characterized by headache, mental status changes, aphasia and focal pyramidal signs. The predilection of virus for ependymal cells may lead to a syndrome of progressive dementia and a gait disturbance with ventricular enhancement on CT or MRI.[53] Pathological findings include inflammation, necrosis and focal vasculitis. Typical owl-eyed inclusion bodies, CMV antigens and CMV DNA are present in infected tissue.

RETINITIS

Progressive CMV retinitis is often seen in AIDS patients. The cotton wool spots and retinal hemorrhages are difficult to distinguish from those seen in syphilis.[54]

MYELITIS

A rare neurological complication of CMV infection is myelitis. Attribution of disease exclusively to CMV is difficult, since both HSV and CMV may be found in the CNS and CSF in AIDS patients who have myelitis.[55]

TREATMENT

Although there is no definitive treatment of non-retinitic CMV complications, many clinicians treat patients with the medications used for CMV retinitis. Intravenous ganciclovir, 5 mg/kg every 12 h for 14–21 days, is followed by lifetime maintenance of 5 mg/kg per day intravenously. Foscarnet is often used with ganciclovir, at a dose of 90 mg/kg intravenously every 12 h for 14–21 days, then 90 mg/kg per day intravenously. Cidofovir may also be used at 5 mg/kg intravenously each week for 2 weeks, then 5 mg/kg intravenously every 2 weeks.[56]

Epstein–Barr virus

More than 90% of adults have antibody to EBV.[57] Despite the ubiquity of EBV infection, neurological complications are rare. Of the eight human herpesviruses, EBV, along with VZV, produces the most diverse neurological complications. Any level of the neuraxis may be involved.

Clinical syndromes

MENINGOENCEPHALITIS

The most common presentation of EBV infection is meningoencephalitis, usually occurring in the setting of acute mononucleosis and complicating less than 1% of cases.[58] Cerebellar ataxia predominates,[59] but athetosis, chorea,[60] stupor and coma[61] may also develop. EBV encephalitis may appear on MRI as increased T2 signal and decreased T1 signal throughout the gray matter and at gray–white junctions.[62,63] A single virologically verified case of EBV encephalitis revealed arcuate fiber demyelination on biopsy.[64] Most EBV encephalitis is self-limited. CSF examination shows a mononuclear pleocytosis and elevated protein.

MYELITIS

The typical features of acute EBV myelopathy (weakness, sensory deficit and sphincter impairment) are associated with enhancing lesions on MRI. A single case report describes successful treatment with intravenous ganciclovir, 10 mg/kg per day for 4 weeks, followed by oral ganciclovir, 60 mg/kg per day for 4 more weeks.[65] Concomitant treatment involved CMV hyperimmune globulin, at 400 mg/kg three times per week for 1 month then twice per week for an additional month. Neurological features and CSF abnormalities resolved completely, and the MRI became normal. There is a single report of encephalomyeloradiculopathy associated with EBV infection.[66]

AUTONOMIC NEUROPATHY

EBV-induced autonomic neuropathy produces paralytic ileus, sicca syndrome, orthostatic hypotension, enlarged pupils and urinary retention.[67,68] One report describes diffuse hyperpathia and burning pain associated with EBV DNA and antibody in the CSF.[69] Treatment with five doses of 20 g of intravenous Ig,[69] bethanechol 0.5 mg/kg/d[68], and L-threo-2,3-dihydroxyphenylserine, 400 mg/day,[67] improves sensory symptoms and dysautonomia but not the pupillary abnormalities.

OPHTHALMOPLEGIA

Diplopia, ptosis, ataxia and facial palsy have been described with acute mononucleosis[70] and with active EBV infection without mononucleosis.[71] Symptoms and signs resolved completely in both cases, whether acyclovir was used or not.

OPTIC NEURITIS

Optic neuritis may develop 2–12 weeks after acute mononucleosis.[72,73] Diagnosis is based on a rising EBV antibody titer. The CSF is either normal or contains a mild mononuclear pleocytosis. MRI is likewise unremarkable. Based on the small number of cases, definitive recommendations for treatment cannot be made.

Human herpesvirus types 6, 7 and 8

Clinical syndromes

Human herpesvirus type 6 (HHV-6) causes roseola infantum. Acute infection has been associated with febrile seizures in childhood[74] as well as with encephalitis.[75] In adults, HHV-6 may produce encephalitis[76] and myelopathy.[77] HHV-6 DNA and antigen have been found in the brains of patients with multiple sclerosis[78,79] and progressive multifocal leukoencephalopathy,[80] perhaps reflecting its presence in blood mononuclear cells that have crossed the blood–brain barrier. Encephalitis patients have been treated with ganciclovir[81] and foscarnet,[82] but controlled studies are lacking.

HHV-7 has been implicated in childhood meningitis and may produce the same spectrum of disease as HHV-6.[83] HHV-8 has been linked to encephalitis in three patients, two of whom were HIV-positive.[84]

RETROVIRUSES

Human immunodeficiency virus

Human immunodeficiency virus (HIV) causes AIDS. The wide spectrum of neurological disease in AIDS patients results from direct HIV infection or from opportunistic infections secondary to the immuno-deficient state (Table 14.1).

Clinical syndromes—direct HIV infection

ASEPTIC MENINGITIS

After a prodromal viral illness, HIV infection may present with cranial nerve palsies,[85] myelopathy,[86] radiculopathy, peripheral neuropathy[87] or spinal myoclonus.[88] Most often, seroconversion is accompanied by aseptic meningitis. CSF findings of a mild mononuclear pleocytosis and protein increase are not specific for HIV nervous system involvement and may be seen in otherwise asymptomatic HIV-infected individuals.[89] After aseptic meningitis, many patients recover.

ENCEPHALOPATHY

Chronic HIV encephalopathy (also known as AIDS dementia complex or HIV encephalitis) can develop after aseptic meningitis. Clinical features include impairment of higher cognitive function and mixed motor deficits (spasticity, rigidity, ataxia, tremor and involuntary movements).[90] Before antiretroviral medications were available, many patients died within 6 months.[91] Anemia, low body-mass index, older age and other constitutional symptoms of HIV infection are associated with a greater incidence of HIV encephalopathy.[92] Brain imaging reveals diffuse, non-enhancing white matter hyper-intensities[91] and cortical atrophy.[93] CT scanning in children with HIV encephalitis may also reveal basal ganglia calcification.[91] The CSF in HIV encephalitis usually contains a mild mononuclear pleocytosis and protein elevation.

Highly active antiretroviral therapy (HAART) regimens have been shown to decrease HIV RNA in the CSF.[94,95] A single report documents improvement of clinical deficit, complete reversal of white matter changes on MRI, decreased CSF burden of HIV RNA, and decreased tumor necrosis factor-alpha (TNF-α), nitric oxide and quinolinic acid concentrations in CSF after treatment with zidovudine, lamivudine and indinavir triple therapy.[96] Another study revealed a decreased incidence of HIV encephalopathy in the AIDS population since HAART became the standard of care in 1997–98,[97] and HAART-treated patients have a 95% reduction

Table 14.1   HIV-related clinical syndromes
Direct HIV infection
Aseptic meningitis
Encephalopathy
Vacuolar myelopathy
Unclear or multiple etiologies
Stroke
Distal symmetric peripheral neuropathy
Polyradiculopathy
Autonomic dysfunction
Diffuse infiltrative lymphocytosis syndrome (DILS)
Myopathy
Opportunistic infections
Viral—cytomegalovirus, varicella zoster virus, herpes simplex virus, JC virus
Bacterial—neurosyphilis, tuberculosis, *Listeria*, *Nocardia*
Fungal—*Cryptococcus*, mucormycosis, histoplasmosis, coccidioidomycosis, *Candida*, *Aspergillus*
Protozoan—toxoplasmosis, pneumocystis
Neoplastic—lymphoma, Kaposi's sarcoma

in the risk of developing HIV encephalopathy compared with untreated AIDS patients.[98] Other studies have shown improvement in motor deficits[99] and MRI findings[100] after HAART. A single trial using lexipafant, a platelet-activating factor antagonist, is also encouraging.[101]

VACUOLAR MYELOPATHY

Spinal cord disease is common in HIV-infected individuals. Myelopathy presents with spastic paraparesis and the pseudoataxia that results from proprioceptive loss. The clinical features indicating impaired function of the lateral corticospinal tract and the posterior columns of white matter (gracile and cuneate fasiculi) are similar to those seen in vitamin B_{12}-deficient individuals. Vacuolar myelopathy usually occurs late in AIDS and is typically progressive. The estimated prevalence at autopsy is 46.5%, compared to 26.8% clinically.[102]

As the neurological signs predict, pathological changes are found mostly in the thoracic spinal cord, predominantly in the posterolateral columns of white matter. Disease typically progresses from the mid-thoracic to the lumbar spine. Microscopic examination reveals myelin loss with relative axonal preservation.[103] HIV is not always found in diseased tissues. MRI changes in the spinal cord include atrophy with diffuse, intramedullary, non-enhancing lesions on T2-weighted imaging. One study of nine patients showed that L-methionine, 3 g twice a day for 6 months, may result in improved strength and bladder and sexual function, and in improved somatosensory evoked potential changes.[104]

Clinical syndromes—unclear or multiple etiologies

STROKE

Two retrospective studies indicated an increased stroke risk in HIV-infected subjects. One study demonstrated an odds ratio of 2.3 for HIV-infected patients even after controlling for risk factors such as cocaine use.[105] After controlling for intravenous drug abuse, the second study defined a stroke rate among AIDS patients of 0.56% compared to 0.025% in the general population.[106] The same study also noted that half of the HIV-infected stroke patients had CNS infections that might predispose to stroke: toxoplasmosis, *Cryptococcus*, tuberculosis and zoster; thus, the exact etiology of HIV-related stroke is unclear. Finally, stroke has been the presenting sign of HIV infection in children as young as 2 months.[107]

POLYNEUROPATHY

A distal, symmetric, axonal polyneuropathy develops in 30% of AIDS patients. Neuropathy is primarily sensory, presenting with pain, paresthesias and dysesthesias, stocking–glove sensory loss and decreased ankle jerks.[108] Clinical and electrophysiological evidence of neuropathy may be present at all stages of HIV infection, but more commonly in late AIDS.[109] The pathological changes are not well defined. Poor nutrition, coinfections and drugs used to treat HIV (ddC, vincristine, isoniazid, thalidomide, d4T, and ddI) may all play a role.[110] Stopping the offending drugs, if possible, can result in symptomatic resolution within 4–16 weeks. Diagnosis is made after other metabolic and infectious causes have been ruled out. Treatment involves pain control with tricyclic antidepressants, carbamazepine, gabapentin, opioids[108] and topical lidocaine.[111]

POLYRADICULOPATHY

HIV-induced axonal polyradiculopathy most commonly presents as a cauda equina syndrome (bilateral lower extremity radiculopathic pain, flaccidity and hyporeflexia). Mild sensory changes with bowel and bladder dysfunction may also be present. This condition develops in immuno-compromised patients with CD4 counts less than 50 cells/mm^3, and progression is rapid. The lumbosacral spine is more commonly involved than the cervical. Besides HIV, CMV, tuberculosis, syphilis, *Cryptococcus* and lymphoma can produce this syndrome. Treatment targets the offending pathogen.

AUTONOMIC DYSFUNCTION

AIDS-related autonomic dysfunction presents with postural hypotension, syncope, post-procedural cardiac arrest and impaired gastrointestinal motility.[112] Dysautonomia occurs at any time during HIV disease, and its prevalence in late AIDS exceeds 60%.[113] The pathology is unknown. Oral florinef 0.1 mg twice daily may produce rapid clinical improvement.[114]

DIFFUSE INFILTRATIVE LYMPHOCYTOSIS SYNDROME

The diffuse infiltrative lymphocytosis syndrome (DILS) mimics most HIV-related neuropathies. Clinical features of neuropathy along with systemic symptoms of dry eyes/dry mouth (sicca syndrome), enlarged parotids and lymphadenopathy alert the clinician to this entity. Typically, CD4 counts are above 200 cells/mm^3.[115] The peripheral CD8 count can be as high as 1400 cells/mm^3, and EMG shows neuropathy.[108] In one study, treatment with zidovudine or steroids improved symptoms and resulted in lowered CD8 counts.[116]

MYOPATHY

HIV-related myopathy produces subacute myalgias, proximal weakness, and esophageal and cardiac dysfunction. EMG demonstrates myopathy. Muscle biopsy reveals an inflammatory infiltrate with CD8-positive cells and immune complexes of macrophages with MHC-1 antigens.[117] A similar myopathy that may develop after 12 months of zidovudine therapy is distinguishable from HIV-induced myopathy only by the presence of ragged red fibers in zidovudine myopathy.[118] Treatment of either HIV- or zidovudine-induced myopathy is with oral prednisone, 40–60 mg daily, although success is variable.

Clinical syndromes—opportunistic infections

HIV depletes the host immune system, predisposing the individual to various opportunistic infections of viral, bacterial, fungal, protozoan and neoplastic etiology which occur at different relative frequencies (Table 14.2).

Table 14.2   Relative frequency of HIV-related opportunistic infections[224,225]

Common	Uncommon	Rare
CMV encephalitis	JC virus/progressive multifocal leukoencephalopathy	HSV encephalitis
Cryptococcal meningitis	VZV encephalitis and vasculitis	*Listeria* meningitis
Tubercular meningitis	Fungal abscess	*Nocardia* rhombencephalitis
Neurosyphilis	Lymphomatous meningitis	*Pneumocystis* meningitis
	CNS tuberculosis	
	VZV, HSV, CMV myelitis	
	Herpes zoster	
	Mononeuritis multiplex	
	CMV polyradiculopathy	
	Toxoplasmosis	

HERPESVIRUSES

Neurological diseases caused by CMV, VZV and HSV are discussed in the section on herpesviruses.

PROGRESSIVE MULTIFOCAL LEUKOENCEPHALOPATHY (PML)

This is the major complication of infection with JC virus. Only 4% of AIDS patients develop PML,[119] despite the high rate (about 70%) of seropositivity for JC virus by adult life.[120] Clinical features include the rapid progression of dementia, focal weakness and visual field defects. Most patients die within 4 months.[120] Meningoencephalitis has also been associated with acute JC virus infection in an immunocompetent host.[121]

MRI reveals non-edematous, non-enhancing white matter lesions. CSF is usually unremarkable. Pathological changes include multifocal demyelination, predominantly in parieto-occipital regions and less often in the cerebellum, brainstem and spinal cord. Oligodendroglia contain hyperchromatic nuclei, and bizarre astrocytes are frequent. JC virus DNA can be amplified in CSF by PCR,[122] or papova virions can be detected by electron microscopy in areas of demyelination. Although there are case reports of PML regression with HAART[123] or cidofovir after HAART has failed,[124] other studies have not confirmed these findings.[125,126] Any apparent success in treating PML seems unrelated to CD4 count or HIV RNA load. One study suggests that higher JC virus load may correlate with treatment failure.[127]

SYPHILIS

Treponema pallidum, a flagellated spirochete, causes syphilis. Neurological complications develop in 4–9% of patients with untreated syphilis[128], and tertiary (cardiovascular or neurological complica-

tions or gummas) disease develops within 1–30 years after primary infection.[129] Meningovascular infarcts,[130] CNS gummas, and myelopathy[131] may occur. Meningovascular syphilis is characterized by headache, fever, stiff neck, and focal neurological deficit. Seizures and cranial nerve deficits, particularly optic neuritis, facial weakness and hearing loss, may also develop. In fact, 20% of syphilis meningitis patients become deaf. Dementia and psychosis characterize general paresis, a late complication of neurosyphilis. The onset of memory loss, delusions of grandeur and dysarthria is insidious. Tabes dorsalis, another late complication, consists of lightning pains in the lower extremities and abdomen, diminished reflexes, severe loss of vibratory and proprioceptive sensation and bilateral Argyll–Robertson pupils (small, irregular pupils that do not react to light, but do accommodate).

Serological analysis, either rapid plasma reagin (RPR) or fluorescent treponemas antibody absorption (FTA-ABS), confirms the diagnosis of syphilis. In neurosyphilis, CSF demonstrates a positive venereal disease research laboratory (VDRL), a mononuclear pleocytosis, slightly elevated protein and usually normal glucose.[128] Neuroimaging may show gummas, which manifest as multifocal ring-enhancing lesions.[132] Brain biopsy material shows endarteritis and periarteritis, with organisms invading blood vessels and producing aneurysms and infarcts. Gummas consist of chronic inflammation with microglial proliferation, increased lymphocytes and multinucleated giant cells.

Neurosyphilis is treated with intravenous penicillin G, 3–4 million units every 4 h for 10–14 days, or a combination of intramuscular procaine penicillin, 2.4 million units every day, and probenecid, 500 mg four times daily, for 10–14 days. Either regimen should be followed by intramuscular benzathine penicillin, 2.4 million units every week for 3 weeks.[133] Unfortunately, failure rates of 5–18% have been documented with these regimens.[134]

MYCOBACTERIA

In 5–10% of AIDS patients,[135] *Mycobacterium tuberculosis* produces meningitis, tuberculomas,[136] hydrocephalus, infarcts[137] or meningomyelitis.[138] *Mycobacterium avium–intracellulare* may also cause meningoencephalitis,[139] encephalopathy[140] or direct CNS invasion without encephalitis or meningitis.[141] Disease results from basilar meningitis and vasculopathy combined with hydrocephalus that develops when meningeal inflammation impairs CSF resorption. Thus, in addition to fever, clinical features of CNS infection are altered mental status and focal deficits. Radiculomyelopathy manifests as back and leg pain with hyporeflexia or hyperreflexia and paraplegia. CNS tuberculosis is suggested by multiple, nodular ring-enhancing lesions with surrounding edema on head CT or MRI. Owing to vasculopathy, infarcts are also commonly seen. CSF frequently shows a monocytic pleocytosis, elevated protein, and depressed glucose. Mycobacteria can be isolated from CSF or brain. CNS lesions contain granulomas and multinucleated giant cells, and show loss of axons and myelin, and reactive astrocytosis. A positive purified protein derivative (PPD) and miliary apical lesions may be seen on chest X-ray, but severely immunocompromised hosts may not mount a PPD response even in active tubercular disease, and CNS tuberculosis may occur in the absence of pulmonary disease. Treatment consists of oral combination therapy: isoniazid 300 mg/day for 9 months, rifampin 300 mg/day for 9 months, pyrazinamide 25 mg/kg per day (maximum 2 g/day) for 2 months, and ethambutol 15–25 mg/kg per day (maximum 2.5 g/day) for 2 months. Additionally, morbidity and mortality may be reduced with intravenous dexamethasone 12 mg/day for 3 weeks followed by a 3-week taper.[142]

LISTERIA

Listeria monocytogenes is a Gram-positive rod that produces both acute and chronic meningoencephalitis. Selective vulnerability of the brainstem to *Listeria* often results in a pontobulbar encephalitis characterized by fever, ataxia and polyneuritis cranialis. Infection occurs most frequently in infants and the elderly, in alcoholics, in patients with CD4 counts below 50 cells/mm³,[143] and in HIV patients taking steroids.[144] In one series of seven HIV-infected patients, the mortality was 29%.[143] Ampicillin 200 mg/kg intravenously every 4 h with gentamicin 5 mg/kg intravenously every 8 h is the treatment of choice. Intravenous trimethoprim–sulfamethoxazole 15 mg/kg per day, divided every 6–8 h, is also a reasonable alternative. Either regimen should continue for 3 weeks in patients with meningitis, or for 6 weeks in patients with abscess or rhombencephalitis.[145]

NOCARDIA

Nocardia asteroides produces cerebral abscesses,[146] characterized by headache, fever, vomiting, seizures, altered mental status, incoordination and focal neurological deficits.[147] Infection is seen in only 0.3% of AIDS patients,[148] but mortality is as high as 85%.[148] Because of technical difficulties in testing *Nocardia's* susceptibility to antibiotics, a clear treatment strategy has not emerged. Intravenous trimethoprim, 2.5–10 mg/kg twice daily, and sulfamethoxazole, 12.5–50 mg/kg twice daily, may be used. Alternatively, two double-strength trimethoprim–sulfamethoxazole tablets may be given orally every 8 h. Treatment should continue for at least 12 months, if not for life.[149] Because of poor abscess penetration by antimicrobial drugs, some abscesses may require surgical debridement before antibiotic use.[146]

CRYPTOCOCCUS

One of the most common opportunistic infections and the most common fungal infection in AIDS patients is cryptococcal meningitis. Infection does not usually occur until the CD4 count is 46 cells/mm³ or less. Mortality approaches 30% within 3 months after diagnosis.[150] CSF India ink staining, CSF and serum cultures and *Cryptococcus* antigen studies all help in diagnosis. Optimal treatment is controversial, because of high failure rates with current protocols. A reasonable approach is intravenous amphotericin B, 0.7–1 mg/kg per day, with or without intravenous flucytosine, 100 mg/kg per day. Therapy should continue for 6–10 weeks, particularly since transient elevation of serum blood urea nitrogen (BUN) or creatinine due to amphotericin nephrotoxicity may require treatment interruption for a day or two. Maintenance therapy with fluconazole, 200–400 mg/day orally, or amphotericin B, 1 mg/kg intravenously 1–3 times per week, is recommended for lifetime suppression.[151] Both appropriate antifungal therapy and a sufficient host immune response are required for adequate treatment of cryptococcal meningitis. Thus, the prognosis is poor in HIV-infected patients who are unable to mount a satisfactory immune response.

OTHER FUNGAL INFECTIONS

Candida albicans,[152] *Coccidioides immitis,*[153] *Histoplasma capsulatum*[154] and mucormycosis[155] may all produce meningoencephalitis. *Aspergillus fumigatus*[156] produces brain abscesses in immunocompromised hosts. Since cultures for fungi are frequently negative, brain biopsy may be needed to reveal pseudohyphae, yeasts and filaments. Despite antifungal treatment, recurrence is frequent. Severe infections may require surgical debridement.

TOXOPLASMA

Toxoplasma gondii is an intracellular protozoan that invades the CNS of patients with CD4 counts below 100 cells/mm^3. Most often, *Toxoplasma* produces focal CNS disease, but diffuse encephalitis and myelopathy also occur.[157] In CNS toxoplasmosis, head CT often shows one or more ring-enhancing lesions.[158] The CSF opening pressure may be high, and the CSF may contain a leukocytosis and elevated protein. PCR can identify *T. gondii* DNA in CSF, and antibody or oligoclonal bands specific for *T. gondii* may also be present.[159] Serum often contains IgG antibody to *T. gondii*, but demonstration of a rising titer is difficult, thus reducing its diagnostic value.[158] Prophylaxis against systemic toxoplasmosis is indicated in AIDS patients with serum IgG against *Toxoplasma* and a CD4 count below 100 cells/mm^3.[160] Prophylaxis consists of trimethoprim–sulfamethoxazole, one double-strength tablet daily, or dapsone–pyrimethamine and folinic acid. Once infection has developed, treatment with pyrimethamine, 200 mg orally once daily, followed by 75–100 mg/day is given along with sulfadiazine, 1–1.5 g orally, every 6 h with folinic acid, 10–15 mg/day, to prevent bone marrow suppression. Treatment continues for 3–6 weeks and is followed by lifetime prophylaxis with pyrimethamine, 25–50 mg daily, sulfadiazine, 500–1000 mg every 6 h, and folinic acid, 10–25 mg daily.[161] Without continuied therapy, recurrence approaches 80%. Response to treatment is so dramatic and rapid that patients who fail to respond clinically and show reduction in CT lesion burden within 7–10 days should undergo brain biopsy to establish a diagnosis.

PNEUMOCYSTIS

Pneumocystis carinii is an intracellular parasite best known for its ability to cause pneumonia, often fulminant in AIDS patients. Hematogenous spread from the lungs rarely produces meningitis, radiculitis[162] or both.[163] Diagnosis is made by visualization of the organism in tissue stained with toluidine blue, Grocott–Gomori methenamine–silver nitrate staining[164] or monoclonal antibody.[163] Treatment of both cerebral and pulmonary infection is with intravenous pentamidine, trimethoprim–sulfamethoxazole, trimethoprim–dapsone, clindamycin–primaquine or trimetrexate. Even with treatment, nearly half of the patients with CNS pneumocystis die.[165]

CNS LYMPHOMA

Lymphoma is the most common tumor found in the CNS of AIDS patients. Clinical features include night sweats and weight loss associated with altered mental status, seizures and focal neurological deficits. Death occurs in 1–2 months without treatment, or in 3–4 months with radiation therapy.[166] CNS lymphoma is the AIDS-defining illness in only 1% of patients,[167] although 20% of AIDS patients eventually develop CNS lymphoma.[168] CNS lymphomas are typically intermediate-grade, diffuse, large cell cancers.[169] Typically, these lymphomas develop in patients with CD4 counts below 50 cells/mm^3. Brain imaging demonstrates homogeneous ring-enhancing lesions, primarily in the corpus callosum and gray matter. CNS lymphoma lesions are usually larger than those in toxoplasmosis.[166] EBV DNA is found in CSF in 87% of patients with primary CNS lymphoma. For this reason, the diagnosis of CNS lymphoma may be made based on the combination of characteristic brain imaging lesions and demonstration of EBV DNA in CSF.[170] Patients with typical lesions in the setting of immunosuppression are treated empirically with anti-*Toxoplasma* medications for 1 week. If there is no improvement in 7–10 days, biopsy is pursued for definitive diagnosis. If the patient is found to have CNS lymphoma, imaging of the entire neuraxis is recommended to identify extracerebral involvement.[166]

LYMPHOMATOUS MENINIGITIS

CNS lymphoma may present as lymphomatous meningitis, a condition characterized by headache, fever, stiff neck and mental status changes with cranial or spinal nerve palsies. CSF white blood cell count, protein and glucose can be normal or elevated. CSF cytological analysis may reveal malignant cells. Brain imaging reveals atrophy with or without meningeal enhancement. The mean survival from the time of diagnosis of lymphomatous meningitis is only 5 weeks. At this stage, treatment is not usually helpful.[171]

KAPOSI'S SARCOMA

Kaposi's sarcoma (KS) is a common HIV-related cancer in skin, lung, adrenal glands and gastrointestinal tract. The cause of KS appears to be

HHV-8.[173] KS may occasionally involve the CNS; symptoms include TIAs, brachial plexopathy, dizziness,[152] tinnitus, lightheadedness or headache.[172] KS limited to dural blood vessels may produce subdural hematoma.[174] Occasionally, KS is not discovered until autopsy.[175] Histologically, the tumor is an anaplastic angiosarcoma characterized by irregular endothelial cells lining the vascular spaces. These endothelial cells contain enlarged, irregular nuclei, frequent mitotic figures and a reticular network surrounding the blood vessels with hemosiderin deposits.[174] Since the advent of antiretroviral therapy in 1996, the incidence of KS has decreased by 36%.[176] Systemic KS may be treated with combination chemotherapy, while isolated tumors are treated with intralesional vinblastine, cryotherapy, radiation, altretinoin gel or laser therapy.[177]

Human T-cell lymphotropic virus type 1

Human T-cell lymphotropic virus type 1 (HTLV-1) infection is seen predominantly in the equatorial regions of southeastern Japan, the Caribbean, Africa, and Central and South America. Its routes of transmission are thought to be sexual, perinatal and by contact with contaminated blood.[178] Most infected individuals remain asymptomatic. Affected patients present with back pain or painless progressive spastic paraparesis with constipation and urinary urgency or incontinence.[179] HTLV-1 myelopathy (HAM), also know as tropical spastic paraparesis (TSP), has a highly variable disease course. Symptoms often stabilize within a few years of onset. Serum ELISA for HTLV-1 may establish the presence of the virus. CSF demonstrates elevated intrathecal synthesis of anti-HTLV-1 IgG. MRI reveals atrophy of the thoracic spinal cord and white matter lesions that can mimic those seen in multiple sclerosis. Although the exact pathogenesis is not well understood, virus particles and virus-infected T- and B-cells have been found in brain and spinal cord parenchyma as well as in perivascular infiltrates. Pathological evaluation shows progressive myelin and axon loss in brain white matter and pyramidal tracts.[180] There is no effective treatment.

OTHER VIRUSES

Many other viruses may cause meningitis, encephalitis or CNS vasculitis. Important diagnostic clues are time of year, self-limited versus recurrent meningitis, and presence or absence of focal deficit. Aseptic (non-bacterial) meningitis is characterized by headache, fever and meningismus. Less common

features include photophobia, sore throat, nausea, vomiting, diplopia and focal sensory changes. While irritability and altered mental state may be present, these symptoms are more often encountered in encephalitis. Encephalitis may appear clinically similar to aseptic meningitis with a few important distinctions. Patients with encephalitis develop insomnia, lethargy, alterations in consciousness, seizures, aphasia and hemiplegia. Imaging may show mild brain swelling or meningeal enhancement, but, more often, imaging is unremarkable.

Diagnosis depends upon CSF examination. White blood cell count is frequently elevated (rarely above 100 cells/mm³) with a polymorphonuclear predominance for 1–2 days followed by lymphocytic predominance. Glucose is typically normal but can be decreased in one-third of patients with enterovirus (coxsackie and echoviruses), mumps and lymphocytic choriomeningitis virus infection. Gram stain and culture are unrevealing. Virus culture is not usually helpful (exceptional instances are described below), but PCR for viral DNA or RNA along with the detection of antiviral antibody can help in diagnosis. Rising serum antibody titers may also be useful. Treatment is supportive. Intravenous fluids, airway protection, balanced nutrition, careful monitoring of serum electrolytes and alertness for a syndrome of inappropriate antidiuretic hormone (SIADH) in some forms of encephalitis are all important. HSV, VZV and CMV warrant specific antiviral therapy (see herpesvirus section).

Enteroviruses

Enteroviruses (coxsackieviruses A and B, echovirus and polioviruses) are the most common cause of aseptic meningitis. Infection takes place primarily in the summer. Fecal–oral spread is the primary mode of transmission. Gastrointestinal symptoms usually precede meningeal symptoms, and fever may be present during both phases of the disease.[181] CSF shows a mononuclear pleocytosis, elevated protein, and normal or low[182] glucose. Viral culture may reveal virus after 18 days' incubation, and PCR may be useful.[183] Antibody against the enteroviruses develops in the CSF after 14 days and may remain for 1 month.

In immunocompetent hosts, CNS infection is self-limited; however, hypo- or agammaglobulinemic patients may develop protracted infection that is frequently fatal.[184] In some cases, treatment with immunoglobulin has been effective.[185]

Although enteroviruses usually cause meningitis, encephalitis may also develop. Presenting symptoms include ataxia, opsoclonus, myoclonus,[186] parkinsonism and rhombencephalitis.[187] Persistent flaccid paralysis,[188] myelitis and cranial or peripheral neuropathy are also possible.

Poliovirus

Since the widespread use of polio vaccines in infants and toddlers, the incidence of acute paralysis due to poliovirus has declined dramatically. Since 1980, there has been no reported poliomyelitis from within the USA, except for sporadic cases of vaccine-associated disease.[189] While most poliovirus infections cause the characteristic myelitis and clinical paralysis, infection resulting in oral–facial dyskinesias and quadriplegia has been described in one case.[190]

Mumps virus

Transmitted among humans by respiratory and oral secretions, mumps virus produces disease during the winter and early spring. The most common systemic features include parotitis, orchitis and mastitis, and, less often, oophoritis, pancreatitis and thyroiditis. Gland or organ tenderness associated with meningeal signs raises the suspicion of mumps. CSF shows a mononuclear pleocytosis that may persist for several months.[191] Mumps is one of the few viruses associated with hypoglycorrachia. Additionally, chronic but usually mild encephalomyelitis may develop.[192]

Influenza viruses

The presence of ataxia, motor deficits and mental status changes associated with systemic flu-like symptoms may indicate influenza virus encephalitis. One series identified CSF lymphocytosis along with rising anti-influenza antibody titers.[193] Although influenza typically strikes during the winter months, it may occur at any time of the year.

Arboviruses

The arthropod-borne (arbo) viruses include togaviruses, bunyaviruses and reoviruses. Transmission from infected animals to humans takes place in the summer or autumn through mosquito or tick vectors. Myalgia is common. Tremor and seizures are frequent features of the encephalitis. Inoculation of the patient's CSF into young mice may produce encephalitis. Antiviral antibody may also be detected in the CSF. The presence of serum IgM or a rising titer of IgG against the particular virus is strong diagnositic evidence.

St Louis encephalitis (SLE)

The most common arbovirus infection is SLE, which occurs most often in the midwestern and southeastern regions of the USA. Infections may be asymptomatic or self-limited, but approximately 5% are fatal. Transmitted by mosquitoes, the SLE virus produces meningitis, encephalitis, opsoclonus, tremulousness[194] and cranial nerve palsies.[195] SIADH may also develop.[196] In approximately 10% of patients, prolonged sequelae include poor memory, fatigue, insomnia, headaches, focal deficits and seizures.

Western equine encephalitis (WEE)

More severe in young children, WEE virus infection is associated with 3–4% mortality. Parkinsonism may present as a transient feature of infection,[197] and mental status changes and seizures may persist, especially in children.[198] This viral disease is most commonly encountered in the western USA during the summer.

California virus encephalitis

La Crosse virus is the most common cause of California encephalitis. Despite its name, viral infection generally occurs in the midwestern and Atlantic USA. Symptoms are generally benign; however, 50% of individuals have seizures, and 20–40% develop focal neurological signs and focal EEG changes.[199] Children are more severely affected than adults, and boys are affected twice as often as girls. Overall mortality is less than 1%.

Eastern equine encephalitis (EEE)

This form of encephalitis is particularly malignant and results in 50–75% mortality. The endemic region is the eastern coast of the USA during the late summer and early autumn. In the majority of survivors, diffuse neurological deficits persist, including mental impairment, seizures, behavioral abnormalities and spastic paralysis.[200] MRI shows basal ganglia and thalamic hyperintensities.[201]

Japanese encephalitis virus

A relative of the St Louis encephalitis virus, Japanese encephalitis virus is found in China, Southeast Asia, India and Sri Lanka. Clinical features range from asymptomatic to mild headache and fever to fulminant encephalitis with tremors, cardiovascular collapse, flaccid upper extremities,[202] coma, seizures and death. Mortality is 20–40%.[203] A vaccine is available in endemic areas.[204]

Colorado tick fever virus

In the Rocky Mountain regions of the USA and Canada, Colorado tick fever virus produces a mild, generally self-limited meningitis. Fevers, headache, myalgias and maculopapular rash are common. Rarely, lethargy, coma, seizures and death may result.

Venezuelan equine encephalitis virus (VEE)

A generally mild encephalitis with a mortality less than 1%, Venezuelan equine encephalitis develops in South and Central America and the Western USA. A viral prodrome is followed by fever and neurological features of encephalitis. The severe forms, including death, occur more often in children.

Tick-borne encephalitis viruses

A broad range of viruses that inhabit the northern hemisphere produce encephalitis of varying severity. Symptoms are likewise varied, but all viruses in this family are transmitted through tick vectors.

Adenoviruses

Adenoviruses frequently cause upper respiratory infections, keratoconjunctivitis and pneumonia. In less than 1% of infections,[205] some strains may cause meningoencephalitis, with mortality between 26% and 38%.[206] One report describes an immunocompromised patient in whom adenovirus produced a focal encephalitis.[207]

Arenaviruses

In the USA, aseptic meningitis or, rarely, fatal meningoencephalitis may result from lymphocytic choriomeningitis virus (LCM) infection. Glandular inflammation may accompany acute infection, similar to mumps.[208] CSF may contain thousands of mononuclear cells and have low glucose. Diagnosis is made when choriomeningitis and seizures develop in mice injected with infected human CSF or when the human host develops anti-LCM antibody in the serum. One atypical case of LCM infection presented as a mimic of systemic lupus erythematosis; both rash and circulating anticoagulant were noted.[209]

Other strains of arenavirus in South America and Africa may produce hemorrhagic fever. Lassa fever virus infection (African strain) presents as multi-organ inflammation, hemorrhage, renal dysfunction and deafness.[210] Between 30% and 66% of patients die. Fevers, facial and thoracic rash, headache, small cutaneous hemorrhages, cerebellar dysfunction and

oculomotor deficits are clues to the South American arenavirus encephalitides. Mortality is 15–30% with the Argentinian Junin virus-induced encephalitis. Other South American viruses that cause similar diseases include the Bolivian Machupo virus,[211] Venezuelan Guanarito virus[212] and Brazilian Sabia virus.[213]

Papovaviruses

BK virus (BKV) is a ubiquitous DNA virus that is typically encountered during childhood. Antibody to BKV is found in 70–80% of adults. BKV becomes latent in the urinary tract and may reactivate in immunocompromised hosts to produce meningo-encephalitis and retinitis.[214] BKV sequences can also be cloned from healthy brain tissue,[215] and there is one case report of BKV encephalitis in an immunocompetent patient.[216] MRI T2-weighted images show diffuse white matter hyperintensities that resolve after acute meningoencephalitis. PCR may amplify BKV DNA transiently in serum.[216] Pathology shows lymphocytic and macrophage invasion of the meninges, mild cortical astrocytosis and ependymal fibrosis.[214] There is no treatment. Infection and the sequelae of JC virus (namely, PML) are discussed in the HIV/AIDS section.

Parvovirus

Parvovirus B19 is another ubiquitous virus that only rarely affects the CNS. During acute infection, which presents as erythema infectiosum in children, aseptic meningitis may develop.[217] Infection most often is benign; however, one case associated with lethargy and convulsions has been reported.[218]

Filoviruses

Extremely virulent forms of encephalitis have been noted with Marburg and Ebola viruses. Both strains appear to be endemic in Africa, where monkeys are the primary hosts. Gastrointestinal upset, fevers, headache and hemorrhage develop first, followed quickly by CNS depression and focal signs. Mortality is about 30% with Marburg and 70–90% with Ebola virus.[219]

Rabies

Contracted from the bite of infected animals, rabies virus invades the local muscle and peripheral nerves. From there, the virus travels transaxonally to the CNS.[220] Encephalitis with features of aggression, lethargy, mydriasis and hydrophobia is characteristic. Another form of CNS rabies, so-called 'dumb rabies,' is characterized by multiple lower cranial nerve palsies, dysarthria and dysphagia and may mimic the polyneuritis cranialis form of the Guillain–Barré syndrome. Early treatment may prevent the onset of clinical rabies. For persons bitten by skunks, raccoons, bats, wild carnivores, or other animals known or suspected to be rabid, the wound should be cleaned with soap and water, and then 20 IU/kg rabies immune globulin injected into the tissue surrounding the wound site. Prophylactic vaccination is accomplished with a 1-ml intramuscular injection on the day of bite exposure as well as 3, 7, 14 and 28 days later.[221] Survival after the onset of clinical rabies is rare.

Measles

There are three forms of encephalitis produced by measles virus. The most common form is a post-infectious encephalomyelitis characterized by the acute onset of headache, fever, stiff neck, seizures and focal deficit, usually within 14 days of rash. Mortality is about 10–20%,[222] and survivors are often left with seizure disorders, impairment of cognitive function and deafness. Pathological changes are found mainly in white matter and are indistinguishable from the inflammatory demyelination seen in fatal cases of post-vaccinial encephalomyelitis due to rabies immunization or smallpox vaccination. Measles virus is not found in the brains of patients who die of measles post-infectious encephalomyelitis.[223]

A less common form of encephalitis is subacute sclerosing panencephalitis (SSPE), a chronic progressive encephalitis that develops years after measles. Dementia, focal deficit and seizures, including myoclonic seizures, characterize the disease. Death usually occurs within a few years. Both gray and white matter are affected, and inclusion bodies, measles virus antigen and RNA as well as para-myxovirus nucleocapsids are abundant in brain. Measles virus vaccination has nearly eradicated both measles post-infectious encephalomyelitis and SSPE.

Finally, a rare form of subacute encephalitis produced by measles virus occurs in immunocompromised individuals. About 50% of such patients have rash in association with severe, usually fatal encephalitis. Measles virus inclusions and viral antigen and RNA are present in brain. Surprisingly, this form of measles virus encephalitis has not emerged as a significant opportunistic virus encephalitis in AIDS patients.

REFERENCES

1. Johnson R. Herpesvirus infections. In: Johnson R, ed. *Viral Infections of the Nervous System*. New York: Raven Press, 1999: 133–168.
2. Whitley RJ, Alford CA, Hirsch MS et al. Vidarabine versus acyclovir therapy in herpes simplex encephalitis. *N Engl J Med* 1986; **314**: 144–149.
3. Weisberg L, Nice C (eds.). Herpes simplex encephalitis. In: *Cerebral Computed Tomography: A Text Atlas*, 3rd edn. Saunders, Philadelphia 1989: 295–297.
4. Schroth G, Gawehn J, Thron A, Vallbracht A, Foigt K. Early diagnosis of herpes simplex encephalitis by MRI. *Neurology* 1987; **37**: 179–183.
5. Westmoreland B. The EEG in cerebral inflammatory processes. In: Niedermeyer E, Lopes daSilva F, eds, *Electroencephalography: Basic principles, clinical applications and related fields*, 2nd edn. Baltimore, Munich: Urban & Schwarzenberg, 1987: 261.
6. Smith J, Westmoreland B, Reagan T, Sandok B. A distinctive clinical EEG profile in herpes simplex encephalitis. *Mayo Clin Proc* 1975; **50**: 469–474.
7. Sage J, Weinstein M, Miller D. Chronic encephalitis possibly due to herpes simplex virus: two cases. *Neurology* 1985; **35**: 1470–1472.
8. Koenig H, Rabinowitz S, Day E, Miller V. Post-infectious encephalomyelitis after successful treatment of herpes simplex encephalitis with adenine arabinoside: ultrastructural observations. *N Engl J Med* 1979; **300**: 1089–1093.
8b. Wang HS, Kuo M-F, Huang S-C, Chou M-L. Choreoathetosis as an initial sign of relapsing of herpes simplex encephalitis. *Pediatr Neurol* 1994; **11**: 341–45.
9. Tedder DG, Ashley R, Tyler KL, Levin MJ. Herpes simplex virus infection as a cause of benign recurrent lymphocytic meningitis. *Ann Intern Med* 1994; **121**: 334–338.
10. Craig C, Nahmias A. Different patterns of neurological involvement with herpes simplex virus types 1 and 2: isolation of herpes virus type 2 from the buffy coat of two adults with meningitis. *J Infect Dis* 1973; **127**: 365–372.
11. Roos K. Encephalitis. *Neurol Clin* 1999; **17**: 813–833.
12. Aurelius E, Johansson B, Skoldenberg B, Forsgren M. Encephalitis in immunocompetent patients due to herpes simplex virus type 1 or 2 as determined by type-specific polymerase chain reaction and antibody assays of cerebrospinal fluid. *J Med Virol* 1993; **39**: 179–186.
13. Oram RJ, Marcellino D, Strauss D et al. Characterization of an acyclovir-resistant herpes simplex virus type 2 strain isolated from a premature neonate. *J Infect Dis* 2000; **181**: 1458–1461.
14. Gilden DH, Kleinschmidt-DeMasters BK, LaGuardia JJ, Mahalingam R, Cohrs R. Neurological complications of the reactivation of varicella-zoster virus. *N Engl J Med* 2000; **342**: 635–645.
15. Thomas M, Robertson W. Dermal transmission of virus as a cause of shingles. *Lancet* 1971; **2**: 1349–1350.
16. Palmer S, Caul E, Donald D, Kwantes W, Tillett W. An outbreak of shingles? *Lancet* 1985; **2**: 1108–1111.
17. Hope-Simpson R. The nature of herpes zoster: a long-term study and a new hypothesis. *Proc R Soc Med* 1965; **58**: 9–20.
18. Thomas J, Howard F. Segmental zoster paresis—a disease profile. *Neurology* 1972; **22**: 459–466.

19. Lapresle J, Lasjaunias P. Cranial nerve ischaemic arterial syndromes: a review. *Brain* 1986; **109**: 207–216.

20. Tyring S, Barbarash RA, Nahlik JE et al. Famciclovir for the treatment of acute herpes zoster: effects on acute disease and postherpetic neuralgia. A randomized, double-blind, placebo-controlled trial. *Ann Intern Med* 1995; **123**: 89–96.

21. Wood MJ, Johnson RW, McKendrick MW, Taylor J, Mandal BK, Crooks J. A randomized trial of acyclovir for 7 days or 21 days with and without prednisolone for treatment of acute herpes zoster. *N Engl J Med* 1994; **330**: 896–900.

22. Eaglstein WH, Katz R, Brown JA. The effects of early corticosteroid therapy on the skin eruption and pain of herpes zoster. *JAMA* 1970; **211**: 1681–1683.

23. Keczkes K, Basheer AM. Do corticosteroids prevent post-herpetic neuralgia? *Br J Dermatol* 1980; **102**: 551–555.

24. Gilden DH, Dueland AN, Cohrs R, Martin JR, Kleinschmidt-DeMasters BK, Mahalingam R. Preherpetic neuralgia. *Neurology* 1991; **41**: 1215–1218.

25. DeMoragas J, Kierland R. The outcome of patients with herpes zoster. *Arch Dermatol* 1957; **75**: 193–196.

26. Rogers RS III, Tindall JP. Geriatric herpes zoster. *J Am Geriatr Soc* 1971; **19**: 495–504.

27. Brown GR. Herpes zoster: correlation of age, sex, distribution, neuralgia and associated disorders. *South Med J* 1976; **69**: 576–578.

28. King RB. Topical aspirin in chloroform and the relief of pain due to herpes zoster and postherpetic neuralgia. *Arch Neurol* 1993; **50**: 1046–1053.

29. Rowbotham M, Harden N, Stacey B, Bernstein P, Magnus-Miller L. Gabapentin for the treatment of postherpetic neuralgia: a randomized controlled trial. *JAMA* 1998; **21**: 1837–1842.

30. Kost RG, Straus SE. Postherpetic neuralgia—pathogenesis, treatment and prevention. *N Engl J Med* 1996; **335**: 32–42.

31. Hall S, Carlin L, Roach ES, McLean WT Jr. Herpes zoster and central retinal artery occlusion. *Ann Neurol* 1983; **13**: 217–218.

32. Ross MH, Abend WK, Schwartz RB, Samuels MA. A case of C2 herpes zoster with delayed bilateral pontine infarction. *Neurology* 1991; **41**: 1685–1686.

33. Fukumoto S, Kinjo M, Hokamura K, Tanaka K. Subarachnoid hemorrhage and granulomatous angiitis of the basilar artery: demonstration of the varicella-zoster virus in the basilar artery lesions. *Stroke* 1986; **17**: 1024–1028.

34. Geny C, Yulis J, Azoulay A, Brugieres P, Saint-Val C, Degos JD. Thalamic infarction following lingual herpes zoster. *Neurology* 1991; **41**: 1846.

35. Hilt DC, Buchholz D, Krumholz A, Weiss H, Wolinsjy JS. Herpes zoster ophthalmicus and delayed contralateral hemiparesis caused by cerebral angiitis: diagnosis and management approaches. *Ann Neurol* 1983; **14**: 543–553.

36. Kuroiwa Y, Kurukawa T. Hemispheric infarction after herpes zoster ophthalmicus: computed tomography and angiography. *Neurology* 1981; **31**: 1030–1032.

37. Elble RJ. Intracerebral hemorrhage with herpes zoster ophthalmicus. *Ann Neurol* 1983; **14**: 591–592.

38. Amlie-Lefond C, Kleinschmidt-DeMasters BK, Mahalingam R, Davis LE, Gilden DH. The vasculopathy of varicella-zoster virus encephalitis. *Ann Neurol* 1995; **37**: 784–790.

39. Horten B, Price RW, Jimenez D. Multifocal varicella-zoster virus leukoencephalitis temporally remote from herpes zoster. *Ann Neurol* 1981; **9**: 251–266.

40. Kleinschmidt-DeMasters BK, Amlie-Lefond C, Gilden DH. The patterns of varicella zoster virus encephalitis. *Hum Pathol* 1996; **27**: 927–938.

41. Gilden DH, Beinlich BR, Rubinstien EM et al. Varicella-zoster virus myelitis: an expanding spectrum. *Neurology* 1994; **44**: 1818–1823.

42. de Silva SM, Mark AS, Gilden DH et al. Zoster myelitis: improvement with antiviral therapy in two cases. *Neurology* 1996; **47**: 929–931.

43. Gilden DH, Wright RR, Schneck SA, Gwaltney JM Jr, Mahalingam R. Zoster sine herpete, a clinical variant. *Ann Neurol* 1994; **35**: 530–533.

44. Dangond F, Engle E, Yessayan L, Sawyer MH. Pre-eruptive varicella cerebellitis confirmed by PCR. *Pediatr Neurol* 1993; **9**: 491–493.

45. Peters AC, Versteeg J, Lindeman J, Bots GT. Varicella and acute cerebellar ataxia. *Arch Neurol* 1978; **35**: 769–771.

46. Alford CA, Stagno S, Pass RF, Britt WJ. Congenital and perinatal cytomegalovirus infections. *Rev Infect Dis* 1990; **12**(suppl 7): S745–753.

47. Dowling P, Menonna J, Cook S. Cytomegalovirus complement fixation antibody in Guillain–Barré syndrome. *Neurology* 1977; **27**: 1153–1156.

48. Griffin J, Li C, Ho T, Xue P, Macko C, Gao C. Guillain–Barré syndrome in northern China: the spectrum of neuropathological changes in clinically defined cases. *Brain* 1995; **118**: 577–595.

49. Wulff EA, Wang AK, Simpson DM. HIV-associated peripheral neuropathy: epidemiology, pathophysiology and treatment. *Drugs* 2000; **59**: 1251–1260.

50. So YT. Clinical subdivision of mononeuropathy multiplex in patients with HIV infection. *Neurology* 1992; **42**(suppl 3): 409.

51. Said G, Lacroix C, Chemouilli P et al. Cytomegalovirus neuropathy in acquired immunodeficiency syndrome: a clinical and pathological study. *Ann Neurol* 1991; **29**: 139–146.

52. Stricker RB, Sanders KA, Owen WF, Kiprov DD, Miller RG. Mononeuritis multiplex associated with cryoglobulinemia in HIV infection. *Neurology* 1992; **42**: 2103–2105.

53. Kalayjian RC, Cohen ML, Bonomo RA, Flanigan TP. Cytomegalovirus ventriculoencephalitis in AIDS: a syndrome with distinct clinical and pathological features. *Medicine* 1993; **72**: 67–77.

54. Young S, Bom S, Lightman S. An unusual case of retinitis. *Lancet* 2000; **355**: 984.

55. Tucker T, Dix RD, Katzen C, Davis RL, Schmidley JW. Cytomegalovirus and herpes simplex virus ascending myelitis in a patient with acquired immune deficiency syndrome. *Ann Neurol* 1985; **18**: 74–79.

56. Tselis A, Lavi E. Cytomegalovirus infection of the adult nervous system. In: Davis LE, Kennedy PG, eds. *Infectious Diseases of the Nervous System*. Oxford: Butterworth-Heinemann, 2000: 109–137.

57. Cohen JI. Epstein–Barr virus infection. *N Engl J Med* 2000; **343**: 481–492.

58. Silverstein A, Steinberg G, Nathanson M. Nervous system involvement in infectious mononucleosis: the heralding and/or major manifestation. *Arch Neurol* 1972; **26**: 353–358.

59. Cleary TG, Henle W, Pickering LK. Acute cerebellar ataxia associated with Epstein–Barr virus infection. *JAMA* 1980; **243**: 148–149.

60. Leavell R, Ray CG, Ferry PC, Minich LL. Unusual acute neurological presentations with Epstein–Barr virus infection. *Arch Neurol* 1986; **43**: 186–188.

61. Friedland R, Yahr MD. Meningoencephalopathy secondary to infectious mononucleosis: unusual presentation with stupor and chorea. *Arch Neurol* 1977; **34**: 186–188.

62. Tolly TL, Wells RG, Sty JR. MR features of fleeting CNS lesions associated with Epstein–Barr virus infection. *J Comput Assist Tomogr* 1989; **13**: 665–668.

63. Donovan WD, Zimmermand RD. Case report: MRI findings of severe Epstein–Barr virus encephalomyelitis. *J Comput Assist Tomogr* 1996; **20**: 1027–1029.

64. Paskavitz JF, Anderson CA, Filley CM, Kleinschmidt-DeMasters BK, Tyler KL. Acute arcuate fiber demyelinating encephalopathy following Epstein–Barr virus infection. *Ann Neurol* 1995; **38**: 127–131.

65. Gruhn B, Meerbach A, Egerer R et al. Successful treatment of Epstein–Barr virus-induced transverse myelitis with gancyclovir and cytomegalovirus hyperimmune globulin following unrelated bone marrow transplantation. *Bone Marrow Transplant* 1999; **24**: 1355–1358.

66. Merelli E, Bedin R, Sola P et al. Encephalomyeloradiculopathy associated with Epstein–Barr virus: primary infection or reactivation? *Acta Neurol Scand* 1997; **96**: 416–420.

67. Kanda F, Uchida T, Jinnai K et al. Acute autonomic and sensory neuropathy: a case report. *J Neurol* 1990; **237**: 42–44.

68. Besnard M, Faure C, Fromont-Hankard G et al. Intestinal pseudo-obstruction and acute pandysautonomia associated with Epstein–Barr virus infection. *Am J Gastroenterol* 2000; **95**: 280–284.

69. Bennett JL, Mahalingam R, Wellish MC, Gilden DH. Epstein–Barr virus-associated acute autonomic neuropathy. *Ann Neurol* 1996; **40**: 453–455.

70. Salazar A, Martinez H, Sotelo J. Ophthalmoplegic polyneuropathy associated with infectious mononucleosis. *Ann Neurol* 1983; **13**: 219–220.

71. Brey RL. Ophthalmoplegic polyneuropathy: another case in association with Epstein–Barr virus. *Ann Neurol* 1984; **15**: 403.

72. Anderson MD, Kennedy CA, Lewis AW, Christensen GR. Retrobulbar neuritis complicating acute Epstein–Barr virus infection. *Clin Infect Dis* 1994; **18**: 799–801.

73. Jones J, Gardner W, Newman T. Severe optic neuritis in infectious mononucleosis. *Ann Emerg Med* 1988; **17**: 361–364.

74. Yamanishi K, Okuno T, Shiraki K et al. Identification of human herpesvirus-6 as a causal agent for exanthem subitum. *Lancet* 1988; **1**: 1065–1067.

75. Asano Y, Yoshikawa T, Kajita Y et al. Fatal encephalitis/encephalopathy in primary human herpesvirus-6 infection. *Arch Dis Child* 1992; **67**: 1484–1485.

76. McCullers JA, Lakeman FD, Whitley RJ. Human herpesvirus 6 is associated with focal encephalitis. *Clin Infect Dis* 1995; **21**: 571–576.

77. Mackenzie IR, Carrigan DR, Wiley CA. Chronic myelopathy associated with human herpesvirus-6. *Neurology* 1995; **45**: 2015–2017.

78. Carrigan DR, Harrington D, Knox KK. Subacute leukoencephalitis caused by CNS infection with human herpesvirus-6 manifesting as acute multiple sclerosis. *Neurology* 1996; **47**: 145–148.

79. Merelli E, Bedin R, Sola P et al. Human herpes virus 6 and human herpes virus 8 DNA sequences in brains of multiple sclerosis patients, normal adults and children. *J Neurol* 1997; **244**: 450–454.

80. Mock DJ, Powers JM, Goodman AD et al. Association of human herpesvirus 6 with the demyelinative lesions of progressive multifocal leukoencephalopathy. *J Neurovirol* 1999; **5**: 363–373.

81. Mookerjee BP, Vogelsang G. Human herpes virus-6 encephalitis after bone marrow transplantation: successful treatment with ganciclovir. *Bone Marrow Transplant* 1997; **20**: 905–906.

82. Bethge W, Beck R, Jahn G et al. Successful treatment of human herpesvirus-6 encephalitis after bone marrow transplantation. *Bone Marrow Transplant* 1999; **24**: 1245–1248.

83. Torigoe S, Koide W, Yamada M, Miyashiro E, Tanaka-Taya K, Yamanishi K. Human herpesvirus 7 infection associated with central nervous system manifestations. *J Pediatr* 1996; **129**: 301–305.

84. Said JW, Tasaka T, de Vos S, Koeffler HP. Kaposi's sarcoma-associated herpesvirus/human herpesvirus type 8 encephalitis in HIV-positive and -negative individuals. *AIDS* 1997; **11**: 1119–1122.

85. Wiselka MJ, Nicholson KG, Ward SC, Flower AJ. Acute infection with human immunodeficiency virus associated with facial nerve palsy and neuralgia. *J Infect* 1987; **15**: 189–190.

86. Denning DW, Anderson J, Ridge P, Smith H. Acute myelopathy with primary infection with human immunodeficiency virus. *BMJ* 1987; **294**: 143–144.

87. Elder G, Dalakas M, Pezeshkpour G, Sever J. Ataxic neuropathy due to ganglioneuronitis after probable acute human immunodeficiency virus infections. *Lancet* 1986; **2**: 1275–1276.

88. Berger JR, Bender A, Resnick L, Perlmutter D. Spinal myoclonus associated with HTLV-III/LAV infection. *Arch Neurol* 1986; **43**: 1203–1204.

89. Hollander H, McGuire D, Burack JH. Diagnostic lumbar puncture in HIV-infected patients: analysis of 138 cases. *Am J Med* 1994; **96**: 223–228.

90. Navia BA, Price RW. The acquired immunodeficiency syndrome dementia complex as the presenting or sole manifestation of human immunodeficiency virus infection. *Arch Neurol* 1987; **44**: 65–69.

91. McArthur JC, Sacktor N, Selnes O. Human immunodeficiency virus-associated dementia. *Semin Neurol* 1999; **19**: 129–150.

92. McArthur JC, Hoover DR, Bacellar H et al. Dementia in AIDS patients: incidence and risk factors. Multicenter AIDS Cohort Study. *Neurology* 1993; **43**: 2245–2252.

93. Di Sclafani V, Mackay RD, Meyerhoff DJ, Norman D, Weiner MW, Fein G. Brain atrophy in HIV infection is more strongly associated with CDC clinical stage than with cognitive impairment. *J Int Neuropsychol Soc* 1997; **3**: 276–287.

94. Gisslen M, Norkrans G, Svennerholm B, Hagberg L. The effect on human immunodeficiency virus type 1 RNA levels in cerebrospinal fluid after initiation of zidovudine or didanosine. *J Infect Dis* 1997; **175**: 434–437.

95. Foudraine NA, Hoetelmans RM, Lange JM et al. Cerebrospinal-fluid HIV-1 RNA and drug concentrations

after treatment with lamivudine plus zidovudine or stavudine. *Lancet* 1998; **351**: 1547–1551.

96. Gendelman HE, Zheng J, Coulter CL et al. Suppression of inflammatory neurotoxins by highly active antiretroviral therapy in human immunodeficiency virus-associated dementia. *J Infect Dis* 1998; **178**: 1000–1007.

97. Maschke M, Kastrup O, Esser S, Ross B, Hengge U, Hufnagel A. Incidence and prevalence of neurological disorders associated with HIV since the introduction of highly active antiretroviral therapy (HAART). *J Neurol Neurosurg Psychiatry* 2000; **69**: 376–380.

98. d'Arminio Monforte A, Duca PG, Vago L, Grassi MP, Moroni M. Decreasing incidence of CNS AIDS-defining events associated with antiretroviral therapy. *Neurology* 2000; **54**: 1856–1859.

99. Sacktor NC, Skolasky RL, Lyles RH, Esposito D, Selnes OA, McArthur JC. Improvement in HIV-associated motor slowing after antiretroviral therapy including protease inhibitors. *J Neurovirol* 2000; **6**: 84–88.

100. Thurnher MM, Schindler EG, Thurnher SA, Pernerstorfer-Schon H, Kleibl-Popov C, Rieger A. Highly active antiretroviral therapy for patients with AIDS dementia complex: effect on MR imaging findings and clinical course. *Am J Neuroradiol* 2000; **21**: 670–678.

101. Schifitto G, Sacktor N, Marder K et al. Randomized trial of the platelet-activating factor antagonist lexipafant in HIV-associated cognitive impairment. Neurological AIDS Research Consortium. *Neurology* 1999; **53**: 391–396.

102. Dal Pan GJ, Glass JD, McArthur JC. Clinicopathologic correlations of HIV-1-associated vacuolar myelopathy: an autopsy-based case–control study. *Neurology* 1994; **44**: 2159–2164.

103. Tan SV, Guiloff RJ, Scaravilli F. AIDS-associated vacuolar myelopathy: a morphometric study. *Brain* 1995; **118**: 1247–1261.

104. Di Rocco A, Tagliati M, Danisi F, Dorfman D, Moise J, Simpson DM. A pilot study of L-methionine for the treatment of AIDS-associated myelopathy. *Neurology* 1998; **51**: 266–268.

105. Qureshi AI, Janssen RS, Karon JM et al. Human immunodeficiency virus infection and stroke in young patients. *Arch Neurol* 1997; **54**: 1150–1153.

106. Engstrom JW, Lowenstein DH, Bredesen DE. Cerebral infarctions and transient neurological deficits associated with acquired immunodeficiency syndrome. *Am J Med* 1989; **86**: 528–532.

107. Visudtibhan A, Visudhiphan P, Chiemchanya S. Stroke and seizures as the presenting sign of HIV infection. *Pediatr Neurol* 1999; **20**: 53–56.

108. Wulff EA, Simpson DM. Neuromuscular complications of the human immunodeficiency virus type 1 infection. *Semin Neurol* 1999; **19**: 157–164.

109. Corral I, Quereda C, Casado JL et al. Acute polyradiculopathies in HIV-infected patients. *J Neurol* 1997; **244**: 499–504.

110. Husstedt IW, Evers S, Reichelt D et al. Screening for HIV-associated distal-symmetric polyneuropathy in CDC-classification stages 1, 2, and 3. *Acta Neurol Scand* 2000; **101**: 183–187.

111. Dorfman D, Dalton A, Khan A et al. Treatment of painful distal sensory polyneuropathy in HIV-infected patients with a topical agent: results of an open-label trial of 5% lidocaine gel. *AIDS* 1999; **13**: 1589–1590.

112. Becker K, Gorlach I, Frieling T, Haussinger D. Characterization and natural course of cardiac autonomic nervous dysfunction in HIV-infected patients. *AIDS* 1997; **11**: 751–757.

113. Welby SB, Rogerson SJ, Beeching NJ. Autonomic neuropathy is common in human immunodeficiency virus infection. *J Infect* 1991; **23**: 123–128.

114. Cohen JA, Miller L, Polish L. Orthostatic hypotension in human immunodeficiency virus infection may be the result of generalized autonomic nervous system dysfunction. *J Acquir Immune Defic Syndr* 1991; **4**: 31–33.

115. Gherardi RK, Chretien F, Delfau-Larue MH et al. Neuropathy in diffuse infiltrative lymphocytosis syndrome: an HIV neuropathy, not a lymphoma. *Neurology* 1998; **50**: 1041–1044.

116. Moulignier A, Authier FJ, Baudrimont M et al. Peripheral neuropathy in human immunodeficiency-virus-infected patients with the diffuse infiltrative lymphocytosis syndrome. *Ann Neurol* 1997; **41**: 438–445.

117. Fuster M, Negredo E, Cadafalch J, Domingo P, Illa I, Clave P. HIV-associated polymyositis with life-threatening myocardial and esophageal involvement. *Arch Intern Med* 1999; **159**: 1012.

118. Dalakas MC, Illa I, Pezeshkpour GH, Laukaitis JP, Cohen B, Griffin JL. Mitochondrial myopathy caused by long-term zidovudine therapy. *N Engl J Med* 1990; **322**: 1098–1105.

119. Berger JR, Kaszovitz B, Post MJ, Dickinson G. Progressive multifocal leukoencephalopathy associated with human immunodeficiency virus infection: a review of the literature with a report of sixteen cases. *Ann Intern Med* 1987; **107**: 78–87.

120. Brown P, Tsai T, Gajdusek C. Seroepidemiology of human papovaviruses. *Am J Epidemiol* 1975; **102**: 331–340.

121. Blake K, Pillay D, Knowles W, Brown DW, Griffiths PD, Taylor B. JC virus associated meningoencephalitis in an immunocompetent girl. *Arch Dis Child* 1992; **67**: 956–957.

122. Weber T, Turner RW, Frye S et al. Specific diagnosis of progressive multifocal leukoencephalopathy by polymerase chain reaction. *J Infect Dis* 1994; **169**: 1138–1141.

123. Inui K, Miyagawa H, Sashihara J et al. Remission of progressive multifocal leukoencephalopathy following highly active antiretroviral therapy in a patient with HIV infection. *Brain Dev* 1999; **21**: 416–419.

124. Brambilla AM, Castagna A, Novati R et al. Remission of AIDS-associated progressive multifocal leukoencephalopathy after cidofovir therapy. *J Neurol* 1999; **246**: 723–725.

125. Tantisiriwat W, Tebas P, Clifford DB, Powderly WG, Fichtenbaum CJ. Progressive multifocal leukoencephalopathy in patients with AIDS receiving highly active antiretroviral therapy. *Clin Infect Dis* 1999; **28**: 1152–1154.

126. Weiner SM, Laubenberger J, Muller K, Schneider J, Kreisel W. Fatal course of HIV-associated progressive multifocal leukoencephalopathy despite successful highly active antiretroviral therapy. *J Infect* 2000; **40**: 100–102.

127. Taoufik Y, Delfraissy JF, Gasnault J. Highly active antiretroviral therapy does not improve survival of patients with high JC virus load in the cerebrospinal

fluid at progressive multifocal leukoencephalopathy diagnosis. *AIDS* 2000; **14**: 758–759.

128. Flood JM, Weinstock HS, Guroy ME, Bayne L, Simon RP, Bolan G. Neurosyphilis during the AIDS epidemic, San Francisco, 1985–1992. *J Infect Dis* 1998; **177**: 931–940.

129. Singh AE, Romanowski B. Syphilis: review with emphasis on clinical, epidemiologic, and some biologic features. *Clin Microbiol Rev* 1999; **12**: 187–209.

130. Tyler KL, Sandberg E, Baum KF. Medial medullary syndrome and meningovascular syphilis: a case report in an HIV-infected man and a review of the literature. *Neurology* 1994; **44**: 2231–2235.

131. Berger JR. Spinal cord syphilis associated with human immunodeficiency virus infection: a treatable myelopathy. *Am J Med* 1992; **92**: 101–103.

132. Horowitz HW, Valsamis MP, Wicher V et al. Brief report: cerebral syphilitic gumma confirmed by the polymerase chain reaction in a man with human immunodeficiency virus infection. *N Engl J Med* 1994; **331**: 1488–1491.

133. Centers for Disease Control and Prevention. 1998 guidelines for the treatment of sexually transmitted diseases. *MMWR* 1998; **47**: 28–49.

134. Malone JL, Wallace MR, Hendrick BB et al. Syphilis and neurosyphilis in a human immunodeficiency virus type-1 seropositive population: evidence for frequent serologic relapse after therapy. *Am J Med* 1995; **99**: 55–63.

135. Shafer RW, Edlin BR. Tuberculosis in patients infected with the human immunodeficiency virus: perspective on the past decade. *Clin Infect Dis* 1996; **22**: 683–704.

136. Lesprit P, Zagdanski AM, de La Blanchardiere A et al. Cerebral tuberculosis in patients with the acquired immunodeficiency syndrome (AIDS): report of 6 cases and review. *Medicine* 1997; **76**: 423–431.

137. Whiteman M, Espinoza L, Post MJ, Bell MD, Falcone S. Central nervous system tuberculosis in HIV-infected patients: clinical and radiographic findings. *Am J Neuroradiol* 1995; **16**: 1319–1327.

138. Woolsey RM, Chambers TJ, Chung HD, McGarry JD. Mycobacterial meningomyelitis associated with human immunodeficiency virus infection. *Arch Neurol* 1988; **45**: 691–693.

139. Malessa R, Diener HC, Olbricht T, Bohmer B, Brockmeyer NH. Successful treatment of meningoencephalitis caused by *Mycobacterium avium intracellulare* in AIDS. *Clin Invest* 1994; **72**: 850–852.

140. Zakowski P, Fligiel S, Berlin GW, Johnson L Jr. Disseminated *Mycobacterium avium-intracellulare* infection in homosexual men dying of acquired immunodeficiency. *JAMA* 1982; **248**: 2980–2982.

141. Dwork AJ, Chin S, Boyce L. Intracerebral *Mycobacterium avium-intracellulare* in a child with acquired immunodeficiency syndrome. *Pediatr Infect Dis J* 1994; **13**: 1149–1151.

142. Girgis NI, Sultan Y, Farid Z et al. Tuberculosis meningitis, Abbassia Fever Hospital—Naval Medical Research Unit No. 3—Cairo, Egypt, from 1976 to 1996. *Am J Trop Med Hyg* 1998; **58**: 28–34.

143. Jurado RL, Farley MM, Pereira E et al. Increased risk of meningitis and bacteremia due to *Listeria monocytogenes* in patients with human immunodeficiency virus infection. *Clin Infect Dis* 1993; **17**: 224–227.

144. Decker CF, Simon GL, DiGioia RA, Tuazon CU. *Listeria monocytogenes* infections in patients with AIDS:

report of five cases and review. *Rev Infect Dis* 1991; **13**: 413–417.

145. Lorber B. Listeriosis. *Clin Infect Dis* 1997; **24**: 1–11.

146. Adair JC, Beck AC, Apfelbaum RI, Baringer JR. Nocardial cerebral abscess in the acquired immunodeficiency syndrome. *Arch Neurol* 1987; **44**: 548–550.

147. LeBlang SD, Whiteman ML, Post MJ, Uttamchandani RB, Bell MD, Smirniotopolous JG. CNS nocardia in AIDS patients: CT and MRI with pathologic correlation. *J Comput Assist Tomogr* 1995; **19**: 15–22.

148. Holtz HA, Lavery DP, Kapila R. Actinomycetales infection in the acquired immunodeficiency syndrome. *Ann Intern Med* 1985; **102**: 203–205.

149. Lerner PI. Nocardiosis. *Clin Infect Dis* 1996; **22**: 891–903.

150. Darras-Joly C, Chevret S, Wolff M et al. *Cryptococcus neoformans* infection in France: epidemiologic features of and early prognostic parameters for 76 patients who were infected with human immunodeficiency virus. *Clin Infect Dis* 1996; **23**: 369–376.

151. Saag MS, Graybill RJ, Larsen RA et al. Practice guidelines for the management of cryptococcal disease. Infectious Diseases Society of America. *Clin Infect Dis* 2000; **30**: 710–718.

152. Levy RM, Pons VG, Rosenblum ML. Central nervous system mass lesions in the acquired immunodeficiency syndrome (AIDS). *J Neurosurg* 1984; **61**: 9–16.

153. Fish DG, Ampel NM, Galgiani JN et al. Coccidioidomycosis during human immunodeficiency virus infection: a review of 77 patients. *Medicine* 1990; **69**: 384–391.

154. Knapp S, Turnherr M, Dekan G, Willinger B, Stingl G, Rieger A. A case of HIV-associated cerebral histoplasmosis successfully treated with fluconazole. *Eur J Clin Microbiol Infect Dis* 1999; **18**: 658–661.

155. Micozzi MS, Wetli CV. Intravenous amphetamine abuse, primary cerebral mucormycosis and acquired immunodeficiency. *J Forensic Sci* 1985; **30**: 504–510.

156. Denning DW, Stevens DA. Antifungal and surgical treatment of invasive aspergillosis: review of 2,121 published cases. *Rev Infect Dis* 1990; **12**: 1147–1201.

157. Cohen BA. Neurologic manifestations of toxoplasmosis in AIDS. *Semin Neurol* 1999; **19**: 201–211.

158. Navia BA, Petito CK, Gold JW, Cho ES, Jordan BD, Price RW. Cerebral toxoplasmosis complicating the acquired immune deficiency syndrome: clinical and neuropathological findings in 27 patients. *Ann Neurol* 1986; **19**: 224–238.

159. Contini C, Fainardi E, Cultrera R et al. Advanced laboratory techniques for diagnosing *Toxoplasma gondii* encephalitis in AIDS patients: significance of intrathecal production and comparison with PCR and ECL-western blotting. *J Neuroimmunol* 1998; **92**: 29–37.

160. USPHS/IDSA Prevention of Opportunistic Infections Working Group. 1999 USPHS/IDSA guidelines for the prevention of opportunistic infections in persons infected with human immunodeficiency virus. *Clin Infect Dis* 2000; **30**(suppl 1): S29–S65.

161. Gilbert DN, Moellering RC, Sande MA eds. *The Sanford Guide to Antimicrobial Therapy.* Hyde Park, VT: Antimicrobial Therapy, 1999: 92.

162. Mayayo E, Vidal F, Alvira R, Gonzalez J, Richart C. Cerebral *Pneumocystis carinii* infection in AIDS. *Lancet* 1990; **336**: 1592.

163. Villanueva JL, Cordero E, Caballero-Granado FJ, Regordan C, Becerril B, Pachon J. *Pneumocystis carinii*

meningoradiculitis in a patient with AIDS. *Eur J Clin Microbiol Infect Dis* 1997; **16**: 940–942.

164. Bartlett JA, Hulette C. Central nervous system pneumocystis in a patient with AIDS. *Clin Infect Dis* 1997; **25**: 82–85.

165. Northfelt DW, Clement MJ, Safrin S. Extrapulmonary pneumocystis: clinical features in human immunodeficiency virus infection. *Medicine* 1990; **69**: 392–398.

166. Ciacci JD, Tellez C, VonRoenn J, Levy RM. Lymphoma of the central nervous system in AIDS. *Semin Neurol* 1999; **19**: 213–221.

167. Lanska DJ. Epidemiology of human immunodeficiency virus infection and associated neurologic illness. *Semin Neurol* 1999; **19**: 105–111.

168. Aboulafia D. Epidemiology and pathogenesis of AIDS-related lymphomas. *Oncology* 1998; **12**: 1068–1081.

169. Jack CR Jr, O'Neill BP, Banks PM, Reese DF. Central nervous system lymphoma: histologic types and CT appearance. *Radiology* 1988; **167**: 211–215.

170. Antinori A, De Rossi G, Ammassari A et al. Value of combined approach with thallium-201 single-photon emission computed tomography and Epstein–Barr virus DNA polymerase chain reaction in CSF for the diagnosis of AIDS-related primary CNS lymphoma. *J Clin Oncol* 1999; **17**: 554–560.

171. Enting RH, Esselink RA, Portegies P. Lymphomatous meningitis in AIDS-related systemic non-Hodgkin's lymphoma: a report of eight cases. *J Neurol Neurosurg Psychiatry* 1994; **57**: 150–153.

172. Levy RM, Bredesen DE, Rosenblum MC. Neurological manifestations of the acquired immunodeficiency syndrome (AIDS): experience at UCSF and review of the literature. *J Neurosurg* 1985; **62**: 475–495.

173. Moore PS, Chang Y. Detection of herpesvirus-like DNA sequences in Kaposi's sarcoma in patients with and without HIV infection. *N Engl J Med* 1995; **332**: 1181–1185.

174. Ariza A, Kim JH. Kaposi's sarcoma of the dura mater. *Hum Pathol* 1988; **19**: 1461–1463.

175. Buttner A, Marquart KH, Mehraein P, Weis S. Kaposi's sarcoma in the cerebellum of a patient with AIDS. *Clin Neuropathol* 1997; **16**: 185–189.

176. Sparano JA, Anand K, Desai J, Mitnick RJ, Kalkut GE, Hanaie LH. Effect of highly active antiretroviral therapy on the incidence of HIV-associated malignancies at an urban medical center. *J Acquir Immune Defic Syndr* 1999; **21**(suppl 1): S18–S22.

177. Dezube BJ. Acquired immunodeficiency syndrome-related Kaposi's sarcoma: clinical features, staging, and treatment. *Semin Oncol* 2000; **27**: 424–430.

178. Cabre P, Smadja O, Cabie A, Newton CR. HTLV-1 and HIV infections of the central nervous system in tropical areas. *J Neurol Neurosurg Psychiatry* 2000; **68**: 550–557.

179. Gomes I, Melo A, Proletti FA et al. Human T lymphotropic virus type I (HTLV-I) infection in neurological patients in Salvador, Bahia, Brazil. *J Neurol Sci* 1999; **165**: 84–89.

180. Romero IA, Prevost MC, Perret E et al. Interactions between brain endothelial cells and human T-cell leukemia virus type 1-infected lymphocytes: mechanisms of viral entry into the central nervous system. *J Virol* 2000; **74**: 6021–6030.

181. Wilfert CM, Lehrman SN, Katz SL. Enteroviruses and meningitis. *Pediatr Infect Dis* 1983; **2**: 333–341.

182. Malcom BS, Eiden JJ, Hendley JO. ECHO virus type 9 meningitis simulating tuberculous meningitis. *Pediatrics* 1980; **66**: 725–726.

183. Rotbart HA, Levin MJ, Villarreal LP. Use of subgenomic poliovirus DNA hybridization probes to detect the major subgroups of enteroviruses. *J Clin Microbiol* 1984; **20**: 1105–1108.

184. McKinney RE Jr, Katz SL, Wilfert CM. Chronic enteroviral meningoencephalitis in agammaglobulinemic patients. *Rev Infect Dis* 1987; **9**: 334–356.

185. Geller TJ, Condie D. A case of protracted coxsackie virus meningoencephalitis in a marginally immunodeficient child treated successfully with intravenous immunoglobulin. *J Neurol Sci* 1995; **129**: 131–133.

186. Kuban KC, Ephros MA, Freeman FL, Laffell LB, Bresnan MJ. Syndrome of opsoclonus-myoclonus caused by Coxsackie B3 infection. *Ann Neurol* 1983; **13**: 69–71.

187. Huang CC, Liu CC, Chang YC, Chen CY, Want ST, Yeh TF. Neurologic complications in children with enterovirus 71 infection. *N Engl J Med* 1999; **341**: 936–942.

188. da Silva EE, Winkler MT, Pallansch MA. Role of enterovirus 71 in acute flaccid paralysis after the eradication of poliovirus in Brazil. *Emerg Infect Dis* 1996; **2**: 231–233.

189. Johnson R. Meningitis, encephalitis and poliomyelitis. In: Johnson R. *Viral Infections of the Nervous System.* New York: Raven Press, 1999: 87–132.

190. Rosenberg RN, Chadwick DL. Oral-facial dyskinesias and quadriplegia associated with poliomyelitis virus type 3. *Am J Dis Child* 1973; **126**: 699–700.

191. Azimi PH, Shaban S, Hilty MD, Haynes RE. Mumps meningoencephalitis: prolonged abnormality of cerebrospinal fluid. *JAMA* 1975; **234**: 1161–1162.

192. Vaheri A, Julkunen I, Koskiniemi ML. Chronic encephalomyelitis with specific increase in intrathecal mumps antibodies. *Lancet* 1982; **2**: 685–688.

193. Horner FA. Neurologic disorders after Asian influenza. *N Engl J Med* 1958; **258**: 983–985.

194. Estrin WJ. The serological diagnosis of St. Louis encephalitis in a patient with the syndrome of opsoclonia, body tremulousness and benign encephalitis. *Ann Neurol* 1977; **1**: 596–598.

195. Kaplan AM, Koveleski JT. St. Louis encephalitis with particular involvement of the brain stem. *Arch Neurol* 1978; **35**: 45–46.

196. Brinker KR, Paulson G, Monath TP, Wise G, Fass RJ. St. Louis encephalitis in Ohio, September 1975: clinical and EEG studies in 16 cases. *Arch Intern Med* 1979; **139**: 561–566.

197. Schultz DR, Barthal JS, Garrett C. Western equine encephalitis with rapid onset of parkinsonism. *Neurology* 1977; **27**: 1095–1096.

198. Earnest MP, Goolishian HA, Calverley JR, Hayse RO, Hill HR. Neurologic, intellectual, and psychologic sequelae following western encephalitis. A follow-up study of 35 cases. *Neurology* 1971; **21**: 969–974.

199. Balfour HH Jr, Siem RA, Bauer H, Quie PG. California arbovirus (La Crosse) infections. I. Clinical and laboratory findings in 66 children with meningoencephalitis. *Pediatrics* 1973; **52**: 680–691.

200. Feemster RF. Equine encephalitis in Massachusetts. *N Engl J Med* 1957; **257**: 701–704.

201. Deresiewicz RL, Thaler SJ, Hsu L, Zamani AA. Clinical and neuroradiographic manifestations of eastern equine encephalitis. *N Engl J Med* 1997; **336**: 1867–1874.

202. Johnson RT, Burke DS, Elwell M et al. Japanese encephalitis: immunocytochemical studies of viral antigen and inflammatory cells in fatal cases. *Ann Neurol* 1985; **18**: 567–573.

203. Bale JF Jr. Viral encephalitis. *Med Clin North Am* 1993; **77**: 25–42.

204. Hoke CH, Nisalak A, Sangawhipa N et al. Protection against Japanese encephalitis by inactivated vaccines. *N Engl J Med* 1988; **319**: 608–614.

205. Meyer HM Jr, Johnson RT, Crawford IP, Dascomb HE, Rogers NG. Central nervous system syndromes of 'viral' etiology: a study of 713 cases. *Am J Med* 1960; **29**: 334–347.

206. Simila S, Jouppila R, Salmi A, Pohjonen R. Encephalomeningitis in children associated with an adenovirus type 7 epidemic. *Acta Paediatr Scand* 1970; **59**: 310–316.

207. Chou SM, Roos R, Burrell R, Gutmann L, Harley JB. Subacute focal adenovirus encephalitis. *J Neuropathol Exp Neurol* 1973; **32**: 34–50.

208. Lews JM, Utz JP. Orchitis, parotitis and meningo-encephalitis due to lymphocytic–choriomeningitis virus. *N Engl J Med* 1961; **265**: 776–780.

209. Schanen A, Gallou G, Hincky JM, Saron MF. A rash, circulating anticoagulant, then meningitis. *Lancet* 1998; **351**: 1856.

210. Cummins D, McCormick JB, Bennett D et al. Acute sensorineural deafness in Lassa fever. *JAMA* 1990; **264**: 2093–2096.

211. Child PL, MacKenzie RB, Valverde LR, Johnson KM. Bolivian hemorrhagic fever: a pathologic description. *Arch Pathol* 1967; **83**: 434–445.

212. Salas R, de Manzione N, Tesh RB et al. Venezuelan haemorrhagic fever. *Lancet* 1991; **338**: 1033–1036.

213. Lisieux T, Coimbra TLM, Nassar ES et al. New arenavirus isolated in Brazil. *Lancet* 1994; **343**: 391–392.

214. Bratt G, Hammarin AL, Grandien M et al. BK virus as the cause of meningoencephalitis, retinitis and nephritis in a patient with AIDS. *AIDS* 1999; **13**: 1071–1075.

215. Elsner C, Dorries K. Evidence of human poliomavirus BK and JC infection in normal brain tissue. *Virology* 1992; **191**: 72–80.

216. Voltz R, Jager G, Seelos K, Fuhry L, Hohlfeld R. BK virus encephalitis in an immunocompetent patient. *Arch Neurol* 1996; **53**: 101–103.

217. Koduri PR, Naides SJ. Aseptic meningitis caused by parvovirus B19. *Clin Infect Dis* 1995; **21**: 1053.

218. Watanabe T, Satoh M, Oda Y. Human parvovirus B19 encephalopathy. Arch Dis Child 1994; **70**: 71.

219. Sanchez A, Ksiazek TG, Rollin PE et al. Reemergence of Ebola virus in Africa. *Emerg Infect Dis* 1995; **1**: 96–97.

220. Lewis P, Fu Y, Lentz TL. Rabies virus entry at the neuromuscular junction in nerve–muscle cocultures. *Muscle Nerve* 2000; **23**: 720–730.

221. Advisory Committee on Immunization Practices (ACIP). Human rabies prevention—United States, 1999. *MMWR* 2000; **49**(RR-8): 21–30.

222. Norrby E, Kristensson K. Measles virus in the brain. *Brain Res Bull* 1997; **44**: 213–220.

223. Gendelman HE, Wolinski JS, Johnson RT, Pressman RT, Pezeshkpour GH, Boisset GF. Measles encephalitis: lack of evidence of viral invasion of the central nervous system and quantitative study of the nature of demyelination. *Ann Neurol* 1984; **15**: 353–360.

224. Masliah E, DeTeresa RM, Mallory ME, Hansen LA. Changes in pathological findings at autopsy in AIDS cases for the last 15 years. *AIDS* 2000; **14**: 69–74.

225. Marra CM. Bacterial and fungal brain infections in AIDS. *Semin Neurol* 1999; **19**: 177–184.

15

Chronic fatigue syndrome and systemic viral infections: current evidence and recent advances

Abhijit Chaudhuri, John Gow and Peter O Behan

INTRODUCTION

Chronic fatigue syndrome (CFS) is a common, potentially disabling condition characterized by the symptoms of overwhelming, relapsing or persistent fatigue in the absence of any other concurrent medical and psychiatric illnesses. This is not a new disease. In the earlier part of the past century, similar illness was recognized in the epidemic forms that was preceded, or followed closely, by attacks of poliovirus infection in the community. It is the sporadic form of the disease that is now common. A significant proportion of current cases, but not all, show evidence of viral infection at the onset of their illness (post-viral fatigue syndrome).[1] There is no real difference in the symptom complex and the natural history of illness between the post-viral and non-viral groups of patients with CFS. From the clinical perspective, the segregation of the post-viral group of CFS patients does not appear to serve any useful purpose. For both diagnosis and research purposes, current CFS case definitions must satisfy the modified CDC criteria (Table 15.1).[2]

FATIGUE AS A SYMPTOM IN CFS

CFS is a true syndrome, not a single disease. As with other neurological syndromes (Parkinsonian, Guillain–Barré or carpal tunnel), the etio-pathogenesis of CFS is diverse, probably multifactorial, with stress and systemic viral infections being the two commonest factors.[3] However, irrespective of the precise pathogenic mechanism of CFS, fatigue symptoms are very similar across all CFS patients and are indistinguishable from the symptoms of fatigue experienced by patients with certain neuro-

logical disorders such as multiple sclerosis (MS) or Parkinson's disease.[4] Fatigue symptoms in MS are very similar to CFS, and there is additional evidence to support a common pathophysiology of fatigue in both these disorders.[5,6] In addition, both MS and CFS patients with fatigue have a significantly lower frequency of psychiatric diagnosis than the depressed controls.[7]

Although fatigue is a common symptom in many diseases encountered in clinical practice (Tables 15.2 and 15.3), its definition and objective evaluation have always been difficult. The physiological definition of fatigue, which is the inability to sustain a specified force output or work rate during exercise, has often been termed 'objective fatigue'.[8] Neuromuscular disorders like myasthenia gravis and metabolic myopathies are the best examples of this type of fatigue. To date, there is insufficient neurophysiological evidence of peripheral neuromuscular failure (involving peripheral nerves, neuromuscular junction or muscles) as the cause of persistent fatigue in CFS patients.[9] Current evidence strongly supports a dominant central mechanism of fatigue in CFS,[10–12] and the oxidative defects in muscle metabolism earlier observed in these patients are likely to be due to impaired bloodflow to the exercising muscles,[13] as a result of dysregulated autonomic control.[14,15] The majority of CFS patients show poor attention span, difficulty in concentration and mild cognitive impairment,[16] supporting the role of an important central mechanism for fatigue in CFS. The specific nature of the central nervous system pathology in CFS has, however, remained elusive. Post-mortem studies of brain in the epidemic or occasional sporadic cases of CFS have not shown any specific diagnostic pathology. Comparison with other neurological disorders

Table 15.1   Modified Centers for Disease Control (CDC) criteria for the diagnosis of CFS

Patients must fulfill the major criteria and four or more minor criteria.[2]

Major criteria:

Clinically evaluated, unexplained, persistent or relapsing chronic fatigue that is of new or definite onset (has not been lifelong); is not the result of ongoing exertion; is not substantially relieved by rest; and results in substantial reduction in previous levels of occupational, educational, social or personal activities; and

Minor criteria:

The concurrent occurrence of four or more of the following symptoms, all of which must have persisted or recurred during six or more consecutive months of the illness and must not have pre-dated the fatigue:

1. self-reported impairment in short-term memory or concentration severe enough to cause a substantial reduction in previous levels of occupational, educational, social or personal activities
2. sore throat
3. tender cervical or axillary lymph nodes
4. muscle pain
5. headaches of new type, pattern or severity
6. unrefreshing sleep
7. post-exertional malaise lasting more than 24 hours
8. multi-joint pain without joint swelling or redness

Other symptoms commonly reported (*not part of the diagnostic criteria*):
Alcohol intolerance, new-onset asthma, chest pain (syndrome X), attacks of sweating, irritable bowel syndrome, body weight changes, vertigo or dysequilibrium, orthostatic intolerance, poor attention span especially affecting the visuospatial tasks, delayed reaction time and difficulty in naming (anomia). The type of headache (a minor criterion) is very similar to migraine

Table 15.2   Classification of chronic fatigue disorders

Idiopathic chronic fatigue syndrome (*cause unknown*):
Defined by the modified CDC criteria in the absence of any other concurrent medical or psychiatric illnesses; symptoms must be present for 6 months or more

Symptomatic chronic fatigue (*secondary to other concurrent diseases*):
Symptoms of chronic fatigue may antedate or appear after the onset of illness; severity of underlying medical disorder may not parallel the severity of fatigue symptoms; fatigue may persist after apparent clinical recovery in many cases
Anaemia (all causes)
Autoimmune diseases and vasculitis (systemic lupus erythematosus, Sjögren's syndrome, giant cell arteritis)
Chronic systemic infection (e.g. HIV, bacterial endocarditis)
Chronic hepatocellular disease (cirrhosis)
Ciguatera fish poisoning
Depression
Drug induced (e.g. alcohol, sedatives, tranquillizers, interferon, HMG-CoA inhibitors)
Endocrine disorders (e.g. Addison's disease, hypothyroidism, hypopituitarism)
Fibromyalgia
Metabolic disorders (diabetes, haemachromatosis)
Neurological disorders (see Table 15.3)
Obesity
Overtrained athlete syndrome
Sarcoidosis
Sleep disorders
Systemic malignancy
Withdrawal syndromes from substance abuse (cocaine, benzodiazepines)

SYSTEMIC VIRAL INFECTIONS AND CFS

Systemic infections, commonly viral, are recognized precipitants for CFS symptoms.[17] The close proximity of poliovirus infection with epidemic CFS[18] (often called 'atypical poliomyelitis' in the literature) also suggested a possible link with viral infection. The symptoms of CFS are also very similar to the post-polio fatigue symptoms (PPFS), the commonest sequel of poliomyelitis.[19,20] There is a long list of

sharing symptoms of CFS-type fatigue suggests a dysfunction of the dopamine-dependent neostriatal–dorsolateral prefrontal network as the final pathway in the genesis of chronic fatigue symptoms.

Table 15.3 Neurological disorders causing symptomatic (secondary) fatigue not due to the peripheral neuromuscular or metabolic muscle dysfunction

Channelopathies

Developmental disorders: cerebral palsy, Chiari malformation

Dysautonomic states

Hypothalamic and pituitary diseases: tumours, granuloma

Intracranial hypertension (chronic)

Intracranial infections: meningitis, encephalitis, HIV encephalopathy

Metabolic and mitochondrial encephalopathy

Migraine

Multiple sclerosis

Neurodegenerative diseases: Parkinson's disease, multiple system atrophy, motor neurone disease, myotonic dystrophy

Paraneoplastic: limbic encephalitis, opsoclonus-myoclonus

Post-encephalitic Parkinsonism

Post-GBS fatigue

Post-viral fatigue, post-polio fatigue

Specific neurosurgery (posterior fossa surgery, pallidotomy)

Vascular diseases affecting prefrontal, subcortical and basal ganglia regions

Table 15.4 Viruses associated with the onset of initial illness leading to the subsequent development of idiopathic CFS

RNA viruses

Enteroviruses (Coxsackie, ECHO, polioviruses)

HTLV-II-related retroviruses

Influenza viruses

Borna disease virus (BDV)

DNA viruses

Herpesviruses (Epstein–Barr virus, cytomegalovirus, VZV, HSV, HHV_6)

'Stealth virus' (simian cytomegalovirus)

viruses associated with the aetiology and initiation of predisposing illness in CFS patients. These include both RNA and DNA (Table 15.4) viruses.[21–26] Research data to date have shown no significant association of the CFS population with any specific RNA viruses, including enteroviruses. Studies on DNA viruses have similarly failed to show any specific association with CFS. Overall, analysis of published data on virological studies show serological evidence of recent infection in less than 20% of patients at the time of, or following, the diagnosis of CFS. In contrast, 80% of patients have a history of 'viral' infection as the initial illness leading to the subsequent development of CFS. There is no single virus that is specific.

For years, the role of a persistent microbial infection as a cause of CFS symptoms has continued to generate research interest and public attention. Historically, both Epstein–Barr virus (EBV) (a DNA virus) and Coxsackie B virus (an RNA enterovirus) were associated with the epidemic outbreak of CFS

in the post-war period. The concept of a persistent systemic viral infection as a cause of CFS was first developed during the 1980s, following the reports of persistent fatiguing illness associated with serological evidence of EBV infection and the description of a cluster of cases in Incline Village, Nevada.[27] It was quickly discovered that EBV serologies did not discriminate outbreak cases from controls, a fact that was borne out in the subsequent studies.[28,29] Indeed, data from multiple studies on virus isolation, genomic detection and lymphocyte transformation generally show no difference between cases and the control population.[30,31] Apart from EBV, a variety of other causative viruses and infective agents have been proposed as models of persistent infection and fatigue in CFS, including enteroviruses, herpesviruses, retroviruses, animal (simian) cytomegalovirus ('stealth virus'), parvovirus, and borna disease-associated viruses (Table 15.5). Besides viruses, persistent systemic infection with *Rickettsia, Borrelia* or *Mycoplasma* has also been espoused as a cause of CFS symptoms.[32] The data regarding the role of bacterial infections in CFS are, however, very thin. There has been no controlled study to properly address the question of atypical

Table 15.5 Persistent virus infection in CFS: agents proposed but none proven

Enteroviruses

Retrovirus (related to HTLV-II)

Borna disease virus

Herpesviruses (EBV, CMV, HHV-6, VZV)

Table 15.6   Viruses known to produce persistent infections in humans

Rubella
Measles
Retroviruses (HIV and HTLV)
Herpesviruses
Papovaviruses
Adenoviruses
Hepatitis B and C

Table 15.7   Diseases postulated to be caused by persistent viral infections

Neurological diseases: MS, MND, AD, HIVE, HAM, SSPE, PRE, CFS and PPFS
Psychiatric diseases: schizophrenia, depression
Autoimmune diseases: SLE, RA, dermatomyositis, PAN
Cardiomyopathy
Crohn's disease
Diabetes
Neoplasms
Paget's disease

MS, multiple sclerosis; MND, motor neuron disease; AD, Alzheimer's disease; HIVE, human immunodeficiency virus-associated encephalopathy; HAM, human T-lymphotrophic virus-associated myelopathy; SSPE, subacute sclerosing panencephalitis; PRE, progressive rubella encephalopathy; CFS, chronic fatigue syndrome; PPFS, post-polio fatigue syndrome; SLE, systemic lupus erythematosus; RA, rheumatoid arthritis; PAN, polyarteritis nodosa.

Table 15.8   Differences between persistent and latent virus infections

Characteristics	Persistent infection	Latent infection
Production of infectious viruses	Yes	No
Viral nucleic acid detectable by in situ hybridization/PCR	Yes	Yes
Viral antigen detected by antibody	Yes	No
Host cell susceptibility to reinfection with the original virus	No	Not known
Potential for extensive virus replication after external stimuli	Not known	Yes

bacterial infection as the cause of CFS symptoms or whether such a phenomenon is merely the marker of an asymptomatic, commensal or opportunistic infection in CFS patients, who are known to have defective natural killer (NK) cell functioin.[33,34]

Certain viruses, however, are known to produce persistent infections in humans (Table 15.6). A number of diseases, including CFS, have been postulated to be caused by persistent viral infections (Table 15.7). In the search for a disease mechanism in CFS, however, it is important to remember that persistence of viruses and latent viral infections are not identical conditions (Table 15.8). It is clear that although an infectious agent is a prime candidate as a precipitant or trigger in the development of CFS, as yet there is no specific agent (bacterial or viral) that can be identified in the majority of patient samples. Despite numerous attempts at viral culture (and success only in a few isolated cases), no conclusive data have emerged. It is nevertheless not inconceivable that the host immune system in CFS is subtly disrupted (suggested by many reports on abnormal NK cell function), and this, in turn, may allow reactivation of common latent viruses such as the herpesvirus family (EBV and HHV$_6$) and also prevent the clearance of endemic viruses such as enteroviruses with normal efficiency. How significant these consequences are in the persistent symptoms of fatigue in CFS is, however, debatable. In this context, it may be relevant to compare the observations made in patients with sarcoidosis, a cause of symptomatic chronic fatigue (Table 15.2). Sarcoidosis patients with fatigue often show extremely high levels of antibodies to herpes-like viruses and EBV that decrease when fatigue subsides, often spontaneously.[35] The significance of possible reactivation of latent viruses awaits a better understanding of the fatigue mechanism in CFS.

CURRENT STATUS OF ANTI-INFECTIVE AND IMMUNE-MODIFYING THERAPY IN CFS

Recent claims have been made about therapeutic successes in CFS patients using long courses of potentially toxic antibiotics[36] and also with the use of immune-modifiers that have putative effects on intracellular antiviral pathways.[37] While 'active' intracellular bacterial infections, e.g. Lyme disease and tuberculosis, can certainly cause chronic fatigue as one of the common symptoms of systemic infections (secondary or symptomatic CFS), the patient with an active bacterial infection does not have CFS by definition, since a confident diagnosis of CFS can only be made after exclusion of all systemic medical causes (Table 15.2). However, unlike antiviral therapy in CFS (although newer antivirals such as pleconaril have not been tested), there has been anecdotal evidence of improvement in a small proportion of CFS patients treated with specific macrolide antibiotics (typically doxycycline, erythromycin or clarithromycin). During the outbreaks of neuromyasthenia in the 1960s, chloramphenicol, another macrolide antibiotic, was believed to be effective in some patients.[38] We do not yet know if this antibiotic-responsive CFS population represents a true cohort of 'chronically' infected patients (and hence cannot be considered as primary CFS by CDC case definition) or whether the antibiotic-associated improvement in fatigue symptoms seen in these patients is related to other pharmacological effects of macrolide antibiotics (i.e. anti-inflammatory effect, effects on ion channels and cell membranes) or purely a placebo effect.

Current data on the antiviral pathway and viral clearance in CFS are equally confusing and contradictory. In theory, it has been proposed that a dysfunction of an intracellular antiviral pathway can lead to inefficient handling and delayed clearance of endemic viral infections. It has been suggested that there may be a possible dysregulation of the interferon-induced 2'–5' A (oligoadenylate) synthetase and PKR (protein kinase RNA) antiviral pathways in CFS patients[39] (Fig. 15.1). In an extension of the same research, a novel low molecular weight (37 kDa) 2'–5' oligoadenylate A-dependent RNase L enzyme protein in the peripheral blood mononuclear cells of the CFS patients was detected.[40] However, this finding cannot yet be accepted as a potential biochemical marker in CFS, because of the design of the study and the absence of appropriately selected control groups (healthy individuals with a recent history of common viral infections). This finding needs to be reduplicated in well-controlled studies by other laboratories before its acceptance as a genuine marker for a subset of CFS patients.

Ampligen, a mismatched synthetic double-stranded RNA preparation, has been claimed to improve the function of the intracellular antiviral pathway with chronic treatment and improve fatigue symptoms in CFS.[37] However, this treatment

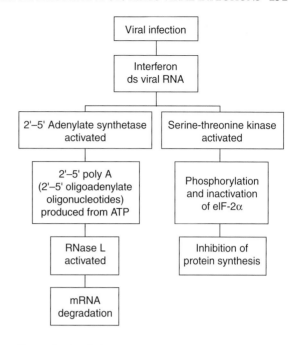

Figure 15.1 2'–5' A synthetase and PKR antiviral pathways. ds, double stranded; 2'–5' oligoadenylates, oligomers of adenylic acid with 2'–5'-phosphodiester linkages and phosphates at 5'-terminus; RNase L, low molecular weight RNase; eIF, eukaryotic initiation factor; mRNA, messenger RNA.

is expensive, and regular use of Ampligen in CFS patients cannot yet be recommended in the absence of appropriately designed, multicentre randomized controlled trial results. Finally, despite initial claims, trials of human intravenous immunoglobulin (IVIg) in CFS have not shown consistent results or sustained improvement in fatigue symptoms. Treatment with high-dose IVIg in CFS patients cannot be advised, especially in view of the high incidence of adverse effects reported by the patients in these trials[41] and the persistence of significant disability due to CFS on long-term follow-up.[42]

CFS: A MODEL OF POST-VIRAL MODIFICATION IN THE FUNCTION OF EXCITABLE TISSUES

Although the possibility of a persistent viral infection as a cause of CFS was first considered and then dismissed, the observation of PPFS that followed years after the clinical attacks of poliomyelitis suggested that the mechanism of fatigue in CFS and PPFS may be similar. Viral injury to the excitable tissues (muscle and nerve) can potentially alter their critical metabolic functions, including ion channel transport, mitochondrial function and the response to the circulating neurotransmitters and neurohormones that may persist well after clinical recovery.

Poliovirus causes selective damage to the midbrain reticular formation, substantia nigra, thalamic, hypothalamic and caudate nuclei, putamen, globus pallidus and locus ceruleus. A recent clinical trial of pyridostigmine failed to improve fatigue symptoms in PPFS patients despite the fact that neuromuscular conduction as measured by the single-fibre EMG had improved.[43] This clearly suggested that the principal mechanism of fatigue in PPFS was not connected with the peripheral neuromuscular changes. The striking similarity in the clinical symptoms, hypothalmic pituitary adrenal (HPA) axis impairment and autonomic dysfunction between PPFS and CFS was a reminder of the historical association that invariably linked epidemics of poliomyelitis with the outbreaks of epidemic CFS or neuromyasthenia ('atypical poliomyelitis'). It is generally accepted that, despite the detection of poliovirus sequence in muscles and cerebrospinal fluid (CSF) in patients, persistent or recurrent infection with poliovirus is not the cause of fatigue in PPFS.[44]

The accumulated research evidence in CFS at present clearly points to a central role of fatigue. We currently believe that basal ganglia pathways are involved in the mechanism of the chronic fatigue that comprises symptoms of both physical and mental fatigue. Basal ganglia are exquisitely sensitive to pro-inflammatory cytokines and also to direct viral invasion (e.g. HIV, various encephalitis viruses, influenza A virus).[45] Post-viral modification of functions affecting the receptors or the neurotransmitter release will induce critical changes in the excitable tissues and affect the facilitatory striato-thalamic input to the prefrontal cortex that may play an important role in the fatigue symptoms in CFS.

RECENT ADVANCES IN UNDERSTANDING THE MECHANISM OF CFS

Basal ganglia are considered to be the neural integrator for the motor and motivational aspects of higher cortical and limbic activities.[46] Dyfunction of the dopamine-dependent neostriatal–thalamic–prefrontal circuit is currently proposed as the neuroanatomical model of the physical and mental fatigue in CFS, while the fluctuations in symptom severity are considered to be the effects of ion channelopathy altering the neurotransmitter signals,[47] affecting the basal ganglia circuitry.

Indeed, the structure of the ion channels (e.g. voltage-gated potassium channel) has been remarkably conserved throughout evolution, and their functions in the excitable tissues can be influenced by viral infections and cell injury.[48] Certain acquired ion channelopathies share identical fatigue symptoms and neuroendocrine changes with CFS, e.g. chronic fatigue after ciguatera fish poisoning (ciguatera toxin chronically inactivates sodium channels in an open mode) and Isaac's syndrome (acquired neuromyotonia, often associated with antibodies to the voltage-gated potassium channels). These observations provide support for the concept of dysfunctional ion channels in CFS.[47] The neurotransmitters that are likely to be involved are serotonin, dopamine and acetylcholine, or, more appropriately, a balance between these three neurotransmitters within the basal ganglia network. The final result is a shift in the neuronal excitability of the cortical, limbic and brainstem areas, giving rise to the characteristic constellation of symptoms seen in CFS. Downregulation of the HPA axis in CFS is probably a secondary phenomenon and an adaptive response to the changes in the neurotransmitter system rather than the primary event responsible for the fatigue symptoms. Immunological dysfunction and aberrant cytokine responses in CFS are likely to be the consequences of this alteration in the HPA axis. The alteration of the neuronal excitability caused by channelopathy may also be the basis of the fluctuating nature of CFS symptoms that is often described by patients as 'good days' and 'bad days'.[47]

CONCLUSION

CFS is a challenging disorder because of its disabling symptoms, poor rate of spontaneous recovery and absence of any successful treatment effective in long-term amelioration of fatigue symptoms. There is no single specific or sensitive diagnostic marker for this illness. The modified CDC criteria are extensively used in the current diagnosis and research of CFS patients, but the need for an improved set of criteria and standardized screening investigations cannot be overemphasized. These are proposed here (Tables 15.9 and 15.10) for consideration and wider consultation.

There is no direct, definitive and credible evidence yet to suggest that persistent systemic infections, viral or bacterial, are responsible for the CFS

Table 15.9 Proposed research criteria for CFS

Essential criteria (*all must be fulfilled*):

1. New onset, persistent or relapsing fatigue lasting for >6 months
2. Failure of rest to improve symptoms
3. Post-exertional malaise lasting for >24 hours
4. Reduced attention span and/or concentration
5. Significant reduction in all levels of activities (personal activities of daily living, professional, social and occupational)
6. Lack of clinical evidence of: any concurrent medical or psychiatric disease; side-effects due to drugs or their withdrawal
7. No past history of somatization disorder

Supportive criteria (*patients must fulfill at least five criteria*):

1. Dysautonomic symptoms (orthostatic intolerance and/or hypotension, dry mouth, temperature changes, fainting and sweating attacks)
2. Vertigo or dysequilibrium (in the absence of orthostatic changes)
3. Unrefreshing sleep or altered sleeping pattern
4. New-onset alcohol intolerance
5. Muscle pain or cramp affecting two or more limbs
6. Any or all of (new onset): daily headache, chest pain (syndrome X), asthma/atopy, recurrent attacks of sore throat, worsening premenstrual symptoms in women of reproductive age
7. Physical evidence of any or all of: abnormal orthostatic changes in heart rate and/or blood pressure, altered sensory threshold to cutaneous sensations, fine distal tremors

Table 15.10 Recommended investigations in suspected CFS patients

1. Mandatory in all patients (*unless tested since the onset of symptoms*):

Full haemogram, erythrocyte sedimentation rate, C-reactive protein, serum ferritin and vitamin B_{12} levels
Glucose, urea and electrolytes, liver function tests (bilirubin, transaminases, GGT) CK, TSH
Morning plasma cortisol or 24-hour urinary cortisol
Autoantibodies for ANA and rheumatoid factor
Urine dipstix for protein
Orthostatic changes in heart rate and blood pressure

2. Optional (*specific indications*):

Short Synacthen (adrenocorticotrophic hormone) test (if plasma or urinary cortisol is low)
Buspirone-induced prolactin test (in adults with depressive symptoms)
Muscle biopsy (if CK is borderline or raised)
MRI of brain (if MS is clinically considered a possibility)
Autonomic functions (if orthostatic changes are present)
Neuropsychological tests (if professional activities are impaired as a result of concentration and attentional problems)

3. Test of unproven value:

Viral tests for reactivation of HHV6

4. Tests of little or no value and which cannot be recommended at present:

Serum angiotensin-converting enzyme (ACE)
Viral serology screen
Low molecular weight (37 kDa) RNase L on PBMC
Serology for *Mycoplasma*, *Rickettsia* or *Borrelia* in the absence of humoral immunodeficiency
Routine chest X-ray, EEG, nerve conduction and EMG studies, CT scan of brain, CSF
Functional neuroimaging (PET, fMRI or SPECT scan) outside the context of a research protocol

GGT, γ-glutamate transferase; CK, creatine kinase; TSH, thyroid stimulating hormone; ANA, antinuclear antibody; PBMC, peripheral blood mononuclear cells; PET, positron emission tomography; fMRI, functional magnetic resonance source imaging; SPECT, single photon emission computed tomography

symptoms. Convincing data are also lacking at present to support the claim that a subgroup of CFS patients may have defective viral clearance mechanisms, especially with the lack of appropriate infected control groups. There is no evidence yet to support the claim that CFS patients would potentially benefit from treatment strategies using antiviral/antibacterial chemotherapy or any of the expensive immune modifiers (Ampligen and IVIg). We are currently investigating the role of the RNase L and PKR pathways in CFS in comparison with healthy controls and asymptomatic subjects with antecedent viral or bacterial infections. Using the technique of reverse-transcriptase polymerase chain reaction (RT-PCR) to estimate the transcribed levels of the RNase L, PKR, RNase L inhibitor and the 2′–5′ A synthetase genes, we found that PKR, RNase L, 2′–5′ A synthetase and RNase L inhibitor gene activities are non-specific markers of recent infections, as demonstrated by their significantly higher levels only in the asymptomatic subjects with previous infections. Our results clearly indicate that CFS patients do not differ from the healthy controls in the activities of these parameters as measured by the RT-PCR.

Our current understanding of CFS is that the mechanism of fatigue is central, possibly related to the dysfunction of the neostriatal–prefrontal cortical network as a consequence of altered neurotransmitter balance and channelopathy that appear to be related to antecedent viral infections, stress and cytokine effect. There is no known therapy at present, either pharmacological, or behavioural, that is effective in curing CFS. Understanding the mechanism of fatigue, the hallmark of CFS, is crucial to the successful development of any treatment strategy. Any therapeutic claims in CFS at present have to be interpreted cautiously and must be tested by well-designed, multicentre, placebo-controlled, randomized trials before recommendations for use in all or a subgroup of CFS patients. Since the symptoms and severity of fatigue in CFS fluctuate, carefully planned treatment designs will be necessary to avoid bias in favour of the treatment due to the phenomenon of regression to mean. There is little doubt, however, that any successful treatment in CFS will have the potential for use in other chronic fatigue disorders in neurology, e.g. MS, PPFS and post-GBS fatigue syndrome.

ACKNOWLEDGEMENT

We gratefully acknowledge the support of the Barclay Trust held in the University of Glasgow and the ME Association in our research work on the chronic fatigue disorders in neurology.

REFERENCES

1. Behan PO, Bakheit AM. Clinical spectrum of post viral fatigue syndrome. *Br Med Bull* 1991; **47**: 793–808.
2. Fukuda K, Strauss SE, Hickie I et al. The chronic fatigue syndrome: a comprehensive approach to case definition and study. *Ann Intern Med* 1994; **121**: 953–956.
3. Chaudhuri A, Behan WMH, Behan PO. Chronic fatigue syndrome. *Proc R Coll Physicians Edinb* 1998; **28**: 150–163.
4. Chaudhuri A, Behan PO. Overlap syndromes of chronic fatigue. *CNS* 1998; **1**(2): 16–20.
5. Vercoulen J, Hommes OR, Swanink C et al. The measurement of fatigue in patients with multiple sclerosis: a multidimensional comparison with patients with chronic fatigue syndrome and healthy subjects. *Arch Neurol* 1996; **53**: 642–649.
6. Hilgers A, Frank J, Bolte P. Prolongation of the central motor conduction time in chronic fatigue syndrome. *J Chronic Fatigue Syn* 1998; **4**(2): 23–32.
7. Pepper CM, Krupp LB, Friedberg F et al. A comparison of neuropsychiatric characteristics in chronic fatigue syndrome, multiple sclerosis and major depression. *J Neuropsychiatr Clin Neurosci* 1993; **5**: 200–205.
8. Layzer RB. Asthenia and chronic fatigue syndrome. *Muscle Nerve* 1998; **21**: 1609–1611.
9. Kent-Braun JA, Sharma KR, Weiner MW et al. Central basis of muscle fatigue in chronic fatigue syndrome. *Neurology* 1993; **43**: 125–131.
10. Bouwer B, Packer T. Corticospinal excitability in patients diagnosed with chronic fatigue syndrome. *Muscle Nerve* 1994; **17**: 1210–1222.
11. Paul L, Wood L, Behan WMH, Maclaren WM. Demonstration of delayed recovery from fatiguing exercise in chronic fatigue syndrome. *Eur J Neurol* 1999; **6**: 63–69.
12. Sacco P, Hope PAJ, Thickbroom GW et al. Corticomotor excitability and perception of effort sustained exercise in chronic fatigue syndrome. *Clin Neurophysiol* 1999; **110**: 1883–1891.
13. McCully KK, Natelson BH. Impaired oxygen delivery to muscle in chronic fatigue syndrome. *Clin Sci* 1999; **97**: 603–608.
14. Bou-Holaigh I, Rowe PC, Kan JS et al. The relationship between neurally mediated hypotension chronic fatigue syndrome. *JAMA* 1995; **274**: 961–967.
15. Schondorf R, Freeman R. The importance of orthostatic intolerance in the chronic fatigue syndrome. *Am J Med Sci* 1999; **317**: 117–123.
16. Smith AP, Behan PO, Bell W et al. Behavioural problems associated with the chronic fatigue syndrome. *Br J Psychol* 1993; **84**: 411–423.
17. Behan PO, Behan WMH. Postviral fatigue syndrome. *CRC Crit Rev Neurobiol* 1988; **4**: 157–178.
18. United States Public Health Service. *The epidemiological study of an epidemic, diagnosed as poliomyelitis, occurring among the personnel of the Los Angeles County General Hospital during the summer of 1934*. Public Health Bulletin No. 240. Washington DC: USPHS, 1938.
19. Parsons PE. *National Health Interview Survey*. Hyattsville, MD: National Center for Health Statistics, 1989.
20. Bruno RL, Frick NM, Crenage SJ et al. Polioencephalitis and the brain fatigue generator model of viral fatigue syndromes. *J Chronic Fatigue Synd* 1996; **2**: 5–27.
21. Behan PO, Behan WMH, Bell EJ. The postviral fatigue syndrome: an analysis of the findings in 50 cases. *J Infect* 1985;. **10**: 211–212.
22. Levine PH, Jacobson S, Pocinki AG et al. Clinical, epidemiologic and virologic studies in four clusters of the chronic fatigue syndrome. *Arch Intern Med* 1992; **152**: 1611–1616.
23. Gow JW, Behan PO. Viruses and chronic fatigue syndrome. *J Chronic Fatigue Synd* 1996; **2**: 67–83.
24. Gow JW, Simpson K, Schliephake A et al. Search for retrovirus in the chronic fatigue syndrome. *J Clin Pathol* 1992; **45**: 1058–1061.
25. Gow JW, Behan WMH, Simpson K et al. Studies on enterovirus in patients with postviral fatigue *Clin Infect Dis* 1994; **18**: S126–S129.

26. Gow JW, de la Torre JC, Behan WMH et al. Borna disease virus in chronic fatigue syndrome. *Neurol Infect Epidemiol* 1997; **2**: 63–66.

27. Barnes DM. Mystery disease at Lake Tahoe challenges virologists and clinicians. *Science* 1986; **234**: 541–542.

28. Holmes GP, Kaplan JE, Stewart JA et al. A cluster of patients with a chronic mononucleosis-like syndrome: is Epstein-Barr virus the cause? *JAMA* 1987; **257**: 2297–2302.

29. Woodward CG, Cox RA. Epstein–Barr virus serology in the chronic fatigue syndrome. *J Infect* 1992; **24**: 133–139.

30. Gold D, Bowden R, Sixbey J et al. Chronic fatigue: a prospective clinical and virologic study. *JAMA* 1990; **264**: 48–53.

31. Swanink CMA, van der Meer JWM, Vercoulen JHMM et al. Epstein–Barr virus (EBV) and the chronic fatigue syndrome: normal virus load in blood and normal immunological reactivity in the EBV regression assay. *Clin Infect Dis* 1995; **20**: 1390–1392.

32. Vojdani A, Franco AR. Multiplex PCR for the detection of *Mycoplasma fermentans*, *M. hominis* and *M. penetrans* in patients with chronic fatigue syndrome, fibromyalgia, rheumatoid arthritis and Gulf War Syndrome. *J Chronic Fatigue Synd* 1999; **5**: 187–197.

33. Behan PO, Behan WMH, Bell EJ. The postviral fatigue syndrome—an analysis of findings in 50 cases. *J Infect* 1985; **10**: 211–222.

34. Morrison LJA, Behan WMH, Behan PO. Changes in killer cell phenotype in patients with viral fatigue syndrome. *Eur Immunol* 1991; **83**: 441–446.

35. Sharma OP. Fatigue and sarcoidosis. *Eur Respir J* 1999; **13**: 713–714.

36. Nicolson GL, Nasralla M, Haier J, Nicolson NL. Diagnosis and treatment of chronic mycoplasmal infections in fibromyalgia and chronic fatigue syndromes: relationship to Gulf War illness. *Biomed Ther* 1998; **16**: 266–271.

37. Strayer DR, Carter WA, Brodsky I et al. A controlled trial with a specifically configured RNA drug Poly(I) Poly(CI2U) in chronic fatigue syndrome. *Clin Infect Dis* 1994; **18S**: S88–S95.

38. Holt GW. Epidemic neuromyasthenia: the sporadic form. *Am J Med Sci* 1965; **249**: 98–112.

39. Suhadolnik RJ, Peterson DL, Cheney PR et al. Biochemical dysregulation of the 2–5A synthetase/RNase L antiviral defense pathway in chronic fatigue syndrome. *J Chronic Fatigue Synd* 1999; **5**: 223–242.

40. De Meirleir K, Bisbal C, Campine I et al. A 37 kDa 2–5A binding protein as a potential marker for chronic fatigue syndrome. *Am J Med* 2000; **108**: 99–105.

41. Peterson PK, Shephard J, Macres M et al. A controlled trial of intravenous immunoglobulin G in chronic fatigue syndrome. *Am J Med* 1990; **89**: 554–560.

42. Rowe KS. Five-year follow up of young people with chronic fatigue syndrome following the double blind randomised controlled intravenous gammaglobulin trial. *J Chronic Fatigue Synd* 1999; **5**: 109–110.

43. Trojan DA, Collet J-P, Shapiro S et al. A multicenter, randomized, double-blind trial of pyridostigmine in postpolio syndrome. *Neurology* 1999; **53**: 1225–1233.

44. Dalakas MC, Bartfield H, Kurkland LT. The postpolio syndrome: advances in the pathogenesis and treatment. *Ann NY Acad Sci* 1995; **753**: 1–411.

45. Pradhan S, Pandey N, Shashank S et al. Parkinsonian symptoms due to predominant involvement substantia nigra in Japanese encephalitis. *Neurology* 1999; **53**: 1781–1786.

46. Nauta WJH. The relationship of basal ganglia to the limbic system. In: Vinken PJ, Bruyn GW eds. *Handbook of Clinical Neurology*, Vol. 49. Amsterdam: Elsevier Science, 1986: 19–32.

47. Chaudhuri A, Behan PO. Chronic fatigue syndrome is an acquired neurological channelopathy. *Hum Psychopharmacol Clin Exp* 1999; **14**: 7–17.

48. Lipton SA. Calcium channel antagonists and human immunodeficiency virus-coat protein mediated neuronal injury. *Ann Neurol* 1991; **31**: 110–114.

16

Bacterial meningitis

Hans-Walter Pfister and Uwe Koedel

CLINICAL ASPECTS OF BACTERIAL MENINGITIS

Bacterial meningitis is clinically characterized by stiff neck, headache, fever, photophobia, malaise, vomiting, alteration of consciousness, seizures, confusion, irritability, and, rarely, acute psychosis. Cerebrospinal fluid (CSF) usually reveals an elevated white blood cell count of more than 1000 white blood cells/µl, consisting of more than 60% polymorphonuclear leukocytes, an elevated total protein content and a decreased CSF/serum glucose ratio. A CSF white blood cell count of less than 1000 cells/µl may be found early in the disease, in partially treated bacterial meningitis, in overwhelming bacterial meningeal infection ('apurulent bacterial meningitis') and in immunosuppressed and leukopenic patients.

With the introduction of antimicrobial agents into clinical practice, the mortality rates of bacterial meningitis were markedly reduced. The mortality rates of meningitis due to *Haemophilus influenzae* type b are less than 7% and those of meningitis due to *Neisseria meningitidis* are 6–14%. With the advent of third-generation cephalosporins, the mortality of Gram-negative bacillary meningitis has decreased from 40–80% to 10–20%. However, despite further progress in antimicrobial therapy and improvements in intensive care medicine, the mortality rate of meningitis due to *Streptococcus pneumoniae*, the organism most often responsible for bacterial meningitis in adults, has remained relatively unchanged during the last decades and is still unacceptably high (approximately 20%). Neurologic and neuropsychologic sequelae resulting from bacterial meningitis are found overall in 10–30% of patients. Cerebral and systemic complications arising during the acute phase of the disease are responsible for both the mortality and the long-term sequelae caused by bacterial meningitis. The major acute complications involving the central nervous system include cerebrovascular insults, brain edema, and hydrocephalus. Cerebrovascular involvement, of both arteries (arteriitis, vasospasm) and veins (septic sinus venous thrombosis), may lead to infarction with severe irreversible cerebral damage and an increase of intracranial pressure due to cytotoxic edema. In addition to edema, increased intracranial blood volume due to disturbed cerebrovascular autoregulation or to septic venous sinus thrombosis may lead to life-threatening elevation of intracranial pressure with the risk of herniation. There is a risk of cortical necrosis when cerebral perfusion pressure (defined as the difference between systemic mean arterial blood pressure and intracranial pressure) decreases as a result of increased intracranial pressure and systemic hypotension. Interstitial edema may occur owing to transependymal movement of CSF from the ventricular system into the surrounding brain parenchyma as a consequence of obstructive hydrocephalus. Systemic complications of bacterial meningitis include sepsis, including septic shock, disseminated intravascular coagulation, adult respiratory distress syndrome, and inappropriate secretion of antidiuretic hormone (ADH).

Recently, high-resolution MRI was used to demonstrate inner ear involvement in adults with bacterial meningitis.[1] The structures most frequently involved were the cochlear nerve, the first cochlear turn, the vestibulum and the semicircular canals. There was a significant correlation between clinical and MRI findings: all patients with cochlear enhancement were deaf (hearing loss, > 90 dB), whereas none of the patients with normal MRI findings had hearing loss of more than 90 dB. This study shows that high-resolution MRI can visualize involvement of vestibulocochlear structures in bacterial meningitis, in both cooperative and consciously impaired patients. These findings suggest a correlation between abnormalities on MRI and the extent of cochlear dysfunction.

GENERAL MANAGEMENT OF A PATIENT WITH BACTERIAL MENINGITIS

In patients with severe, life-threatening meningitis, the most important aspect of management is the immediate institution of empirical antibiotic therapy (Fig. 16.1; Table 16.1). We recommend that patients suspected of having bacterial meningitis, who present with a rapidly progressive course and severe alteration of mental status/coma, receive an initial antibiotic dose immediately after the drawing of a single blood culture, prior to any other diagnostic procedures. In less acutely ill patients with clinical signs and symptoms suggesting acute bacterial meningitis, and in the acutely ill patient after initiation of therapy, a lumbar puncture should be performed immediately after the initial clinical examination. In patients who are unconscious and have focal neurologic deficits, a CT scan should be performed prior to lumbar puncture. Contraindications to lumbar puncture are clinical signs of cerebral herniation (e.g. unconsciousness, a unilaterally dilated and unreactive pupil, decerebrate movements) or a focal mass lesion (e.g. large, space-occupying brain abscess) on CT. The presence of a parameningeal infectious focus such as sinusitis or mastoiditis should also be investigated by CT, including the bone window technique. In addition, clinical examination by an otolaryngologist should be performed. If a parameningeal focus (e.g. otitis, mastoiditis, sinusitis) is identified as a possible origin of bacterial meningitis, an operation is required as soon as possible. In contrast, surgical correction of

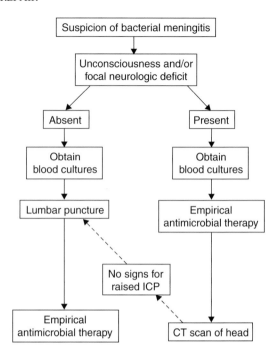

Figure 16.1 Algorithm for initial management of a patient with bacterial meningitis.

CSF dural leaks (e.g. in patients with previous head trauma) is usually performed when the meningeal infection is treated, typically after 10–14 days, rather than during the very acute stage of meningitis. If the patient's clinical condition does not improve despite

Table 16.1 Empirical antibiotic therapy of bacterial meningitis		
Age	**Typical pathogens**	**Therapy**
<1 month	Gram-negative Enterobacteriaceae Streptococci (group B streptococci) *Listeria monocytogenes*	Cefotaxime + ampicillin
Children	*Haemophilus influenzae*[a] *Neisseria meningitidis* *Streptococcus pneumoniae*, other streptococci	Cephalosporin
Adults	*Neisseria meningitidis* *Streptococcus pneumoniae, H. influenzae, Listeria*, staphylococci, Gram-negative Enterobacteriaceae	Cephalosporin + ampicillin

[a]The incidence has dramatically decreased since the introduction of the *H. influenzae* vaccine.

antibiotic therapy, the possibility of complications of bacterial meningitis should be investigated (e.g. repeated CT or MRI scanning), and additional sources of infection sought (e.g. endocarditis). Importantly, the sensitivity of the causative pathogen to the antibiotic regimen administered must be confirmed by in vitro testing, and antibiotic coverage must be adjusted to the sensitivity results. If the causative organism has not been isolated, broadening of the antibiotic coverage should be considered in patients who fail to respond to the initial therapy.

INITIAL EMPIRICAL ANTIBIOTIC THERAPY

If antibiotic therapy has to be started without microbiological confirmation, empirical therapy is initiated with regard to the patient's age, predisposing factors, underlying diseases, and the most probable meningeal pathogens (Table 16.1). Repeat lumbar punctures should be performed within 24 h if the patient fails to respond promptly to antibiotic therapy.

The initial antibiotic treatment of healthy, immunocompetent adults for community-acquired bacterial meningitis, most often caused by *S. pneumoniae* or *N. meningitidis*, consists of a combination of a third-generation cephalosporin (most commonly ceftriaxone or cefotaxime) and ampicillin, the latter being added to cover *Listeria monocytogenes*. CSF isolates of *S. pneumoniae* or *N. meningitidis* should be tested for penicillin G and cephalosporin susceptibility. In recent years, an increasing number of penicillin-resistant strains of *S. pneumoniae* have been reported from several countries around the world, particularly Spain, Hungary, Australia, New Guinea, South Africa, and some areas of the USA. Furthermore, penicillin-resistant strains of *N. meningitidis* are also emerging in some regions of the world (e.g. Spain, South Africa). For penicillin-resistant meningococci or relatively penicillin-resistant pneumococci, a third-generation cephalosporin is recommended. Highly resistant pneumococci typically also have reduced sensitivity or resistance to third-generation cephalosporins, and in areas where these highly resistant organisms are commonly isolated, the addition of vancomycin (or rifampin) is recommended, until the organism and its antibiotic susceptibilities are known.

DURATION OF ANTIBIOTIC TREATMENT

Treatment of bacterial meningitis due to *S. pneumoniae*, *N. meningitidis*, *H. influenzae* and group B streptococci usually consists of intravenous administration of antibiotics for 10–14 days. However, some clinical observations have suggested that shorter courses of 7, 5, or even 4 days may be adequate for uncomplicated meningococcal meningitis. For antibiotic treatment of meningitis due to *L. monocytogenes* and Gram-negative Enterobacteriaceae, a treatment duration of 3–4 weeks may be required.

PATHOPHYSIOLOGY

An unfavorable clinical outcome is predominantly due to intracranial complications, including cerebrovascular insults, raised intracranial pressure, hydrocephalus and brain edema. During recent years, experimental studies using animal models (Table 16.2) and cell culture systems have substantially increased our knowledge of the complex pathophysiologic mechanisms underlying the development of intracranial complications and brain injury during bacterial meningitis.[2] Once the bacteria reach the CSF, they are likely to survive, because immunoglobulin concentrations in the CSF are very low and complement components appear to be virtually absent ('regional host immunodeficiency'). The host immune response to bacteria (Fig. 16.2) seems to be induced by a direct interaction with subcapsular cell wall components generated by bacterial autolysis or during antimicrobial treatment (e.g., peptidoglycans and lipoteichoic acids of Gram-positive pathogens and lipopolysaccharides of Gram-negative pathogens) with host Toll-like receptors (TLR), especially with TLR-2 and TLR-4.[3]. Additionally, microbial toxins, such as H_2O_2 and pneumolysin, can act as powerful triggers of the

Table 16.2 Animal models of experimental meningitis	
Early pathogenic mechanism	Inoculation of pathogens
Infant rat model of *Haemophilus influenzae* and *Escherichia coli* meningitis	Intranasal/intraperitoneal (hematogenous)
Pathophysiologic alterations	
Adult rabbit model	Intracisternal
Adult rat model	Intracisternal
Adult mouse model	Lumbar, intracerebral, intracisternal (secondary hematogenous)

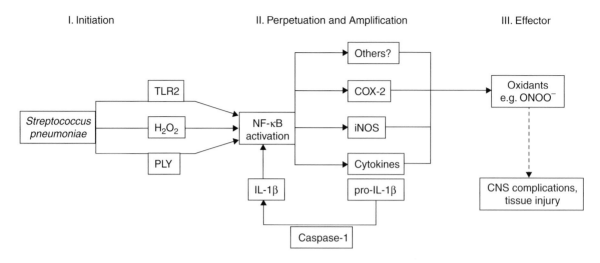

Figure 16.2 Pathogenic mechanisms during bacterial meningitis. PLY, pneumolysin; ONOO⁻, peroxynitrite; COX, cyclooxygenase

host immune response (Fig. 16.2: initiation phase). A hallmark of the inflammatory reaction in bacterial meningitis seems to be an increased and prolonged activation of nuclear factor (NF)-κB. NF-κB is a transcriptional activator of many genes that encode proteins/host factors involved in the pathogenesis of bacterial meningitis including pro-inflammatory cytokines (e.g. interleukin-1β (IL-1β), tumor necrosis factor-alpha (TNF-α), chemokines, and adhesion molecules.[4] IL-1β is synthesized as an inactive precursor pro-IL-1β that is processed to its mature, pro-inflammatory form by the intracellular cysteine protease caspase-1 (Casp1, also known as IL-1β-converting enzyme, ICE).[5] The mature form of IL-1β is a potent trigger of activation of NF-κB. Thus, Casp1, by activating pro-IL-1β, may contribute to an exaggerated activation of NF-κB, leading to uncontrolled expression of pro-inflammatory mediators (Fig. 16.2: perpetuation and amplification phase). This process is paralleled by increased expression of adhesion molecules, both on the endothelium and on neutrophils, resulting in leukocyte–endothelial interactions (rolling, sticking, and finally adhesion) and subsequently in massive influx of leukocytes into the CSF. Leukocytes in the subarachnoid space are thought to be more harmful than beneficial. Because of the lack of opsonins, they are ineffective in the eradication of the microbial pathogens in the CSF. However, activated leukocytes release a complex assortment of potentially cytotoxic agents, including reactive oxygen species (ROS, such as superoxide) and reactive nitrogen intermediates (RNI, such as nitric oxide). The simultaneous

production of both nitric oxide and superoxide favors the production of a potentially even more toxic species, the strong oxidant peroxynitrite. Oxidants such as peroxynitrite may contribute to the development of intracranial complications and brain damage during bacterial meningitis via a variety of independent mechanisms (Fig. 16.2: effector phase). One of these pathways involves attack on polyunsaturated fatty acids, thus initiating lipid peroxidation which can ultimately lead to loss of cellular membrane function and integrity.[6] An alternative pathway involves oxidant-induced DNA strand breakage and subsequent poly ADP-ribase polymerase (PARP) activation, thus initiating an energy-consuming intracellular cycle which can ultimately result in cellular energy depletion and death.[6] Both mechanisms contribute to endothelial cell injury during bacterial meningitis. Endothelial dysfunction leads to loss of (1) cerebrovascular autoregulation, (2) carbon dioxide reactivity of cerebral vessels, and (3) integrity of the blood–brain barrier. Vasogenic brain edema is considered to be the major cause of the increase in ICP during bacterial meningitis. Elevated ICP is potentially harmful to patients with bacterial meningitis, either by causing cerebral herniation or by decreasing cerebral perfusion (due to a reduction in cerebral perfusion pressure and/or a loss of cerebravascular autoregulation) which can ultimately lead to cortical necrosis and hippocampal apoptosis.[7] From the experimental data described above, it can be deduced that agents which interfere with the production of oxidants, with lipid peroxidation and/or PARP activation may represent novel therapeutic strategies to limit meningitis-associated intracranial complications and brain damage, and thus to improve the outcome of this serious disease.

ADJUNCTIVE THERAPY

Dexamethasone has shown beneficial effects in animal models of bacterial meningitis. It inhibits the synthesis or release of inflammatory mediators involved in the pathophysiologic processes of bacterial meningitis. It may be most beneficial to administer the first dexamethasone dose several minutes before the first antibiotic dose in order to achieve maximal inhibition of the inflammatory cascade, which is initiated by antibiotic-induced bacteriolysis and the release of cell wall components.

Recently, a meta-analysis of 11 randomized clinical trials carried out since 1988 using dexamethasone as adjunctive therapy in bacterial meningitis was performed.[8] In *H. influenzae*-meningitis in children, dexamethasone reduced severe hearing loss overall. In pneumococcal meningitis, only studies in which dexamethasone was given early suggested protection, which was significant for severe hearing loss and approached significance for any neurologic or hearing deficit. Outcomes were similar in studies that used 2 versus more than 2 days of dexamethasone therapy. The incidence of gastrointestinal tract bleeding increased with longer duration of dexamethasone treatment.

In a recent multicenter, double-blind, randomized trial in France and Switzerland, the clinical benefit of early adjunctive dexamethasone therapy (10 mg q.i.d. for 3 days) was investigated in adults with bacterial meningitis.[9] Unfortunately, the study had to be stopped prematurely, because of a new national recommendation of experts to use a third-generation cephalosporin and vancomycin as a result of the increasing rate of penicillin-resistant *S. pneumoniae* in France. The difference of rate of cured patients without any neurologic sequelae was not statistically significant between the dexamethasone group (74.2%; $n = 31$) and the placebo group (51.7%; $n = 29$).

In January 2000, 241 adult patients were included in the multicenter, placebo-controlled, double-blind, European Dexamethasone in Bacterial Meningitis Study (Principal Investigator: Jan de Gans, Amsterdam). The calculated number of patients in this trial is 300.

In animal models of penicillin- and cephalosporin-resistant pneumococcal meningitis, the penetration of both ceftriaxone and vancomycin into the CSF was reduced with dexamethasone therapy, resulting in a delay in CSF sterilization. When rifampin was used with ceftriaxone, bacteriologic cure occurred promptly, irrespective of therapy with dexamethasone. Thus, it was recommended that in areas with high rates of resistant pneumococcal strains, initial empirical therapy should include two antibiotics, ceftriaxone and either rifampin or vancomycin. When dexamethasone is used in this situation, ceftriaxone combined with rifampin is preferred.

Experimental or clinical data have not proven the efficacy of dexamethasone in meningococcal meningitis. Corticosteroids are not recommended for the therapy of meningitis following infective endocarditis, or in newborns with bacterial meningitis.

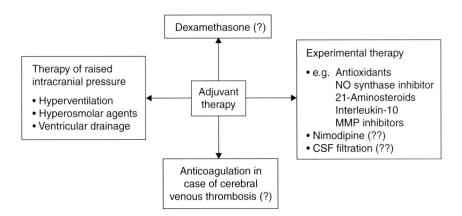

Figure 16.3 Adjuvant therapeutic approaches in bacterial meningitis. MMP, matrix metalloproteinase.

Increased intracranial pressure may be managed by elevation of the head of the bed to 30°, hyperventilation to maintain a pCO_2 concentration between 25 and 30 torr, and the intravenous administration of hyperosmolar agents (e.g. 20% mannitol; Fig. 16.3). Stuporous or comatose patients may benefit from intracranial pressure monitoring to control this therapy. If meningitis-associated hydrocephalus is diagnosed by CT, CT scan follow-up investigations or ventricular drainage should be performed, depending on the patient's level of consciousness and the degree of ventricular dilatation on CT. Anticoagulation of septic venous sinus thrombosis in bacterial meningitis is controversial. There are no prospective controlled clinical studies, but anticoagulation with dose-adjusted intravenous heparin should be considered in patients with meningitis-associated septic venous sinus thrombosis proven by MRI or cerebral angiography. Anticonvulsants are given to treat seizures, e.g. rapid intravenous phenytoin administration (e.g. 20 mg/kg, no faster than 50 mg/min in adults). Sterile subdural effusion usually resolves spontaneously and does not require surgical therapy. CT-guided stereotactic aspiration is recommended initially for cases of subdural empyema, but open surgical procedures may be necessary.

Experimental approaches

Previous angiographic studies in patients with bacterial meningitis and focal neurologic deficits revealed vasospasm of the large arteries at the base of the brain resembling vasospasm following subarachnoid hemorrhage. Likewise, transcranial Doppler sonography may show changes of blood flow velocity in basal cerebral arteries. In these patients, nimodipine (e.g. 1–2 mg/h i.v. in adults) therapy should be investigated systematically in clinical trials. Currently, there exist no data which justify the experimental procedure of CSF filtration in patients with bacterial meningitis.

Several therapeutic agents which may limit meningeal inflammation have shown beneficial effects in animal models of bacterial meningitis (in particular of the rat and the rabbit). Aside from dexamethasone, these anti-inflammatory agents include non-steroidal anti-inflammatory drugs (e.g., indomethacin), pentoxifylline, antagonists of leukocyte–endothelial cell adhesion molecules, monoclonal antibodies against cytokines, platelet-activating factor receptor antagonists, free radical scavengers and NOS inhibitors. Apart from dexamethasone, these agents have not yet been investigated in humans with bacterial meningitis, but some show promising beneficial effects in experimental models. Further experimental studies are needed to clarify whether some of these approaches may be applied to clinical practice.

REFERENCES

1. Dichgans M, Jäger L, Mayer T et al. Bacterial meningitis in adults: demonstration of inner ear involvement using high-resolution MRI. *Neurology* 1999; 52: 1003–1009.
2. Koedel U, Pfister HW. Models of experimental meningitis. Role and limitations. *Infect Dis Clin North Am* 1999; **13**: 549–577.
3. Wright SD. Toll, a new piece in the puzzle of innate immunity. *J Exp Med* 1999; **189**: 605–609.
4. Baldwin AS Jr. The NF-kappaB and IkappaB proteins: new discoveries and insights. *Annu Rev Immunol* 1996; **14**: 649–683.
5. Dinarello CA. Interleukin-1 beta, interleukin-18, and the interleukin-1 beta converting enzyme. *Ann NY Acad Sci* 1998; **856**: 1–11.
6. Koedel U, Pfister HW. Oxidative stress in bacterial meningitis. *Brain Pathol* 1999; **9**: 57–67.
7. Pfister HW, Borasio GD, Dirnagl U, Bauer M, Einhäupl KM. Cerebrovascular complications of bacterial meningitis in adults. *Neurology* 1992; **42**: 1497–1504.
8. McIntyre PB, Berkey CS, King S et al. Dexamethasone as adjunctive therapy in bacterial meningitis. *JAMA* 1997; **278**: 925–931.
9. Thomas R, Le Tulzo Y, Bouget J et al. Trial of dexamethasone treatment for severe bacterial meningitis in adults. Adult Meningitis Study Group. *Intensive Care Med* 1999; **25**: 475–480.

17

Human prion diseases

Amos D Korczyn

INTRODUCTION

Prion diseases are a group of unusual diseases affecting humans and animals (Table 17.1), which involve only the central nervous system (CNS) and always lead to a fatal outcome. The unique nature of prion diseases includes their pathogenesis, mode of transmission, and neuropathology. These diseases can be transmitted by a small fraction from the brain of a diseased individual. The 'prion hypothesis', advanced by Prusiner[1] and recently reviewed by him,[1] is now widely accepted. It maintains that the 'infectious' agent is an abnormal conformation of a naturally occurring protein. This harmless prion protein (PrP^c) may transform into a protease-resistant form (PrP^{Sc} or PrP^{res}), which is strongly linked to disease pathogenesis. Although most workers accept the 'protein-only' theory, others present data which they interpret as demonstrating that nucleic acids, or other unidentified agents, are also involved in the transmission of these diseases.[2–6]

The terminology of the diseases is still changing. The term 'spongiform encephalopathy' is inadequate, since in patients with fatal familial insomnia (FFI) as well as in those with dementia and spastic paraparesis (P1O5L) spongiosis is not seen. The term 'transmissible encephalopathies' is also problematic, since it is not always easy to demonstrate transmissibility. The term 'prion diseases' is preferable, because it concentrates on the unique features of these diseases and the central role played by prions in the pathogenesis (which may, however, be different in sporadic, transmitted and genetic cases).

EPIDEMIOLOGY AND RISK FACTORS

Creutzfeld–Jakob disease (CJD) is the most common of the human prion diseases, with an annual incidence of about one per million population.[7,8] In some countries, only a very few cases have been identified; recently, cases were first reported in

Table 17.1 Prion diseases

Human diseases

Creutzfeld–Jakob disease (CJD)
- Sporadic
- Genetic
- Iatrogenic
- Transmitted

Gerstmann–Straussler–Scheinker disease (GSS)
- Genetic

Kuru
- Transmitted

Prion dementia without characteristic pathology

Dementia with spastic paraparesis

Animal diseases

Scrapie

Transmissible mink encephalopathy

Chronic wasting disease of mule and deer

Bovine spongiform encephalopathy (BSE, mad cow disease)

Oman[9] and Iran.[10] The apparently low prevalence in these countries is probably related to the small number of practicing neurologists rather than to the rarity of the disease compared to Western societies. A recent epidemiological study in Austria demonstrated an increasing incidence of CJD, probably reflecting greater awareness of prion diseases.[11]

Some indications support the notion that CJD may be underdiagnosed and under-reported. Reviewing about 1000 necropsy cases of demented subjects from the Corsellis Collection, Bruton et al[12] identified 19 cases of spongiform encephalopathy. Since only 11 had been diagnosed clinically, the authors concluded that CJD may be considerably more common than usually thought. It is notable that several of the undiagnosed patients had a dementing process of long duration (3–6 years) without specific distinguishing features like a cerebellar syndrome or myoclonic jerks. This may also point to the possibility that prion disease may present as a non-specific dementing process. Nevertheless, a study from the USA suggests that death certificates may be an efficient way to study the epidemiology of CJD.[13]

The intense epidemiological surveillance of CJD in the UK was rewarded by the identification of a new variant of the disease,[14–16] in which psychiatric features predominate. Several enigmas still surround the BSE epidemic and its relationship to humans. It is generally accepted that the transmission in cattle is through the food chain, and particularly because offal, originating in diseased animal brain, was allowed to be recycled using modern food technology. There is no direct support for the assumption that BSE was first introduced to cows by the use of scrapie-infected sheep brain. The well-known species barrier to the transmission of prion diseases makes this assumption somewhat unlikely. It is possible, however, that sporadic occurrence of the disease in a single cow resulted in the epidemic, by analogy to the origin and transmission of kuru. The evidence supporting the transmission from cow to humans, resulting in vCJD (see below) is stronger. Because of the difficulties in collecting data on exposure to BSE, and the long incubation time of prion diseases, it is, however, at present impossible to predict how many new cases will appear, and when.[17,18]

High prevalence rates of CJD have been reported in populations with a genetic predisposition. The best studied is the population of Jewish immigrants from Libya to Israel, in which the incidence is about $100 : 10^6$. This high frequency is related to a mutation in the PRNP gene (E200K), first identified by us.[19]

Genetic forms of prion diseases behave as autosomal dominant traits. The age of onset is highly variable, not only from one genetic form to another but also within the same genetic mutation. For example, with the E200K mutation, some patients develop clinical disease in their thirties, whereas others survive into their ninth decade without expressing neurological dysfunction. Two analyses of the Libyan Jewish cluster[20,21] have demonstrated that the mutation has an almost complete penetrance by age 80. In Chile, where the E200K mutation is also common, an 88-year-old normal subject was shown to carry the mutation.[22] A very important remaining question is whether environmental factors are responsible for the age at which the disease occurs. This is particularly important, since in the Slovak cluster of E200K mutation carriers a much lower penetrance of CJD was reported.[23] The fact that in genetically predisposed individuals CJD may appear very late in life underscores the view that CJD should not be included among the 'presenile dementias' (although in individual cases the onset may be as early as in their thirties).

In a recent reanalysis of four case–control studies in Europe and the USA, the main risk factor identified was a family history of CJD.[24] A small excess of dementia among first-degree relatives may have been related to undiagnosed prion disease in genetic CJD. An additional risk factor was a previous psychotic episode (possibly in the initial stages of CJD), while exposure to cows or sheep was of borderline significance (but might reflect recall bias, since CJD is not more common in countries where scrapie exists).

CLINICAL FEATURES

There is a wide scope of clinical phenomenology in human prion diseases, regarding the age of onset, presenting features, rate of progression and appearance of other clinical manifestations. The recent description of *dementia without distinguishing features, dementia without characteristic pathology*[25] and *dementia associated with spastic paraparesis*,[26] the latter associated with a PRNP point mutation, and possibly also of mental illness without neurological signs,[27] extend the clinical heterogeneity of prion diseases even further.

CJD

Clinically, CJD usually presents with *cortical manifestations*, mainly subacute cognitive decline, although this is frequently heralded by non-specific affective and other psychiatric symptoms, as well as sleep disturbances. Memory loss is an early complaint, but cases have been reported who presented with focal manifestations imitating strokes,[28] such as hemisensory deficit,[29] hemianopia,[30] aphasia,[31,32] or myoclonic alien hand.[33] As the disease progresses, other cortical manifestations appear, such as blindness, optic ataxia and generalized tonic–clonic seizures. In the *Heidenhain variety*, CJD presents with cortical blindness. *Movement disorders* are common. They may include parkinsonian features, mainly bradykinesia and rigidity. Cerebellar ataxia may be very disabling.[34] Towards the final stages of the disease,

Table 17.2	Diagnostic criteria for sporadic CJD

I   Rapidly progressive dementia

II A Pyramidal or extrapyramidal features
    B Visual or cerebellar problems
    C Myoclonus
    D Akinetic mutism

III A Typical EEG
    B Positive 14–3–3

Definite: Neuropathological/immunocytochemically
            confirmed
Probable: I + 2 of II + III A or III B
Possible: I + 2 of II and duration <2 years

patients develop myoclonic seizures. These are initially driven by auditory (sometimes visual or tactile) stimuli (stimulus-sensitive myoclonus), but later become spontaneous, at a rate of about 1 Hz, which may or may not be symmetrical.

Clinical criteria have been formulated for CJD. Some of these, not yet published formally, are presented in Table 17.2. While these criteria are very important for epidemiological studies, they are less useful for clinical decisions on individual cases, particularly early on in the course of the disease. Myoclonus and akinetic mutism usually appear late in the disease, and the EEG may also not show typical features initially. Finally, the duration of the disease is unknown in a living patient, and can exceed 2 years in some cases. The value of akinetic mutism as a classification criterion for the diagnosis of CJD has recently been discussed.[35]

Originally it was assumed that inherited prion diseases due to different mutations of the PRNP gene will each result in a unique clinical phenotype. Remarkably, recent descriptions of patients with the E200K mutation have shown marked clinical heterogeneity even within this single point mutation.[36] For example, one E200K patient demonstrated clinical and pathological features reminiscent of FFI[37] (see below). Cerebellar onset also occurs.[34] We have recently described three patients with this mutation who suffered from severe pruritus.[38] The pathogenesis of the pruritus is unknown, but it is probably analogous to that of scrapie in goats and sheep. Another large kindred with the E200K mutation had dementia and ataxia, but with additional supra-

nuclear palsy developing early in the disease.[39] Although prion diseases are essentially limited to the CNS, a notable exception is demyelinating peripheral neuropathy in patients with CJD associated with the E200K mutation.[40,41] The pathogenesis of the neuropathy is unclear, since deposition of PrP^{Sc} was not demonstrated in peripheral nerves, although it was clearly seen in the CNS of these patients.[41]

CJD is assumed to be primarily a neuronal disease (although electron microscopy reveals changes not only of neurons but also of glia cells). As a neuronal disease, it affects primarily gray matter—cortical, basal ganglionic, cerebellar, etc. However, a rare panencephalopathic form is also recognized.[42] The main clinical hallmark of this form is a slow progressive course leading to a vegetative state. Pathologically, this variant is characterized by extensive demyelination and gemistocytic gliosis, the latter suggesting that the white matter degeneration is an active destructive process rather than secondary to axonal damage. In two recently described patients with the panencephalopathic form,[42] the thalami were also severely involved, similar to that which is observed in FFI (see below). On neuroimaging, symmetrical involvement of the centrum semiovale was observed, and this was confirmed pathologically. Since the internal capsule is relatively spared, the process seems to affect mainly hemispheric U fibers.

Recently, a new variant of CJD (termed vCJD) has been described in the United Kingdom.[14–16] Clinically, it affects relatively young adults (15–42 years at onset) with initial psychiatric symptomatology leading to a progressive cerebellar syndrome, usually within months. An early onset of CJD is very rare (although it was common in kuru). Moreover, the clinical onset was atypical for the usual adult-type CJD, because of the prominence of psychiatric symptomatology and ataxia rather than cognitive decline. Again, this picture is reminiscent of kuru. Finally, a unique pathological picture emerged. The spongiform changes are concentrated in the basal ganglia and thalamus. 'Kuru-type' amyloid plaques are widely distributed, and may have features distinguishing them from the plaques formed in other prion diseases.

Gerstmann–Strussler syndrome

GSS is much less common than CJD. Its onset is in the third to sixth decades of life, and the presenting symptom is cerebellar ataxia, with the gradual appearance of cognitive impairment and sometimes pyramidal symptomatology. The evolution of GSS is typically considerably longer than that of CJD. All cases of GSS described to date have been associated with specific mutations of the PRNP gene.

GSS is classically associated with a P102L mutation of the PRNP gene. Dementia develops insidiously and death occurs in about 10 years. Other point mutations of the PRNP gene were also associated with the GSS genotype, involving codons 105, 117, 145, 198 and 217. The pathological phenotype of GSS is defined as the occurrence of multicentric amyloid plaques in the CNS composed largely of prion protein. Nevertheless, in the largest family with the codon 102 mutation, some patients presented not with ataxia but rather with dementia. Patients with the A117V point mutation can also present with either dementia or ataxia.

Fatal familial insomnia (FFI)

Hypersomnia or insomnia are well known to occur in CJD, and were reported by Heidenhain in one of his original cases. Nevertheless, a new disease was later described, in which the insomnia was very severe.[44] These patients also had autonomic symptoms such as hypertension, tachycardia, hyperhydrosis and hyperthermia. Dysarthria, dysphagia, ataxia and myoclonus developed later. Because of the predominance of the sleep abnormalities, this variant of prion disease was termed fatal familial insomnia. The pathological features include severe destruction of the thalamic nuclei with astrogliosis, but without spongiform changes or amyloid deposits.

The disease is transmitted as a dominantly inherited disorder and was linked to a mutation at codon 178 of the PRNP. Interestingly, the same mutation may cause CJD, and which phenotype develops depends on a polymorphism at codon 129 of the PRNP gene, with homozygosity leading to FFI and heterozygosity to CJD. It was suggested that in both cases the disease is initiated by a conversion, in the thalamus, of the cellular form of PrP (PrP^c) into a β-pleated, protease-resistant, isoform (PrP^{res}). If the patients are homozygous at codon 129, further local rapid transformation occurs, leading to the clinical picture of FFI, whereas in patients who are heterozygous at 129, a more widespread distribution of PrP^{res} throughout the brain will occur, with the consequence of the development of CJD rather than FFI.[45,46]

A detailed examination of the behavioral cognitive features of patients with FFI demonstrated: (1) early impairment of attention and vigilance; (2) memory deficits, mainly of working memory; (3) impairment of temporal ordering of events; and (4) a progressive dream-like state with neuropsychological and behavioral features of a confusional state.[47]

Kuru

The clinical features of kuru have included, in many cases, childhood onset of ataxia and spasticity which have progressed and led to death within a few years. The disease was transmitted by ritualistic cannibalism and it is now mainly of historical interest.

Kuru is perhaps the most stereotypic of the human prion diseases, and the elucidation of the transmitted nature of the disease by Gajdusek was the breakthrough leading to the understanding of basic mechanisms related to prion diseases. It is of scientific interest, however, that although ritualistic cannibalism has presumably not been practiced in New Guinea for 30 years or more, very few new cases still occur in the region. None of these occur in children (who had been most frequently affected in the past when kuru was prevalent), pointing to the very long incubation period which may occur in kuru and other prion diseases.

DIAGNOSTIC METHODS

Pathology

Until recently, a firm diagnosis of prion diseases was based on pathological examination of brain tissues. The typical pathology of prion diseases, in humans and in animals, consists of spongiform changes, remarkable gliosis, and deposition of protein amyloid plaques. The distribution of these changes in the brain differs in the various diseases. For example, in CJD, 'status spongiosus' is mainly cortical, while the amyloid plaques are meager. In GSS, the degenerative changes occur mainly in the cerebellum, and plaques are abundant. However, spongiotic changes may occasionally be seen in other degenerative brain diseases. Staining for prion protein is obviously the only truly specific microscopic verification for prion disease, and is probably the earliest sign.[48] A monoclonal antibody was developed[49] which is specific to PrP^{Sc}.

The availability of brain tissue is obviously limited, and the diagnosis is frequently established only after death. In vivo brain biopsies are limited, and the biopsied site may not necessarily represent changes occurring elsewhere in the brain (e.g. the thalamus or the cerebellum). Neuropathological diagnostic criteria for prion diseases were recently proposed.[50]

Recent evidence suggests that PrP may exist in tonsilar tissue in vCJD,[51] and possibly in other reticulolymphoid tissues.

Transmissibility

Inoculation of brain tissue removed from a diseased individual intracerebrally into an experimental animal is a specific method to demonstrate the existence of prion disease. It is technically difficult and can only be performed in laboratories which specialize in this area. Another disadvantage of this method is that results are only observed after prolonged periods, depending, among other factors, on the species barrier and the exact type of PrP[res] which is injected. Recently, FFI was also transmitted to rodents.[52]

Neuroimaging

The main changes observed with CT and MRI in CJD reflect the atrophic changes, although these appear relatively late in the course of the disease. Because of their non-specific nature, these will not assist in the diagnosis except when atrophy progresses within a few months, since this is unlikely to be seen in other degenerative brain diseases.[53-55] The occurrence of hyperdense lesions in brain CT and of high signals in the basal ganglia (and sometimes cortically) on T2-weighted images on the MRI has been observed in iatrogenic, genetic and sporadic CJD. Occasional enhancement after gadolinium has also been seen.[56-63] These MRI changes are suggestive of CJD, and occurred in 23 of 29 consecutive CJD patients in a recently described series.[61] Another series[57] suggested that the site of hyperintensity on MRI correlates with clinical features, e.g. that patients with basal ganglia hyperintensities have extrapyramidal features. Their pathogenesis is unknown, but possibly reflects the combination of gliosis with iron deposition.

Magnetic resonance diffusion abnormalities have also been described in CJD.[58]

EEG

Early in the course of the disease, EEG shows non-specific slowing consistent with the cognitive impairment. As the disease progresses, triphasic waves appear leading to the characteristic periodic spikes occurring at a rate of approximately 1 Hz. These discharges are not metronomic and, if myoclonic contractions occur, they do not necessarily coincide with the myoclonus. These EEG changes are not specific and may occur in various metabolic encephalopathies and may be due to toxic effects of drug,[64,65] but have not been described in other neurodegenerative diseases. Therefore, in the right context, their occurrence constitutes strong evidence favoring the diagnosis of CJD.[66] Interestingly, patients with E200K CJD are less likely than sporadic cases to exhibit this phenomenon. Occasionally, the complexes appear as periodic lateralized epileptiform complexes. In GSS and FFI, EEG slowing may occur but periodic sharp wave discharges have not been reported. The pathogenesis of the pseudo-periodic EEG discharges in CJD is unclear.[68] The assumption that they originate from simultaneous cortical activation by deep structures, perhaps the thalamus, is not supported by data. In fact, using microcomputer brain-mapping techniques, the generalized discharges were shown not to be strictly generalized in onset, nor bilaterally symmetrical, suggesting that multifocal areas of onset trigger the discharges.[69]

The degenerative process is reflected by a progressive deterioration of brainstem auditory evoked potentials in CJD.[70]

Cerebrospinal fluid

The cerebrospinal fluid (CSF) in prion diseases is usually normal, except for a mild to moderate hyperproteinorrhachia in some cases. There is no evidence of an inflammatory reaction. In 1986 Harrington et al demonstrated that the CSF of CJD patients contains abnormal protein fractions.[71] The amino acid sequence of these proteins matched that found in a brain protein known as 14-3-3.[62] A simple rapid radioimmunoassay which was developed proved 14-3-3 to be a sensitive and relatively specific marker for prion diseases in humans and animals, although false-positive results occur in patients with encephalitis or a recent stroke.[72] The reliability of the test in the early detection of prion disease remains to be established.[73] The widespread use of this test may help in the estimation of the prevalence of prion disease in patients with dementia who do not have other clinical markers of the disease.

Neuron-specific enolase (NSE) was also confirmed to be elevated in the CSF of most patients with CJD,[73] but the relevance of this assay in the early diagnosis of CJD is unknown. Glial proteins such as S-100 may also be helpful.[74,75] It is quite likely that a combination of all these markers together may be quite specific (but probably less sensitive) for the diagnosis of CJD.[76]

TRANSMISSIBILITY OF PRION DISEASES TO HUMANS

Human-to-human transmission of CJD has been repeatedly demonstrated,[77–79] although it always invoked iatrogenic procedures rather than direct case-to-case transmission. A previous claim for conjugal CJD was recently withdrawn.[80] Nevertheless, secure disinfection procedures of instruments used, particularly in neurosurgery, must be ensured. Inactivation by high-temperature (134 °C) moist-heat sterilization has been suggested.[81]

The practical issues involved in handling the tissues for patients with established or suspected prion diseases have been addressed in a consensus report by Budka et al.[82] When following the recommended guidelines, autopsy or biopsy can be safely performed.

REFERENCES

1. Prusiner SB. Human prion diseases and neurodegeneratior. *Curr Topics Microbiol Immunol* 1996; **207**: 1–17.
2. Manuelidis L, Sklaviadis C, Akowitz A, Fritch W. Viral particles are required for infection in neurodegenerative Creutzfeldt–Jakob disease. *Proc Natl Acad Sci USA* 1995; **92**: 5124–5128.
3. Manuelidis L, Fritch W. Infectivity and host responses in Creutzfeldt–Jakob disease. *Virology* 1996; **216**: 46–59.
4. Lasmezas C, Deslys J-P, Robain O et al. Transmission of the BSE agent to mice in the absence of detectable abnormal prion protein. *Science* 1997; **275**: 402–404.
5. Korczyn AD. Prion disease. *Curr Opin Neurol* 1997; **10**: 273–281.
6. Aguzzi A, Weissmann C. Prion research: the next frontiers. *Nature* 1997; **389**: 795–798.
7. Holman RC, Khan AS, Kent J, Strine TW, Schonberger LB. Epidemiology of Creutzfeldt–Jakob disease in the United States, 1979–1990: analysis of national mortality data. *Neuroepidemiology* 1995; **14**: 174–181.
8. Alperovitch A. Epidemiology of Creutzfeldt–Jakob disease—past and present uncertainties. *Eur J Neurol* 1996; **3**: 500–506.
9. Scrimgeour EM, Chand PR, Kimbra K, Brown P. Creutzfeldt–Jakob disease in Oman: report of two cases. *J Neurol Sci* 1996; **142**: 148–150.
10. Masullo C, Brown PW, Macchi G. Creutzfeldt–Jakob disease in an Iranian: the first clinico-pathologically described cases. *Clin Neuropathol* 1996; **15**: 26–29.
11. Hainfellner JA, Jellinger K, Diringer H et al. Creutzfeldt–Jakob disease in Austria. *J Neurol Neurosurg Psychiatry* 1996; **61**: 139–142.
12. Bruton CJ, Bruton RK, Gentleman SM, Roberts GW. Diagnosis and incidence of prion (Creutzfeldt–Jakob) disease: a retrospective archival survey with implications for future research. *Neurodegeneration* 1995; **4**: 357–368.
13. Davanipour Z, Smoak C, Bohr T, Sobel E, Liwnicz B, Chang S. Death certificates: an efficient source for ascertainment of Creutzfeldt–Jakob disease cases. *Neuroepidemiology* 1995; **14**: 1–6.
14. Will RG, Ironside JW, Zeidler M et al. A new variant of Creutzfeldt–Jakob disease in the UK. *Lancet* 1996; **347**: 921–925.
15. Zeidler M, Stewart GE, Barraclough CR et al. New variant Creutzfeldt–Jakob disease: neurological features and diagnostic tests. *Lancet* 1997; **350**: 903–907.
16. Zeidler M, Johnstone EC, Bamber RWK et al. New variant Creutzfeldt–Jakob disease: psychiatric features. *Lancet* 1997; **350**: 908–910.
17. Korczyn AD. Bovine spongiform encephalopathy and Creutzfeldt–Jakob disease—a beefy problem? *Singapore Med J* 1996; **37**: 245–246.
18. Cousens SN, Vynnycky E, Zeidler M, Will RG, Smith RG. Predicting the CJD epidemic in humans. *Nature* 1997; **385**: 197–198.
19. Goldfarb LG, Korczyn AD, Brown P, Chapman J, Gajdusek DC. Mutation in codon 200 of scrapie amyloid precursor gene linked to Creutzfeldt–Jakob disease in Sephardic Jews of Libyan and non-Libyan origin. *Lancet* 1990; **336**: 637–638.
20. Chapman J, Ben-Israel J, Goldhammer Y, Korczyn AD. The risk of developing Creutzfeldt–Jakob disease in subjects with the PRNP gene codon 200 point mutation. *Neurology* 1994; **44**: 1683–1686.
21. Spudich S, Mastrianni JA, Wrensch M et al. Complete penetrance of Creutzfeld–Jakob disease in Libyan Jews carrying the E200K mutation in the prion protein gene. *Mol Med* 1995; **6**: 607–613.
22. Salvatore M, Pocchiari M, Cardone F et al. Codon 200 mutation in a new family of Chilean origin with Creutzfeldt–Jakob disease. *J Neurol Neurosurg Psychiatry* 1996; **61**: 111–123.
23. Goldfarb LG, Brown P, Mitrova B et al. Creutzfeldt–Jakob disease associated with the PRNP codon 200Lys mutation: an analysis of 45 families. *Eur J Epidemiol* 1991; **7**: 477–486.
24. Wientjens DPWM, Davanipour Z, Hofman A et al. Risk factors for Creutzfeldt–Jakob disease: a re-analysis of case–control studies. *Neurology* 1996; **46**: 1287–1291.
25. Collinge J, Owen F, Poulter M et al. Prion dementia without characteristic pathology. *Lancet* 1990; **336**: 7–9.
26. Kitamoto T, Amano N, Terao Y et al. A new inherited prion disease (PrP-P105L mutation) showing spastic paraparesis. *Ann Neurol* 1993; **34**: 808–813.
27. Samaia HB, Mari J de J, Vallada HP, Moura RP, Simpson AJG, Brentani RR. Prions linked to mental illness. *Nature* 1997; **390**: 241.
28. McNaughton HK, Will RG. Creutzfeldt–Jakob disease presenting acutely as stroke; an analysis of 30 cases. *Neurol Infect Epidemiol* 1997; **2**: 19–24.
29. Kothbauer-Margreiter I, Baumgartner RW, Bassetti C, Mathis J. Hemisensory deficit in a patient with Creutzfeld–Jakob disease. *Eur Neurol* 1996; **36**: 108–109.
30. Vargas ME, Kupersmith MJ, Savino PJ, Petito F, Frohman LP, Warren FA. Homonymous field defect as the first manifestation of Creutzfeld–Jakob diseases. *Am J Ophthalmol* 1995; **119**: 497–504.
31. Mandell M, Alexander MP, Carpenter S. Creutzfeldt–Jakob disease presenting as isolated aphasia. *Neurology* 1989; **39**: 55–58..
32. Kirk A, Ang LC. Unilateral Creutzfeldt–Jakob disease presenting as rapidly progressive aphasia. *Can J Neurol Sci* 1994; **21**: 350–352.
33. MacGowan DJL, Delantry N, Petito F, Edgar M, Mastrianni J, DeArmond SL. Isolated myoclonic alien hand as the sole presentation of pathologically established Creutzfeldt–Jakob disease: a report of two patients. *J Neurol Neurosurg Psychiatry* 1997; **63**: 404–407.

34. Kott B, Bornstein B, Sandbank U. Ataxic form of Creutzfeldt-Jakob disease: its relation to subacute spongiform encephalopathy. *J Neurol Sci* 1967; **5**: 107–113.

35. Otto A, Zerr I, Lantsch M, Weidehaas K, Riedemann C, Poser S. Akinetic mutism as a classification criterion for the diagnosis of Creutzfeldt–Jakob disease. *J Neurol Neurosurg Psychiatry* 1998; **64**: 524–528.

36. Chapman J, Brown P, Goldfarb LG, Arlazaroff A, Gajdusek DC, Korczyn AD. Clinical heterogeneity and unusual presentations of Creutzfeldt–Jakob disease in Jewish patients with PRNP codon 200 mutation. *J Neurol Neurosurg Psychiatry* 1993; **56**: 1109–1112.

37. Chapman J, Arlazoroff A, Goldfarb LG et al. Fatal insomnia in a case of familial Creutzfeldt–Jakob disease with the codon 200(Lys) mutation. *Neurology* 1996; **46**: 758–761.

38. Shabtai H, Nisipeanu P, Chapman J, Korczyn AD. Pruritus in Creutzfeldt–Jakob disease. *Neurology* 1996; **46**: 940–941.

39. Bertoni M, Brown P, Goldfarb LG, Rubenstein R, Gajdusek C. Familial Creutzfeldt–Jakob disease (Codon 200 mutation) with supranuclear palsy. *JAMA* 1992; **268**: 2413–2415.

40. Neufeld M, Josiphov J, Korczyn D. Demyelinating peripheral Creutzfeld–Jakob disease. *Muscle Nerve* 1992; **15**: 1234–1239.

41. Antoine JC, Laplanche JL, Mosnier JF, Beaudry P, Chatelain J, Michel D. Demyelinating peripheral neuropathy with Creutzfeldt–Jakob disease and mutation at codon 200 of the prion protein gene. *Neurology* 1996; **46**: 1123–1126.

42. Carota A, Pizzolato GP, Gailloud P et al. A panencephalopathic type of Creutzfeldt–Jakob disease with selective lesions of the thalamic nuclei in 2 Swiss patients. *Clin Neuropathol* 1996; **15**: 125–134.

43. Mastrianni JA, Curtis MT, Oberholtzer JC et al. Prion disease (PrP-A117V) presenting with ataxia instead of dementia. *Neurology* 1995; **45**: 2042–2050.

44. Medori R, Tritschler H-J, LeBlanc A et al. Fatal familial insomnia, a prion disease with a mutation at codon 178 of the prion protein gene. *N Engl J Med* 1992; **326**: 444–449.

45. Hauw J-J, Sazdovitch V, Seilhean D et al. The nosology and neuropathology of human conditions related to unconventional infectious agents or prions. *Eur J Neurol* 1996; **3**: 487–499.

46. Gambetti P. Fatal familial insomnia and familial Creutzfeldt–Jakob disease: a tale of two diseases with the same genetic mutations. *Curr Topics Microbiol Immunol* 1996; **207**: 19–25.

47. Gallassi R, Morreale A, Montagna P et al. Fatal familial insomnia: behavioral and cognitive feature. *Neurology* 1996; **46**: 935–939.

48. Castellani R, Parchi P, Stahl J, Capellari S, Cohen M, Gambetti P. Early pathologic and biochemical changes in Creutzfeldt–Jakob disease: study of brain biopsies. *Neurology* 1996; **46**: 1690–1693.

49. Korth C, Stierli B, Streit P et al. Prion (PrP^Sc)-specific epitope defined by a monoclonal antibody. *Nature* 1997; **390**: 74.

50. Budka H, Aguzzi A, Brown P et al. Neuropathological diagnostic criteria for Creutzfeldt–Jakob disease (CJD) and other human spongiform encephalopathies (prion diseases). *Brain Pathol* 1995; **5**: 459–466.

51. Hill AF, Zeidler M, Ironside J, Collinge J. Diagnosis of new variant Creutzfeldt–Jakob disease by tonsil biopsy. *Lancet* 1996; **347**: 921–925.

52. Tateishi J, Brown P, Kitamoto T, Hoque ZM, Cervenkov L, Gajdusek DC. First experimental transmission of fatal familial insomnia. *Nature* 1995; **375**: 434–435.

53. Garcia Santos JM, Lopez Corbalan JA, Martinez-Lage JF, Sicilia Guillon J. CT and MRI in iatrogenic and sporadic Creutzfeldt–Jakob disease: as far as imaging perceives. *Neuroradiology* 1996; **38**: 226–231.

54. Hunter R, Gordon A, McLuskie R et al. Gross regional cerebral hypofunction with normal CT scan in Creutzfeldt–Jakob disease. *Lancet* 1989; **333**: 214–215.

55. Ishida S, Sugino M, Koizumi N et al. Serial MRI in early Creutzfeldt–Jakob disease with a point mutation of prion protein at codon 180. *Neuroradiology* 1995; **37**: 531–534.

56. Finkenstaedt M, Szudra A, Zerr I et al. MR imaging of Creutzfeldt–Jakob disease. *Radiology* 1996; **199**: 793–798.

57. Urbach H, Klisch J, Wolf HK, Brechtelsbauer D, Gass S, Solymosi L. MRI in sporadic Creutzfeld–Jakob disease: correlation with clinical and neuropathological data. *Neuroradiology* 1998; **40**: 65–70.

58. Bahn MM, Kido DK, Lin W, Pearlman AL. Brain magnetic resonance diffusion abnormalities in Creutzfeldt–Jakob disease. *Arch Neurol* 1997; **54**: 1411–1415.

59. Almond JW, Brown P, Gore SM et al. Creutzfeldt–Jakob disease and bovine spongiform encephalopathy: magnetic resonance imaging may have a role in diagnosing Creutzfeldt–Jakob diseas. *BMJ* 1996; **312**: 180–181.

60. Yoon SS, Chan S, Chin S, Lee K, Goodman RR. MRI of Creutzfeldt–Jakob disease: asymmetric high signal intensity of the basal ganglia. *Neurology* 1995; **45**: 1932–1933.

61. Horng-Huei L, Hou-Chang C, Hon-Man L. Abnormal enhancement of the left putamen on brain MRI in a case of proven Creutzfeldt–Jakob disease. *Eur Neurol* 1996; **36**: 107–108.

62. Ogawa T, Inugami A, Fujita H et al. Serial positron emission tomography with fludeoxyglucose F18 in Creutzfeldt–Jakob disease. *Am J Neuroradiol* 1995; **16**(suppl): 978–981.

63. Matochik JA, Molchan SE, Zametkin AJ, Warden DL, Sunderland T, Cohen RM. Regional cerebral glucose metabolism in autopsy-confirmed Creutzfeldt–Jakob disease. *Acta Neurol Scand* 1995; **91**: 153–157.

64. Fear CF. Drug-induced Creutzfeldt–Jakob like syndrome: a review. *Human Psychopharmacol* 1992; **7**: 89–95.

65. Koponen H, Honkonen S, Partanen J, Riekkinen PJ. Epileptic attack, delirium and a Creutzfeldt–Jakob-like syndrome during mianserin treatment. *Neuropsychobiology* 1990; **23**: 164–168.

66. Steinhoff BJ, Rucker S, Herrendorf G et al. Accuracy and reliability of periodic sharp wave complexes in Creutzfeldt–Jakob disease. *Arch Neurol* 1996; **53**: 162–166.

67. Au WJ, Gabor AJ, Vijayan N, Markand ON, Periodic lateralized epileptiform complexes (PLEDs) in Creutzfeldt–Jakob disease. *Neurology* 1980; **30**: 611–617.

68. Shibasaki H, Motomura S, Yamashita Y, Shii H, Kuroiwa Y. Periodic synchronous discharge and myoclonus in Creutzfeldt–Jakob disease: diagnostic application of jerk-locked averaging method. *Ann Neurol* 1981; **9**: 150–156.

69. Neufeld MY, Korczyn AD. Topographic distribution of the periodic Creutzfeldt–Jakob disease (CJD). *Brain Topography* 1992; **4**: 201–206.

70. Pollak L, Klein C, Giladi R, Kertesz J, Arlazoroff A. Progressive deterioration of brainstem auditory evoked potentials in Creutzfeldt–Jakob disease: clinical and electroencephalographic correlation. *Clin Electroencephalogr* 1996; **27**: 95–99.

71. Harrington MG, Merril CR, Asher DM, Gajdusek DC. Abnormal proteins in the cerebrospinal fluid of patients with Creutzfeldt–Jakob disease. *N Engl J Med* 1986; **315**: 279–283.

72. Zerr I, Bodemer M, Gefeller O et al. Detection of 14-3-3 protein in the cerebrospinal fluid supports the diagnosis of Creutzfeldt–Jakob disease. *Ann Neurol* 1998; 32–40.

73. Zerr I, Bodemer M, Rocker, Grosche S, Poser S. Cerebrospinal fluid concentration of neuron-specific enolase in diagnosis of Creutzfeldt–Jakob disease. *Lancet* 1995; **345**: 1609–1610.

74. Otto M, Stein H, Szudra A et al. S-100 protein concentration in the cerebrospinal fluid of patients with Creutzfeld–Jakob disease. *J Neurol* 1997; **244**: 566–570.

75. Otto M, Wiltfang J, Schutz F et aI. Diagnosis of Creutzfeldt–Jakob disease by measurement of S100 protein in serum: prospective case–control study. *BMJ* 1998; **316**: 577–582.

76. Weber T, Otto M, Bodemer M, Zerr I. Diagnosis of Creutzfeldt–Jakob disease and related human spongiform encephalopathies. *Biomed Pharmacother* 1997; **51**: 381–387.

77. Holmes SJ, Ironside JW, Shalet SM. Neurosurgery in a patient with Creutzfeldt–Jakob disease after pituitary derived growth hormone therapy in childhood. *J Neurol Neurosurg Psychiatry* 1996; **60**: 333–335.

78. Collins SJ, Masters CL. Transmissibility of Creutzfeldt–Jakob disease and related disorders. *Sci Prog* 1995; **78**(Pt 3): 217–227.

79. Brown P. The risk of bovine spongiform encephalopathy ('Mad Cow Disease') to human health. *JAMA* 1997; **278**: 1008–1011.

80. Hainfellner JA, Jellinger K, Budka H. Testing for prion protein does not confirm previously reported conjugal CJD. *Lancet* 1996; **347**: 616–617.

81. van Asten JAAM, Geertsma RE, Dorpema J-W. Prions and hospital infections. *Lancet* 1996; **347**: 966–967.

82. Budka H, Aguzzi A, Brown P et al. Tissue handling in suspected Creutzfeldt–Jakob disease (CJD) and other human spongiform encephalopathies (prion diseases). *Brain Pathol* 1995; **5**: 319–322.

18

Neurologic manifestations of lymphoproliferative disorders

Tali Siegal

INTRODUCTION

Neurologic manifestations of lymphoproliferative disorders can be categorized into those related to a specific disorder (Table 18.1) or by the way in which the disorder may affect the nervous system (Table 18.2).

Many patients with either direct or indirect involvement of the nervous system may present with clinical symptoms that are similar to each other. For example, parenchymal brain infiltration and metabolic encephalopathy can all appear as delirium, pointing to the brain as the site of the lesion but giving no clue as to the nature of the lesion. Similarly, spinal cord compression, radiation-induced myelopathy and

---

Table 18.1 Neurologic manifestations of lymphoproliferative disorders

Neurologic manifestations of plasma cell dyscrasias
Paraproteinemias
  Neoplastic
  Benign (MGUS)
Plasmacytoma
  Solitary or multiple plasmacytomas
  Typical osteolytic
  Osteosclerotic
Multiple myeloma
  Typical osteolytic
  Osteosclerotic

Neurologic manifestations of lymphomas
Primary central nervous system lymphomas (NHL)
  B-cell type
  T-cell type
Systemic lymphomas
  Non-Hodgkin's lymphomas (B-cell, T-cell type)
  Hodgkin's lymphoma

Neurologic manifestations of leukemias
ALL
AML
CLL
Others

NHL, non-Hodgkin's lymphoma.

Table 18.2 Classification of neurologic complications of the neoplastic process

Direct effects of the neoplastic process on the nervous system
Intracranial
Spinal
Leptomeningeal
Nerves (cranial nerves, peripheral nerves, plexuses, nerve roots)
Muscle (rare)

Indirect neurologic complications of the neoplastic disorder (non-metastatic or paraneoplastic)
Vascular disorders
Infections
Metabolic and nutritional disorders
Side-effects of therapy
  Chemotherapy
  Radiation therapy
  Surgery and other diagnostic or therapeutic procedures
  Bone marrow transplantation
Paraneoplastic syndromes

paraneoplastic myelopathy can all present with similar symptoms. Because such situations arise commonly in neuro-oncologic manifestations of lymphoproliferative disorders, it is useful to determine the site of the lesion first and then to consider the various neuro-oncologic disorders that may cause it. This approach is outlined in Table 18.3, which lists the common causes of neuro-oncologic disorders found in lymphoproliferative processes, and localizes them to specific portions of the central and peripheral nervous systems.

The scope of neurologic complications of lymphoproliferative disorders is too large to be covered in this chapter. Therefore, I have decided to discuss

Table 18.3 Neurologic complications by site in patients with lymphoproliferative disorder	
Site	**Neurologic problem**
Brain	Infiltration (metastases)
	Leptomeningeal involvement (metastases)
	Metabolic encephalopathy
	Toxic encephalopathy (e.g. HD-Arac, fludarabine, procarbazine)
	Leukoencephalopathy (delayed, treatment-induced)
	Nutritional deficiency (e.g. thiamine)
	Infections (meningitis, brain abscess)
	Radiation encephalopathy (acute, subacute, delayed)
	Cerebral hemorrhage, infarction (DIC, NBTE, intravascular lymphoma)
	Sinus thrombosis (hyperviscosity, L-asparaginase coagulopathy)
	Subdural hemorrhage (thrombocytopenia, lumbar punctures, neoplastic)
	Paraneoplastic (encephalopathy, cerebellar degeneration)
Spinal cord and cauda equina	Neoplastic epidural compression (± spinal instability)
	Leptomeningeal metastases (intradural compression, cord infiltration, root infiltration)
	Intramedularry mass involvement (metastatic)
	Epidural abscess or hematoma
	Radiation myelopathy
	Myelopathy secondary to intrathecal chemotherapy
	Paraneoplastic myelopathy
Cranial and peripheral nerves	Extrinsic compression by tumor or other mass (e.g. hematoma)
	Direct infiltration by tumor
	Drug toxicity (e.g. vinca alkaloids)
	Varicella zoster infection
	Radiation plexopathies
	Paraneoplastic neuropathy
	Autoimmune-mediated demyelination (Guillain–Barré syndrome)
	Nutritional deficiency (e.g. thiamine)
Neuromuscular	Corticosteroid-induced myopathy
	Cachectic myopathy
	Paraneoplastic disorders (myasthenia gravis)
	Drugs (cramps, malaise, aminoglycoside)

DIC, disseminated intravascular coagulation; NBTE, non-bacterial thrombotic endocarditis.

two common neurologic complications that affect patients with lymphoproliferative disorders: (1) epidural spinal cord and cauda equina compression, and (2) leptomeningeal and intraparenchymal metastatic involvement of the central nervous system (CNS). By discussing the rationale for treatment options and the associated early and delayed complications, insight may be gained into the complexity of issues involved in neuro-oncology.

EPIDURAL SPINAL CORD AND CAUDA EQUINA COMPRESSION

Hematologic malignancies that may cause disorders of the spine or an epidural compression with neurologic compromise include plasma cell dyscrasias, lymphomas and, infrequently, leukemias. In most series, lymphomas and myeloma are listed among the five most common malignancies causing epidural spinal compression.[1] The epidural invasion in lymphoproliferative disorders results from diverse modes of neoplastic spread, which should be recognized for appropriate diagnostic work-up and educated selection of therapeutic modalities.

Multiple myeloma is the most common primary tumor of bone. Bone lesions are the major manifestations in both solitary plasmacytomas and multiple myelomas and therefore they frequently present with vertebral destruction and spinal cord compression (SCC).[1] On the other hand, vertebral lesions are detected in less than 30% of patients with SCC due to lymphoma, and are rarely present in leukemia presenting an epidural mass.[1]

Plasmacytomas and multiple myeloma

Solitary plasmacytomas of bone (SPB) account for 5% of malignant plasma cell disorders.[2] The spine is a frequent site of involvement, representing 25–60% of all SPB.[1,3,4] A high incidence of SCC is reported in SPB, ranging between 43% and 71% of the cases.[1,5,6] In contrast, in multiple myeloma, where spinal involvement is always present, the reported incidence of SCC varies between 10% and 16%.[1,7,8] In many cases, SCC is the presenting manifestation of the disease, although the majority of spinal lesions are asymptomatic. Back pain and radicular pain usually precede signs of SCC by several weeks to months in about 80% of patients. The pain may be related to bone destruction, nerve root compression or dural impingement. Neurologic signs relate to the level of the lesion(s). The most affected spinal area is the thoracic spine, followed by the lumbar, while cervical involvement is uncommon.[1]

Diagnosis

Radiographically, the lesions are mainly osteolytic, although occasional osteosclerotic lesions are reported. Bone scan may be normal or may show reduced uptake, and therefore CT and MRI should be used to detect vertebral involvement and extra-osseous (epidural or paraspinal) extension.[9–11] It is important to delineate whether the tumor or bone fragments are the cause of SCC, and the whole length of the spinal canal should be investigated, since multilevel involvement is common. Therapeutic decisions and treatment planning should take into account the full extent of spinal and/or epidural disease. When SCC is the first manifestation of the disease, the diagnosis of multiple myeloma is usually not difficult, since most patients show signs of a more generalized disease process. However, in SPB, tissue diagnosis is often required to establish the nature of the lesion. The tumor is hypervascular, and needle biopsy may be associated with extensive epidural bleeding. Therefore, once the diagnosis is suspected, spinal angiography and presurgical embolization should be considered in order to obliterate the tumor blood supply prior to surgery.

Treatment

The efficacy of treatment depends on the radiosensitivity of the tumor, the patient's neurologic status at the time treatment is initiated, and maintenance of spinal stability. Myeloma and SPB are highly radiosensitive tumors, and therefore radiation therapy is currently the primary treatment of choice. The ambulation rate in patients with radiosensitive tumors approaches 80–90% following radiotherapy, and even the presence of a complete paraplegia has not prevented full recovery in 30% of the patients.[12] The role of surgery in myeloma is limited. When pain and neurologic deficit result from spinal instability and impingement of bone fragments on the neural elements, surgery may be required and considered for effective decompression and for spinal stabilization. Spine involvement in myeloma presents a particularly difficult surgical problem. Surgery may be hazardous because of poor general condition and hemostatic abnormalities. In addition, attempts at spinal stabilization may fail, as anchorage of instrumentation on the diffusely affected vertebrae may not be feasible. Preoperative MRI of the whole spine is imperative, since it demonstrates the extent of marrow involvement and facilitates treatment planning for both radiotherapy and surgery.

For SPB, radiation therapy is the treatment of choice, although many patients still undergo surgical procedures either at the time of diagnosis or for spinal stabilization. Plasmacytomas may cause enough vertebral destruction to leave the spine unstable, even when radiotherapy has eradicated all active disease. The manifestations of instability include failure to achieve pain control and progressive evolution of neurologic deficit. Prompt stabilization is then indicated, using an anterior or a posterior approach.[13] If instability is present at diagnosis or is expected after a planned surgical procedure, the best strategy is to combine tumor resection with spinal stabilization. Patients with SPB are potentially long-term survivors (50% alive at 10 years)[1,4] and therefore consideration of any further therapy should take into account long-term adverse effects. The role of adjuvant chemotherapy in the absence of residual disease is not clear, and treatment with alkylating agents is associated with a high rate of late secondary leukemia (AML): 27% in plasmacytomas after 5 years.[1,6] The evolution of plasmacytomas to myeloma or the risk for dissemination appears to depend upon several prognostic factors, listed in Table 18.4. In such patients the benefit of chemotherapy should be weighed against the risk of late complications.[1,14]

Table 18.4 Prognostic factors related to dissemination of a solitary plasmacytoma of bone

Soft tissue extension

Multiple plasmacytomas

Poorly differentiated plasma cells

Presence/persistence of paraprotein

Spinal involvement

Older age (?)

Lymphomas

SCC occurs less frequently in lymphomas than in plasma cell dyscrasias. Generally, I shall discuss the lymphomas as one group, because the clinical picture is similar. The reported incidence of SCC in malignant lymphomas varies in different series. The overall incidence for Hodgkin's disease (HD) is about 4%, and that for non-Hodgkin's lymphomas (NHL) is 2.5–4.5%.[1,15] Yet lymphomas are disproportionally represented in series of SCC when it occurs as the initial manifestation of malignancy.[1,16] Lymphomas may reach the epidural space by three routes: (1) extension from involved paravertebral

lymph nodes through the intervertebral foramina into the spinal canal; (2) extension from a lesion in the vertebral body; and (3) as isolated deposits in the epidural space or fat tissue (primary epidural lymphoma—stage IE).[17] Extension of a paravertebral tumor into the spinal canal is the most frequent modality of spread, followed by bone lesions, which are observed in 30% at diagnosis of SCC. Therefore, in adults presenting with SCC as the first manifestation of malignancy, the presence of a paravertebral mass with no bone destruction should place lymphoma high in the differential diagnosis.

Treatment

Malignant lymphomas are radio- and chemosensitive neoplasms that respond rapidly to both these modalities and only rarely cause vertebral destruction leading to spinal instability. Therefore, surgical intervention has only a limited role in the management of SCC in lymphomas. Surgery must be employed when the diagnosis has not been established and a biopsy of the mass is not possible.

Epidural metastases are likely (but not certain) to respond to chemotherapy, like the rest of the systemic tumor, particularly early in the course of the disease. Unfortunately, this effect has drawn little investigative interest. The response of certain spinal lymphomas to corticosteroid treatment[18] may serve as an example. The usual policy is not to use specific chemotherapy alone as the primary treatment of patients with SCC, because of the uncertainty of its response and the irreversibility of severe spinal cord dysfunction. Whenever possible, specific chemotherapy is combined with other therapeutic modalities. Several reports suggest that good recovery of neurologic function can be obtained by chemotherapy alone in lymphoma.[1,15] However, published experience with such a therapeutic approach is still limited, and not even one large-scale study is available. Therefore, specific chemotherapy should be considered for treating epidural tumors in the following settings. (1) When SCC is the presenting manifestation of malignancy, or when it is recognized during evaluation of the extent of disease, particularly in patients with mild neurologic dysfunction and no sign of rapid deterioration, chemotherapy should be used first. (2) A patient with SCC previously irradiated and who is not a candidate for further radiation or surgical therapy should be considered for chemotherapy. (3) In the acute treatment of symptomatic SCC, chemotherapy probably should be used in conjunction with either surgery or radiotherapy. Once a decompressive procedure has established the diagnosis and has been followed by a satisfactory neurologic recovery, then the use of radiotherapy may be postponed and chemotherapy can be administered instead. It is unclear whether radiotherapy should still follow in a patient with a complete response. However, most physicians use routine postoperative radiotherapy.

Corticosteroids and SCC

Many clinicians use high doses of steroids in SCC, although no clear-cut advantage over conventional doses has been demonstrated.[18–20] Therefore, the associated side-effects that can arise with the use of corticosteroids should be kept in proper perspective. The following recommendations apply for the use of steroids: (1) for patients with imaging evidence of SCC, but without signs of myelopathy, dexamethasone does not need to be given during treatment by radiotherapy,[20,21] (2) patients with SCC and moderate pain, but without myelopathy, may be treated with a standard dose (16 mg/day) of dexamethasone for pain relief and (3) symptomatic patients with SCC should be treated initially with high doses of dexamethasone to increase their chance of post-treatment ambulation.[13] This comes with moderate probability of high toxicity (up to 11%), which has to be accepted in view of the expected benefit. The drug should be tapered as soon as treatment with definitive modalities has been initiated.

CNS INVOLVEMENT BY SYSTEMIC LYMPHOMA

Metastatic involvement of the CNS is frequently diagnosed in patients with NHL, as opposed to its rarity in Hodgkin's disease. Table 18.5 shows the data related to the frequency of CNS involvement. Risk factors for CNS involvement were retrospectively analyzed by univariant and multivariant analysis in two large recent series.[22,23] The results are presented in Tables 18.6 and 18.7. The cumulative risk of CNS relapse at 4 years was 39% for high-grade, 20% for intermediate-grade and 7% for low-grade lymphomas.[23] CNS relapse occurred within a median of 8.5–12 months from initial diagnosis, with an interval ranging between 1 month and 8 years. As a rule, CNS relapse is soon followed by a systemic relapse in patients achieving a previous systemic response. Based on the high risk of CNS involvement in lymphoblastic histology and Burkitt's lymphoma, some form of prophylaxis for CNS disease is always included in their standard chemotherapeutic regimens. For stage IV B disease of intermediate and high-grade lymphomas, the issue of prophylaxis is still controversial, but routine initial staging should include cytologic evaluation of cerebrospinal fluid (CSF). There are no indications that peripheral or cutaneous T-cell lymphomas need special prophylactic measures compared to B-cell NHL. The influence of prophylaxis on survival in intermediate-grade and stage IV B disease will be limited, as only a few will develop an isolated CNS relapse (10% of all CNS

Table 18.5 CNS involvement in NHL	
Overall rate of involvement	5%
Lymphoblastic lymphoma and small-cell non-cleaved (Burkitt's)	20–30%
Immunoblastic and large-cell NHL	5–8%
Low- and intermediate-grade NHL	3%[a]

[a]Low grade: after transformation to high-grade disease.

Table 18.6 Risk factors for CNS involvement (univariant analysis)	
Danish series[22] n = 498	**Dutch series[23]** n = 532
Lymphoblastic histology (including Burkitt's lymphoma)	High grade
Age < 35 years	Age < 30 years
B symptoms	
Stage IV	Stage III–IV
Testis involvement	Testis involvement
Bone marrow (+)	Bone marrow (+)
	Progression on Tx

Table 18.7 Risk factors for CNS involvement (multivariant analysis)	
Danish series[22] n = 498	**Dutch series[23]** n = 532
Lymphoblastic histology	Intermediate grade
Stage IV disease	High grade
B symptoms	Stage IV

Table 18.8 Sites of CNS involvement in NHL

Author	Year	No. of patients	LM (%)	Parenchymal (%)	Combined (%)
Lossos et al[34]	1999	23	50	30	18
van Biesen et al[37]	1998	24	62	NA	38
Bollen et al[23]	1997	66	32	42	26
Keldsen et al[22]	1996	27	33	56	11
Bashir et al[38]	1991	14	79	21	0
Wolf et al[39]	1985	44	52	45	2
Johnson et al[40]	1984	29	79	10	10
Levitt et al[41]	1980	52	85	15	0
Herman et al[42]	1979	50	80	18	2
Litam et al[43]	1979	31	84	13	3
Young et al[44]	1979	20	80	10	10

LM, leptomeningeal metastases; NA, not available.

relapses). Whether prophylaxis reduces neurologic morbidity is unclear, and the issue of possible delayed neurotoxicity of prophylactic regimens in adults has never been studied systematically. The simultaneous development of systemic and CNS disease as observed in most patients has important therapeutic implications, as will be discussed later.

Clinical manifestations

Symptoms and signs of CNS involvement are caused by either leptomeningeal or parenchymal infiltration and by CSF flow obstruction with a resulting increase in intracranial pressure. Table 18.8 summarizes the sites of CNS involvement, and Table 18.9 delineates the signs and symptoms described in a large series of CNS involvement by NHL. It is clear that in recent years parenchymal involvement has been recognized more frequently with the routine use of MRI for staging of the CNS disease. Parenchymal involvement may be present in more than 50% of patients with CNS disease, and this recognition has important therapeutic implications.

As the whole neuroaxis may be involved, symptoms and signs are variable, depending on the localization of tumor cells. Characteristically, there are symptoms and signs at several levels of the neuroaxis.

Diagnosis

A high index of suspicion is important in order to diagnose patients at early presentation of CNS

Table 18.9 Signs and symptoms in 90 patients with CNS involvement by NHL[45]

Symptoms/signs	% of patients
Positive cytology—asymptomatic	11
Headaches	23
Cranial nerve involvement	36
VII	18
III	11
V	8
VI	7
IX, X	4
XII	4
II, IV, VIII	3
Encephalopathy, altered cognitive function	42
Seizures	3
Spinal cord symptoms and signs	44

involvement. Any patient with a history of NHL who develops neurologic symptoms must be suspected for CNS involvement. The diagnosis rests on positive CSF cytology and on typical MRI findings. In most patients, CSF is diagnostic and MRI verifies parenchymal infiltration, which is often asymptomatic. Repeated CSF studies may be required to prove the diagnosis, since the first spinal tap is positive in

Table 18.10   Complementary tests in patients with persistent negative CSF cytology and suspected CNS seeding

Cisternal or ventricular CSF evaluation

Immunocytochemical studies of CSF cells with monoclonal antibodies (polyclonality does not rule out tumor)

Biochemical markers (non-specific)

  β_2-Microglobulin

  LDH isoenzymes (IV and V)

Flow cytometry (occasionally helpful)

PCR

  Ig gene rearrangement (B-cells)

  T-cell receptor

Enhanced MRI of the whole neuroaxis (suggestive, non-specific)

LDH, lactate dehydrogenase.

50–80% of patients and diagnostic certainty increases with repeated taps and approaches 90%. Still, in some patients, CSF cytology remains negative and in less than 5% of patients with LM the CSF is entirely normal. Table 18.10 lists the methods which may help in the presence of persistently negative cytology. It should be recognized that none of the listed methods can absolutely exclude the presence of an atypical infection, like toxoplasmosis, which may mimic CNS involvement by the primary neoplasm, or may coexist with asymptomatic seeding of the CNS.

Treatment and complications

In primary CNS lymphoma (which is a NHL), which has a high propensity for subarachnoid dissemination, standard therapy usually includes systemic chemotherapy, high-dose chemotherapy and various combinations of radiotherapy.[24,25] Recent evidence indicates that intensive systemic chemotherapy schedules probably reduce the need to fortify treatment with high doses of radiation therapy delivered to extended fields of the CNS. Favorable outcomes can be obtained by systemic chemotherapy alone, by limited use of radiotherapy and intra-CSF therapy.[26-28] A similar approach is being adopted and employed in the effort to prevent or treat CNS seeding by systemic lymphoproliferative neoplasms.[29] Efforts to establish effective therapy for leptomeningeal metastases have had a dramatic effect only in childhood acute lymphoblastic leukemia with the addition of prophylactic therapy.

Prophylactic therapy treats subclinical leptomeningeal seeding and includes various combinations of intra-CSF chemotherapy and irradiation. Yet, CNS prophylaxis can be successfully obtained by treatment protocols that use systemic high doses of methotrexate (MTX) or cytosine arabinoside (Ara-C), eliminating the need to apply radiation therapy to the CNS, or alternatively by combining intra-CSF chemotherapy with cranial irradiation. The use of high doses of either MTX or Ara-C leads to therapeutic levels within the CNS[29,30] and offers concomitant treatment to other sanctuaries located outside the CNS (systemic disease).

Conventional therapy for overt meningeal leukemia or lymphomas consists of intrathecal or intraventricular chemotherapy (mainly with MTX and/or Ara-C) plus radiation therapy applied to the cranial, craniospinal or symptomatic regions of the CNS. This approach is effective in clearing the CSF of malignant cells and in obtaining an initial clinical response in about 80% of patients. However, it is limited in both leukemias and lymphomas by the short duration of remission due to successive CNS, bone marrow and systemic relapses. Review of the survival data of patients with leptomeningeal lymphomas reveals a dismal prognosis, despite the high rate of initial response. The median survival ranges between 2 and 6 months and the 1-year survival is between 12% and 23% (Table 18.11).

Table 18.11   Survival of patients with CNS involvement by systemic NHL

Author	Year	No. of patients	Median survival (months)	1-year survival (%)
Young et al[44]	1979	38	1.5	16
Mackintosh et al[46]	1982	105	2.2	12
Wolf et al[39]	1985	44	3.2	17
Recht et al[45]	1988	96	4.0	12
Pfeffer et al[47]	1988	36	8.0	23
Liang et al[48]	1989	44	6.0	14
Bashir et al[38]	1991	14	8.0 (?)	NA
Grossman et al[49]	1993	10	3.8	NA
Keldsen et al[22]	1996	27	4.5	> 20
Chamberlain and Kormanik[33]	1996	22	10	NA
van Beisen et al[37]	1998	24	NA	25
Lossos et al[34]	1999	23	6	34

Table 18.12   Complications associated with treatment of CNS involvement by NHL

Type of complication	Frequency
Ommaya reservoir placement	About 1%
Hemorrhage	
Misplacement	
Malfunction	
Infections (ventriculitis/meningitis)	About 5%
Chemotherapy	
Acute complications	
Corticosteroid encephalopathy/psychosis/others	About 20%
Aseptic meningitis	
Intra-CSF MTX	10–50%
Intra-CSF Ara-C	
Myelopathy (after intra-CSF chemotherapy	Rare
Acute encephalopathy	
High-dose MTX	
High-dose Ara-C	
Chronic encephalopathy	
Diffuse leukoencephalopathy	> 50% (with XRT) after > 4–6 months
Intra-CSF MTX	
Intra-CSF Ara-C	
IV high-dose MTX/Ara-C	
Radiotherapy	
Acute encephalopathy	
Subacute encephalopathy	
Subacute myelopathy	10% between 2 and 6 months post-XRT
Delayed cognitive dysfunction	> 50% after > 6 months
Delayed vasculopathy	
Delayed myelopathy	

MTX, methotrexate; Ara-C, cytosine arabinoside.

Death is often related to the concomitant relapse of CNS and systemic disease. Therefore, concurrent CNS and systemic therapy is needed to treat overt active disease as well as sanctuary sites inside and outside the CNS. Such an approach may be either alternative or complementary to direct CNS therapy and is currently exemplified by systemic administration of high doses of MTX and/or Ara-C. The advantage of this approach over intra-CSF therapy is related to a more uniform distribution of the drug throughout the neuroaxis, with therapeutic concentrations obtained in brain and spinal cord tissues and deep perivascular spaces.[31,32] Such therapeutic levels are acquired regardless of the frequent presence of CSF flow obstruction.[33] Despite the clear logic and potential advantages of this approach, it has not been evaluated systematically. The limited published experience in which meningeal leukemia or lymphoma were treated by systemic high doses of Ara-C indicates that a complete CNS response was obtained in 86% of the patients, often after the first course of treatment.[29] Only 24% of these patients manifested a persistent residual extraneural disease. The median duration of complete CNS response correlated with the presence or absence of residual systemic disease, and was 8 months for no systemic residua and 4 months for patients with extraneural disease. We have treated 23 patients with CNS relapse, with a protocol based on systemic high-dose MTX as an initial modality.[34] An initial response was obtained in all the patients and addition of radiotherapy has not significantly increased the overall rate of complete response. Yet, most patients relapsed systemically and patients with parenchymal involvement did worse. It is clear that this approach needs to be combined with more intensive or additional treatment aimed at eradicating systemic disease (like high-dose chemotherapy with peripheral stem cell rescue). The best schedule and sequencing of high-dose therapy with other drugs that have more limited access to the CNS is not yet determined and is awaiting further investigation.

The systemic approach for treatment of CNS relapse offers the greatest advantage to patients with isolated CNS relapse who survive for prolonged periods or may even be cured of their disease.[29,35,36] We followed 13 patients with leptomeningeal lymphoma for a median follow-up period of 61 months after treatment withdrawal.[35,36] These patients comprised 29% of a larger group of patients with leptomeningeal lymphoma treated by radiotherapy, intra-CSF therapy and systemic chemotherapy. In these patients, the potential elimination of radiotherapy from their treatment scheme may reduce the rate of delayed neuropsychological deterioration, similar to the experience gained in brain lymphoma.[26–28] Although we did not follow our patients with formal neuropsychological testing, it is clear that all our long-term survivors have significant diffuse white matter abnormalities observed on surveillance MR imaging and 67% of them do function at home but are unemployed.

Table 18.12 lists complications observed with current modalities of therapy in use, namely intra-CSF chemotherapy, radiotherapy and systemic chemotherapy. The overall rate of complication is not negligible for both the early phase of treatment and for long-term survivors. This should be taken into account while specific treatment is offered to an individual patient with different prognostic parameters.

REFERENCES

1. Siegal T, Siegal T. Spinal epidural involvement in haematological tumors: clinical features and therapeutic options. *Leuk Lymphoma* 1991; **5**: 101–110.
2. Conklin R, Alexanian R. Clinical classification of plasma cell myeloma. *Arch Intern Med* 1975; **135**: 139–143.
3. Corwin J, Lindberg RD. Solitary plasmacytoma of bone vs. extramedullary plasmacytoma and their relationship to multiple myeloma. *Cancer* 1979; **43**: 1007–1013.
4. Bataille R, Sany J. Solitary myeloma: clinical and prognostic features of a review of 114 cases. *Cancer* 1981; **48**: 845–851.
5. Valderrama JA, Bullough PG. Solitary myeloma of the spine. *J Bone Joint Surg [Br]* 1968; **50**: 82–90.
6. Delauche-Cavallier MC, Laredo JD, Wybier M et al. Solitary plasmacytoma of the spine. Long-term clinical course. *Cancer* 1988; **61**: 1707–1714.
7. Brenner B, Carter A, Tatarsky I, Gruszkiewicz J, Peyser E. Incidence, prognostic significance and therapeutic modalities of central nervous system involvement in multiple myeloma. *Acta Haematol* 1982; **68**: 77–83.
8. Camacho J, Arnalich F, Anciones B et al. The spectrum of neurological manifestations in myeloma. *J Med* 1985; **16**: 597–611.
9. Kim RY, Smith JW, Spencer SA, Meredith RF, Salter MM. Malignant epidural spinal cord compression associated with a paravertebral mass: its radiotherapeutic outcome on radiosensitivity. *Int J Radiat Oncol Biol Phys* 1993; **27**: 1079–1083.
10. Kim HJ, Ryu KN, Choi WS, Choi BK, Choi JM, Yoon Y. Spinal involvement of hematopoietic malignancies and metastasis: differentiation using MR imaging. *Clin Imaging* 1999; **23**: 125–133.
11. Albertyn LE, Croft G, Kuss B, Dale B. The perivertebral collar—a new sign in lymphoproliferative malignancies. *Australas Radiol* 1992; **36**: 214–218.
12. Benson WJ, Scarffe JH, Todd ID, Palmer M, Crowther D. Spinal-cord compression in myeloma. *BMJ* 1979; **1**: 1541–1544.
13. Sundaresan N, Steinberger AA, Moore F et al. Indications and results of combined anterior–posterior approaches for spine tumor surgery. *J Neurosurg* 1996; **85**: 438–446.
14. Bacci G, Savini R, Calderoni P, Gnudi S, Minutillo A, Picci P. Solitary plasmacytoma of the vertebral column. A report of 15 cases. *Tumori* 1982; **68**: 271–275.
15. Wong ET, Portlock CS, O'Brien JP, DeAngelis LM. Chemosensitive epidural spinal cord disease in non-Hodgkins lymphoma. *Neurology* 1996; **46**: 1543–1547.
16. Schiff D, O'Neill BP, Suman VJ. Spinal epidural metastasis as the initial manifestation of malignancy: clinical features and diagnostic approach. *Neurology* 1997; **49**: 452–456.
17. Mora J, Wollner N. Primary epidural non-Hodgkin lymphoma: spinal cord compression syndrome as the initial form of presentation in childhood non-Hodgkin lymphoma. *Med Pediatr Oncol* 1999; **32**: 102–105.
18. Posner JB, Howieson J, Cvitkovic E. 'Disappearing' spinal cord compression: oncolytic effect of glucocorticoids (and other chemotherapeutic agents) on epidural metastases. *Ann Neurol* 1977; **2**: 409–413.
19. Greenberg HS, Kim JH, Posner JB. Epidural spinal cord compression from metastatic tumor: results with a new treatment protocol. *Ann Neurol* 1980; **8**: 361–366.
20. Loblaw DA, Laperriere NJ. Emergency treatment of malignant extradural spinal cord compression: an evidence-based guideline. *J Clin Oncol* 1998; **16**: 1613–1624.
21. Maranzano E, Latini P, Beneventi S et al. Radiotherapy without steroids in selected metastatic spinal cord compression patients. A phase II trial. *Am J Clin Oncol* 1996; **19**: 179–183.

22. Keldsen N, Michalski W, Bentzen SM, Hansen KB, Thorling K. Risk factors for central nervous system involvement in non-Hodgkins lymphoma—a multivariate analysis. *Acta Oncol* 1996; **35**: 703–708.

23. Bollen EL, Brouwer RE, Hamers S et al. Central nervous system relapse in non-Hodgkin lymphoma. A single-center study of 532 patients. *Arch Neurol* 1997; **54**: 854–859.

24. Abrey LE, DeAngelis LM, Yahalom J. Long-term survival in primary CNS lymphoma. *J Clin Oncol* 1998; **16**: 859–863.

25. DeAngelis LM, Yahalom J, Thaler HT, Kher U. Combined modality therapy for primary CNS lymphoma. *J Clin Oncol* 1992; **10**: 635–643.

26. Cher L, Glass J, Harsh GR, Hochberg FH. Therapy of primary CNS lymphoma with methotrexate-based chemotherapy and deferred radiotherapy: preliminary results. *Neurology* 1996; **46**: 1757–1759.

27. Dahlborg SA, Henner WD, Crossen JR et al. Non-AIDS primary CNS lymphoma: first example of a durable response in a primary brain tumor using enhanced chemotherapy delivery without cognitive loss and without radiotherapy. *Cancer J Sci Am* 1996; **2**: 166.

28. Freilich RJ, Delattre JY, Monjour A, DeAngelis LM. Chemotherapy without radiation therapy as initial treatment for primary CNS lymphoma in older patients. *Neurology* 1996; **46**: 435–439.

29. Morra E, Lazzarino M, Brusamolino E et al. The role of systemic high-dose cytarabine in the treatment of central nervous system leukemia. Clinical results in 46 patients. *Cancer* 1993; **72**: 439–445.

30. Lopez JA, Nassif E, Vannicola P, Krikorian JG, Agarwal RP. Central nervous system pharmacokinetics of high-dose cytosine arabinoside. *J Neurooncol* 1985; **3**: 119–124.

31. Balis FM, Blaney SM, McCully CL, Bacher JD, Murphy RF, Poplack DG. Methotrexate distribution within the subarachnoid space after intraventricular and intravenous administration. *Cancer Chemother Pharmacol* 2000; **45**: 259–264.

32. Blaney SM, Balis FM, Poplack DG. Current pharmacological treatment approaches to central nervous system leukaemia. *Drugs* 1991; **41**: 702–716.

33. Chamberlain MC, Kormanik PA. Prognostic significance of [111]indium-DTPA CSF flow studies in leptomeningeal metastases. *Neurology* 1996; **46**: 1674–1677.

34. Lossos A, Lossos I, Bokstein F, Siegal T. CNS involvement by systemic non-Hodgkin's lymphomas: results of treatment with high-dose methotrexate-based combination chemotherapy. *Neurology* 1999; **52**: A281.

35. Siegal T. Leptomeningeal metastases: rationale for systemic chemotherapy or what is the role of intra-CSF-chemotherapy? *J Neurooncol* 1998; **38**: 151–157.

36. Siegal T, Lossos A, Pfeffer MR. Leptomeningeal metastases: analysis of 31 patients with sustained off–therapy response following combined-modality therapy. *Neurology* 1994; **44**: 1463–1469.

37. van Besien K, Ha CS, Murphy S et al. Risk factors, treatment, and outcome of central nervous system recurrence in adults with intermediate-grade and immunoblastic lymphoma. *Blood* 1998; **91**: 1178–1184.

38. Bashir RM, Bierman PJ, Vose JM, Weisenburger DD, Armitage JO. Central nervous system involvement in patients with diffuse aggressive non-Hodgkin's lymphoma. *Am J Clin Oncol* 1991; **14**: 478–482.

39. Wolf MM, Olver IN, Ding JC, Cooper IA, Liew KH, Madigan JP. Non-Hodgkin's lymphoma involving the central nervous system. *Aust NZ J Med* 1985; **15**: 16–21.

40. Johnson GJ, Oken MM, Anderson JR, O'Connell MJ, Glick JH. Central nervous system relapse in unfavourable-histology non-Hodgkin's lymphoma: is prophylaxis indicated? *Lancet* 1984; **2**: 685–687.

41. Levitt LJ, Dawson DM, Rosenthal DS, Moloney WC. CNS involvement in the non-Hodgkin's lymphomas. *Cancer* 1980; **45**: 545–552.

42. Herman TS, Hammond N, Jones SE, Butler JJ, Byrne GE Jr, McKelvey EM. Involvement of the central nervous system by non-Hodgkin's lymphoma: the Southwest Oncology Group experience. *Cancer* 1979; **43**: 390–397.

43. Litam JP, Cabanillas F, Smith TL, Bodey GP, Freireich EJ. Central nervous system relapse in malignant lymphomas: risk factors and implications for prophylaxis. *Blood* 1979; **54**: 1249–1257.

44. Young RC, Howser DM, Anderson T, Fisher RI, Jaffe E, DeVita VT Jr. Central nervous system complications of non-Hodgkin's lymphoma. The potential role for prophylactic therapy. *Am J Med* 1979; **66**: 435–443.

45. Recht L, Straus DJ, Cirrincione C, Thaler HT, Posner JB. Central nervous system metastases from non-Hodgkin's lymphoma: treatment and prophylaxis. *Am J Med* 1988; **84**: 425–435.

46. MacKintosh FR, Colby TV, Podolsky WJ et al. Central nervous system involvement in non-Hodgkin's lymphoma: an analysis of 105 cases. *Cancer* 1982; **49**: 586–595.

47. Pfeffer MR, Wygoda M, Siegal T. Leptomeningeal metastases—treatment results in 98 consecutive patients. *Isr J Med Sci* 1988; **24**: 611–618.

48. Liang RH, Woo EK, Yu YL et al. Central nervous system involvement in non-Hodgkin's lymphoma. *Eur J Cancer Clin Oncol* 1989; **25**: 703–710.

49. Grossman SA, Finkelstein DM, Ruckdeschel JC, Trump DL, Moynihan T, Ettinger DS. Randomized prospective comparison of intraventricular methotrexate and thiotepa in patients with previously untreated neoplastic meningitis. Eastern Cooperative Oncology Group. *J Clin Oncol* 1993; **11**: 561–569.

Part 3

Vascular and traumatic events: Pathogenesis and repair

19

Cerebrovascular disorders: therapeutic strategies and repair

Jorge Moncayo Gaete and Julien Bogousslavsky

INTRODUCTION

The last decades of this century have witnessed new and fundamental insights into the pathophysiology of brain ischaemia. As a result, fresh concepts and novel pharmacological interventions have been developed, modifying the popularly held assumption that acute stroke is a discouraging condition for which little can be done. Exciting recent results from research in the acute-stroke field suggest that delivering treatment within the first few hours after onset changes the panorama of expectations. Certain acute therapeutic strategies which to date have shown no solid positive effects continue under development and are expected to provide promising results in the near future. Additionally, interest in secondary stroke prevention has grown owing to the increasing possibilities of stroke survival.

This chapter focuses on the most encouraging therapeutic medical strategies for the acute phase of ischaemic stroke and on repair mechanisms after an event. Outstanding aspects of secondary stroke prevention are also summarized.

POTENTIAL TARGETS FOR INTERVENTION IN ACUTE STROKE

Brain ischaemia is a dynamic and complex process involving simultaneous or sequential physiological, biochemical and pathological changes.[1,2] Once it is produced, it becomes of prime importance to minimize its severity, duration and extent, to prevent the development of cerebral infarction. Current therapeutic medical strategies in the acute phase of stroke are directed towards re-establishing the bloodflow in an occluded vascular territory (thrombolysis), limiting the neuronal injury produced by metabolic and biochemical events that occur in ischaemic brain cascade (neuroprotection),

and preventing early stroke recurrence and progression of stroke (antithrombotics).[3-5] Treatments directed to restoring circulation and neuroprotection that are applied soon after stroke can salvage the functionally silent but potentially viable tissue lying in the periphery of the core of ischaemia (the 'ischaemic penumbra').

Based on animal models of brain ischaemia, the therapeutic window for both thrombolysis and neuroprotection is no longer than 3 h.[6-8] Nevertheless, a direct extrapolation of the therapeutic window in animal models cannot be made to stroke in human beings. Moreover, penumbral tissue in humans can remain potentially viable for about 48 h after onset of brain ischaemia.[9,10] Finally, considering that the reperfusion and cytoprotective therapeutic windows do not necessarily overlap, the total therapeutic window in human stroke is probably at least 6 h before irreversible damage occurs.[11,12]

Another potential strategy of intervention is the blocking or limiting of post-ischaemic events occurring after reperfusion, which may aggravate neuronal damage through the expression of inflammatory mediators,[13] suppression of normal protein synthesis,[14] and expression of immediate early genes.[15,16]

THROMBOLYTIC THERAPY

Arterial occlusion in the appropriate distribution of brain infarction has been observed angiographically in 75–80% of patients within 8 h of onset of symptoms.[17-19] Spontaneous clot lysis, probably resulting from activation of an endogenous plasminogen activator, occurs from the first to the seventh day after onset of stroke in 14–73% of patients,[17,19,20] but is usually not accompanied by clinical improvement.[17]

Trials of intravenous thrombolysis with different designs carried out prior to 1995 provided no conclusive evidence of its benefits.[21–27] Five years ago, however, National Institute of Neurological Disorders and Stroke investigators reported for the first time a convincing benefit of intravenous tissue plasminogen activator (t-PA) when administered within 3 h after stroke onset in selected patients with brain infarction.[28] A trend to neurological improvement, as measured by the median NIHSS score, was observed 24 h after thrombolysis in the t-PA-treated group. Outcome at 90 days favoured thrombolysis in each of the four assessment scales, regardless of presumed ischaemic stroke subtype. In absolute terms, 11–13% of the t-PA-treated patients had minimal or no disability compared with the placebo group at 3 months. However, there was no statistical difference in the mortality rate at 3 months between the t-PA-treated and placebo-treated patients.[28]

The efficacy of early intravenous thrombolysis (< 3 h) was corroborated in a cohort of 87 patients (14% of the total) enrolled in the ECASS trial who received t-PA within the first 3 h after stroke onset (Fig. 19.1). Improvement in functional outcome was found in all three outcome scales assessed, although only the NIHSS score was significant.[29]

The improved outcome found in the NINDS t-PA trial was at the expense of a high rate of both symptomatic intracranial haemorrhages and fatalities, in comparison with the placebo group, within 36 h after thrombolysis.[28] Two years after the initial report on t-PA efficacy, these investigators reported that severity of neurological deficit at baseline, oedema or mass effect on baseline CT had been independently associated with increased risk of

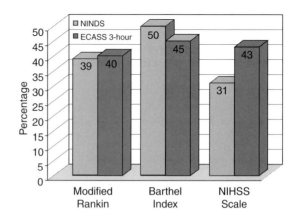

Figure 19.1 Comparison of favourable outcome between NINDS trial and ECASS 3-h cohort.

intracerebral haemorrhage after t-PA thrombolysis, although in their opinion these findings should not necessarily exclude patients for thrombolysis if administered within 3 h of stroke onset.[30]

Ancrod, a viper venom, when delivered by intravenous infusion for 5 days (in most instances begun within 3 h after stroke onset), significantly favoured a better functional outcome at 90 days in comparison with placebo. This outcome persisted even when ancrod was administered more than 3 h after stroke onset. As in other early thrombolysis trials, ancrod increased both symptomatic intracranial haemorrhage and mortality.[31]

Intravenous thrombolysis with t-PA given within 5–6 h after onset of stroke did not provide clear benefits (Table 19.1).[26,32,33] Failure of thrombolysis

Table 19.1 Favourable outcome with rt-PA intravenous thrombolysis beyond 3 h

Endpoints	ECASS II[a]			ATLANTIS[b]		
	rt-PA	Placebo	P	rt-PA	Placebo	P
mRS (0 or 1)	40.3%	36.6%	0.277	41.7%	40.5%	0.97
Barthel Index	49.9%	45.8%	0.258	54.1%	54.6%	0.9
NIHSS (0 or 1)	NA	NA	–	34.5%	34%	0.89
GOS (= 1)	NA	NA	–	46.3%	46.1%	0.97

[a]ECASS: European Cooperative Acute Stroke Study.[32]
[b]ATLANTIS: Alteplase Thrombolysis for Acute Non-interventional Therapy in Ischemic Stroke.[33]
Favourable outcome defined as: scores of < 1 on MRS; 95 or 100 on Barthel Index, < 1 on NIHSS; and 1 on GOS.
mRS, modified Rankin scale; NIHSS, National Institute Health Study Scale, GOS, Glasgow Outcome Scale; NA, not available.

administered within this time frame may be due to early spontaneous recanalization or, in some instances, to the occurrence of severe irreversible brain injury before therapy is applied. Nevertheless, applying the methodology of the NINDS trial in a post hoc, non-predefined analysis of the intention-to-treat data set of the ECASS I trial, intravenous t-PA was found to significantly improve the outcome at 90 days when the endpoint statistic measure was considered. This result should be interpreted cautiously, however.[34] In the ECASS II trial (using lower doses of t-PA than ECASS I), a non-significant trend to favourable outcome was observed in t-PA-treated patients. Nevertheless, in a post hoc analysis considering outcome in a dichotomized fashion for dependency, a significant absolute reduction of 8.3% in the rate of dependence at 3 months was observed in the t-PA-treated patients.[32] On the other hand, symptomatic intracerebral haemorrhage was two or three times more frequent (ECASS I and II) and mortality at day 90 tended to be higher in t-PA-treated patients than in the placebo group.[26,32,33]

Currently, one-fifth of patients arrive at emergency rooms between 3 and 6 h after stroke onset,[35] and some may respond favourably to thrombolysis administered beyond a 3-h period. In these instances, magnetic resonance imaging (MRI) may be useful to identify a subset of patients with potentially salvageable tissue.[36]

Local intra-arterial thrombolysis (LIAT) can achieve higher rates of recanalization with lower doses of thrombolytics compared with the intravenous approach.[37–42] Recanalization shows a direct relationship to the size of the occluded artery.[42] This therapeutic approach enhances the recanalization rate and provides an opportunity for favourable outcome in patients with basilar thrombosis.[42–44] Good outcome at 3 months occurred in 60% of patients treated with LIAT.[42] Recently, age < 75 years, NIHSS < 20 at baseline and the following day, recanalization grade and residual cerebral bloodflow evaluated by SPECT before thrombolysis were all found to be predictors of good outcome at 6 months.[45] The rate of intracranial haemorrhage is similar to that seen with intravenous thrombolysis. LIAT may be performed within a longer time window, but the downside is that it requires an interventional team and has a higher cost. To date, a direct comparison of the efficacy of LIAT and intravenous thrombolysis has not been conducted.

Higher rates of recanalization were found with early intravenous thrombolysis followed by LIAT compared with LIAT alone in 35 patients enrolled in a pilot study, but functional outcome was no different between the combined thrombolysis and the LIAT approach.[46]

To date, intravenous thrombolysis with t-PA is the only approved treatment for acute ischaemic stroke in the USA and Canada. It is recommended within 3 h after onset for patients with brain infarction who have no contraindications for thrombolysis, including intracranial haemorrhage, which should be ruled out by neuroimaging studies. Nevertheless, no more than 6% of ischaemic-stroke patients get to medical facilities within this time and would be able to benefit from early intravenous thrombolysis.[47,48]

CYTOPROTECTIVE THERAPY

A plethora of potential neuroprotective drugs acting at several different levels in the ischaemic cascade has been tested in experimental and clinical settings. To date, positive effects of neuroprotective therapy have been established in animal models of stroke,[49–53] but unfortunately unequivocal evidence of their benefit in well-designed clinical trials still remains elusive.[54,55]

Some circumstances might explain the lack of efficacy in clinical trials, such as species differences and incompatibility of animal stroke models to the human condition. Neuroprotective drugs have been administered with different therapeutic windows, in some instances beyond the 24 h after stroke onset. Therefore, probably a neuroprotectant could not be demonstrated to be an efficient drug. Heterogeneity of stroke patients enrolled in clinical trials may dilute the positive effects of neuroprotection. Outcome measures and follow-up periods used are probably not able to detect the efficacy of the therapeutic intervention, especially in patients with mild stroke. Finally, the neuroprotective agent may act only in one step of the ischaemic cascade, without arresting entirely the other biochemical mechanisms triggered by ischaemia.

Recently, several clinical trials have revealed encouraging results of neuroprotective agents (Table 19.2). Nimodipine administered within 12 h after ischaemic stroke significantly improved the functional outcome in 3719 patients.[56] Lubeluzole, through presynaptic inhibition of glutamate release, was related to a significant favourable outcome at 3 months in patients treated within 6 h of the onset of ischaemic stroke.[57]

Piracetam is the prototype nootropic agent with membrane cell-modulating properties. No significant difference in outcome between piracetam-treated and placebo-treated patients was established within a 12-h window, but those treated early

Table 19.2   Results of recent trials of cytoprotective agents

Agent	Mode of action	Results
Nimodipine[56]	Voltage-dependent Ca^{2+} channel antagonists	Significant improvement if given < 12 h
Lubeluzole[57]	Presynaptic inhibition of glutamate release	Benefit if given < 6 h
Piracetam[58]	Membrane cell modulator	No overall benefit
		Improves outcome if given < 7 h
Clomethiazole[59]	GABA$_A$ agonist	No overall benefit
		Significant improvement in large cortical strokes
Ebselen[60,61]	Lipid peroxidation inhibition	Contradictory results
Citicoline[62]	Reduction of free radical generation	No overall benefit
		Improves outcome in patients with NIHSS > 8
Magnesium[63]	Glutamate antagonist	IMAGES study underway
	Voltage-dependent Ca^{2+} antagonist	
Glycine[64]	Antagonism of NMDA receptor	Phase III planned
G19C89[65]	Sodium channel blocker	Phase III planned
Aptiganel[66]	Non-competitive NMDA antagonist	Safety CNS concerns
Selfotel[67]	Competitive NMDA antagonist	Increased mortality
		Abandoned

NMDA, *N*-methyl-D-aspartate; CNS, central nervous system.

(< 7 h), particularly with moderate and severe stroke, have a better neurological score.[58] Clomethiazole, which enhances GABA$_A$ receptor activity, showed no benefit in 1354 patients, but it can be useful in patients with large strokes of the carotid territory within 12 h of stroke onset.[59]

A trend to benefit in functional outcome at 1 month but not at 3 months was found in 151 patients treated orally with ebselen (a seleno-organic compound that inhibits lipid peroxidation) within 48 h after onset of ischaemic stroke. Therapy started in the first 24 h carried a significantly better outcome at 1 month and a marginal significance at 3 months.[60] However, a non-significant trend to improve good outcome was found in ebselen-treated patients within 12 h.[61]

Citicoline stabilizes cell membranes and reduces free radical generation. Recently, it has not shown overall benefit. However, patients with baseline NIHSS > 8 had a significantly better outcome than the placebo group.[62]

Studies of safety and tolerability have been recently completed for parenteral magnesium (with non-competitive antagonism of the glutamate receptor and non-specific antagonism of voltage-sensitive channel properties[63]), a glycine antagonist of the NMDA receptor,[64] and a sodium channel blocker.[65]

Therefore, clinical trials of efficacy will be launched soon.

On the other hand, aptiganel, a non-competitive NMDA receptor antagonist, showed an excess of hypertension and central nervous system adverse effects.[66] Recently, selfotel, a competitive antagonist of the NMDA receptor, increased mortality at 8 and 30 days, particularly in patients with severe stroke, and therefore the clinical trial was abandoned prematurely.[67]

The rationale for a combined approach, a neuroprotectant coupled with a thrombolytic agent, is excellent. The former may extend the therapeutic window for thrombolysis, and the latter may enhance the neuroprotectant's concentration.[68] Another form of this 'cocktail approach' might consist of several neuroprotective agents, given simultaneously or in succession, acting at different levels of the brain cascade.

ANTITHROMBOTIC THERAPY

Anticoagulation with heparin in the acute phase of ischaemic stroke has been in use despite a lack of net benefit.[69] Low molecular weight heparin given within 48 h of stroke onset reduced the rate of death or disability at 6 months compared with placebo, but only high doses reached significance.[70] Two other trials of heparin and heparinoid administered within the first hours of stroke failed to find benefit in the outcome at 3 and 6 months.[47,71] Likewise, no evidence has emerged of the benefit of immediate anticoagulation after ischaemic stroke with a variety of regimens in 23 374 patients.[72] On the other hand, heparin significantly reduced the rate of early stroke recurrence,[47] but heparinoid therapy did not carry benefit.[71] Anticoagulant therapy was not safe and was associated with an increase in the rate of haemorrhagic complications.[47,71]

Two recent studies have addressed the efficacy of aspirin (160–300 mg/day) administered within a few hours of stroke onset.[47,73] In these trials, aspirin reduced the rate of recurrent strokes. A small reduction in the rate of death or disability with aspirin was observed at 6 months, and an excess of extracranial bleeds did not outweigh this benefit.[47] Considering together the results of the two trials, aspirin produces a small reduction of about 9 per 1000 patients treated for the combined outcome of death or non-fatal recurrences during the first weeks after stroke.[5]

The results of the first trial of intravenous abciximab administered no longer than 24 h after stroke onset have recently been published.[74] Abciximab is a monoclonal antibody directed against the platelet glycoprotein IIb/IIIa receptor, producing blockade of the glycoprotein Ib/IIIa receptor, reduction of ADP-induced platelet aggregation, and prolongation of the bleeding time.[75] Doses of abciximab were similar to those used in the treatment of coronary artery disease.[74] Functional outcome at 3 months was improved by abciximab. Asymptomatic parenchymal haemorrhages were more common in abciximab-treated patients, but the frequency of non-neurological bleedings was not different between the treated and placebo groups.[74] Moderate thrombocytopenia occurred in 7% of abciximab patients.[74] Based on preliminary encouraging results obtained with this antiplatelet agent, further trials are planned.

Acute anticoagulation does not confer a benefit in ischaemic-stroke patients, although judicious use is justified in some patients at high risk of early recurrence after a cardioembolic stroke.[76] Antiplatelet agents may be an acute therapeutic option for a great proportion of patients who are not candidates for thrombolysis or for whom it is not available.

REPAIR

Plastic functional and biochemical changes take place after ischaemic injury in lower species and in the human cortex.[77] Cortical motor reorganization

allowing recovery of hemiparesis after focal ischaemic stroke has shown several patterns identified by means of non-invasive functional neuroimaging techniques. Subcortical infarction produced an increase in ipsilateral motor cortex activation as well as recruitment of the adjacent inferior parietal cortex and the anterior aspects of the insula.[78,79] Activation of homologous areas in the non-damaged hemisphere soon after stroke has been documented;[80,81] in other cases, bilateral activation of sensorimotor areas has occurred.[82–84] Patients recovering from aphasia showed activation of ipsilateral cortex beginning some days after brain infarct, and this persisted for several months.[85]

Short-term mechanisms involved in cortical reorganization after brain injury include activation of latent synapses and increases in synaptic strength,[86] whereas axonal sprouting and formation of new synaptic connections develops later.[77,86,87]

Astrocytes and microglia play an important role in both the development and repair of neuronal damage after ischaemia. Reactive astrocytes upregulate the expression of neurotrophic factors involved in the repair of injured neurons.[88] Experimental evidence exists showing that basic fibroblast growth factor and, particularly, insulin-like growth factor-1 play a role in axonal sprouting, directing the territorial expansion of innervation into the deafferented fields.[89] Additionally, some studies have demonstrated new synapse formation in areas surrounding the infarct and in the contralateral hemisphere within a short interval after an event, and this mechanism has persisted over a period of several weeks.[90,91] Monoamine agonists, particularly amphetamines, can enhance immunoreactivity to synaptic protein after brain ischaemia,[92] and an amphetamine coupled with intensive physical therapy improved motor recovery in a small cohort of patients given treatment within 2–4 weeks after brain infarct.[93]

Animal studies with growth factors have provided promising results,[94,95] and an initial study of basic fibroblast growth factor conducted on human beings has also produced encouraging findings.[96] Therefore, therapeutic strategies targeted to promote repair mechanisms have begun to constitute important areas of research.

SECONDARY STROKE PREVENTION

The risk of symptomatic recurrence after any first event ranges between 4% and 14%, and is especially high during the first year.[97,98] Prevention of recurrences for patients after a first-ever event must include the identification and modification of risk factors. In most instances, data on the potential benefits of risk-factor management for secondary stroke prevention have been extrapolated from studies focused on primary prevention. In the last few years, however, a body of evidence has shown that antihypertensive therapy decreases recurrences by one-third among subjects who have already suffered a first stroke.[99–101] Cigarette smoking increases the risk of stroke 1.5-fold and should be intensely discouraged.[102] Although specific evidence regarding the benefits of secondary stroke prevention is still lacking, it has been suggested that statins may reduce the incidence of first stroke by 30% in patients with symptomatic coronary artery disease or hypercholesterolaemia, and a similar efficacy might be expected to occur in patients with prior stroke.[103] Nevertheless, there is still a large gap between the benefits of risk-factor control in reducing recurrences as reported by several studies and its application in routine clinical practice.[104,105]

Platelet activation is involved in the pathophysiology of most strokes, thus providing the rationale for the use of antiplatelet agents in secondary prevention. A large meta-analysis of aspirin in the mid-1990s showed conclusively that aspirin reduces the risk of a further brain event by one-fifth and that in subjects with previous ischaemic infarct it reduces the risk of all vascular events by a quarter. Moreover, high and medium doses were equally effective.[106] In particular, bleeding complications and gastrotoxicity—the main concerns in aspirin use—were clearly dose dependent, favouring the trend to the use of either low or medium doses.[107,108] Hence, optimal aspirin dosage is still a matter of controversy, and a well-controlled trial designed to resolve this issue is needed.

Antiplatelet aggregation with adenosine receptor antagonists (ticlopidine and clopidogrel) has been found to be slightly more effective than aspirin in preventing vascular events.[109,110] In effect, ticlopidine (500 mg/day) was found to be 20% more efficacious than high doses of aspirin in the relative reduction of fatal or non-fatal stroke, and this benefit was particularly high in the first year after the qualifying event.[109] Unfortunately, diarrhoea, rash and, principally, severe neutropenia were more common in ticlopidine patients.[109] These adverse effects, plus its high cost, limited its broader use. To date, only one large randomized trial of clopidogrel (75 mg/day) versus aspirin (325 mg/day) has been performed.[110] Clopidogrel significantly reduced the rate of ischaemic stroke, myocardial infarction or vascular death by an additional 8.7% versus aspirin in the

whole population studied, and it also provided a non-significant 7% additional reduction of further stroke in 6431 patients.[110] Clopidogrel is much better tolerated than ticlopidine and does not produce significant adverse haematological effects.[111]

Interest in dipyridamole has recently re-emerged. Modified-release dipyridamole was more effective than placebo in reducing the risk of stroke recurrence and/or death;[112] however, this antiplatelet agent administered alone in high doses or in combination with low doses of aspirin was not found to be superior to aspirin alone in high doses.[113]

At present, aspirin in doses of 50–325 mg once a day is still the first-line choice for patients after atherothrombotic stroke, whereas adenosine-receptor antagonists, especially clopidogrel, are the preferred option for patients who either cannot tolerate aspirin or in whom it is ineffective. Aspirin may also be of benefit in patients with atrial fibrillation in whom anticoagulation is contraindicated, and in patients with low-risk cardiac sources of embolism.[114,115]

Anticoagulation may be useful in approximately 20% of patients with a first-ever ischaemic stroke caused by embolus from the heart. Long-term anticoagulation with warfarin (target INR 2.0 to 3.0) is indicated in patients with high-risk cardiac sources for recurrent embolism, including atrial fibrillation, rheumatic mitral valve disease, dilated cardiomyopathies, left ventricular thrombus, left atrial spontaneous echocontrast and left ventricular dyskinesia.[114,116,117] Prosthetic heart valves require high-intensity anticoagulation with a target INR between 3.0 and 4.0.[117] Long-term anticoagulation may be useful in selected stroke patients with paradoxical embolism who refuse the surgical option. It is also indicated for those with no other demonstrated cause of brain infarct who have at least one of the following factors: massive right-to-left shunt, recurring clinical brain infarcts or multiple silent ischaemic lesions on brain MRI, patent foramen ovale associated with atrial septal aneurysm, or Valsalva manoeuvre preceding onset of stroke.[115]

Based on the benefits proven by two large-scale studies, a skilfully performed carotid endarterectomy is strongly recommended for symptomatic patients with high-grade internal carotid stenosis (70–99%) and a recent non-disabling ischaemic stroke.[118,119] Carotid endarterectomy significantly lowered the risk of ipsilateral stroke in both the North American and European studies.[118,119] To date, there has been no substantial benefit of carotid endarterectomy in symptomatic patients with 30–69% stenosis.[120]

CONCLUSION

Substantial advances have occurred in acute ischaemic-stroke treatment in the last 5 years. The beneficial functional effects of early intravenous thrombolysis, the only currently approved acute treatment for brain infarct, are unfortunately restricted to a small group of patients. Safety and feasibility in routine clinical practice are the major concerns regarding thrombolysis. This therapeutic approach, delivered beyond the presently recommended time frame of 3 h, may also be beneficial based on a proper selection of patients.

The search for a safe neuroprotective agent, or combination of agents, with a convincing benefit remains an ongoing challenge, but success appears to be not very far off. Acute antiplatelet therapy and other envisioned treatment strategies represent fertile ground for research and promising options for the future. Secondary stroke prevention depends upon optimal control of risk factors and a proper selection of medical or surgical alternatives.

REFERENCES

1. Pulsinelli W. Pathophysiology of acute ischemic stroke. *Lancet* 1992; **339**: 533–536.
2. Scheinberg P. The biologic basis for the treatment of acute stroke. *Neurology* 1991; **41**: 1867–1873.
3. Adams HP Jr, Brott TG, Crowell RM et al. Guidelines for the management of patients with acute ischemic stroke. A statement for healthcare professionals from a special writing group of the Stroke Council, American Heart Association. *Stroke* 1994; **25**: 1901–1914.
4. The European Ad Hoc Consensus Group. Neuroprotection as initial therapy in acute stroke. Third Report of an Ad Hoc Consensus Group Meeting. *Cerebrovasc Dis* 1998; **8**: 59–72.
5. Hill MD, Hachinski V. Stroke treatment: time is brain. *Lancet* 1998; **352**(suppl III): 10–14.
6. Jones TH, Morawetz RB, Crowell RM et al. Thresholds of focal cerebral ischemia in awake monkey. *J Neurosurg* 1981; **54**: 773–782.
7. Kaplan B, Brint S, Tanabe J, Wang X, Pulsinelli W. Temporal thresholds for neocortical infarction in rats subjected to reversible focal cerebral ischemia. *Stroke* 1991; **22;** 1032–1039.
8. Yip PK, He Y, Hsu CY, Garg N, Marangos P, Hogan EL. Effect of plasma glucose on infarct size in focal cerebral ischemia–reperfusion. *Neurology* 1991; **41**: 899–905.
9. Heiss W-D, Huber M, Fink GR et al. Progressive derangement of periinfarct viable tissue in ischemic stroke. *J Cereb Blood Flow Metab* 1992; **12**: 193–203.
10. Marchal G, Beaudouin V, Rioux P et al. Prolonged persistence of substantial volumes of potentially viable brain tissue after stroke: a correlative PET-CT study with voxel-based data analysis. *Stroke* 1996; **27**: 599–606.
11. Pulsinelli W. The therapeutic window in ischemic brain injury. *Curr Opin Neurol* 1995; **8**: 3–5.

12. Zivin JA. Factors determining the therapeutic window for stroke. *Neurology* 1998; **50**: 599–603.
13. DeGraba TJ. The role of inflammation after acute stroke. Utility of pursuing anti-adhesion molecule therapy. *Neurology* 1998; **51**(suppl 3): S62–S68.
14. Araki T, Kato H, Inoue T, Kogure K. Impairment of protein synthesis following brief cerebral ischemia in the gerbil. *Acta Neuropathol* 1991; **79**: 501–505.
15. Ann G, Lin TN, Liu JS, Xue JJ, He YY, Hsu CY. Expression of c-fos and c-jun family genes after focal cerebral ischemia. *Ann Neurol* 1993; **33**: 457–464.
16. Kinouchi H, Shar FR, Chan PH, Koistinaho J, Sagar SM, Yoshimoto T. Induction of c-fos, junB, c-jun, and hsp70 mrNA in cortex, thalamus, basal ganglia and hippocampus following middle cerebral artery occlusion. *J Cereb Blood Flow Metab* 1994; **14**: 808–817.
17. Fieschi C, Argentino C, Lenzi GL, Sachetti ML, Toni D, Bozzao L. Clinical and instrumental evaluation of patients with ischemic stroke within first six hours. *J Neurol Sci* 1989; **92**: 311–322.
18. Wolpert SM, Bruckmann H, Greenlee R, Weschler L, Pessin M, del Zoppo GJ for the rt-PA Acute Stroke Study Group. Neuroradiologic evaluation of patients with acute stroke treated with recombinant tissue plasminogen activator. *Am J Neuroradiol* 1993; **14**: 3–13
19. del Zoppo GJ, Higashida RT, Furlan AJ et al. The Prolyse in Acute Cerebral Thromboembolism Trial (PROACT): results of 6 mg dose tier. *Stroke* 1996; **27**: 164.
20. Mori E, Yoneda Y, Tabuchi M et al. Intravenous recombinant tissue plasminogen activator in acute carotid artery territory stroke. *Neurology* 1992; **42**: 976–982.
21. Abe T, Kazama M, Naito I et al. Clinical evaluation for efficacy of tissue cultured urokinase (TCUK) on cerebral thrombosis by mean of multi-centre double blind study. *Blood Vessel* 1981; **12**: 321–341.
22. Atarashi I, Ohtomo E, Araki G, Itoh E, Togi H, Matsuda T. Clinical utility of urokinase in the treatment of acute stage cerebral thrombosis: multi-center double blind study in comparison with placebo. *Clin Eval* 1985; **13**: 659–709.
23. Ohtomo E, Araki G, Itoh E et al. Clinical efficacy of urokinase in the treatment of cerebral thrombosis: multi-centre double-blind study in comparison with placebo. *Clin Eval* 1985; **15**: 711–731.
24. Haley EC, Brott TG, Shepard GL et al. Pilot randomized trial of tissue plasminogen activator in acute ischemic stroke. *Stroke* 1993; **24**: 1000–1004.
25. Morris AD, Ritchie C, Grosset DG, Adams FG, Lees KM. A pilot study of streptokinase for acute cerebral infarction. *Q J Med* 1995; **88**: 727–731.
26. Hacke W, Kaste M, Fieschi C et al. Intravenous thrombolysis with recombinant tissue plasminogen activator for acute hemispheric stroke. *JAMA* 1995; **274**: 1017–1025.
27. Multicenter Acute Stroke Trial: Italy (MAST-I) Group. Randomised controlled trial of streptokinase, aspirin, and combination of both in treatment of acute ischaemic stroke. *Lancet* 1995; **346**: 1509–1514.
28. The National Institute of Neurological Disorders and Stroke rt-PA Stroke Study Group. Tissue plasminogen activator for acute ischemic stroke. *N Engl J Med* 1995; **333**: 1581–1587.
29. Steiner T, Bluhmki E, Kaste M et al. The ECASS 3-Hour Cohort. Secondary analysis of ECASS data by time stratification. *Cerebrovasc Dis* 1998; **8**: 198–203.

30. The NINDS t-PA Stroke Study Group. Intracerebral hemorrhage after intravenous t-pA therapy for ischemic stroke. *Stroke* 1997; **28**: 2109–2118.

31. Sherman DG, Atkinson RP, Chippendale T et al. Intravenous ancrod for treatment of acute ischemic stroke. The STAT study: a randomized controlled trial. *JAMA* 2000; **283**: 2395–2403.

32. Hacke W, Kaste M, Fieschi C et al. Randomised double-blind placebo-controlled trial of thrombolytic therapy with intravenous alteplase in acute ischemic stroke (ECASS II). *Lancet* 1998; **352**: 1245–1251.

33. Clark WM, Wissman S, Albers GW, Jhamandas JH, Madden KP, Hamilton S, for the ATLANTIS Study Investigators. Recombinant tissue-type plasminogen activator (alteplase) for ischemic stroke 3 to 5 hours after symptoms onset. The ATLANTIS Study: a randomized controlled trial. *JAMA* 1999; **282**: 2019–2026.

34. Hacke W, Bluhmki E, Steiner T et al. Dichotomized efficacy end points and global end-point analysis applied to the ECASS intention-to-treat data set: post hoc analysis of ECASS I. *Stroke* 1998; **29**: 2073–2075.

35. Zweifler RM, Brody ML, Graves GC et al. Intravenous t-PA for acute ischemic stroke: therapeutic yield of a stroke code system. *Neurology* 1998; **50**: 501–503.

36. Albers GW. Expanding the window for thrombolytic therapy in acute stroke. The potential role of acute MRI for patient selection. *Stroke* 1999; **30**: 2230–2237.

37. Ezura M, Kagawa S. Selective and superselective infusion of urokinase for embolic stroke. *Surg Neurol* 1992; **38**: 353–358.

38. Barnwell SL, Clark WM, Nguyen TT, O'Neill OR, Wynn ML, Coull BM. Safety and efficacy of delayed intra-arterial urokinase therapy with mechanical clot disruption for thromboembolic stroke. *AJNR* 1994; **15**: 1817–1822.

39. Sasaki O, Takeuchi S, Koike T, Koizumi T, Tanaka R. Fibrinolytic therapy for acute embolic stroke: intravenous, intracarotid, and intra-arterial local approaches. *Neurosurgery* 1995; **36**: 246–253.

40. del Zoppo GJ, Higashida RT, Furlan AJ et al. PROACT: A phase II randomized trial of recombinant pro-urokinase by direct arterial delivery in acute middle cerebral artery stroke. *Stroke* 1998; **29**: 4–11.

41. Furlan A, Higashida R, Weschler L et al. Intra-arterial prourokinase for acute ischemic stroke. The PROACT II Study: a randomized controlled trial. *JAMA* 1999; **282**: 2003–2011.

42. Gönner F, Remonda L, Mattle H et al. Local intra-arterial thrombolysis in acute ischemic stroke. *Stroke* 1998; **29**: 1894–1900.

43. Brandt T, von Kummer R, Muller-Kuppers M, Hacke W. Thrombolytic therapy of acute basilar artery occlusion: variables affecting recanalization and outcome. *Stroke* 1996; **27**: 875–881.

44. Zeumer H, Freitag HJ, Zanella F, Thie A, Arning C. Local intra-arterial fibrinolytic therapy in patients with stroke: urokinase versus recombinant tissue plasminogen activator (r-TPA). *Neuroradiology* 1993; **35**: 159–162.

45. Ueda T, Sakaki S, Kumon Y, Ohta S. Multivariable analysis of predictive factors related outcome at 6 months after intra-arterial thrombolysis for acute ischemic stroke. *Stroke* 1999; **30**: 2360–2365.

46. Lewandowski CA, Frankel M, Tomsick TA et al. Combined intravenous and intra-arterial r-TPA versus intra-arterial therapy for acute ischemic stroke. Emergency management of stroke (EMS) Bridging Trial. *Stroke* 1999; **30**: 2598–2605.

47. International Stroke Trial Collaborative Group. The International Stroke Trial (IST): a randomised trial of aspirin, subcutaneous heparin, both or neither among 19,435 patients with acute ischaemic stroke. *Lancet* 1997; **349**: 1569–1581.

48. Chiu D, Krieger D, Villar-Cordova C et al. Intravenous tissue plasminogen activator for acute ischemic stroke. Feasibility, safety, and efficacy in the first year of clinical practice. *Stroke* 1998; **29**: 18–22.

49. Sauer D, Allegrini PR, Cosenti A, Pataki A, Amacker H, Fagg CE. Characterization of the cerebroprotective efficacy of the competitive NMDA receptor antagonist CGP 40116 in a rat model of focal cerebral ischemia: an in vivo magnetic resonance imaging study. *J Cereb Blood Flow Metab* 1993; **13**: 595–602.

50. Takasago T, Peters EE, Graham DI, Masayasu H, Macrae IM. Neuroprotective efficacy of ebselen, and anti-oxidant with anti-inflammatory actions, in a rodent model of permanent middle cerebral artery occlusion. *Br J Pharmacol* 1997; **122**: 1251–1256.

51. Sydserff SG, Cross AJ, West KJ, Green AR. The effect of chlormethiazole on ischaemic neuronal damage in a model of transient focal ischaemia. *Br J Pharmacol* 1995; **114**: 1631–1635.

52. Kakihana M, Fukuda N, Suno M, Nagaoka A. Effects of CDP choline on neurologic deficits and cerebral glucose metabolism in a rat model of cerebral ischemia. *Stroke* 1988; **19**: 217–222.

53. Aronowski J, Strong R, Grotta JC. Treatment of experimental focal ischemia in rats with lubeluzole. *Neuropharmacology* 1996; **35**: 689–693.

54. Silver B, Weber J, Fisher M. Review: medical therapy for ischemic stroke. *Clin Neuropharmacol* 1996; **19**: 101–128.

55. Devuyst G, Bogousslavsky J. Clinical trial update: neuroprotection against acute ischemic stroke. *Curr Opin Neurol* 1999; **12**: 73–79.

56. Mohr JP, Orgogozo JM, Harrison MJG et al. Meta-analysis of oral nimodipine trials in acute ischemic stroke. *Cerebrovasc Dis* 1994; **4**: 197–203.

57. Grotta J, for the US and Canadian Lubeluzole Ischemic Stroke Study Group. Lubeluzole treatment of acute ischemic stroke. *Stroke* 1997; **28**: 2338–2346.

58. De Deyn PP, De Reuck J, Deberdt W, Vlietinck R, Orgogozo J-M, for Members of the Piracetam in Acute Stroke Study (PASS) Group. Treatment of acute ischemic stroke with piracetam. *Stroke* 1997; **28**: 2347–2352.

59. Wahlgren NG, Ranasinha KW, Rosolacci T et al. Clomethiazole Acute Stroke Study (CLASS). Results of a randomized, controlled trial of clomethiazole versus placebo in 1360 acute stroke patients. *Stroke* 1999; **30**: 21–28.

60. Yamaguchi T, Sano K, Takakura K et al. Ebselen in acute ischemic stroke: a placebo-controlled, double-blind clinical trial. *Stroke* 1998; **29**: 12–17.

61. Ogawa A, Yoshimoto T, Kikuchi H et al. *Cerebrovasc Dis* 1999; **9**: 112–118.

62. Clark WM, Williams BJ, Selzer KA, Zweifler RM, Sabounjian LA, Gammans RE, for the Citicoline Stroke Study Group. A randomized efficacy trial of citicoline in patients with acute ischemic stroke. *Stroke* 1999; **30**: 2592–2597.

63. Muir KW, Lees KR. Dose optimization of intravenous magnesium sulfate after acute stroke. *Stroke* 1998; **29**: 918–923.

64. The North American Glycine Antagonist in Neuroprotection (GAIN) Investigators. Phase II studies of the glycine antagonist GV 150526 in acute stroke. *Stroke* 2000; **31**: 358–365.

65. Muir KW, Hamilton SJC, Lunnon MW, Hobbiger S, Lees KR. Safety and tolerability of 619C89 after acute stroke. *Cerebrovasc Dis* 1998; **8**: 31–37.

66. Dyker AG, Edwards KR, Fayad PB, Hormes JT, Lees KR. Safety and tolerability study of aptiganel hydrochloride in patients with an acute ischemic stroke. *Stroke* 1999; **30**: 2038–2042.

67. Davis SM, Lees KR, Albers GW et al. Selfotel in acute ischemic stroke. Possible neurotoxic effects of an NMDA antagonist. *Stroke* 2000; **31**: 347–354.

68. Grotta JC. Acute stroke therapy at the millennium: consuming the marriage between the laboratory and bedside: the Feinberg Lecture. *Stroke* 1999; **30**: 1722–1728.

69. Marsh EE III, Adams HP Jr, Biller J et al. Use of antithrombotic drugs in the treatment of acute ischemic stroke. A survey of neurologists in practice in the United States. *Neurology* 1989; **39**: 1631–1634.

70. Kay R, Wong KS, Yu YL et al. Low-molecular-weight heparin for the treatment of acute ischemic stroke. *N Engl J Med* 1995; **333**: 1588–1593.

71. The Publications Committee for the Trial of ORG 10172 in Acute Stroke Treatment (TOAST) Investigators. Low molecular weight heparinoid, ORG 10172 (Danaparoid), and outcome after acute ischemic stroke. A randomized controlled trial. *JAMA* 1998; **279**: 1265–1272.

72. Sandercock PA, Gubitz G, Counsell C, Signorini D. Immediate anticoagulant therapy for acute ischaemic stroke Part I: A systematic review of 21 randomised trials of anticoagulant vs control, including 23,374 patients. *Stroke* 1999; **30**: 248.

73. CAST (Chinese Acute Stroke Trial) Collaborative Group. CAST: randomised placebo-controlled trial of early aspirin use in 20,000 patients with acute ischaemic stroke. *Lancet* 1997; **349**: 1641–1649.

74. The Abciximab in Ischemic Stroke Investigators. Abciximab in acute ischemic stroke. A randomized, double blind, placebo-controlled, dose-escalation study. *Stroke* 2000; **31**: 601–609.

75. Mascelli MA, Lance ET, Damajaru L, Wagner CL, Weisman HF, Jordan RE. Pharmacodynamic profile of short-term abciximab treated demonstrates prolonged platelet inhibition with gradual recovery from GP IIb/IIIa receptor blockade. *Circulation* 1998; **97**: 1680–1688.

76. Chamorro A, Vila N, Ascaso C, Blanc R. Heparin in acute stroke with atrial fibrillation. *Arch Neurol* 1999; **56**: 1098–1102.

77. Hallet M. The plastic brain. *Ann Neurol* 1995; **38**: 4–5.

78. Chollet F, DiPiero V, Wise RJS, Brooks DJ, Dolan RJ, Frackowiack RSJ. The functional anatomy of motor recovery after stroke in humans: a study with positron emission tomography. *Ann Neurol* 1991; **29**: 63–71.

79. Weiller C, Chollet F, Friston KJ, Wise RJS, Frackowiack RSJ. Functional reorganization of the brain in recovery from striatocapsular infarction in man. *Ann Neurol* 1992; **31**: 463–472.

80. Silvestrini M, Troisi E, Matteis M, Cupini LM, Caltagirone C. Involvement of the healthy hemisphere in recovery from aphasia and motor deficit in patients with cortical ischemic infarction: a transcranial Doppler study. *Neurology* 1995; **45**: 1815–1820.

81. Caramia MD, Iani C, Bernardi G. Cerebral plasticity after stroke as revealed by ipsilateral responses to magnetic stimulation. Neuroreport 1996; **7**: 1756–1760.

82. Shibasaki H, Sadato N, Lyshkow H et al. Both primary motor cortex and supplementary motor area play a role in complex finger movement. *Brain* 1993; **116**: 1387–1398.

83. Silvestrini M, Cupini LM, Placidi F, Diomedi M, Bernardi G. Bilateral hemispheric activation in the early recovery of motor function after stroke. *Stroke* 1998; **29**: 1305–1310.

84. Cao Y, D'Olhaberriague L, Vikingstad EM, Levine SR, Welch KMA. Pilot study of functional MRI to assess cerebral activation of motor function after poststroke hemiparesis. *Stroke* 1998; **29**: 112–122.

85. Thulborn KR, Carpenter PA, Just MA. Plasticity of language-related brain function during recovery from stroke. *Stroke* 1999; **30**: 749–754.

86. Sell FJ. Recovery and repair issues after stroke from the scientific perspective. *Curr Opin Neurol* 1997; **10**: 49–51.

87. Mano Y, Nakamuro T, Tamura R et al. Central motor reorganization after anastomosis of the musculocutaneous and intercostal nerves following cervical root avulsion. *Ann Neurol* 1995; **38**: 15–20.

88. Eddleston E, Mucke L. Molecular profile of reactive astrocytes. Implications for their role in neurologic disease. *Neuroscience* 1993; **54**: 15–36.

89. Guthrie KM, Nguyen T, Gall CM. Insulin-like growth factor-1 mRNA is increased in deafferented hippocampus: spatiotemporal correspondence of a trophic event with axon sprouting. *J Comp Neurol* 1995; **352**: 147–160.

90. Stroemer RP, Kent TA, Hulsebosch CE. Neocortical neural sprouting synaptogenesis, and behavioral recovery after neocortical infarction in rats. *Stroke* 1995; **26**: 2135–2144.

91. Jones TA, Kleim JA, Greenough WT. Synaptogenesis and dendritic growth in the cortex opposite unilateral sensorimotor cortex damage in adult rats: a quantitative electron microscopic examination. *Brain Res* 1996; **733**: 142–148.

92. Stroemer RP, Kent TA, Hulsebosch CR. Enhanced neocortical neural sprouting, synaptogenesis, and behavioral recovery with d-amphetamine therapy after neocortical infarction in rats. *Stroke* 1998; **29**: 2381–2385.

93. Walker-Batson D, Smith P, Curtis S, Unwin H, Greenlee R. Amphetamine paired with physical therapy accelerates motor recovery after stroke—further evidence. *Stroke* 1995; **26**: 2254–2259.

94. Nudo RJ, Wise BM, SiFuentes F, Milliken GW. Neural substrate for the effects of rehabilitative training on motor recovery after ischemic infarct. *Science* 1996; **272**: 1791–1794.

95. Kawamata T, Dietrich WD, Schaller TT, Finklestein SP. Intracisternal basic fibroblast growth factor (bFGF) enhances functional recovery and upregulates the expression of a molecular marker of neuronal sprouting following focal cerebral infarction. *Proc Natl Acad Sci USA* 1997; **94**: 8179–8184.

96. Fisher M, Bogousslavsky J. Further evolution toward effective therapy for acute ischemic stroke. Special communication. *JAMA* 1998; **279**: 1298–1303.

97. Sacco RL, Foulkes MA, Mohr JP, Wolf PA, Hier DB, Price TR. Determinants of early recurrence of cerebral infarction: Stroke Data Bank. *Stroke* 1989; **20**: 983–989.

98. Easton JD. Epidemiology of stroke recurrence. *Cerebrovasc Dis* 1997; **7**(suppl 1): 2–4.

99. Gueyffier F, Boutitie F, Boissel JP et al. INDANA: a meta-analysis on individual patient data in hypertension. Protocol and preliminary results. *Thérapie* 1995; **50**: 353–362.

100. PATS Collaborating Group. Post-stroke Antihypertensive Treatment Study. A preliminary result. *Chin Med J* 1995; **108**: 710–717.

101. Gueyffier F, Boissel JP, Boutitie F et al. The INDANA (INdividual Data ANalysis of Antihypertensive intervention trials) Project Collaborators. Effect of antihypertensive treatment in patients having already suffered from stroke. Gathering the evidence. *Stroke* 1997; **28**: 2557–2562.

102. Jamrozik K, Broadhurst RJ, Anderson CS, Stewart-Wyne EG. The role of lifestyle factors in the etiology of stroke: a population-based case–control study in Perth, Western Australia. *Stroke* 1994; **25**: 51–59.

103. Blauw GJ, Lagaay AM, Smelt AHM, Westendorp RGJ. Stroke, statins and cholesterol: a meta-analysis of randomized, placebo-controlled, double-blind trials with HMG-CoA reductase inhibitors. *Stroke* 1997; **28**: 946–950.

104. Joseph LN, Babikian VL, Allen NC, Winter MR. Risk factor modification in stroke prevention. The experience of a stroke clinic. *Stroke* 1999; **30**: 16–20.

105. Klungel OH, Kaplan RC, Heckbert SR et al. Control of blood pressure and risk of stroke among pharmacologically treated hypertensive patients. *Stroke* 2000; **31**: 420–424.

106. Antiplatelet Trialists' Collaboration. Collaborative overview of randomised trials of antiplatelet therapy—I. Prevention of death, myocardial infarction, and stroke by prolonged antiplatelet therapy in various categories of patients. *BMJ* 1994; **308**: 81–106.

107. UK-TIA Study Group. The United Kingdom transient ischemic attack (UK-TIA) aspirin trial: final results. *J Neurol Neurosurg Psychiatry* 1991; **54**: 1044–1054.

108. The Dutch Trial Study Group. A comparison of two doses of aspirin (30 mg vs 283 mg a day) in patients after a transient ischemic attack or minor ischemic stroke. *N Engl J Med* 1991; **325**: 1261–1266.

109. Hass WK, Easton JD, Adams HP Jr et al. A randomized trial comparing ticlopidine hydrochloride with aspirin for the prevention of stroke in high-risk patients. *N Engl J Med* 1989; **321**: 501–507.

110. CAPRIE Steering Committee. A randomized, blinded trial of clopidogrel versus aspirin in patients at risk of ischaemic events. *Lancet* 1996; **348**: 1329–1339.

111. Bousser MG, Roberts RS, Gent M. Ticlopidine and clopidogrel in secondary stroke prevention. *Cerebrovasc Dis* 1997; **7**(suppl 6): 17–23.

112. Diener HC, Cunha L, Forbes C, Sivenius J, Smets P, Lowenthal A. European Stroke Prevention Study 2. Dipyridamole and acetylsalicylic acid in the secondary prevention of stroke. *J Neurol Sci* 1996; **143**: 1–13.

113. Dyken ML. Aspirin with and without dipyridamole. *Cerebrovasc Dis* 1997; **7**(suppl 6): 10–16.

114. European Atrial Fibrillation Trial Study Group. Secondary prevention of vascular events in patients with nonrheumatic atrial fibrillation and recent transient ischemic attack or minor ischemic stroke. *Lancet* 1993; **342**: 1255–1262.

115. Devuyst G, Bogousslavsky J. Status of patent foramen ovale, atrial septal aneurysm, atrial septal defect and aortic arch atheroma as risk factors for stroke. *Neuroepidemiology* 1997; **16**: 217–223.

116. Hart RG, Sherman DG, Easton JD, Cairns JA. Prevention of stroke in patients with nonvalvular atrial fibrillation. *Neurology* 1998; **51**: 674–681.

117. Poole RM, Chimowitz MI. Cardiac sources of embolism: diagnosis, management and prevention. In: Batjer HH, Caplan LR, Friberg L, Greenlee RG Jr, Kopitinik TA, Young WL, eds. *Cerebrovascular Disease*. Philadelphia: Lippincot-Raven Publishers, 1997: 377–383.

118. North American Symptomatic Carotid Endarterectomy Trial Collaborators. Beneficial effect of carotid endarterectomy in symptomatic patients with high-grade carotid stenosis. *N Engl J Med* 1991; **325**: 445–453.

119. European Carotid Surgery Trialists' Collaborative Group. MRC European carotid surgery trial: interim results for symptomatic patients with severe (70–99%) or with mild (0–29%) carotid stenosis. *Lancet* 1991; **337**: 1235–1243.

120. European Carotid Trialists' Collaborative Group. Endarterectomy for moderate symptomatic carotid stenosis: interim results from the MRC European Carotid Surgery Trial. *Lancet* 1996; **347**: 1591–1593.

20

Vasculitis of the nervous system

Aksel Siva

INTRODUCTION

Vasculitis refers to the inflammation of blood vessels with or without vessel wall necrosis. Both the central nervous system (CNS) and peripheral nervous system (PNS) may be involved. This type of involvement is considered as primary nervous system vasculitis, when it is restricted to the nervous system. However, the clinical behaviour and neuroimaging, as well as the histopathology, are not uniform in all such cases. This variation is likely to point to a spectrum, depending on the type and extent of the vascular involvement within the CNS, covering a group of disorders, rather than a single disease, which may explain the different prognosis and response to treatments.

Nervous system vasculitic syndromes are classified as secondary when they occur in the setting of a known systemic vasculitis and other disorders known to cause inflammatory vasculopathy, such as connective tissue disorders and systemic infections. Such disorders may present initially with vasculitic involvement of the CNS or PNS. Some infectious agents or other systemic disorders may also cause a vasculitis confined to the CNS or PNS, without similar involvement at other sites. Altogether, a broad variety of diseases are known to cause vasculitis in the nervous system with a similarly broad variety of pathogenetic mechanisms.

VASCULITIS OF THE CNS

'Vasculitis of the CNS' is often included in the differential diagnosis of many neurological diseases. It is not uncommon for a physician to see a patient with non-specific neurological symptoms and signs and an imaging modality, usually an MRI, that is reported to have changes suggestive of a vasculitic disorder. The diagnostic and therapeutic challenges of such cases are wide, and in this chapter a brief clinical review of how to identify vasculitic syndromes and to differentiate primary and secondary CNS vasculitides, and their treatment will be found.

EPIDEMIOLOGY

Giant cell arteritis is the most common of the primary systemic vasculitides in the Western world. Its annual incidence is 42–270 per million in adults aged 50 years or older.[1] This disease is very rare in the east and Far East, with an estimated incidence of 1 per million.[1] Some other systemic vasculitides, such as Wegener's granulomatosis, also show similar geographical and ethnic differences, whereas Takayasu arteritis has the reverse trend. The overall annual incidences of most other systemic vasculitic diseases are reported to be <1–42 per million.[1] However, there are no exact figures for the incidence rates of either the primary or secondary vasculitides of the CNS, and we are left only with estimates.

Although the clinical features of vasculitis are related to vascular pathology, a stroke-like onset is rare, and this observation is valid for both primary and most secondary vasculitides of the CNS.[2–4] These disorders have a broad variety of CNS involvement patterns. Therefore, they need to be considered in the differential diagnosis of patients who present with severe headache, and focal or multifocal neurological dysfunction, especially in the presence of symptoms and signs of diffuse neurological dysfunction, such as altered cognition or consciousness, and a non-specific imaging study.

PRIMARY ANGIITIS OF THE CNS

Primary angiitis of the central nervous system (PACNS), also known as isolated CNS angiitis and granulomatous angiitis of the CNS, was initially described as a non-infectious granulomatous angiitis with a predilection for leptomeningeal and intraparenchymal arteries of the CNS.[5] However, with the increasing number of reported cases based on pathological studies, it has been demonstrated that granulomatous changes, necrosis of the vessel wall and involvement of the leptomeningeal arteries were not uniform findings or could not be detected in all cases.[6-10] PACNS involves both small and medium-sized leptomeningeal, cortical and subcortical arteries, and to a lesser degree veins and venules. Its hallmark is a striking inflammatory alteration of the affected vessel wall. The perivascular brain parenchyma may show infarct and haemorrhages, as well as loss of myelin and axonal degeneration.[7] Either leptomeningeal or parenchymal arteries may dominate the pathology or be involved almost completely. The distribution is focal and segmental, explaining why only 66–75% of biopsies are diagnostic.[6-8,10,11]

PACNS can be seen at any age, but it occurs predominantly in the fourth to sixth decades.[7,10,12] In earlier series males predominated, but recent studies show an equal sex ratio,[10,12] and if angiographically documented so-called 'benign' cases are included, then the gender dominance reverses in favour of females.

The most common presentation is headache with encephalopathy accompanied by multifocal signs. Neurocognitive deficits, in the form of intermittent confusion or progressive dementia with or without behavioural and psychiatric symptoms, are not uncommonly reported in histologically verified cases. Cranial neuropathies, spinal cord disease and seizures may occur. Stroke-like episodes, as mentioned before, are uncommon. However, intra-cerebral or subarachnoid haemorrhages and atypical presentations suggestive of a mass lesion or chronic meningitis have been noted.[6,7,10] Patients may complain of mild malaise and low-grade fever, together with myalgias and even muscle weakness at the time of presentation.

The average time from disease onset to diagnosis was reported to be 1.5–4.5 months in angiographically diagnosed cases, and about 6 months in histologically.[6,7,13] This clearly shows that, in most patients, the onset is subacute or insidious with a remitting or progressive course and the diagnosis is somehow delayed. An acute onset is less likely, and the wide spectrum of the clinical presentation with non-specific laboratory and imaging findings may cause confusion in some cases.

A progressive course with fluctuations, resulting in permanent disability or death, was reported in earlier studies, and aggressive treatment with immunosuppressants was advocated. However, as the number of reported cases, diagnosed with various methods, increased, it became clear that cases of 'PACNS' were not uniform. Patients with limited signs and symptoms, with improvement and a relapsing course probably represent an intermediate group. On the other extreme stands the 'benign' subgroup, with single episodes of mild CNS involvement and no recurrences or progression, who do not require long-term therapy. However, as we proceed, from the 'severe' end to the 'mild', the number of cases with pathological verification decreases. This limits our understanding of the 'behaviour of the disease', as well as a full evaluation of the reported so-called PACNS cases. The clinical presentation, the course and outcome show a wide variation, suggesting that we are most likely dealing not with a single disease, but with a group of related (or unrelated?) disorders. In accordance with this observation, the histopathology is also heterogeneous.

Calabrese et al analysed their population and reviewed the literature to assess cases that had received a diagnosis of PACNS with angiography alone and compared them with cases in which a histological verification was made in addition to imaging studies. Their subgroup analysis showed that among the angiographically documented cases there was a clinically distinctive subset that had a better clinical course and outcome.[6,14] These cases were more likely to be female, and had a clinical picture dominated by headache, with or without focal neurological dysfunction of a relatively acute onset. Diffuse neurological dysfunction and spinal cord involvement were uncommon, their cerebrospinal fluid (CSF) examination did not show significant changes, and, most importantly, recurrences were not expected, and overall the prognosis was benign.

As angiographic findings of vasculitis are non-specific and may not reflect inflammation and the underlying pathological changes, Calabrese et al proposed the term 'angiopathy' instead of 'angiitis' and suggested that such patients should be included in a subgroup called 'benign angiopathy of the CNS'.[6,14] However, in their retrospectively studied series of angiographically defined PACNS patients, Woolfenden et al challenged this assumption by showing that these cases did not always have a benign outcome and a monophasic course.[13] They could not identify any predictors of a benign course and suggested that immunosuppressive treatment should be considered in these patients as well. One of the decisions they made was to reserve biopsy for patients in whom diagnosis remains uncertain, who have a normal angiogram and who deteriorate despite aggressive immunosuppressive treatment. However, it should not be forgotten that histological verification is not only to confirm the vasculitis, but to exclude other diagnoses which may mimic vasculitic syndromes, such as multiple sclerosis or its variants, primary brain lymphoma, infectious encephalitis, amyloid angiopathy, vasculopathy due to hypertension and/or athersclerosis.[8,15–17] Therefore, histological verification is necessary in patients who are evaluated for the differential diagnosis of vasculitis. In addition, tissue diagnosis is important in these patients before initiating long-term immunosuppressive treatment that is known to have significant complications. Although limited in number, it has been our experience to see patients who presented with relatively acute onset of multifocal neurological signs and symptoms, who had changes consistent with vasculitis on their MRIs and angiographies, and in whom brain biopsy disclosed non-specific ischaemic changes or was not diagnostic. After treating the acute episode, we withheld long-term immunosuppressive treatment and followed these patients, who either improved or were left with some neurological sequel. We have not observed new episodes or progression during their follow-up period, which ranged from 1 to 14 years. Our experience with such cases gave us the impression that there might be another subgroup of patients with a self-limited episode of CNS vasculitis. In these patients, who may be placed within the 'intermediate group', the clinical presentation may not be so benign, the brain biopsy is not diagnostic— but significant in excluding other causes—and they are not expected to have further disease activity, and therefore do not require long-term treatment.

There are also reports on the coxistence of PACNS and cerebral amyloid angiopathy in the same patient, but whether their co-occurrence was simply coincidental or somehow aetiogically or pathophysiologically related was unclear.[18,19]

It is a common practice to include 'vasculitis of the CNS' within the differential diagnosis of many neurological disorders, despite the fact that it is seen quite infrequently. Many cases who have intermediate or mild CNS symptomatology are referred because of an MRI study disclosing lesions consistent with a non-specific 'vasculopathy'. On the other hand, there are also cases who have a complex neurological picture, with an MRI disclosing multiple lesions of an uncertain nature. The difficulty arises from the limitations in diagnosing CNS vasculitis, especially the primary type, as it has neither a characteristic clinical manifestation, nor a definite non-invasive diagnostic method. The work-up of patients with suspected PACNS, after a careful detailed history and complete physical and neurological examination, will include the following laboratory/serological tests to exclude systemic diseases: MRI, CSF study, cerebral angiography and, finally, a brain biopsy.

Laboratory studies in PACNS

There are no diagnostic laboratory/serological tests for PACNS. However, several routine biochemical and serological tests should be requested in patients suspected to have PACNS, in order to exclude systemic diseases.

Complete blood count, erythrocyte sedimentation rate (ESR), coagulation screen and standard biochemistry are routine tests to be performed. An elevated ESR will favour a diagnosis of systemic vasculitis or other systemic disease, but does not rule out PACNS. Some studies report an elevated ESR in PACNS, but it is not clear if infections and other systemic causes were completely excluded in these patients. In the absence of symptoms and signs of systemic vasculitis, serological testing is rarely helpful.

C-reactive protein, complement levels, cryoglobulins, immune complexes, anti-neutrophil cytoplasmic antibodies (c- and p-ANCA), anti-SS-A (Ro), anti-SS-B (La), rheumatoid factor, angiotensin-converting enzyme and anti-cardiolipin antibodies should be negative.[7] Antinuclear antibodies are also required to be negative; however, their presence in low titres does not exclude PACNS, provided that the other above-mentioned tests are negative. Serum protein electrophoresis is expected to be normal.

CNS vasculitides, diagnosed as PACNS, are reported to occur in patients with viral and to a lesser extent with bacterial and other infections, both in immunocompromised and immunocompetent patients. The most commonly encountered infections associated with CNS vasculitis are varicela-zoster virus (VZV), HIV, cytomegalovirus (CMV) and, rarely, *Mycobacterium tuberculosis*, *Borrelia burgdorferi* and *Treponema pallidum*. Several fungal and rickettsial infections have also been reported in association with vasculitis of the nervous system.[6,7] Hence, serological studies should be carried out to exclude these infections as well as hepatitis B and hepatitis C virus infections, which are known to be associated with systemic vasculitic syndromes.[20]

Imaging in PACNS

CT

CT scan is abnormal in one-third to two-thirds of cases. Because of its low sensitivity for the diagnosis of PACNS, it may only be applied to exclude other diagnoses when MRI is not available, or to rule out early haemorrhage.[6,7,21]

MRI

MRI is sensitive, but not specific. MRI sensitivity has been reported to vary between 50% and 100%.[22] It approaches 100% in histologically confirmed cases, but there are no pathognomonic findings.[6,22,23] Lesions suggestive of ischaemic and inflammatory changes, involving both the cortex and the white matter, have been reported. Some of these lesions are within known arterial territories,[23–25] but this is not the rule, and it is also not uncommon for veins to be involved by the inflammatory process.[26] However, it is not always possible to confine these abnormalities to well-known vascular territories. The lesions are commonly bilateral and supratentorial,[6,22,23,25] but brainstem and cerebellar lesions have also been recorded.[26] It has, however, been observed that infratentorial lesions always occur in the presence of supratentorial lesions at all times.[25]

The lesions of PACNS can show enhancement with intravenous gadopentetate dimeglumine. Enhancing linear lesions, accepted to correspond to the inflammation of the perforating arteries, have also been reported.[26] There may be meningeal enhancement as well.[6] Occasionally, intracerebral or subarachnoid haemorrhage may be seen.[23–25] MRI features resembling demyelinating diseases, including bilateral diffuse white matter involvement, can cause confusion in diagnosis.[16,24,27–29] Mass lesions suggestive of tumours, such as low-grade gliomas, have also been observed.[6,23]

MRI may remain normal in a few cases, despite an abnormal angiogram and a biopsy consistent with CNS vasculitis.[24] Most patients with PACNS, however, will show abnormalities in their MRIs, but these may not always be in correspondence with the angiographic abnormalities.[25]

Considering that MRI is abnormal in most cases with PACNS, the combination of a normal MRI and CSF findings has a strong negative value and will exclude the possibility of CNS vasculitis in many patients.[6]

Magnetic resonance angiography (MRA)

Currently, the resolution of MRA remains insufficient to disclose fine vascular abnormalities frequently seen with CNS vasculitis.

Angiography

Cerebral angiography is considered to be the most sensitive imaging study for the diagnosis of CNS vasculitis, but the findings are not pathognomonic.[12,24] Among pathologically documented cases of PACNS, angiography was reported to remain normal in up to 44% of the patients in one study.[4] However, when a combination of different diagnostic methods is used to reach a final diagnosis of PACNS, the sensitivity of angiography is increased to 100%.[22] The wide range of sensitivity for the angiographic findings may be explained by the heterogeneity of the inflammatory pathology, as well as different predilections for the sizes and types of vessel involved. Furthermore, the modest correlation of angiographic lesions with MRI findings[25] indicates that all vascular changes do not cause parenchymal injury. Similarly, many lesions seen on MRI that do not have corresponding angiographic changes are probably the results of the involvement of small vessels, which are not demonstrable on angiography.

Common findings include single or multiple areas of segmental narrowings and dilatations along the course of a vessel, vascular occlusions, hazy vessel margins, and collateral formation, often with a prolonged circulation time in the affected vascular distributions.[10,12,24] A considerable number of cases have only small-vessel disease, and in some cases who show abnormalities on angiography, the findings are indistinguishable from vasospasm. When abnormalities suggestive of vasculitis are seen, the diagnosis of PACNS can be strongly supported, and potential biopsy sites may be identified in combination with the MRI results.

As with CT and MRI, angiography is not specific for PACNS. Similar abnormalities may be seen not only with secondary CNS vasculitides, but also with non-inflammatory vasculopathies. Findings suggestive of vasculitis on angiography are known to occur in hypertensive vasculopathy, atherosclerosis, non-bacterial thrombotic endocarditis, radiation vasculopathy, CNS infections and vasospasm due to various conditions.[6,22–24,30] Vasospasm has been reported with the use of drugs such as ergotamine and sympathomimetics. Migraine, non-aneurysmal thunderclap headache, subarachnoid haemorrhage, eclampsia, phaeochromocytoma, sarcoidosis and neoplasia are other conditions known to present with vasospasm on angiography.[6,23,31] Cyclosporin neurotoxicity is well known, and as it is related to a vasculopathy similar to hypertensive encephalopathy,[32] it can be expected to demonstrate similar changes and therefore it may be included in the clinical imaging differential diagnosis of cases suggestive of CNS vasculitis.

Table 20.1   Non-vasculitic conditions diagnosed pathologically in patients referred for brain biopsy with a presumptive diagnosis of 'nervous system vasculitis'[8,15,16]

Vasculopathy due to hypertension and atherosclerosis

Multiple sclerosis or its variants

Sarcoidosis

Primary brain lymphoma and other lymphoproliferative diseases

Primary or metastatic brain tumours

Infectious encephalitis

    Neurocysticercosis

    Cytomegalovirus

    Herpes simplex

    Fungal infections

    Progressive multifocal leukoencephalopathy

    Creuzfeldt–Jacob disease

Partial or complete healing of areas of segmental narrowing by angiography along the course of the disease has been observed, and it was suggested that angiography may be used in the follow-up of patients and treatment effects.[24] Improvement of the abnormalities could be detected on early repeat angiographic studies, whereas completely reversible areas of narrowing were less likely to occur later in the course of the disease.[24] The increase in stenotic narrowing over time was associated with scarring, rather than inflammation, and detection of non-progressive fixed deficits after treatment was considered an indication to discontinue immunosuppressive treatment.[24] The absence of inflammation demonstrated at autopsy after long-term cyclophosphamide treatment in a patient who had serial angiographies was consistent with this conclusion.[33] However, the use of serial angiography has its limitations, and its value in follow-up of treatment is not established; therefore, a combination of MRI with advanced MRA may be preferred for such a purpose in the future.

The combination of normal MRI and CSF, as previously mentioned, is a very powerful negative predictor of CNS vasculitis and may obviate the need for angiography, although rare exceptions can occur.[6,10]

Other imaging techniques

Functional imaging of the brain with single photon emission computed tomography (SPECT) and positron emission tomography (PET) may show diffuse perfusion abnormalities coupled with multifocal perfusion defects in patients with various forms of CNS vasculitis, but they are neither specific nor sensitive for this group of disorders. However, they may add to our understanding of the neurological and psychiatric behaviour of these patients in academic settings.

Cerebrospinal fluid in PACNS

CSF is reported to be abnormal in 80–90% of pathologically documented cases of PACNS.[6] An elevated protein level and lymphocytic pleocytosis are commonly found. The mean CSF protein was reported to be 177 mg% (median 100 mg%) and the mean number of cells 77/mm³ (median 55 cells/mm³).[6] Increased IgG synthesis and the presence of oligoclonal bands are detected in some patients, but this finding has no diagnostic value. Normal CSF findings are accepted to have a high negative predictive value.

CSF analysis should include appropriate stains, cultures, serological tests to search for CNS infections, and cytology to exclude malignancy.

Serial CSF studies in a patient with PACNS were reported to show changes consistent with the CNS inflammation, such as an elevated level of albumin and increased immunoglobulin synthesis, that responded to treatment and correlated with the favourable clinical course.[34] The authors suggested that this method be used for monitoring response to therapy, but no further reports confirmed this observation.

Brain biopsy in PACNS

Histological confirmation is the gold standard for the diagnosis of PACNS. As mentioned before, brain biopsy is important not only to confirm the diagnosis, but also for the exclusion of a number of other conditions which may mimic vasculitis. Vasculopathy due to hypertension and atherosclerosis, multiple sclerosis or its variants, sarcoidosis, primary brain lymphoma and other lymphoproliferative diseases, primary or metastatic brain tumours, and infectious encephalitis such as neurocysticercosis, cytomegalovirus, herpes simplex, fungal infections, progressive multifocal leukoencephalopathy and Creuzfeldt–Jacob disease were some of the diagnoses found in patients referred for a brain biopsy with a suspected clinical diagnosis of PACNS (Table 20.1).[8,15,16]

The biopsy site is selected on the basis of an abnormality on MRI. The biopsy from enhancing lesions improves the sensitivity of the procedure.[6] In the absence of any focal abnormality, the biopsy should be taken from the anterior tip of the non-dominant temporal lobe. It is also essential to obtain tissue samples for staining and culture purposes.[6] The biopsied sample should include the leptomeninges, together with cortical and subcortical tissues, in order to increase the diagnostic sensitivity.[8,11,22,35] In a recent pathology study, however, parenchymal involvement was found to be more frequent than leptomeningeal involvement, contradicting some earlier reports, and it was also shown in this study that there was no significant difference in the diagnostic yield between open and stereotactic biopsies.[15]

The typical biopsy reveals segmental inflammation of small arteries and arterioles, intimal proliferation and fibrosis, with sparing of the media, and, in some cases, multinucleate giant Langerhan's cells.[9,11] Although PACNS is considered to be a diffuse disease, it is segmental in vascular involvement; hence a false-negative rate of at least 25% can be expected, but correlating the site of biopsy with neuroimaging findings may improve the histopathological diagnosis. False-positive biopsy results, although rare, have also been reported, which make it a necessity to interpret the biopsy in the light of the entire clinical picture, CSF and imaging findings of the patient.[6]

The morbidity of brain biopsy in patients with suspected vasculitis was found to be 3.3%, a much lower rate than the significant side-effects associated with immunosuppressive therapy.[8] As up to 50% of patients referred for a brain biopsy, with a presumptive diagnosis of PACNS, are found to have other diagnoses,[8,15] some necessitating totally different treatment modalities, histopathological confirmation is highly recommended in most cases of suspected PACNS.

Diagnosis

The diagnosis of PACNS depends on a combination of clinical, imaging (MRI and then angiography) and histological features. Laboratory exclusion of systemic diseases and infections is essential, and CSF findings are supportive. Table 20.2 summarizes the modified criteria for the diagnosis of PACNS, suggested by Moore.[12] This set of criteria, which covers a step-by-step use of diagnostic methods, is aimed at excluding other possibilities which may mimic CNS vasculitis, and finally confirm the diagnosis by biopsy.

Table 20.2 Criteria for the diagnosis of PACNS[a]

Clinical features consistent with a multifocal or diffuse CNS disease with a recurrent or progressive course[a] (clinical evidence)

Exclusion of an underlying systemic inflammatory process or infection by appropriate laboratory studies (laboratory/blood evidence)

A CSF study consistent with CNS inflammation (elevated protein and pleocytosis) and excluding infection and neoplasia (laboratory/CSF evidence)

An MRI study suggestive of CNS vasculitis and excluding other alternative diagnoses; followed by a cerebral angiogram that is consistent with vasculitis (imaging evidence)

A brain biopsy confirming the presence of vascular inflammation and excluding infection, neoplasia or alternative causes of vasculopathy (histological evidence)

For a definite clinical diagnosis of PACNS, patients must fulfill all of the above.
[a] Modified from Moore[12]
[b] Clinical features may suggest focal CNS involvement in some patients, but imaging studies are expected to reveal more widespread disease

---

Treatment of PACNS

There are no controlled trials of therapy in PACNS. Furthermore, the clinical, imaging and histological heterogeneity of the disease, as well as the various methods used in its diagnosis in published reports, makes it very difficult to evaluate treatment options in this disorder. The standard recommendation for treatment involves the combination of glucocorticoids and cyclophosphamide (CYC). However, this approach, which is based on earlier reports documenting a very high mortality rate, should now be reserved for patients who have a progressive course with histological verification. The morbidity associated with the long-term use of glucocorticoids and cytotoxic drugs is significant. Therefore, when a complete evaluation of the clinical features, including the course of the disease, combined with the CSF, MRI and angiographic studies, suggests a diagnosis of PACNS, a brain biopsy should be performed prior to treatment. There will be some cases in whom the clinical and imaging features will strongly suggest PACNS, but their biopsies will reveal non-specific or only ischaemic changes. When other diagnoses mimicking vasculitis are ruled out, it becomes essential to observe closely the disease activity in these patients, not only clinically, but also by CSF and imaging studies, in order to detect subclinical activity. When the disease remains limited and does not progress, we choose to continue to follow the patients, without putting them on long-term therapy. However, in cases with either clinical, biological or imaging evidence of progression, we re-evaluate all the data we have or consider re-biopsy. When the clinician and the pathologist are confident that the other diagnoses listed in Table 20.1 are ruled out, and the biopsy specimen was obtained from a site that correlated well with an abnormal area seen both on the MRI and angiography, or the patient declines a second biopsy, then we prefer to start immunosuppressive therapy.

There are several therapeutic regimens that combine glucocorticoids and cytotoxic drugs. They vary with regard to dose, route of administration, duration and types of combined agents.[36,37] The most common treatment regimen used in vasculitis of the CNS is high-dose intravenous methylprednisolone (IVMP), 1 g/day for 3–7 days, followed by oral prednisolone 60 mg, together with oral CYC (2–2.5 mg/kg per day), or intravenous CYC. Pulsed intravenous CYC is given at a dosage of 500–1000 mg/m² of body surface. It is administered every second week for the first three times, and then at monthly intervals[21,36] Oral CYC administration is accepted to be more potent in its immunosuppressive properties, but it has more side-effects as well.[21] The optimal duration of treatment is unknown, but, following clinical remission, a period of 6–12 months is the minimum required. The 12 months of therapy was reported to correspond to a relapse rate lower than 10%.[12]

Azathioprine (AZA) and methotrexate (MTX) are generally recommended as glucocorticoid-sparing drugs. AZA can be an alternative therapy in patients with a diagnosis suggestive of PACNS, but in whom histological verification could not be obtained. However, it was also used with success as the first-line therapy in PACNS.[34] The use of antiplatelet agents has been recommended by some as additional maintenance therapy.[37]

Serial CSF analysis and angiography have been used to monitor treatment response,[24,34] but, as discussed above, they have limitations and are invasive methods. The clinical response with serial MRI studies done with intravenous contrast, may serve as an alternative way to follow patients and their response to treatment.

New drugs, such as the immunosuppressant mycophenolate mofetil and the immunomodulatory lefunamide, were shown to be effective in experimental models of autoimmune diseases, and had also shown some efficacy in systemic vasculitides such as Wegener's granulomatosis and vasculitis of rheumatoid arthritis.[37,38] There are no known reports on their use in PACNS. Interferon alpha (IFN-α) was shown to be effective in hypereosinophilic syndromes and in some hepatitis C virus-associated vasculitic disorders.[20,38] These drugs might be of interest in the treatment of PACNS, as might intravenous immunoglobulins (IVIg), which were reported to have efficacy in several vasculitides, either in small series or case reports.[39,40] However, not all reports on IVIg use in vasculitic disorders are promising, and currently the use of IVIg therapy cannot be recommended for the treatment of systemic vasculitis other than Kawasaki disease.[21] Campath-1H, a humanized monoclonal antibody directed against the CD52 antigen, was used in systemic vasculitis in combination with another monoclonal antibody against CD4, and had shown sustained benefit, but there are no reports on its use in CNS vasculitis.[36] Plasmapheresis and antiviral chemotherapy also have no proven efficacy in PACNS.

SECONDARY VASCULITIDES OF THE NERVOUS SYSTEM

Vasculitides of the nervous system secondary to a known cause or underlying disease are more commonly seen than the primary vasculitides confined to the nervous system in clinical practice. They may affect the CNS or the PNS, or both. These 'secondary vasculitides' can be further subclassified into two separate groups according to the extent of their known vasculitic involvement. Interestingly, in some systemic disorders and infections known to cause inflammatory vasculopathy, the vasculitis may remain confined to the nervous system without evidence of systemic vasculitis, whereas in many there will be a more widespread vasculitis, involving many non-neural systems. This selectivity currently is not completely understood.

Nervous system vasculitis secondary to infections and related conditions

Infections due to viruses, bacteria, fungi, and protozoa may all cause vascular inflammation within the nervous system.[6,41] These organisms are also associated with systemic vasculitis, and it is not uncommon for them to induce either focal or diffuse cerebral vasculitis and present with neurological manifestations in the absence of clinical evidence of systemic involvement. In many instances, the responsible organism may be angio-invasive, but in some the vascular inflammation is related to alterations in host defences, resulting in secondary damage to host tissues.[6] The production of immune complexes and the initiation of cytotoxic and cell-mediated immune mechanisms may account for some of the systemic manifestations and cause the vasculitis.[41] The most common pathogens associated with nervous system vasculitis are listed in Table 20.3 and some will be briefly reviewed here.

Varicella-zoster virus infections
VZV causes a variety of neurological disorders.[42] Both the central and peripheral nervous systems are affected, and the documentation of cases with VZV infections involving the nervous system without rash emphasizes the importance of its consideration in the differential diagnosis of several neurological disorders, including vasculitis. Encephalitis resulting from VZV is now recognized to be a vasculopathy that affects large or small vessels.[42] The large-vessel encephalitis is the result of large-vessel vasculitis (granulomatous arteritis) and is characterized by stroke-like acute focal deficit, developing after zoster of contralateral trigeminal distribution.[42] This complication of VZV infection generally occurs in immunocompetent patients, whereas the encephalitis due to small-vessel vasculitis is more likely to occur in immunodeficient patients, though this is not a rule. The clinical picture of small-vessel encephalitis consists of a progressive encephalopathy of an acute–subacute onset, with features such as headache, fever, seizures, and focal or multifocal deficits.[42,43] The MRI shows multiple areas of ischaemic and haemorrhagic infarcts of varying size, involving both the grey and white matter.

The diagnosis of nervous system vasculitis secondary to VZV infection is extremely important. Such cases may receive a clinical diagnosis of 'CNS vasculitis', unknown to be due to VZV infection, and be treated mistakenly with immunosuppressants.[44] However, its diagnosis is not always easy, even in cases where brain tissue is available. The histopathological study of the brain in some cases has shown that both the inflammatory process and the detection of the VZV antigen were focal, consistent with the tendency of vasculitis to be patchy from one artery to another, as well as within a given artery.[43] Furthermore, in some vessels, despite the pathologi-

Table 20.3   Microorganisms associated with nervous system vasculitis

Viruses
  Herpes simplex, VZV, CMV
  HIV
  Hepatitis C virus; hepatitis B virus; hepatitis A virus
Bacteria
  Mycobacterium tuberculosis (tuberculosis)
  Haemophilus influenzae, pneumococcus, meningococcus
Rickettsia
  Rocky Mountain spotted fever, typhus
Spirochetes
  Treponema pallidum (syphilis)
  Borrelia burgdorferi (Lyme)
Fungi
  Aspergillus, coccidioides, mucomycoses, *Histoplasma capsulatum*
Protozoa
  Malaria, *Toxoplasma*

cal demonstration of inflammation, the virus could not be detected. These observations clearly show the necessity of studying multiple sites and arteries before rejecting such a diagnosis.

The diagnosis depends on PCR analysis and antibody testing of CSF for VZV. The demonstration of VZV DNA, antibodies to VZV, or both in CSF supports the diagnosis.[42] Analysis of the serum is of no value, as antibodies to VZV are detected in most adults.

The treatment of nervous system VZV infection consists of antiviral therapy with acyclovir, with or without a short course of glucocorticoids.[42]

Human immunodeficiency virus infection
Both central and peripheral nervous system complications are common in HIV infection and may be due to opportunistic infections or HIV itself. HIV infection can cause a vasculitis affecting the CNS manifested as encephalitis, stroke or myelopathy. PNS vasculitides due to HIV infection, causing peripheral neuropathies, also occur and are seen more commonly than CNS vasculitis.[45] These neurological syndromes are frequently seen as the presenting features of HIV infection, but also occur after acquired immunodeficiency syndrome (AIDS) has developed.[45]

Vasculitis affecting the CNS, without evidence of vasculitis outside the CNS, has been reported with HIV infection. The histopathology is heterogeneous, and granulomatous angiitis, eosinophilic vasculitis and necrotizing vasculitis have all been described in HIV infection, as well as vascular inflammation with transmural infiltration but no other features in asymptomatic HIV-positive people.[45,46] In a large number of patients the vasculitis may be secondary to opportunistic infections such as CMV vasculitis, VZV small-vessel encephalitis and *Toxoplasma*-related vasculitis. Syphilitic cerebral vasculitis should also be considered in HIV-infected patients.

The pattern of neuropathy in vasculitic peripheral neuropathy associated with HIV infection varies and can be seen as a distal symmetrical sensory neuropathy, as a symmetrical or asymmetrical sensorimotor polyneuropathy or as mononeuritis multiplex.[45,47] Most occur early, are not associated with multisystem involvement, can be painful and have a monophasic course.[45,47] Cryoglobulinaemia, which may be associated with vasculitis, has also been described in patients with HIV infection and mononeuritis multiplex, in the absence of co-infection with hepatitis B or C viruses.[45] Secondary infections and lymphoproliferative diseases also need to be considered in the differential diagnosis of PNS vasculitis in HIV infection, as their treatment protocols are different.

Hepatitis viruses

Neurological complications resulting from infection with the hepatitis viruses are relatively uncommon, and when they occur they are either directly or indirectly related to infection with the viral agent causing hepatitis. These neurological complications of the hepatitis viruses are diverse, involving either the PNS or the CNS, separately or in combination. In general, they develop in the setting of multiple extrahepatic manifestations of viral hepatitis, but nervous system involvement may occasionally occur in isolation, may precede the hepatitis, or may occur with anicteric hepatitis.[20,48–50]

An isolated mononeuritis, a mononeuritis multiplex syndrome, a generalized sensorimotor polyneuropathy, an acute inflammatory demyelinating polyneuropathy indistinguishable from Guillain–Barré syndrome, a chronic inflammatory demyelinating polyneuropathy and a subacute inflammatory myopathy all were observed as PNS manifestations of viral hepatitis infections.[20,49,50] An autoimmune vasculitis involving the vasa nervorum or a mixed cryoglobulinaemia induced during infection are among the responsible mechanisms that have been

suggested.[49] The detection of hepatitis C virus (HCV) RNA in the nerves and muscles of patients with HCV-associated neuropathy was reported to be inconstant, but an association between the detection of positive HCV RNA in nerve and necrotizing arteritis was observed.[51]

Cranial neuropathies, including optic neuritis and facial nerve palsy, transverse myelitis, and an encephalopathy or focal deficits resulting from a virus-induced vasculitis that involves the brain, are among the CNS manifestations reported to be associated with viral hepatitis infections.[20,48–50]

Of the two conditions associated with persistent hepatitis B or C antigenaemia, and nervous system vasculitis, polyarteritis nodosa is reviewed with the primary systemic vasculitides and cryoglobulinaemia will be briefly mentioned here.

Cryoglobulinaemia

Cryoglobulinaemia is an immune-mediated disorder that can develop during or after viral hepatitis C and to a lesser extent with hepatitis B infection.[49] The neurological complications seen in cryoglobulinaemia are the consequences of either a vasculitis related to the deposition of immune complexes or a hyperviscosity syndrome, although the vasculitis is not uniformly demonstrated in CNS involvement.[36,41] Vasculitic complications are more common with type II and type III cryoglobulinaemias, whereas peripheral thrombotic and ischaemic complications due to a hyperviscosity syndrome or precipitation of immunoglobulins are more likely to occur in type I, which may be associated with myeloproliferative diseases, and sometimes with type II.[36,41] Hepatitis C virus genotypes lb and 3 were reported to produce cryoglobulins that are more likely to be associated with neuropathy, whereas infection with genotype 2 produces cryoglobulins that result in skin disease.[52]

Mononeuritis or mononeuritis multiplex presenting as motor and sensory deficits that occur suddenly in the distribution of a single nerve, often accompanied by severe pain, were noted to be the commonest phenotypes seen in vasculitic involvement, but a painful sensorimotor polyneuropathy has also been reported.[20,36,49,53] Recently, in a large series, however, it was found that cryoglobulinaemic neuropathy presented predominantly as a sensory peripheral neuropathy associated with purpuric skin lesions, commonly axonal in nature, and most likely due to vasculitis, which appeared prior to or concurrently with the onset of neuropathic symptoms or findings.[54]

Vasculitic CNS involvement in chronic hepatitis C infection is rare, but does occur. Stroke-like episodes or progressive encephalopathy with bilateral white matter lesions on MRI, suggesting microangiopathic brain disease, have been reported.[20,55]

Immunosuppression with glucocorticosteroids, and immunomodulation with IFN-α, are the currently accepted therapies in patients with nervous system vasculitis secondary to hepatitis C infection and cryoglobulinaemia.[20] The nucleoside analogue ribavirin might be of value as an add-on therapy, with its expected effect of eliminating the HCV. The combination of prednisone with other immunosuppressants such as cyclophosphamide for treating acute episodes and then for long-term use has also been reported.[49,50]

Nervous system vasculitis associated with lymphoproliferative diseases and other malignancies

CNS vasculitis, although uncommon, has been reported in association with Hodgkin's lymphoma, non-Hodgkin's lymphoma, hairy-cell leukaemia, neoplastic angioendotheliamatosis and premalignant lymphomatoid granulomatosis,[22,36,56,57] making it a necessity to include such disorders in the differential diagnosis of CNS vasculitis.

Paraneoplastic vasculitis of the PNS is a rare disorder, characterized by a subacute vasculitic neuropathy, usually presenting as a mononeuropathy multiplex with progressive dysfunction of several nerves, but a symmetrical polyneuropathy has also been observed.[56,58] The cases reported are limited in number and most were seen in association with small cell lung cancer and lymphoma, and there were single cases with renal cell, gastric, bile duct, prostate and endometrial cancers.[56,58] An anti-Hu antibody association was also noted in a few cases. Its verification with nerve biopsy is crucial, as it may respond to anticancer chemotherapy and immunotherapy for vasculitis.[58]

Nervous system vasculitis secondary to drugs and substance abuse

CNS vasculitis has been reported in association with exposure to a variety of drugs, including amphetamines and related sympathomimetic agents, cocaine and opioids. Recreational drug users are at increased risk for CNS vascular complications that cover a wide spectrum, including vasospasm, non-vasculitic occlusive and haemorrhagic strokes and vasculitis. Cerebral angiography may reveal changes consistent with a vasculitic appearance in these patients, who present with cerebral vascular events. But, as noted earlier, such changes are not always due to vasculitis. The underlying mechanism responsible for the vascular events related to drug use or substance abuse may be platelet and coagulation factor abnormalities, accelerated atherosclerosis, foreign body embolism, cerebral vasospasm, hypertension, and rarely endocarditis and meningitis.[59]

Recreational drug abusers are known to have higher incidences of coexisting infections, such as hepatitis B, HIV, and syphilis, all independently associated with nervous system vasculitides. However, CNS vasculitis secondary to drug and substance abuse has been histologically verified in users of cocaine, amphetamines and related drugs such as phenylpropanolamine, metamphetamine, and methylphenidate, as well as in abusers of multiple drugs unrelated to such infections.[22,41,59] Phenylpropanolamine, which was present in appetite suppressants and in some over-the-counter cough and cold remedies, was recently reported to be an independent risk factor for haemorrhagic stroke in women in a case–control study.[60] Subsequently, the FDA issued a public health advisory concern on this risk, and many products containing phenylpropanolamine were withdrawn from the market. However, the relationship between this vasoconstrictor drug and cerebrovascular events, including vasculitis, is not new.[41,61,62]

The exact nature of the cerebral vasculopathy causing stroke related to heroin use is not clear.[59] Phencyclidine, ergotamine, LSD, barbiturates and cyclosporin are other drugs reported to be associated with CNS vasculopathy, but also lack histological confirmation of inflammatory changes consistent with vasculitis.[32,59]

Nervous system vasculitis associated with primary systemic vasculitides

Vasculitides of the nervous system, in association with primary systemic vasculitides and connective tissue disorders, form another group. Both the PNS and the CNS can be affected to different extents. The PNS involvement is more common and occurs earlier than the CNS involvement in most such disorders. Since the purpose of this chapter is not to cover all vasculitic disorders, the primary vasculitides will be briefly reviewed without detail, and connective tissue disorders will only be mentioned.

Primary systemic vasculitides

Many attempts have been made to classify the primary systemic vasculitides, according to: the size of the vessels involved; or aetiological factors; the presence

Table 20.4 Classification of (primary) systemic vasculitides[1,63,64]

Size of the dominant vessels involved	Granulomatous	Non-granulomatous	p/cANCA association
Large	Giant cell artentis Takayasu's arteritis		
Medium		Classic polyarteritis nodosa Kawasaki disease	±
Small	Wegener's granulomatosis Churg–Strauss syndrome		+++ ++
		Microscopic polyangiitis Henoch–Schönlein purpura Cutaneous leukocytoclastic v. Essential cryoglobulinaemia	++

or absence of antineutrophil cytoplasmic autoantibodies (ANCAs); and treatment responses (Table 20.4).[1,10,63,64] Despite its shortcomings, the classification based on the size of the vessels is commonly used. But it should be kept in mind that most vasculitic syndromes do not respect vessel size boundaries, and recently the classification based on ANCA association has also gained wide approval.[1,63] A similar difficulty is seen with the terminology, as some primary vasculitic disorders are known to be associated with some infectious agents, and hence may not be primary! Some of the polyarteritis nodosa (PAN) cases, which have been associated with hepatitis B and epidemic Kawasaki disease, are such examples. Such an association may also be operative for some of the other vasculitides, but as this issue has yet not been classified, the current terminology of 'primary vasculitides' will be used throughout the text.

Giant cell (temporal) arteritis
Giant cell (temporal) arteritis (GCA) is the most common primary systemic vasculitis, and is defined as a granulomatous arteritis of the aorta and its major branches, with a predilection for the extracranial branches of the carotid artery. It often involves the temporal artery and usually occurs in patients older than 50. It is often associated with polymyalgia rheumatica. Visual symptoms related to retinal ischaemia, ischaemic optic neuropathy and diplopia secondary to ischaemia of the extraocular muscles are the most common neurological complications. Stroke is an uncommon vasculitic complication, but when it occurs, it is secondary to the involvement of

the arteries of the posterior intracranial circulation. PNS involvement in peripheral neuropathy and mononeuritis multiplex are reported as well.[65,66] Isolated psychiatric symptoms with psychotic features can be a presenting feature of temporal arteritis, and therefore sudden onset of psychosis in the elderly may raise its diagnostic possibility.[67]

Ocular motor paresis, unilateral visual loss or both will develop in half of the untreated patients. Following the onset of visual loss, up to one-third of the patients will lose vision in the other eye within 3 weeks if left untreated.[68] The visual loss is almost always a result of retinal or optic nerve ischaemia; however, a visual disturbance can rarely result from infarction of the visual cortex. A constant or intermittent non-specific pain, over the superficial temporal artery, is common. However, as the incidence of headache in temporal arteritis was reported to be around 80% in large series, it should be kept in mind that its absence will not rule out the diagnosis.[67] The temporal artery can be swollen and it is often tender to touch. Jaw claudication should raise the suspicion of temporal arteritis, as should the observation of tongue and scalp ischaemia.[67]

Polymyalgia rheumatica (PMR) may precede the onset of GCA, and symptoms such as backache, proximal muscle and periarticular pain, morning stiffness, fever, anorexia and weight loss are common. A tumour-like presentation in GCA has been reported and its association with ovarian pseudotumour has been emphasized.[69]

The laboratory investigation is non-specific, and the most frequently used tests for the diagnosis of temporal arteritis include ESR, C-reactive protein (CRP) and plasma electrophoresis.[67,68] The ESR shows a marked increase but may be relatively normal in at least 10% of presenting patients. An increased CRP value is common, and its combination with an elevated ESR, in a patient suspected to have GCA, will give the best diagnostic specificity (97%).[67] The temporal artery biopsy is diagnostic but has a low sensitivity. Its positivity varies according to the segmental nature of the disease, the length of the segment biopsied and the duration of steroid treatment prior to the biopsy.[35] Choroidal bloodflow studies using ocular plethysmography, or timed fluorescein angiography, as well as Doppler sonography of the temporal arteries, are techniques used recently in the diagnosis of GCA.[67]

Elevation of anti-cardiolipin antibodies in GCA has attracted considerable attention for following the biological activity of the disease, besides ESR and CRP.[67] Recently, it was also demonstrated that plasma interleukin-6 (IL-6) was more sensitive than ESR for indicating disease activity in untreated and treated GCA patients.[70]

GCA is a self-limited disease, in general, that typically persists for several months up to 3 years. The disease usually becomes quiescent within 1 year. When GCA is suspected, corticosteroids are administered immediately, at a daily dose that varies between 60 mg and 120 mg of prednisone, according to the presence or absence of visual involvement.[67,68] If administered acutely (within 24 h), high-dose intravenous methylprednisolone 500–1000 mg every 12-24 h may reverse acute visual loss.[67,68] This dose is maintained for up to 7 days and is then followed by standard high doses (80–100 mg) of oral prednisone or an equivalent corticosteroid. The dose of corticosteroid is maintained until the CRP and the ESR normalize or demonstrate a significant trend towards normalization, and the systemic complaints remit. After 1 month, the dose is gradually reduced as long as the ESR is stable and the symptoms are quiescent.[68]

Despite its relatively good prognosis, an increased incidence of aortic aneurysms, mainly of the thoracic aorta, has been observed in patients with GCA as a late complication, and was associated with increased mortality,[71] making it necessary to follow closely these patients.

Takayasu's arteritis

Takayasu's arteritis is a granulomatous arteritis of the aorta and its major branches. It is considered together with temporal arteritis as a GCA, but, despite identical histopathology, it has a tendency to affect primarily the aorta and proximal portions of its major branches, whereas the symptomatology of temporal arteritis is more likely related to the involvement of the distal cranial branches of the aorta. Takayasu's arteritis usually occurs in patients younger than 50, is more common in females and affects Asians more frequently than Caucasians. CNS involvement is seen in up to one-third of the cases and is secondary to carotid artery stenosis, cerebral hypoperfusion and subclavian steal syndrome.[10]

Polyarteritis nodosa

PAN is the classic systemic necrotizing vasculitis that affects medium and small vessels. It has been associated with HBsAg-positive hepatitis in up to 70% of patients, and recently it was reported in mixed cryoglobulinaemia associated with hepatitis C infection.[10,12,49] However, a significant decrease in the number of HBV-related cases has also been noted with the development and widespread use of vaccines against viral hepatitis B.[72]

A PAN-like syndrome has also been described in patients with HIV infection, and cases of PAN following other infections such as parvovirus B19, hepatitis A, CMV and human T-cell leukaemia lymphoma virus-1 have been reported, but none of these agents has been associated consistently with PAN.

Neurologically, both central and peripheral nervous system involvement occur in PAN, but neuropathy is more frequent and accompanies PAN in 50–75% of cases, and occurs earlier.[10,12,49,72] Mononeuritis multiplex is the commonest and earliest neurological manifestation of PAN, but polyneuropathy, plexopathy and radiculopathy may also occur.[10,72] Asymmetrical sensory and/or motor dysfunction affecting limbs in the distribution of different nerves is characteristic. Pain may precede motor deficit, which in turn may precede sensory loss. Rarely, the patient presents with symmetrical distal polyneuropathy. Vascular inflammation in the vasa nervosum and active axonal degeneration with asymmetrical involvement and vasculitic infarction of the nerve are observed histologically.[10,12]

CNS involvement is seen in up to 40% of patients with PAN, and has a tendency to occur relatively late.[10,12] With regard to the extent and size of affected vessels and sites involved, CNS manifestations of PAN are diverse. A diffuse encephalopathy with cognitive decline and seizures related to the involvement of small arteries, or stroke-like episodes with focal or multifocal findings secondary to vasculitic involvement of medium-sized arteries, may occur.[10] Spinal cord involvement resulting from vasculitis of the spinal arteries, although rare, has been reported. Cranial nerve palsies are present in less than 2% of patients.[72] Intracerebral or subarachnoid haemorrhages may be seen. PAN is usually a multisystem disease; however, disease limited to a single organ has been described. Examples are vasculitis limited to the PNS and cutaneous PAN.

The treatment protocols of PAN without hepatitis B infection differ from the protocols of HBV-related PAN.[72] The initial management of PAN without HBV starts with IVMP 1 g/day for at least 3 days, followed by oral prednisone at 1–1.5 mg/kg per day until the clinical status of the patient improves and the ESR returns to normal.[72] The prednisone dose is then tapered gradually, and oral or monthly pulse cyclophosphamide therapy is instituted. In cases of HBV-associated PAN, early treatment with antiviral agents such as IFN-α or vidarabine in combination with glucocorticoids is preferred. Initial glucorticoid treatment to control severe multisystem manifestations of PAN, followed by abrupt stoppage of steroids to enhance hepatitis B early antigen to anti-hepatitis B early antigen antibody seroconversion, has been suggested in these patients.[40] The addition of an antiviral agent was shown to be effective in viral clearance, and plasma exchanges were reported to control the course of HBV-related PAN, without the addition of immunosuppressive therapy.[72] However, the approach of treating the different forms of PAN separately has not gained universal acceptance.

Microscopic polyangiitis

Microscopic polyangiitis (MPA), accepted to be a variant of PAN, is a necrotizing non-granulomatous vasculitis, with few or no immune deposits, affecting small vessels (i.e. capillaries, venules, or arterioles), but involvement of small- to medium-sized vessels may be present as well.[41,72] Renal involvement is a major feature of MPA and is characterized by rapidly progressive glomerulonephritis. Pulmonary involvement with haemorrhagic complications is also frequent. Involvement of the PNS is less common than in PAN, and is seen in 10–20% of patients with MPA. Relapses after remission are more common in MPA. ANCAs are detected in the majority of patients (50–80%), most being pANCA antimyeloperoxidase, and some disclosing the cANCA pattern, and evidence of HBV infection is usually unexpected.[41,72]

Kawasaki disease

Kawasaki disease is an acute febrile vasculitis involving predominantly medium-sized arteries, but large and small arteries are also affected. Its aetiology is unknown, but its occurrence in epidemic forms and other reported associations suggest an infectious cause.[1,73] It generally affects infants and young children, and is associated with a mucocutaneous lymph node syndrome, bilateral conjunctivitis, a strawberry tongue, diffuse oropharyngeal reddening and injection, skin changes in the distal part of the extremities and coronary artery disease. Neurological symptoms include seizures, facial palsy, and, rarely, cerebral infarction. CSF pleocytosis can be documented in some cases. Aspirin and high-dose intravenous immunoglobulins are both recommended for children and adults with Kawasaki disease.[74]

Wegener's granulomatosis

Wegener's granulomatosis is an inflammatory multisystem disorder characterized by necrotizing granulomas in the upper and lower respiratory tract, with or without focal segmental glomerulonephritis and a systemic necrotizing vasculitis, affecting small- to medium-sized vessels.[41,75] The orbits, heart, skin, and joints are also frequently involved. It can occur at any age, but the peak incidence is in the fourth and fifth decades, without a clear gender preference. A positive test for cANCA, with proteinase 3 specificity, and the absence of antinuclear antibodies is highly diagnostic in patients with appropriate clinical signs and symptoms suggestive of Wegener's granulomatosis. However, a biopsy from the involved upper respiratory tract may be needed for confirmation when clinical and laboratory features are ambiguous.

Neurological involvement has been reported to occur in 22–54% of cases in large series.[41,75,76] However, with the introduction of effective treatment regimens, this rate now remains close to the lower end of the range.[41] The most common neurological manifestation which is related to vasculitis is mononeuritis multiplex, followed by distal symmetrical sensorimotor neuropathy.[41,75,76] Neuropathy occurs in approximately 16% and may be more common in cases with renal disease.[76] Involvement of the brain and meninges is seen in less than 10% of patients. The spectrum of the vascular involvement of the CNS in Wegener's granulomatosis is broad, and is manifested as intracerebral or subarachnoid haemorrhage, or as cerebral arterial or venous thrombosis.[75,76] Some of these cerebral vascular complications are secondary to inflammatory vasculitis, but arterial occlusion secondary to direct invasion from nasal or paranasal sites into the skull base, emboli from marantic endocarditis, infarct secondary to hypertension, and other causes unrelated to Wegener's granulomatosis, have also been reported.[77,78] Facial weakness, diplopia, visual and hearing loss secondary to granulomatous meningitis or bony erosion of the skull base may occur, as well as diabetes insipidus due to granulomatous involvement of the hypothalamo-pituitary axis.

MRI is highly sensitive in demonstrating the wide spectrum of findings of CNS involvement in patients with Wegener's granulomatosis, which include: diffuse linear or focal dural thickening and enhancement contiguous with orbital, nasal or paranasal disease; infarcts; non-specific white matter changes; an enlarged pituitary gland with infundibular thickening and enhancement; and granulomatous lesions and atrophy.[77,78]

The current standard therapeutic regimen includes combined therapy with glucocorticoids and cyclophosphamide. Oral cyclophosphamide is continued for at least 1 full year at a dose of 2 mg/kg per day after remission is achieved, but prednisone, 1 mg/kg per day, is given for a shorter duration and is slowly tapered after 2–4 weeks. Complete remission in 75–93% of patients was reported with this regimen, with a mean duration of remission of 48 months.[79] In severe cases, sulphonamides in conjunction with these protocols, and new drugs such as mycophenolate moteil and lefunamide, are emerging as alternative maintenance therapies for use in ANCA-associated vasculitides.[80] Other protocols such as pulsed-dose treatment with cyclophosphamide, intravenous immunoglobulin, methotrexate, cyclosporin A, and trimethoprim-sulphamethoxazole have been tried, but have not been shown to be superior to the above-mentioned standard therapeutic regimen; however, they may be used when standard therapy is failing, or causes considerable toxicity.

Churg–Strauss syndrome

Churg–Strauss syndrome, originally designated as allergic granulomatosis and angiitis, is characterized with eosinophil-rich and granulomatous inflammation involving the respiratory tract, and necrotizing vasculitis affecting small- to medium-sized vessels, associated with asthma and eosinophilia. A positive test for cANCA, with myeloperoxidase specificity, is found in up to 60% of patients.

Clinical and pathological involvement in Churg–Strauss syndrome may be widespread (classic form) or isolated (limited form).[9] Pulmonary infiltrates are a central feature of this syndrome and may occur in up to 90% of patients.[80] The development of vasculitis may be preceded by many years of allergic disease, consisting of allergic rhinitis and nasal polyposis and asthma.[80] A cutaneous eruption occurs in up to 70% of patients, and gastrointestinal manifestations in about half. Cardiac involvement is observed and accounts for half of all deaths due to the syndrome. Neurological involvement is common, with 60–70% of patients having peripheral neuropathies, in the form of mononeuritis multiplex or polyneuropathy, which can be very painful. PNS involvement is related to vasculitis affecting the vasa nervosum. The CNS is affected in 25% of patients, with most developing cranial neuropathies, but encephalopathy or stroke-like presentations may be observed.[10,80] Ischaemic optic neuropathy is followed by involvement of motor ocular nerves, facial paresis and hearing loss.

Nervous system vasculitis associated with connective tissue disorders

Systemic lupus erythematosus, Sjögren's syndrome, rheumatoid vasculitis, scleroderma and dermatomyositis are among the connective tissue disorders associated with nervous system vasculopathies resulting in CNS and PNS manifestations. The diagnostic studies in patients with clinical signs and symptoms suggestive of systemic inflammatory disease, including connective tissue disorders with nervous system involvement, are summarized in Table 20.5.

Other forms of vasculitis with nervous system involvement and some other diseases mimicking vasculitis

Behçet's diease (BD)

As BD is relatively less known and is among the major interests of the author, it will be reviewed more lengthily. BD is a multisystem, vascular inflammatory disease of unknown origin. The classical triad of oral and genital ulcerations with uveitis was originally described by the Turkish dermatologist Hulusi Behçet in 1937.[81] Other systems reported to be involved throughout the course of the disease are the cardiovascular, pulmonary, gastrointestinal and central nervous systems. Currently, the most widely used diagnostic criteria are those of the International Study Group, according to which a definitive diagnosis requires recurrent oral ulcerations plus two of the following: recurrent genital ulcerations, skin lesions, eye lesions and a positive pathergy test.[82]

The major causes of morbidity and mortality in BD result from ocular, major vascular or

Table 20.5 Diagnostic studies in patients with clinical signs and symptoms suggestive of systemic inflammatory diseases with nervous system involvement

	Initial diagnostic approach to confirm the systemic disease	Advanced diagnostic procedure to confirm nervous system involvement
Connective tissue disorders	Serological studies for related antibodies, clinical and laboratory evidence of non-neural involvement	CSF analysis (cell count, protein, glucose, OCB) CT and MRI for CNS, cerebral angiography to rule out coincidental cardiovascular disease or other causes EMG and NCS for PNS involvement
SLE	ANA, anti-dsDNA, anti-Smab	As above
RA, Sjögren	RF, anti-Ro, anti-La, ANA	As above
Scleroderma	Anti-scl70	As above
Systemic vasculitides	pANCA, cANCA, anti-PR3, anti-MPO extraneuronal biopsy	As above
Wegener's granulomatosis	cANCA, extraneuronal biopsy (from paranasal sinuses, lung, kidney)	As above
Churg–Strauss	Eosinophilia, extraneuronal biopsy	As above
PAN	Biopsy of muscle, testes, peripheral nerves and visceral angiography, HbsAg, anti-HCV	As above
Giant cell	Elevated ESR with typical clinical findings, Doppler ultrasonography of temporal artery	Temporal arterial biopsy
Behçet's disease Others	HLA B5, pathergy test	Cranial MRI; CSF analysis
Cogan's syndrome	Clinical—ininflammatory eye disease (interstitial keratitis) and vestibuloauditory dysfunction/associated systemic vasculitis	Cranial MRI
Susac syndrome	Clinical—retinopathy, hearing loss, encephalopathy	Cranial MRI Cerebral angiography Brain biopsy

SLE, systemic lupus erythematosus; CSF, cerebrospinal fluid; OCB, oligoclonal bands; CNS, central nervous system; ANA, antinuclear antibody; RA, rheumatoid arthritis; RF, rheumatoid factor; PAN, polyarteritis nodosa.

neurological involvement. Despite a broadened clinical understanding of this disease, the aetiological factors remain obscure and speculative; viral agents, immunological factors, genetic causes, bacterial factors and fibrinolytic defects have all been implicated. It is postulated that an autoimmune reaction is triggered by infectious (viral or bacterial) or other antigens in genetically predisposed individuals, resulting in the basic pathological process of BD, which is vasculitis.[83]

Neuro-Behçet syndrome (NBS)
Patients with BD may present with different neurological problems, related either directly or indirectly to the disease. Cerebral venous sinus thrombosis, CNS involvement secondary to vascular inflammation, and the neuro-psycho-Behçet variant, in which an organic psychotic syndrome is prominent, are direct effects. A non-structural recurrent vascular-type headache that starts after the onset of the systemic manifestations of BD, and is sometimes

associated with their exacerbations, is relatively common. Tension-type headache, depression and neurological complications of BD treatments are among the indirect neuropsychiatric consequences of the disease.[77] PNS involvement is extremely rare, despite the fact that neurophysiological studies may demonstrate non-specific findings in some patients.

The reported incidence of NBS in BD patients varies between 2.2% and 49%, and was found to be 4.8% in our non-selected series from the Behçet's Disease Research Centre, with the mean age of onset for BD and NBS being 26.7 ± 8.0 and 32.0 ± 8.7 years, respectively,[84] consistent with other series.[85,86] Neurological complications in BD occur more commonly in males.

NBS may be manifested in the form of either CNS involvement or cerebral venous sinus thrombosis, the two major neurological presentations of BD. There is a tendency to designate only CNS parenchymal involvement as NBS, and to include cerebral venous sinus thrombosis within the spectrum of so-called vasculo-Behçet.[87,88] However, as both have neurological consequences, they may be identified as 'intra-axial NBS' and 'extra-axial NBS', respectively.

Clinical and neuroimaging evidence also confirms this subclassification of NBS. CNS NBS or intra-axial NBS is due to small-vessel disease and causes the focal or multifocal CNS involvement manifested in the majority of patients. The second form, cerebral venous thrombosis (CVT) or extra-axial NBS, which is due to large-vessel disease in the form of cerebral venous sinus thrombosis, has limited symptoms, a better prognosis and generally an uncomplicated outcome.[84] These two types of involvement occur in the same individual very rarely, and presumably have a different pathogenesis. Many of the CNS NBS patients with small-vessel inflammation have a relapsing–remitting course initially, with some ultimately developing a secondary progressive course later, and a few will have a progressive CNS dysfunction from the onset. In our series the rate of CNS NBS was 75.6%, and CVT 12.2%, with the remaining cases having other or indefinite diagnoses.[84]

The most common neurological symptom among patients with BD is headache. A substantial number of patients with BD may report a severe headache of recent onset not consistent with a primary headache or ocular inflammatory pain. These patients require further evaluation even if they do not have neurological signs, as such a symptom may indicate the onset of NBS. In addition to headache alone, NBS may present with focal or multifocal CNS dysfunction with or without headache. The most common symptoms detected at onset in our series of 164 patients were: headache (61.6%), weakness of the upper motor neuron type (53.7%), brainstem and cerebellar (49%), and cognitive/behavioural (16%).[84] Rare presentations include isolated optic neuritis, psychiatric manifestations referred to as neuro-psycho-Behçet syndrome, aseptic meningitis, intra-cerebral haemorrhage due to ruptured aneurysms, extrapyramidal syndromes and peripheral neuropathy.

Neuroimaging studies in CNS NBS have shown that cranial MRI is both specific and more sensitive than computerized tomography in demonstrating the typical reversible inflammatory parenchymal lesions. Lesions are generally located within the brainstem, occasionally with extension to the diencephalon, or within the periventricular and subcortical white matter.[89] The pattern of parenchymal lesions is suggestive of small-vessel vasculitis,[89] but the pathology in CNS NBS is not always uniform and covers a wide spectrum that includes vasculitis, a low-grade inflammation, demyelination and degenerative changes. A definite vasculitis is not observed in all cases.[90] With the exception of the rarely occurring lesions only affecting periventricular and subcortical white matter, cranial MRIs in CNS NBS are rarely confused with multiple sclerosis. The cranial MRI findings of CNS NBS are also dissimilar from those of thrombotic or embolic stroke.

If performed during the acute stage, CSF studies usually show inflammatory changes in most cases of CNS NBS.[85,86] CSF in patients with CVT may be under increased pressure, but the cellular and chemical composition is usually normal.

Neurological involvement in BD is a remarkable cause of morbidity, and approximately 50% of the CNS NBS patients are moderately to severely disabled after 10 years of disease.[84] Onset with cerebellar symptoms and a progressive course were unfavourable factors, while onset with headache and a diagnosis of CVT was favourable. An elevated protein level and pleocytosis in the CSF were also reported to be associated with a poorer prognosis.[85]

Neurological involvement in BD is heterogeneous and it is difficult to predict its course and prognosis, and response to treatment. Acute attacks of CNS NBS are treated with either oral prednisolone (1 mg/kg for up to 4 weeks, or until improvement is observed) or with high-dose IVMP (1 g/day) for 5–7 days. Both forms of treatment should be followed with an oral tapering dose of glucocorticoids over 2–3 months in order to prevent early relapses.[91]

Immunosuppressive agents such as azathioprine, cyclosporin A, cyclophosphamide and chlorambucil that are given as long-term treatments for various systemic manifestations of BD do not seem to prevent the development of the neurological involvement of the disease, or its exacerbations, or stop its progression.[91] Immunomodulatory treatments such as IFN-α and thalidomide have been shown to be effective in treating some of the systemic manifestations of BD, but there is no information on their effect on the development and progression of CNS NBS. Dural venous sinus thrombosis in BD is treated with heparin or low molecular weight heparins given together with a short course of steroids, despite the fact that theraupetic evidence for such treatment is weak.

Graft-versus-host disease

Both a vasculitic neuropathy in the form of a sensory multiple mononeuropathy and an angiitis-like syndrome of the CNS have been reported in patients who have undergone bone marrow transplantation.[92,93]

There are two 'vasculopathic' disorders that have clinical similarities, as, in both, ocular and audiovestibular symptoms are prominent and nervous system involvement can occur. These are Cogan's syndrome and Susac syndrome. A systemic vasculitis that may involve the nervous system has been reported in the first, whereas Susac syndrome is the result of a non-inflammatory vasculopathy.

Cogan's syndrome (CS)

This syndrome is characterized by cochleovestibular symptoms clinically indistinguishable from Meniere's disease and loss of vision due to interstitial keratitis. There is uveitis but rarely retinal vasculitis. The diagnosis of CS requires clinical signs of both eye and inner ear inflammation.[94] Almost three-quarters of the patients develop systemic manifestations, and a vasculitis involving large vessels, similar to Takayasu's arteritis, or involving medium vessels, resembling periarteritis nodosa, may develop in 10–15% of patients.[41,94,95] Neurological involvement is not common, and a true vasculitis has been documented in only a minority of the reported cases. The spectrum of the neurological manifestations is wide, and includes headache, psychosis, stroke, cerebral sinus thrombosis, seizures, encephalopathy, myelopathy, cranial neuropathies, mononeuropathies and polyneuropathy.[41,94,95] Cogan's syndrome should be considered when neurological deficits are accompanied by eye, ear and systemic symptoms.

Susac syndrome

Susac syndrome is a non-inflammatory vasculopathy causing small infarcts in the retina, the cochlea and the brain, resulting in the clinical triad of retinopathy, hearing loss, and encephalopathy.[96] Most of the patients do not have the clinical triad at the onset of symptoms, and recurrences of one or more of the components of the triad are generally observed. Headache and cognitive and psychiatric disturbances are the most frequent manifestations of the encephalopathy, and neurological signs are diffuse and multifocal and may progress during the course of the disease.[96,97]

Familial mediterranean fever (FMF) and some pseudovasculitic conditions may mimic vasculitis, and therefore need to be included in its differential diagnosis.

Familial mediterranean fever

FMF is an autosomal recessive disorder characterized by intermittent attacks of fever with peritonitis, pleuritis, and synovitis, affecting certain ethnic groups originating from the Mediterranean region and Middle East, with a tendency for amyloidosis to develop in untreated patients.[98] A close association between FMF and some vasculitic conditions, such as PAN, has been noted.[98] Nervous system involvement is rare, but coincidental multiple sclerosis or multiple sclerosis-like neurological manifestations, as well as CNS complications of PAN-type vasculitis, have been reported.[99]

Pseudovasculitic conditions

Many disorders may cause obstruction of blood vessels or vasculopathies without inflammation of the vessel wall, mimicking vasculitis. Some examples with neurological complications are: the antiphospholipid syndrome, sickle-cell disease, thrombotic thrombocytopenic purpura, amyloidosis, embolism from myxoma, infective endocarditis and cholesterol embolism.[91,98]

REFERENCES

1. Watts RA, Scott DGI. Classification and epidemiology of vasculitides. *Baillière's Clin Rheumatol* 1997; **11**(2): 335–355.
2. Ferro JM. Vasculitis of the central nervous system. *J Neurol* 1998; **245**: 766–776.
3. Montalban JI, Rio J, Khamastha M et al. Value of immunologic testing in stroke patients: a prospective multi-center study. *Stroke* 1994; **25**: 2412–2415.
4. Vollmer TL, Guamaccia I, Harrington W, Pacia SV, Petroff OAC. Idiopathic granulomatous angiitis of the central nervous system; diagnostic challenges. *Arch Neurol* 1993; **50**: 925–930.

5. Cravioto H, Feigin I. Noninfectious granulomatous angiitis with a predilection for the nervous system. *Neurology* 1959; **9**: 599–609.

6. Calabrese LH, Duna GF, Lie JT. Vasculitis in the central nervous system. *Arthritis Rheum* 1997; **40**: 1189–1201.

7. Goldberg JW. Primary angiitis of the central nervous system. In: Rolak LA, Harati Y, eds. *Neuroimmunology for the Clinician.* Butterworth-Heinemann, Boston 1997: 177–186.

8. Chu TC, Gray L, Goldstein B, Hulette CM. Diagnosis of intracranial vasculitis: a multidisciplinary approach. *J Neuropathol Exp Neurol* 1998; **57**: 30–38.

9. Lie JT. Classification and histopathologic spectrum of central nervous system vasculitis. *Neurol Clin* 1997; **15**: 805–819.

10. Newman GC. CNS *Vasculitis, Clinical Neuroimmunology,* Education Syllabus, AAN, 1998: FC.005–143–FC.005–174.

11. Parisi JE, Moore PM. The role of biopsy in vasculitis of the central nervous system. *Semin Neurol* 1994; **14**: 341–348.

12. Moore P. Neurology of vasculitides and connective tissue diseases. *J Neurol Neurosurg Psychiatry* 1998; **65**: 10–22.

13. Woolfenden AR, Tong DC, Marks MP et al. Angiographically defined primary angiitis of the CNS. Is it really benign? *Neurology* 1998; **51**: 183–188.

14. Calabrese LH, Grag LA, Furlan AJ. Benign angiopathy: a distinct subset of angiographically defined primary angiitis of the central nervous system. *J Rheumatol* 1993; **20**: 2046–2050.

15. Alrawi A, Trobe JD, Blaivas M, Musch DC. Brain biopsy in primary angiitis of the central nervous system. *Neurology* 1999; **11**(53): 858–860.

16. Finelli PF, Onykie HC, Uphoff DF. Idiopathic granulomatous angiitis of the CNS manifesting as diffuse white matter disease. *Neurology* 1997; **49**: 1696–1699.

17. Goldstein LB, Chu CT, Gray L, Hulette CM. Angiographically defined primary angiitis of the CNS: Is it really benign? *Neurology* 1999; **52**: 1302–1303.

18. Fountain NB, Eberhard DA. Primary angiitis of the CNS associated with cerebral amyloid angiopathy: report of two cases and review of the literature. *Neurology* 1996; **46**: 190–197.

19. Fountain NB, Lopes MB. Control of primary angiitis of the CNS associated with cerebral amyloid angiopathy by cyclophosphamide alone. *Neurology* 1999; **52**: 660–662.

20. Heckmann JG, Kayser C, Heuss D et al. Neurological manifestations of chronic hepatitis C. *J Neurol* 1999; **246**: 486–491.

21. Calabrese LH. Therapy of systemic vasculitis. *Neurol Clin* 1997; **15**: 973–991.

22. Calabrese LH, Duna GF. Evaluation and treatment of central nervous system vasculitis. *Curr Opin Rheumatol* 1995; **7**: 37–44.

23. Greenan TJ, Grossman RI, Goldberg HI. Cerebral vasculitis: MR imaging and angiographic correlation. *Radiology* 1992; **182**: 65–72.

24. Alhalabi M, Moore P. Serial angiography in isolated angiitis of the central nervous system. *Neurology* 1994; **44**: 1221–1226.

25. Pomper MG, Miller TJ, Stone JH et al. CNS vasculitis in autoimmune disease: MR imaging findings and correlation with angiography. *Am J Neuroradiol* 1999; **20**: 75–85.

26. Shoemaker EI, Zwu-Shin L, Rae-Grant AD, Little B. Primary angiitis of the CNS: unusual MR appearance. *AJNR* 1994; **15**: 331–334.

27. Berger JR, Wei T, Wilson D. Idiopathic granulomatous angiitis of the CNS manifesting as diffuse white matter disease. *Neurology* 1998; **51**: 1774–1775.

28. (No authors listed) Case records of the MGH, case 33–1995. *N Engl J Med* 1995; **333**: 1135–1143.

29. Ehsan T, Hasan S, Powers J. Serial magnetic resonance imaging in isolated angiitis of the central nervous system. *Neurology* 1995; **45**: 1462–1465.

30. Vassallo R, Remstein ED, Parisi JE, Huston J 3rd, Brown RD Jr. Multiple cerebral infarctions from nonbacterial thrombotic endocarditis mimicking cerebral vasculitis. *Mayo Clin Proc* 1999; **74**: 798–802.

31. Dodick DW, Brown RD Jr, Britton JW, Huston J 3rd. Nonaneurysmal thunderclap headache with diffuse, multifocal, segmental, and reversible vasospasm. *Cephalalgia* 1999; **19**: 118–123.

32. Schwartz RB, Bravo SM, Klufas R et al. Cylosporin neurotoxicity and its relation to neuropathy: CT and MR findings in 16 cases. *Am J Roentgenol* 1995; **165**: 627–631.

33. Riemer G, Lamszus K, Zschaber R et al. Isolated angiitis of the central nervous system: lack of inflammation after long-term treatment. *Neurology* 1999; **52**: 196–199.

34. Oliveira V, Povoa P, Costa A, Ducla-Soares J. Cerebrospinal fluid and therapy of isolated angiitis of the central nervous system. *Stroke* 1994; **25**: 1693–1695.

35. Lie JT. Biopsy diagnosis of systemic vasculitis. *Baillière's Clin Rheumatol* 1997; **11**(2): 219–236.

36. Scolding N. Cerebral vasculitis. In: Scolding N, ed. *Immunological and Inflammatory Disorders of the Central Nervous System.* Butterworth-Heinemann, 1999: 210–257.

37. Zivkovic S, Moore PM. Systemic and central nervous system vasculitides. *Curr Treatment Options Neurol* 2000; **2**: 459–472.

38. Gross WL. New concepts in treatment protocols for severe systemic vasculitis. *Curr Opin Rheumatol* 1999; **11**: 41–46.

39. Boman S, Ballen JL, Seggev JS. Dramatic responses to intravenous immunoglobulin in vasculitis. *J Intern Med* 1995; **238**: 375–377.

40. Lockwood CM. Intravenous immunoglobulin for the treatment of vasculitides. In: Kazatchkine MD, Morell A, eds. *Intravenous Immunoglobulin Research and Therapy.* New York: The Parthenon Publishing Group, 1996: 143–145.

41. Nadeau SE. Neurologic manifestations of vasculitis and connective tissue diseases. In: Joynt RJ, Griggs RC, eds. *Baker's Clinical Neurology on CD Rom 2000.*

42. Gilden DH, Kleinscmidt-deMasters BK, LaGuardisa JJ et al. Neurologic complications of the reactivation of varicella zoster virus. *N Engl J Med* 2000; **342**: 635–645.

43. Gilden DH, Kleinscmidt-deMasters BK, Wellish M et al. Varicella zoster virus, a cause of waxing and waning vasculitis. *The New England Journal of Medicine* 1996; case 5-1995 revisited. *Neurology* 1996; **47**: 1441–1446.

44. Case records of the MGH, case 5-1995 *N Engl J Med* 1995; **332**: 452–459.

45. Brannagan III TH. Retroviral-associated vasculitis of the nervous system. *Neurol Clin* 1997; **15**: 927–944.

46. Gray F, Lescs MC, Keohane C et al. Early brain changes in HIV infection: neuropathological study of 11 HIV seropositive, non-AIDS cases. *J Neuropathol Exp Neurol* 1992; **51**: 177–185.

47. Bradley WG, Verma A. Painful vasculitic neuropathy in HIV-1 infection. Relief of pain with prednisone therapy. *Neurology* 1996; **47**: 1446–1451.

48. Dawson TM, Starkebaum G. Isolated central nervous system vasculitis associated with hepatitis C infection. *J Rheumatol* 1999; **26**: 2273–2276.

49. Irani DN. Neurological complications of the hepatitis viruses. In: Gilman S, ed. *Neurobase 3rd 2000 edition*. Ann Arbor Publishing, 2000.

50. Tembl JI, Ferrer JM, Sevilla MT et al. Neurologic complications associated with hepatitis C virus infection. *Neurology* 1999; **53**: 861–864.

51. Authier FJ, Payan Ch, Guillevin L, Belec L, Gherardi RK. Detection of genomic but not replicative hepatitis C virus RNA in nerve and muscle of patients with HCV-associated neuropathy. *Neurology* 2000; **54** (supp 3): A385.

52. Origgi L, Vanoli M, Lunghi G et al. Hepatitis C virus genotypes and clinical features in hepatitis C virus-related mixed cryoglobulinemia. *Int J Clin Lab Res* 1998; **28**: 96–99.

53. Authier FJ, Pawlotsky JM, Viard JP, Guillevin L, Degos JD, Gherardi RK. High incidence of hepatitis C infection in patients with cryoglobulinemic neuropathy. *Ann Neurol* 1993; **34**: 749–750.

54. Klein CM, Suarez GA. The natural history of peripheral neuropathy associated with cryoglobulinemia. *Neurology* 2000; **54** suppl 3: A385.

55. Petty GW, Duffy J, Huston J. Cerebral ischemia in patients with hepatitis C virus infection and mixed cryoglobulinemia. *Mayo Clin Proc* 1996; **71**: 671–678.

56. Poser JB. *Neurological Complications of Cancer*. Philadelphia: FA Davis Company, 1995.

57. Rosen CL, DePalma L, Morita A. Primary angiitis of the central nervous system as a first presentation in Hodgkin's disease: a case report and review of the literature. *Neurosurgery* 2000; **46**: 1504–1508.

58. Oh SJ. Paraneoplastic vasculitis of the peripheral nervous system. *Neurol Clin* 1997; **15**: 849–863.

59. Brust JCM. Vasculitis owing to substance abuse. *Neurol Clin* 1997; **15**: 945–957.

60. Kernan WN, Viscoli CM, Brass LM et al. Phenylpropanolamine and the risk of hemorrhagic stroke. *N Engl J Med* 2000; **343**: 1826–1832.

61. Fallis RJ, Fisher M. Cerebral vasculitis and hemorrhage associated with phenylpropanolamine. *Neurology* 1985; **35**: 405–407.

62. Glick R, Hoying J, Cerullo L, Perlman S. Phenylpropanolamine: an over the counter drug causing central nervous system vasculitis and intracerebral hemorrhage. Case report and review. *Neurosurgery* 1987; **20**: 969–974.

63. Savage COS, Harper L, Adu D. Primary systemic vasculitis. *Lancet* 1997; **349**: 535–558.

64. Jennette JC, Falk RJ, Andrassy K et al. Nomenclature of systemic vasculitides. Proposal of an international consensus conference. *Arthritis Rheum* 1994; **37**: 187–192.

65. Wilke WS. Large vessel vasculitis. *Baillière's Clin Rheumatol* 1997; **11**: 285–314.

66. Zeidler M, Hughes T, Zeman A. Confused by arteritis. *Lancet* 2000; **355**: 374–375.

67. Goodwin J. Temporal arteritis. In: Gilman S, ed. *Neurobase 4th 2000 edition*. Ann Arbor Publishing, 2000.

68. Kupersmith MJ, Carlow T. Giant cell arteritis—what the neurologist needs to know. In: *American Academy of Neurology, 52nd Annual Meeting, 2000*, Syllabi on CD-ROM, 2BS.006-1–2BS.006–18.

69. Kariv R, Sidi Y, Gur H. Systemic vasculitis presenting as a tumorlike lesion. Four case reports and an analysis of 79 reported cases. *Medicine (Baltimore)* 2000; **79**: 349–359.

70. Weyand CM, Fulbright JW, Hunder GG, Evans JM, Goronzy JJ. Treatment of giant cell arteritis: interleukin-6 as a biologic marker of disease activity. *Arthritis Rheum* 2000; **43**: 1041–1049.

71. Evans JM, O'Fallon WM, Hunder GG. Increased incidence of aortic aneurysm and dissection in giant cell (temporal) arteritis. A population-based study. *Ann Intern Med* 1995; **122**(7): 502–507.

72. Guillevin L, Lhote F, Gherardi R. Polyarteritis nodosa, microscopic angiitis, and Churg–Strauss syndrome: clinical aspects, neurologic manifestations, and treatment. *Neurol Clin* 1997; **15**: 865–886.

73. Cohen Tervaert JW, Popa E, Bos NA. The role of superantigens in vasculitis. *Curr Opin Rheumatol* 1999; **11**: 24–33.

74. Burns JC, Capparelli EV, Brown JA, Newburger JW, Glode MP. Intravenous gamma-globulin treatment and retreatment in Kawasaki disease. US/Canadian Kawasaki Study Group. *Pediatr Infect Dis* 1998; **17**: 1144–1148.

75. Drachman DA. Neurological complications of Wegener's granulomatosis. *Arch Neurol* 1963; **8**: 145–155.

76. Nishino H, Rubino FA, DeRemee RA et al. Neurological involvement in Wegener's granulomatosis: an analysis of 324 consecutive patients at the Mayo Clinic. *Ann Neurol* 1993; **33**: 4–9.

77. Murphy JM, Gomez-Anson B, Gillard JH et al. Wegener granulomatosis: MR imaging findings in brain and meninges. *Radiology* 1999; **213**: 794–799.

78. Provenzale JM, Allen NB. Wegener granulomatosis: CT and MR findings. *AJNR* 1996; **17**: 785–792.

79. Hoffman GS. Wegener's granulomatosis. *Curr Opin Rheumatol* 1993; **5**: 11–17.

80. Gross WL. Systemic necrotizing vasculitis. *Baillière's Clin Rheumatol* 1997; **11**(2): 259–284.

81. Behçet H. Uber residivierende, aphtöse, durch ein virus verursachte Geschwüre am Mund, am Auge und an den Genitalien. *Derm Woschenscr* 1937; **105**: 1152–1157.

82. International Study Group for Behçet's disease. Criteria for diagnosis of Behçet's disease. *Lancet* 1990; **335**: 1078–1080.

83. Sakane T, Takeno M, Suzuki N, Inaba G. Behçet's disease. *N Engl J Med* 1999; **341**: 1284–1291.

84. Siva A, Kantarci OH, Saip S et al. Behçet's disease: diagnostic and prognostic aspects of neurological involvement. *J Neurol* 2001; **248**: 95–103.

85. Akman-Demir G, Serdaroğlu P, Taşçı B. Clinical patterns of neurological involvement in Behçet's disease: evaluation of 200 patients. *Brain* 1999; **122**: 2171–2181.

86. Kidd D, Steuer A, Denman AM, Rudge P. Neurological complications in Behçet's syndrome. *Brain* 1999; **122**: 2183–2194.

87. Serdaroğlu P. Behçet's disease and the nervous system. *J Neurol* 1998; **245**: 197–205.

88. Wechsler B, Vidailhet M, Bousser MG et al. Cerebral venous sinus thrombosis in Behçet's disease: long-term follow-up of 25 cases. *Neurology* 1992; **42**: 614–618.

89. Koçer N, Işlak C, Siva A et al. CNS involvement in Neuro-Behçet's syndrome: an MR study. *AJNR* 1999; **20**: 1015–1024.

90. Hadfield MG, Aydin F, Lippman HR, Sanders KM. Neuro-Behçet's disease. *Clin Neuropathol* 1997; **16**: 55–60.

91. Siva A, Fresko I. Behçet's dease. *Curr Treatment Options Neurol* 2000; **2**: 435–447.

92. Padovan CS, Bise K, Hahn J et al. Angiitis of central nervous system after allogeneic bone marrow transplantation. *Stroke* 1999; **30**: 1651–1656.

93. Gabriel CM, Goldman JM, Lucas S, Hughes RA. Vasculitic neuropathy in association with chronic graft-versus-host disease. *J Neurol Sci* 1999; **168**: 68–70.

94. St Clair EW, McCallum RM. Cogan's syndrome. *Curr Opin Rheumatol* 1999; **11**: 47–52.

95. Nazarian S. Cogan's syndrome. In: Gilman S, ed. *Neurobase 4th 2000 edition*. Arbor Publishing, 2000.

96. Susac JO. Susac's syndrome. The triad of microangiopathy of the brain and retina with hearing loss in young women. *Neurology* 1994; **44**: 591–593.

97. O'Halloran HS, Pearson PA, Lee WB, Susac JO, Berger JR. Microangiopathy of the brain, retina, and cochlea (Susac syndrome). A report of five cases and a review of the literature. *Ophthalmology* 1998; **105**: 1038–1044.

98. Hamuryudan V, Özdoğan H, Yazıcı H. Vasculitis. Other forms of vasculitis and pseudovasculitis. *Baillière's Clin Rheumatol* 1997; **11**(2): 335–355.

99. Topçuoğlu MA, Karabudak R. Familial Mediterranean fever and multiple sclerosis. *J Neurol* 1997; **244**: 510–512.

21

Brain vasculitis and antiphospholipid syndrome

Lubica Rauova, Joab Chapman and Yehuda Shoenfeld

ANTIPHOSPHOLIPID SYNDROME AND ANTIPHOSPHOLIPID ANTIBODIES

Antiphospholipid syndrome (APS) is an autoimmune disorder characterized by recurrent venous and arterial thrombosis, fetal loss and thrombocytopenia in association with elevated titers of circulating auto-antibodies directed against phospholipids, including lupus anticoagulant.[1] Antiphospholipid antibodies (aPL) are crucial for diagnosis and represent a very heterogeneous group, as multiple specificities against various phospholipids are found. The anti-cardiolipin ELISA assay, introduced in 1983, is the most established and standardized method for detecting aPL, since other aPL directed to phosphatidylserine, phosphatidylethanolamine, phosphatidylcholine, phosphatidylglycerine, phosphatidylinositol and recently lysobisphosphatidic acid[2] have been investigated less frequently. Moreover, in 1990 three independent groups reported the requirement of a protein cofactor, β_2 glycoprotein I (β_2-GPI), for efficient binding of 'autoimmune' antibodies to the phospholipids, in contrast to 'infectious' aPL recognizing phospholipids alone. Since then, the anti-β_2-GPI antibodies have been defined as a population overlapping but distinct from aPL and have been found to be significantly associated with thrombosis and thrombocytopenia occurring in APS. β_2-GPI alone was found to be capable of inducing full-blown APS in a mouse model and was consequently proposed as an autoantigen in APS.[4]

The syndrome is predominantly associated with systemic lupus erythematosus (SLE) or with other autoimmune disorders as secondary APS, or can exist in isolation as primary antiphospholipid syndrome (pAPS). APS manifests with microvascular thrombosis as well as large-vessel occlusion with acute thrombotic episodes, which may involve all organ systems. Involvement of the central nervous system (CNS) is common in patients with pAPS (Table 21.1). The high frequency of neurologic involvement in APS might be due to vulnerability of the cerebral vasculature, where the thrombotic event is more likely to be symptomatic than in the periphery.[5] Neurologic complications such as transient ischemic attack and ischemic stroke have been described as typical features since the first report.[1] Seizure, transverse myelopathy, migraine, chorea, cognitive dysfunction ranging from mild neurocognitive disorders to more severe vascular dementia, depression and psychosis are also associated with APS. Also, CNS involvement in SLE patients is closely associated with the presence of IgG-aPL[6–8] as well as with the clinical features of APS, mainly history of arterial thrombosis and recurrent fetal loss.[9]

Table 21.1 Neurologic complications in APS	
Focal ischemic	**Diffuse**
Transient ischemic attack[1,57]	Seizures[58]
Recurrent stroke[1,57]	Transverse myelopathy[59]
Multi-infarct dementia[30]	Chorea[60]
Cerebral venous thrombosis[61]	Neurocognitive dysfunction[32,62–65]
Migraine[66]	Dementia[31]
Ocular ischemia[25]	Transient visual disturbances[67]
	Depression[53]
	Psychosis[68]
	Guillain–Barré syndrome[69,70]
	Multiple sclerosis[71,72]

VASCULITIS VERSUS VASCULOPATHY

Although CNS involvement in APS has been recognized for more than 15 years, its exact etiopathology is still not well defined. The strong association of neuropsychiatric lupus (NPSLE) with cutaneous vasculitis[9,10] may imply an underlying vasculitic process in the CNS, particularly in APS secondary to SLE. However, the most common neuropathologic findings in autopsy studies of NPSLE as well as in pAPS are thrombosis and small-vessel non-inflammatory proliferative vasculopathy.[11–13] APS is mostly characterized as a thrombotic microangiopathy with endothelial cell swelling and thrombosis, depositions of fibrin and/or platelets and proliferation of myointimal cells, without immunoglobulin (Ig) or complement deposition and the cell infiltrate usually found in classical systemic autoimmune vasculitis. The vasculopathy in NPSLE is characterized by hyalinization, occasionally associated with occlusion, pericapillary microglia, microinfarcts and microhemorrhages. Vasculitis of the brain vessel with typical cell infiltration in the vessel wall has been documented in 7–15% of NPSLE autopsy cases,[9] and in a small number of patients with APS secondary to SLE systemic and cerebral vasculitis may coexist with disseminated coagulopathy.[14] In primary APS, thrombosis, and not vasculitis, is postulated as the pathologic basis of vaso-occlusive disease. Vasculopathy can mimic vasculitis clinically and is not distinguishable in angiography. Cerebral angiography is neither sensitive for detecting inflammatory vascular disease nor specific for differentiating it from non-inflammatory vasculopathy. The distinction between vasculitis and vasculopathy is feasible only histologically by the absence of a typical cellular infiltrate in vessel wall; however, brain biopsy is characterized by poor sensitivity. Some controversy exists, because organized thrombus with recanalization may have a meager residual cellular infiltrate, which can be misinterpreted as healed vasculitis. There is also confusion between reactive perivascular cell infiltrates and true vasculitis. Considering all the controversies, thrombotic microangiopathy along with true vasculitis was described recently in two patients with pAPS.[15] However, vasculitis is generally not accepted as a primary pathologic feature of APS. The specific form of vasculopathy related to the presence of aPL might be triggered by the occurrence of vasculitis and the reaction of incident aPL with phospholipids flipped to the outer leaflet of endothelial cells.[16]

THE ROLE OF ANTIPHOSPHOLIPID ANTIBODIES

The association between the clinical manifestations of APS and the elevated levels of aPL raises the question of whether these antibodies are really pathogenic or secondary to other pathogenic processes and serve only as markers of a thrombotic syndrome. The direct pathogenic role of the aPL has been strengthened by experiments where the fully expressed syndrome was induced in naive BALB/c mice following passive infusion of monoclonal or polyclonal mouse and human aPL.[17–19] Moreover, in experimental APS induced in BALB/c mice by active immunization with monoclonal anti-cardiolipin (aCL), APS mice displayed behavioral and neurologic deficits along with elevated levels of aPL, anti-endothelial cell (AECA) and anti-β_2-GPI anti-antibodies, and other clinical manifestations of APS.[20] Anti-cardiolipin antibodies have also been shown to possess thrombogenic properties in mice.[21,22] One animal model for spontaneously occurring APS is the MRL/MPJ–lpr/ lpr (MRL/lpr) mouse, which develops a high titer of aPL at 2–3 months of age. These mice develop cognitive and neurologic defects which cannot be explained by multiple infarcts. They have mononuclear infiltrates in the chorioid plexus, in contrast to control strains without aPL.[23]

There is, in addition, a debate on whether aPL cause brain dysfunction by purely vascular mechanisms or have direct effects on neuronal structures. The most often suggested mechanism is cerebrovascular thrombosis resulting from aPL-mediated interference with platelet–endothelial cell interactions.[12,24,25] Although the mechanisms are unclear, aPL are implicated in the pathogenesis of the thrombotic events that characterize APS. Indeed, focal infarcts are the commonest MRI abnormalities found in patients with APS with CNS symptoms, and small-vessel thrombi have been described in several organs, including brain, in patients with APS. However, brain atrophy and diffuse white matter hyperintense lesions can also be found in a high percentage of cases.[26,27] aPL were found to react with almost all components of the coagulation system: platelets, anticoagulation proteins, humoral factors and endothelial cells. Thromboembolism, due to the procoagulant state exerted by the aPL, is considered to be the main pathophysiologic process. In experimental studies, aPL have been shown to cause enhanced thrombus formation in an in vivo thrombosis model,[27] and to activate monocytes in vitro.[28] The most common arterial thrombotic manifestations associated with aPL are recurrent ischemic stroke and thromboembolic events in patients younger than 50 years.[29] Repeated episodes of cerebral infarction, demonstrated also by computed tomographic (CT) scan, may lead to the development of dementia.[30]

On the other hand, there is much evidence from clinical and pathologic studies that not all brain damage is accompanied by vasculopathy and ischemia and there is an alternative mechanism for aPL-mediated dysfunction. aPL may cause silent damage to the cerebral microcirculation as well as affect psychological function, since cognitive defects can be found in elderly patients with aPL without demonstrable MRI iesions.[5] Mosek et al[31] found a significant association of aPL with apparently diffuse brain disease in elderly patients with dementia. In another study,[32] persistently elevated IgG aCL levels were associated with a reduction in psychomotor speed and suggested to predict subtle deterioration in cognitive function in some patients with SLE. Thus thrombosis can explain only part of the neurologic clinical manifestations, and a direct interaction between aPL and brain tissue phospholipids has also been proposed. This suggests a complementary hypothesis, that aPL may have direct effects on neuronal or astrocytic function. aPL were shown to interfere with astrocyte proliferation and functioning,[33] and to bind to the myelin, chorioidal and ependymal epithelial cilia[34] and to neuronal membranes, inducing depolarization of synaptoneurosomes.[35] Additionally, anti-β_2-GPI antibodies have also been shown to bind to the CNS, in particular to astrocytes, neurons and cerebral vascular endothelium. This reactivity was specific for anti-β_2-GPI, independent from aCL, since aCL + a-β_2-GPI-negative antibodies did not bind to these cells.[36] Anti-β_2-GPI antibodies probably contribute mostly to the CNS damage in pAPS as well as APS secondary to SLE.[37] Anti-neuronal antibodies involved in NPSLE are not present in significantly higher levels in APS with CNS involvement.[38]

Currently available attitudes combine both vascular and non-vascular mechanisms in the pathologic process. The blood–brain barrier (BBB) creates a relatively immunoprotected state in the brain and blocks entry of most cells and large molecules into the parenchyma of the CNS.[39] Therefore, CNS injury could only occur if antibodies or immunocompetent cells gained entry through an altered BBB. If circulating aPL interact with vascular endothelial or chorioidal epithelial BBB components, the resultant BBB compromise may allow antibody access to CNS targets. This may occur in the presence of thrombosis

or inflammation or both.[34] Cellular entry is controlled by the expression of adhesion molecules on vascular endothelium. Recent studies have shown that aPL are able to induce enhanced expression of adhesion molecules on endothelial cells.[40–42] Affinity-purified aPL from patients with APS upregulated expression of intercellular adhesion molecule-1 (ICAM-1), vascular adhesion molecule-1 (VCAM-1) and E-selectin in vitro, and these effects correlated with enhanced thrombosis and leukocyte adhesion in vivo.[43] We have shown recently[44] that the upregulation of ICAM-1, VCAM-1 and E-selectin on HUVEC in vitro by certain murine anti-β_2-GPI monoclonal antibodies correlates with the capability to induce in vivo clinical signs of APS (increased fetal resorptions, reduced platelet counts, and prolonged activated partial thromboplastin time). The upregulated expression of adhesion molecules on endothelial cell membranes is associated with an increased turnover of their soluble isoforms released into the circulation. Indeed, soluble ICAM-1, VCAM and P-selectin were found to be elevated in the plasma of patients with APS and thrombosis.[45]

Conversion of the normal antithrombotic endothelial phenotype to a prothrombotic state may be a primary pathophysiologic event. After the monocyte adhesion to E-selectin expressed on activated endothelium, monocytes undergo a phenotypic transformation that includes surface expression of tissue factor,[46] and enhanced tissue factor activity on blood monocytes and/or vascular endothelial cells contributes further to the hypercoagulability in APS. In addition, adhesion molecules such as ICAM-1, VCAM-1 and P-selectin act as mediators in the pathogenic effects of aPL and are necessary for thrombotic complications mediated by aPL. Both activation of endothelial cells and enhanced thrombus formation induced by affinity-purified aPL are impaired in ICAM-1-knockout and ICAM-1/P-selectin double-knockout mice.[47] Moreover, treatment with anti-ICAM-1 monoclonal antibody early in life resulted in significant improvement in motor coordination (Fig. 21.1) and, to a lesser extent, also cognitive dysfunction (Fig. 21.2) in β_2-GPI-induced experimental APS in BALB/c mice.[48] It also protects against an expected dramatic decline in neurologic functioning with age, along with suppression of inflammatory lesions in skin and peripheral nerve, but not kidney or chorioid plexus, of MRL/lpr mic.[49]

CONCLUSION

Hence, though there is no definite pathologic evidence of vasculitis in APS, recent data support the

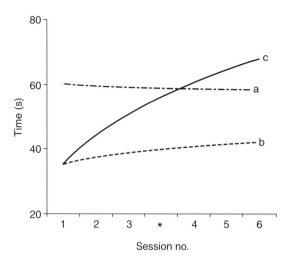

Figure 21.1 ROTA-ROD performance (regression curves) by control BALB/c mice (a), BALB/c mice immunized with β_2-GPI (b) and BALB/c mice treated with ICAM monoclonal antibody (c). Non-treated β_2-GPI-immunized mice showed motor incoordination, displaying a shorter mean duration on the rotating bar and difficulties in learning tasks ($P <0.05$ ANOVA with repeated measures), while β_2-GPI-immunized anti-ICAM-treated mice exhibited significant improvement in performance of the task, reaching the performance level of the controls (immunized with BSA).

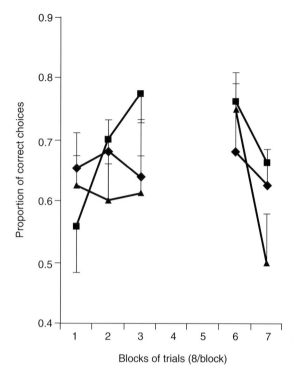

Figure 21.2 T-maze performance by control BALB/c mice (■), BALB/c immunized with β_2-GPI (▲) a BALB/c mice treated with a-ICAM monoclonal antibody (◆). The mean of correct choices displayed by the mice is depicted. Mice immunized with β_2-GPI demonstrated a significant deficit choosing the correct arm on the choice trials, compared to the controls, which were immunized with BSA. A trend for improvement in performance of the task was achieved in the anti-ICAM-treated mice.

hypothesis that aPL can induce a procoagulant and pro-inflammatory endothelial phenotype. Anti-β_2-GPI antibodies bind to endothelial cells and activate them to an extent which is inadequate to induce significant Ig deposition or cell infiltration. However, they induce expression of adhesion molecules and interleukin-6 production.[50] Complement activation occurs in patients with aPL-associated cerebral ischemia as well.[51] Patients with APS possess circulating β_2-GPI-specific Th1 cells producing the pro-inflammatory cytokine interferon gamma.[52]

Unraveling the kind of pathology associated with neurologic disease in APS is crucial for choosing the appropriate form of drug treatment for the patients. Therapeutic approaches today are mainly restricted to conventional thrombosis therapy. Corticosteroid therapy has not been beneficial in preventing recurrent thrombotic events.[53] Several immunomodulations were tried in animal models of SLE and were found to be highly effective in the amelioration of clinical, serologic and histologic manifestations of APS (review: Krause et al[54]). The most promising potential for application may represent therapy with high-dose intravenous immunoglobulins. IVIg was successful in in vitro inhibition of anti-cardiolipin antibodies and lupus anticoagulant[55] and in the amelioration of experimental APS.[56] The most recent research supports the future inhibition of expression of adhesion molecules.

ACKNOWLEDGEMENT

This work was supported by a research grant from Sir David Alliance, UK.

REFERENCES

1. Hughes GR. Thrombosis, abortion, cerebral disease, and the lupus anticoagulant. *BMJ Clin Res Ed* 1983; **287**: 1088–1089.

2. Kobayashi T, Stang E, Fang KS, de Moerloose P, Parton RG, Gruenberg J. A lipid associated with the antiphospholipid syndrome regulates endosome structure and function. *Nature* 1998; **392**: 193–197.

3. Blank M, Faden D, Tincani A et al. Immunization with anticardiolipin cofactor (beta-2-glycoprotein I) induces experimental antiphospholipid syndrome in naive mice. *J Autoimmune* 1994; **7**: 441–455.

4. Shoenfeld Y, Gharavi A, Koike T. Beta2GP-I in the anti phospholipid (Hughes') syndrome—from a cofactor to an autoantigen—from induction to prevention of antiphospholipid syndrome. *Lupus* 1998; **7**: 503–506.

5. Hess DC. Models for central nervous system complications of antiphospholipid syndrome. *Lupus* 1994; **3**: 253–257.

6. Harris EN, Gharavi AE, Asherson RA, Boey ML, Hughes GR. Cerebral infarction in systemic lupus: association with anticardiolipin antibodies. *Clin Exp Rheumatol* 1984; **2**: 47–51.

7. Toubi E, Khamashta MA, Panarra A, Hughes GR. Association of antiphospholipid antibodies with central nervous system disease in systemic lupus erythematosus. *Am J Med* 1995; **99**: 397–401.

8. Tincani A, Brey R, Balestrieri G et al. International survey on the management of patients with SLE. II. The results of a questionnaire regarding neuropsychiatric manifestations. *Clin Exp Rheumatol* 1996; **14**(suppl 16); S23–S29.

9. Karassa FB, Ioannidis JP, Touloumi G, Boki KA, Moutsopoulos HM. Risk factors for central nervous system involvement in systemic lupus erythematosus. *Q J Med* 2000; **93**: 169–174.

10. Alarcon Segovia D, Perez Vazquez ME, Villa AR, Drenkard C, Cabiedes J. Preliminary classification criteria for the antiphospholipid syndrome within systemic lupus erythematosus. *Semin Arthritis Rheum* 1992; **21**: 275–286.

11. Baker WH, Potthoff WP, Biller J, McCoyd K. Carotid artery thrombosis associated with lupus anticoagulant. *Surgery* 1985; **98**: 612–615.

12. Briley DP, Coull BM, Goodnight SH Jr. Neurological disease associated with antiphospholipid antibodies. *Ann Neurol* 1989; **25**: 221–227.

13. Levine SR, Deegan MJ, Futrell N, Welch KM. Cerebrovascular and neurologic disease associated with antiphospholipid antibodies: 48 cases. *Neurology* 1990; **40**: 1181–1189.

14. Lie JT, Kobayashi S, Tokano Y, Hashimoto H. Systemic and cerebral vasculitis coexisting with disseminated coagulopathy in systemic lupus erythematosus associated with antiphospholipid syndrome. *J Rheumatol* 1995; **22**: 2173–2176.

15. McCarthy GA. Vascular pathology of the antiphospholipid antibody syndrome. In: Khamashta MA, ed. *Hughes Syndrome: Antiphospholipid Syndrome*. London: Springer Verlag: 2000: 263–280.

16. Alarcon Segovia D, Cardiel MH, Reyes E. Antiphospholipid arterial vasculopathy. *J Rheumatol* 1989; **16**: 762–767.

17. Blank M, Cohen J, Toder V, Shoenfeld Y. Induction of anti-phospholipid syndrome in naive mice with mouse lupus monoclonal and human polyclonal anti-cardiolipin antibodies. *Proc Natl Acad Sci USA* 1991; **88**: 3069–3073.

18. Yodfat O, Blank M, Krause I, Shoenfeld Y. The pathogenic role of anti-phosphatidylserine antibodies: active immunization with the antibodies leads to the induction of antiphospholipid syndrome. *Clin Immunol Immunopathol* 1996; **78**: 14–20.

19. Branch DW, Dudley DJ, Mitchell MD. Immunoglobulin G fractions from patients with antiphospholipid antibodies cause fetal death in BALB/c mice: a model for autoimmune fetal loss. *Am J Obstet Gynecol* 1990; **163**: 210–216.

20. Ziporen L, Shoenfeld Y, Levy Y, Korczyn AD. Neurological dysfunction and hyperactive behavior associated with antiphospholipid antibodies. *J Clin Invest* 1997; **100**: 613–619.

21. Olee T, Pierangeli SS, Handley HH et al. A monoclonal IgG anticardiolipin antibody from a patient with the antiphospholipid syndrome is thrombogenic in mice. *Proc Nati Acad Sci USA* 1996; **93**: 8606–8611.

22. Pierangeli SS, Liu SW, Anderson G, Barker JH, Harris EN. Thrombogenic properties of murine anti-cardiolipin antibodies induced by beta 2 glycoprotein 1 and human immunoglobulin G antiphospholipid antibodies. *Circulation* 1996; **94**: 1746–1751.

23. Hess DC, Taormina M, Thompson J et al. Cognitive and neurologic deficits in the MRL/lpr mouse: a clinicopathological study. *J Rheumatol* 1993; **20**: 610–617.

24. Brey RL, Coull BM. Antiphospholipid antibodies: origin, specificity, and mechanism of action. *Stroke* 1992; **23**: I15–I18.

25. Levine SR, Brey RL. Neurological aspects of antiphospholipid antibody syndrome. *Lupus* 1996; **5**: 347–353.

26. Rovaris M, Viti B, Ciboddo G et al. Brain involvement in systemic immune mediated diseases: magnetic resonance and magnetisation transfer imaging study. *J Neurol Neurosurg Psychiatry* 2000; **68**: 170–177.

27. Pierangeli SS, Barker JH, Stikovac D et al. Effect of human IgG antiphospholipid antibodies on an in vivo thrombosis model in mice. *Thromb Haemost* 1994; **71**: 670–674.

28. Kornberg A, Blank M, Kaufman S, Shoenfeld Y. Induction of tissue factor-like activity in monocytes by anticardiolipin antibodies. *J Immunol* 1994; **153**: 1328–1332.

29. Brey RL. Stroke prevention in patients with antiphospholipid antibodies. *Lupus* 1994; **3**: 299–302.

30. Asherson RA, Mercey D, Phillips G et al. Recurrent stroke and multi-infarct dementia in systemic lupus erythematosus: association with antiphospholipid antibodies. *Ann Rheum Dis* 1987; **46**: 605–611.

31. Mosek A, Yust I, Treves TA, Vardinon N, Korczyn AD, Chapman J. Dementia and antiphospholipid antibodies. *Dement Geriatr Cogn Disord* 2000; **11**: 36–38.

32. Hanly JG, Hong C, Smith S, Fisk JD. A prospective analysis of cognitive function and anticardiolipin antibodies in systemic lupus erythematosus. *Arthritis Rheum* 1999; **42**: 728–734.

33. Sun KH, Liu WT, Tsai CY, Liao TS, Lin WM, Yu CL. Inhibition of astrocyte proliferation and binding to brain tissue of anticardiolipin antibodies purified from lupus serum. *Ann Rheum Dis* 1992; **51**: 707–712.

34. Kent MN, Alvarez FJ, Ng AK, Rote NS. Ultrastructural localization of monoclonal antiphospholipid antibody binding to rat brain. *Exp Neurol* 2000; **163**: 173–179.

35. Chapman J, Cohen Armon M, Shoenfeld Y, Korczyn AD. Antiphospholipid antibodies permeabilize and depolarize brain synaptoneurosomes. *Lupus* 1999; **8**: 127–133.

36. Caronti B, Pittoni V, Palladini G, Valesini G. Anti-beta 2-glycoprotein I antibodies bind to central nervous system. *J Neurol Sci* 1998; **156**: 211–219.

37. Caronti B, Calderaro C, Alessandri C et al. Serum anti-beta2-glycoprotein I antibodies from patients with antiphospholipid antibody syndrome bind central nervous system cells. *J Autoimmun* 1998; **11**: 425–429.

38. Tishler M, Alosachie I, Chapman Y et al. Anti-neuronal antibodies in antiphospholipid syndrome with central nervous system involvement: the difference from systemic lupus erythematosus. *Lupus* 1995; **4**: 145–147.

39. Hickey WF, Hsu BL, Kimura H. T-lymphocyte entry into the central nervous system. *J Neurosci Res* 1991; **28**: 254–260.

40. Simantov R, LaSala JM, Lo SK et al. Activation of cultured vascular endothelial cells by antiphospholipid antibodies. *J Clin Invest* 1995; **96**: 2211–2219.

41. Del Papa N, Guidali L, Spatola L et al. Relationship between anti-phospholipid and anti-endothelial cell antibodies III: beta 2 glycoprotein I mediates the antibody binding to endothelial membranes and induces the expression of adhesion molecules. *Clin Exp Rheumatol* 1995; **13**: 179–185.

42. Blank M, Shoenfeld Y, Cabilly S et al. Prevention of experimental antiphospholipid syndrome and endothelial cell activation by synthetic peptides. *Proc Natl Acad Sci USA* 1999; **96**: 5164–5168.

43. Pierangeli SS, Colden Stanfield M, Liu X, Barker JH, Anderson GL, Harris EN. Antiphospholipid antibodies from antiphospholipid syndrome patients activate endothelial cells in vitro and in vivo. *Circulation* 1999; **99**: 1997–2002.

44. George J, Blank M, Levy Y et al. Differential effects of anti-beta2-glycoprotein I antibodies on endothelial cells and on the manifestations of experimental antiphospholipid syndrome. *Circulation* 1998; **97**: 900–906.

45. Kaplanski G, Cacoub P, Farnarier C et al. Increased soluble vascular cell adhesion molecule 1 concentrations in patients with primary or systemic lupus erythematosus-related antiphospholipid syndrome: correlations with the severity of thrombosis. *Arthritis Rheum* 2000; **43**: 55–64.

46. Lo SK, Cheung A, Zheng Q, Silverstein RL. Induction of tissue factor on monocytes by adhesion to endothelial cells. *J Immunol* 1995; **154**: 4768–4777.

47. Pierangeli SS, Gharavi AE, Harris EN. Experimental thrombosis and antiphospholipid antibodies: new insights. *J Autoimmun* 2000; **15**: 241–247.

48. Ziporen L, Rauova L, Chapman J, Brey R, Korczyn AD, Shoenfeld Y. Anti-ICAM Ab partially improve neurologic dysfunction in mice with experimental APS. *J Autoimmun* 2000; **15**: A27 (abst).

49. Brey RL, Amato AA, Kagan-Hallet K, Rhine CB, Stallworth CL. Anti-intracellular adhesion molecule-1 (ICAM-1) antibody treatment prevents central and peripheral nervous system disease in autoimmune-prone mice. *Lupus* 1997; **6**: 645–651.

50. Del Papa N, Guidali L, Sala A et al. Endothelial cells as target for antiphospholipid antibodies. Human polyclonal and monoclonal anti-beta 2-glycoprotein I antibodies react in vitro with endothelial cells through adherent beta 2-glycoprotein I and induce endothelial activation. *Arthritis Rheum* 1997; **40**: 551–561.

51. Davis WD, Brey R. Antiphospholipid antibodies and complement activation in patients with cerebral ischemia. *Clin Exp Rheumatol* 1992; **10**: 455–460.

52. Visvanathan S, McNeil HP. Cellular immunity to beta 2-glycoprotein-1 in patients with the antiphospholipid syndrome. *J Immunol* 1999; **162**: 6919–6925.

53. Brey RL, Escalante A. Neurological manifestations of antiphospholipid antibody syndrome. *Lupus* 1998; **7**(suppl 2): S67–S74.

54. Krause I, Blank M, Shoenfeld Y. Immunomodulation of experimental APS: lessons from murine models. *Lupus* 1996; **5**: 458–462.

55. Caccavo D, Vaccaro F, Ferri GM, Amoroso A, Bonomo L. Anti-idiotypes against antiphospholipid antibodies are present in normal polyspecific immunoglobulins for therapeutic use. *J Autoimmun* 1994; **7**: 537–548.

56. Krause I, Blank M, Kopolovic J et al. Abrogation of experimental systemic lupus erythematosus and primary antiphospholipid syndrome with intravenous gamma globulin. *J Rheumatol* 1995; **22**: 1068–1074.

57. Brey RL. Differential diagnosis of central nervous system manifestations of the antiphospholipid antibody syndrome. *J Autoimmun* 2000; **15**: 133–138.

58. Verrot D, San-Marco M, Dravet C et al. Prevalence and significance of antinuclear and anticardiolipin antibodies in patients with epilepsy. *Am J Med* 1997; **103**: 33–37.

59. Kovacs B, Lafferty TL, Brent LH, DeHoratius RJ. Transverse myelopathy in systemic lupus erythematosus: an analysis of 14 cases and review of the literature. *Ann Rheum Dis* 2000; **59**: 120–124.

60. Cervera R, Asherson RA, Font J et al. Chorea in the antiphospholipid syndrome. Clinical, radiologic, and immunologic characteristics of 50 patients from our clinics and the recent literature. *Medicine* 1997; **76**: 203–212.

61. Carhuapoma JR, Mitsias P, Levine SR. Cerebral venous thrombosis and anticardiolipin antibodies. *Stroke* 1997; **28**: 2363–2369.

62. Denburg SD, Carbotte RM, Ginsberg JS, Denburg JA. The relationship of antiphospholipid antibodies to cognitive function in patients with systemic lupus erythematosus. *J Int Neuronsychol Soc* 1997; **3**: 377–386.

63. Fukui T, Kawamura M, Hasegawa Y, Kato T, Kaga B. Multiple cognitive impairments associated with systemic lupus erythematosus and antiphospholipid antibody syndrome: a form of progressive vascular dementia? *Eur Neurol* 2000; **43**: 115–116.

64. Schmidt R, Auer Grumbach P, Fazekas F, Offenbacher H, Kapeller P. Anticardiolipin antibodies in normal subjects. Neuropsychological correlates and MRI findings. *Stroke* 1995; **26**: 749–754.

65. Jacobson MW, Rapport LJ, Keenan PA, Coleman RD, Tietjen GE. Neuropsychological deficits associated with antiphospholipid antibodies. *J Clin Exp Neuropsychol* 1999; **21**: 251–264.

66. Cuadrado MJ, Khamashta MA, Hughes GRV. Migraine and stroke in young women. *Q J Med* 2000; **93**: 317–318.

67. Gelfand YA, Dori D, Miller B, Brenner B. Visual disturbances and pathologic ocular findings in primary antiphospholipid syndrome. *Ophthalmology* 1999; **106**: 1537–1540.

68. Schwartz M, Rochas M, Weller B et al. High association of anticardiolipin antibodies with psychosis. *J Clin Psychiatry* 1998; **59**: 20–23.

69. Brey RL, Gharavi AE, Lockshin MID. Neurologic complications of antiphospholipid antibodies. *Rheum Dis Clin North Am* 1993; **19**: 833–850.

70. Gilbird B, Stein M, Tomer Y et al. Autoantibodies to phospholipids and brain extract in patients with the

Guillain–Barré syndrome: cross-reactive or pathogenic? *Autoimmunity* 1993; **16**: 23–27.

71. Ijdo JW, Conti-Kelly AM, Greco P et al. Anti-phospholipid antibodies in patients with multiple sclerosis and MS-like illnesses: MS or APS? *Lupus* 1999; **8**: 109–115.

72. Cuadrado MJ, Khamashta MA, Ballesteros A, Godfrey T, Simon MJ, Hughes GR. Can neurologic manifestations of Hughes (antiphospholipid) syndrome be distinguished from multiple sclerosis? Analysis of 27 patients and review of the literature. *Medicine* 2000; **79**: 57–68.

22

Neuronal protection in cerebral ischemia—from lessons of the past to a brighter future

Ronen R Leker

INTRODUCTION

Cerebral ischemia results from atherothrombosis, emboli, hypoperfusion or a variety of other causes that impair cerebral bloodflow (CBF) and lead to deprivation of both oxygen and glucose. When persistent and critical, such impairment in blood flow may eventually lead to neuronal death.[1-4] Cells at the center of the ischemic focus, the ischemic core, may be especially vulnerable and may die within minutes of ischemic onset.[3] Surrounding the ischemic core is an area of reduced perfusion in which cells are still viable, the ischemic penumbra.[1,2,5-11] Cells in the ischemic penumbra are subjected to various pathological processes that may lead to their demise, and their survival is only possible for a limited amount of time.[10,12-15] Spontaneous reperfusion usually occurs in the set-up of cerebral ischemia.[16] While this process may reverse the ischemic damage when occurring early enough (e.g. transient ischemic attacks), it usually takes place at a much later time point when most penumbral cells have died. Essentially, the goal of neuronal protection therapies is to keep penumbral cells from dying until such time when spontaneous reperfusion occurs and surviving cells regain their functional capabilities.[17]

THE ISCHEMIC PENUMBRA

The ischemic penumbra may be characterized by CBF values or by neurochemical and electrical properties. In general, it is assumed that brain areas perfused at a rate of less than 12 ml/100 g per min are destined to die and represent the ischemic core.[2,5,11,18,19] A rim of viable tissue that is perfused at a suboptimal rate surrounds the ischemic core. The area closest to the core is critically hypoperfused at a rate of 15–18 ml/100 g per min and is at danger of dying, as the evolving infarct may grow into it.[2] The zone immediately surrounding this primary penumbral tier is less likely to die, as its perfusion is somewhat better, although it is usually well below the minimal normal rate of 55 ml/100 g per min. At a perfusion rate of 15–18 ml/100 g per min, the cells are electrically silent, because of malfunction of the membrane Na^+/KA^+ ion pumps. The survival of penumbral cells is generally believed to be around 6 h.[1,2,5,10] This may hold true for only some cases, as it has become clearer that different brain areas have different susceptibilities to ischemia.[1] For example, brainstem neurons are more resilient to ischemic changes and may survive for up to 24 h before reperfusion occurs, while cortical neurons appear to be more vulnerable.[20] Furthermore, even within the same penumbral zones, different cell types have different susceptibilities to ischemia. These differences may be explained by differences in cell connections, neurochemical properties and the amount of growth factors the cells are exposed to.[20]

The ischemic penumbra may be visualized in different experimental paradigms in both animals and humans. Positron emission tomography studies have shown the relative hypoperfusion of the penumbral zone and may be used as a surrogate marker for determining final infarct volume and prognosis.[5,21,22]

More recently, magnetic resonance imaging (MRI)-based techniques such as diffusion- and perfusion-weighted imaging (DWI and PWI respectively) have been advocated for penumbral demonstration in both animals and humans.[8,9,11,23] DWI MRI may be especially sensitive for detecting irreversible tissue damage, while PWI MRI reflects the perfusion deficits.[24-28] Most early scans in ischemia show a mismatch between the two methods, with a larger PWI lesion and a smaller DWI lesion.[24-28] By subtracting the DWI lesion volume from the PWI volume, it is possible to represent the penumbral volume. Demonstrating the actual presence of a penumbra is suggested to be of the utmost importance, since it may be used as a guide to whether thrombolytic therapy should be used in a given patient. Thus, if a penumbra cannot be demonstrated (i.e. PWI lesion volume is smaller than or equal to the DWI volume), then no salvageable tissue is thought to be present and no thrombolytic therapy should be given.[18,24]

PATHOGENESIS OF CELL DAMAGE IN ISCHEMIA

Cells in the ischemic penumbra are subject to various pathological processes that can lead to their death (Table 22.1). These include the following.

Excitotoxicity

Glutamate and aspartate are excreted in large quantities in ischemic areas. Glutamate activates NMDA and AMPA receptors, which trigger the entry of calcium, sodium and water into the cells of the ischemic region.[19,29-32] This results in cytotoxic edema and massive intracellular calcium overflow, since the mechanisms of sodium and calcium excretion are

Table 22.1 Pathological mechanisms leading to cell death in ischemia

Mechanism	Mediators/Pathway
Excitotoxicity	Glutamate (NMDA, AMPA) leading to intracellular calcium overflow
Free radicals	Reactive oxygen species, metal radicals etc.
Inflammation	ICAM, VCAM, cytokines (TNF-α, IL-1β), polymorphonuclears, lymphocytes
Apoptosis	Cytochrome C leading to caspase formation and DNA cleavage

TNF, tumor necrosis factor; IL, interleukin; NMDA, N-methyl-D-aspartate; AMPA, alpha-methyl-propionic acid; ICAM, intracellular adhesion molecule; VCAM, vascular cell adhesion molecule.

energy dependent and energy is lacking in the penumbral region. Intracellular calcium activates various intracellular enzymes such as lipases, proteases and endonucleases. These enzymes may damage DNA, and various cell proteins and lipids, thus leading to cellular death. Binding of glutamate to its AMPA receptors and binding of aspartate to its respective receptors have also been shown to contribute to excitotoxic damage.[33] Inhibition of excitatory amino acid release from presynaptic terminals or blocking of their binding to their corresponding receptors have been shown to be cerebroprotective in various experimental paradigms.[34-39]

Nitric oxide and reactive oxygen species

Nitric oxide (NO) is a gaseous, ubiquitous neurotransmitter with multiple functions in the central nervous system (CNS). It is produced from arginine by three distinct forms of NO synthase (NOS).[40] Neuronal NOS (nNOS) is a calcium-dependent, constitutive neuronal enzyme, encoded by a gene located on chromosome 12.[41] It is especially prevalent in brain areas irrigated by the middle cerebral artery that are susceptible to becoming the ischemic core under ischemic conditions.[42] During ischemia, nNOS is upregulated and the NO produced reacts with reactive oxygen species (ROS) to produce radicals that have deleterious effects on neuronal survival.[42-45] Inducible NOS (iNOS) is a calcium-dependent enzyme encoded by a gene located on chromosome 17.[40] It is upregulated under various stressful conditions and can be produced by macrophages and a variety of other cells. The NO produced by iNOS is also believed to have deleterious effects on neuronal survival in ischemia, since it causes mitochondrial and cellular dysfunction.[43,44,46] Endothelial NOS (eNOS) is a calcium-dependent, constitutive enzyme of endothelial cells encoded by a gene located on chromosome 7.[41] In contrast to the other NOS isoenzymes, its actions under ischemic conditions are thought to be cerebroprotective because of a possible vasodilating effect that improves cerebral perfusion.[41,47] Thus, blocking eNOS and nNOS activity with non-specific inhibitors such as L-nitro-arginine (L-NAME) leads to larger infarcts, while blocking nNOS activity with specific inhibitors such as 7-nitroindazole (7-NI) causes smaller infarcts.[45,48,49] Furthermore, eNOS-knockout mice experience larger infarcts than wild-type mice,[45,48-52] and nNOS-knockout mice experience smaller infarcts than wild-type mice.[50] The cerebroprotective effect of eNOS may be mediated by several mechanisms. As NO is a small, diffusible molecule, it could exert a paracrine, vasodilatatory effect on surrounding blood vessels.[43,47,53,54] It may diffuse to adjacent penumbral regions, where it can inhibit platelet aggregation[55,56] in penumbral capillaries and leukocyte infiltration into the parenchyma.[57,58] In addition, penumbral vascular endothelial growth factor (VEGF) production may induce eNOS expression,[59–61] leading to the formation of new blood vessels in the penumbra.[61] A neuroprotective effect of NO produced by eNOS may also be related to its role in modifying presynaptic signals that result in increased GABA release.[62] Such alterations in presynaptic signals by eNOS-derived NO may be important in the context of neuronal plasticity and recovery.[63–65] NO produced by eNOS may reduce apoptotic neuronal death. It has been shown[66] that eNOS can protect motor neurons from apoptotic death by a cGMP-related mechanism.

Inflammation

The presence of inflammatory cells in the ischemic region may increase cellular damage. Polymorphonuclear cells may cause tissue damage by the effects of their toxic enzymes such as myeloperoxidase, which can further damage cell membranes.[67,68] Inflammatory cytokines such as TNF-α, IL-1 and IL-6 appear to be activated and secreted as early as 1 h after the ischemic insult.[69–72] These cytokines may induce an inflammatory reaction and also act as chemoattractants to leukocytes. Adhesion molecules such as ICAM and endothelial leukocyte adhesion molecule (ELAM) and tissue metalloproteinases are also expressed early after the insult and facilitate penetration of leukocytes through the blood–brain barrier.[12,73]

Endothelins may also be of importance in causing tissue damage, because of their vasoconstricting effects, which may exacerbate ischemia.[47,74–76] Indeed, an upregulation in endothelin levels was also observed after ischemic onset and persisted for a considerable amount of time thereafter.[74,77]

Other immunomodulatory cytokines such as IL-10, which downregulates the immune system, may, on the other hand, have a cytoprotective role.[78]

Apoptosis

It is currently believed that apoptosis may be responsible for up to 50% of cellular death in ischemia.[79] The mechanisms leading to apoptotic death in ischemia are intricate and involve several possible

pathways, including an NFκB-dependent pathway,[80,81] and activation of inducible proapoptotic members of the *bcl* family (e.g. *bad, bax*).[82,83] Induction of these factors leads to the formation of the caspases, which are present in cells as proenzymes and are cleaved to their active form by other caspases.[84–87] The pathway of caspase activation entails release of cytochrome c from mitochondria and activation of procaspase 9. Following this step, a cascade of caspase activation is generated that culminates in the formation of caspase 3 (effector caspase).[87–91] Caspase 3 in turn activates DNA-breaking enzymes (e.g. endonucleases) and energy-consuming DNA repair enzymes such as PARP (poly-ADP-ribose polymerase), leading eventually to breakdown of DNA and cell death.[87–91]

ENDOGENOUS PROTECTIVE MECHANISMS

Not all mediators induced in the ischemic penumbra necessarily contribute to cellular death. Thus, protective compounds such as the heat shock proteins,[10,92] anti-inflammatory cytokines[70,78] and growth factors[93–99] are all induced in the early hours following ischemia (Table 22.2). These mediators possess anti-ischemic properties and represent endogenous efforts to counteract ischemic damage and improve neuronal repair. Unfortunately, the secretion of such survival-promoting agents is limited both in time and space and usually cannot completely counteract the overwhelming death-promoting processes mentioned above.

Table 22.2   Self-protective mechanisms in ischemia

Heat shock proteins
Growth factors
Anti-inflammatory cytokines (e.g. IL-10)
Antioxidants (glutathione)

NEUROPROTECTION IN ISCHEMIA

Previous research in neuronal protection has mainly focused on individual damage-producing mechanisms. Numerous studies have tried to counteract excitotoxicity by blocking NMDA[17,37,39,100–106] or AMPA receptors,[34,35,38,39] preventing excitatory amino acid release from presynaptic terminals or altering postsynaptic effects of these mediators. These studies have usually shown promising results in animal models with improved functional capabilities and reduced infarct volumes. The prototype agent representing this category is the NMDA antagonist MK-801.[36,37,102,103] However, none of these agents have proven clinical efficacy in humans. Some studies were terminated early because of toxic side-effects, and others demonstrated no advantage over placebo.[36,100,107]

Studies employing antioxidants for cerebral protection have also yielded promising results in laboratory animals but have failed to produce clinically significant improvements in humans.[108–110] Likewise, studies employing anti-inflammatory agents showed very promising results in laboratory animals but very disappointing results in clinical practice, including a study that reported excess mortality in patients treated with a monoclonal anti-ICAM antibody.[12,67,70,72,111–113] Furthermore, it has been repeatedly shown that apoptotic death can be prevented by manipulations of the steps that lead to activation of the caspase cascade or by direct inhibition of caspases.[86,114–116] However, no clinical data regarding the efficacy of such agents in humans are currently available. Endothelin antagonists have also been shown to reduce ischemic damage in animal models, probably by improving perfusion to the ischemic zone.[117,118] However, no clinical human data on the use of these agents are currently available.

There are many possible reasons for the discrepancies between preclinical studies, which usually show very promising results with neuroprotective drugs, and the clinical practice, which is very disappointing. These include inadequate animal models for stroke,[119] inadequate drug delivery, use of a too short and non-realistic time window in the animal studies that cannot be duplicated in humans and inadequate study designs.[20,107,119–121] However, the most important reason for the failure of early trials may be related to the fact that all these studies concentrated on blocking just one of the individual death-related processes in ischemia, leaving the door open for the other processes to produce cellular death. Thus, it was elegantly shown by Choi et al that, after blocking of all excitotoxic activity, cells will die of apoptosis instead of excitotoxicity.[31,79] Likewise, it is probable that blocking apoptotic death may change the dying process from apoptotic death to other forms of cellular death.[29,81,91]

One possible solution for these problems would be using drug combinations with compounds active against individual mechanisms. Indeed, several investigators have shown that such drug combination strategies are possible.[39,104,122,123] Thus, Grotta et al have shown that the combination of diacetylsalicylate

and an NMDA antagonist is more efficacious than either agent alone.[124] Furthermore, caspase inhibition was proved to be synergistic with anti-excitotoxic and anti-inflammatory measures of reducing infarct volume.[86–104]

Another therapeutic option would be to identify single agents active against more than just one mechanism of tissue damage. In a previous report we found that administration of the synthetic cannabinoid dexanabinol (HU-211, (+)-(3S,4S)-7-hydroxy-Δ^6-tetrahydrocannabinol-1,1-dimethylheptyl) confers significant neuroprotection.[125] It is a novel drug that has been shown to be a non-competitive antagonist of the NMDA glutamate receptor in both traumatic and ischemic conditions. Unlike other NMDA antagonists, dexanabinol seems to be a safe drug, and devoid of psychotropic side-ffects. The drug may also have some properties as a free radical scavenger, thus exerting an antioxidant effect, although, as shown previously, it probably does not involve nNOS-related free radical generation. Dexanabinol has been recently shown to abrogate the effects of TNF-α. Indeed, we were able to demonstrate that it reduces infarct volume significantly when given to rats 1 h after the induction of cerebral ischemia, i.e. in a way similar to treatment of human patients.[125] Dexanabinol may be taken as an example of a new class of multipotent drugs effective against more than one ischemia-related damaging process.

Another promising neuroprotective perspective is the use of hypothermia. Several studies have previously documented the neuroprotective effects of mild hypothermia, which may completely abrogate the ischemic changes.[126–129] Similarly to multipotent agents, hypothermia appears to convey protection by acting via several mechanisms.[129] Furthermore, a combination of hypothermia with putative cerebroprotective drugs shows synergistic effects as compared to either drug therapy or hypothermia alone.[130] Postulated mechanisms of action of hypothermia include lowering excitatory amino acid secretion and downregulation of glutamate receptors,[131,132] diminished production of ROS and reduced consumption of tissue antioxidants,[133,134] and reduced inflammatory response.[135,136] Other postulated mechanisms include a non-specific lowering of cerebral metabolic rate,[137] and changes in cerebral bloodflow.[138]

Another promising neuroprotective strategy would be to enhance the self-defense mechanisms. Indeed, previous studies have reported promising results with animals overexpressing heat shock proteins[10,92,139] and with viral vectors for induction of heat shock protein.[140]

Exogenous administration of growth factors may be used to enhance recovery, but this is usually limited clinically because these compounds do not normally cross the blood–brain barrier.[93–95,97,98,141–152] One possible way of overcoming this obstacle, besides administration into the ventricles,[141,146,153] is to administer molecular mimickers of these growth factors.[30] Amother potential option would be to induce over-expression of endogenous growth factors.[154,155]

The combination of reperfusion by either thrombolytic (e.g. tissue plasminogen activation (TPA)) or fibrinolytic (e.g. Ancrod) agents with neuroprotectants may offer significant advantages to the singular use of each strategy.[124] Thus, reperfusion may be associated with excessive production of ROS in the previously ischemic areas, and this may contribute to further tissue damage.[42,156] The adjuvant neuroprotective agents may be able to reduce such damage, and therefore increase the therapeutic gain of reperfusion.[112] Furthermore, reperfusion may enhance the therapeutic effect of neuroprotective agents because of better delivery into the ischemic region. Indeed, Zhang et al have shown that combining an antiadhesion molecule antibody with TPA is more effective than either agent alone.[157]

Finally, as noted above, growth factors may have significant uses in cerebral ischemia, and their combination with more conventional neuroprotective agents may represent another therapeutic breakthrough, as they may enhance neuronal repair after stroke. The addition of a reperfusing agent to this package may also be advantageous for the reason noted above.[123]

FUTURE DIRECTIONS

It appears that the vast amount of knowledge accrued concerning neuronal protection from ischemic injury will soon start to pay off. Future studies would probably concentrate more on combinations of drugs active against individual damaging mechanisms. Moreover, current knowledge of the time course of penumbral zone survival calls for more prolonged and repetitive dosing of neuroprotectants in order to achieve a durable effect. Furthermore, combining neuroprotective, thrombolytic and neurotrophic agents into a therapeutic cocktail appears to be more feasible now than ever. Such cocktails may have synergistic effects on cell survival and neuronal reorganization and plasticity, and would increase the hope of bringing a brighter future for stroke victims.

REFERENCES

1. Aronowski J, Cho KH, Strong R, Grotta JC. Neurofilament proteolysis after focal ischemia; when do cells die after experimental stroke? *J Cereb Blood Flow Metab* 1999; **19**: 652–660.
2. Back T. Pathophysiology of the ischemic penumbra—revision of a concept. *Cell Mol Neurobiol* 1998; **18**: 621–638.
3. Kaufmann AM, Firlik AD, Fukui MB, Wechsler LR, Jungries CA, Yonas H. Ischemic core and penumbra in human stroke. *Stroke* 1999; **30**: 93–99.
4. Kempski O, Seiwert T, Otsuka H, Heimann A, Nakase H. Modelling of the ischemic penumbra. *Acta Neurochir Suppl Wien* 1999; **73**: 41–44.
5. Baron J. Mapping the ischaemic penumbra with PET: implications for acute stroke treatment. *Cerebrovasc Dis* 1999; **9**: 193–201.
6. Christensen T, Balchen T, Bruhn T, Diemer NH. Double-tracer autoradiographic study of protein synthesis and glucose consumption in rats with focal cerebral ischemia. *Neurol Res* 1999; **21**: 687–694.
7. Dijkhuizen RM, de Graaf RA, Garwood M, Tulleken KA, Nicolay K. Spatial assessment of the dynamics of lactate formation in focal ischemic rat brain. *J Cereb Blood Flow Metab* 1999; **19**: 376–379.
8. Grohn OH, Lukkarinen JA, Oja JM et al. Noninvasive detection of cerebral hypoperfusion and reversible ischemia from reductions in the magnetic resonance imaging relaxation time, T2. *J Cereb Blood Flow Metab* 1998; **18**: 911–920.
9. Karonen JO, Vanninen RL, Liu Y et al. Combined diffusion and perfusion MRI with correlation to single-photon emission CT in acute ischemic stroke. Ischemic penumbra predicts infarct growth. *Stroke* 1999; **30**: 1583–1590.
10. Kogure T, Kogure K. Molecular and biochemical events within the brain subjected to cerebral ischemia (targets for therapeutical intervention). *Clin Neurosci* 1997; **4**: 179–183.
11. Schlaug G, Benfield A, Baird AE et al. The ischemic penumbra: operationally defined by diffusion and perfusion MRI. *Neurology* 1999; **53**: 1528–1537.
12. del Zoppo G, Ginis I, Hallenbeck JM, Iadecola C, Wang X, Feuerstein GZ. Inflammation and stroke: putative role for cytokines, adhesion molecules and iNOS in brain response to ischemia. *Brain Pathol* 2000; **10**: 95–112.
13. Feuerstein GZ, Wang X, Barone FC. The role of cytokines in the neuropathology of stroke and neurotrauma. *Neuroimmunomodulation* 1998; **5**: 143–159.
14. Iadecola C, Ross ME. Molecular pathology of cerebral ischemia: delayed gene expression and strategies for neuroprotection. *Ann NY Acad Sci* 1997; **835**: 203–217.
15. Kato H, Kogure K. Biochemical and molecular characteristics of the brain with developing cerebral infarction. *Cell Mol Neurobiol* 1999; **19**: 93–108.
16. Kidwell CS, Saver JL, Mattiello J et al. Thrombolytic reversal of acute human cerebral ischemic injury shown by diffusion/perfusion magnetic resonance imaging. *Ann Neurol* 2000; **47**: 462–469.
17. Hickenbottom SL, Grotta J. Neuroprotective therapy. *Semin Neurol* 1998; **18**: 485–492.
18. Heiss WD, Graf R, Grond M, Rudolf J. Quantitative neuroimaging for the evaluation of the effect of stroke treatment. *Cerebrovasc Dis* 1998; **8**(Suppl 2): 23–29.

19. Dirnagl U, Iadecola C, Moskowitz MA. Pathobiology of ischaemic stroke: an integrated view. *Trends Neurosci* 1999; **22**: 391–397.

20. Zivin JA. Factors determining the therapeutic window for stroke. *Neurology* 1998; **50**: 599–603.

21. Heiss WD, Kracht L, Grond M et al. Early [(11)C]Flumazenil/H(2)O positron emission tomography predicts irreversible ischemic cortical damage in stroke patients receiving acute thrombolytic therapy. *Stroke* 2000; **31**: 366–369.

22. Stevens H, Jansen HM, De Reuck J et al. 55Co-PET in stroke: relation to bloodflow, oxygen metabolism and gadolinium-MRI. *Acta Neurol Belg* 1997; **97**: 172–177.

23. Hatazawa J, Shimosegawa E, Toyoshima H et al. Cerebral blood volume in acute brain infarction: a combined study with dynamic susceptibility contrast MRI and 99mTC-HMPAO-SPECT. *Stroke* 1999; **30**: 800–806.

24. Baird AE, Warach S. Magnetic resonance imaging of acute stroke. *J Cereb Blood Flow Metab* 1998; **18**: 583–609.

25. Minematsu K, Li L, Fisher M, Sotak CH, Davis MA, Fiandaca MS. Diffusion-weighted magnetic resonance imaging: rapid and quantitative detection of focal brain ischemia. *Neurology* 1992; **42**: 235–240.

26. Mintorovitch J, Yang GY, Shimizu H, Kucharczyk J, Chan PH, Weinstein PR. Diffusion-weighted magnetic resonance imaging of acute focal cerebral ischemia: comparison of signal intensity with changes in brain water and Na+,K(+)-ATPase activity. *J Cereb Blood Flow Metab* 1994; **14**: 332–336.

27. Moseley ME, Cohen Y, Kucharczyk J et al. Diffusion-weighted MR imaging of anisotropic water diffusion in cat central nervous system. *Radiology* 1990; **176**: 439–445.

28. Warach S, Chien D, Li W, Ronthal M, Edelman RR. Fast magnetic resonance diffusion-weighted imaging of acute human stroke [published erratum appears in *Neurology* 1992; **42**(11): 2192]. *Neurology* 1992; **42**: 1717–1723.

29. Martin LJ, Al Abdulla NA, Brambrink AM, Kirsch JR, Sieber FE, Portera Cailliau C. Neurodegeneration in excitotoxicity, global cerebral ischemia, and target deprivation: a perspective on the contributions of apoptosis and necrosis. *Brain Res Bull* 1998; **46**: 281–309.

30. Mattson MP. Neuroprotective signal transduction: relevance to stroke. *Neurosci Biobehav Rev* 1997; **21**: 193–206.

31. Lee JM, Zipfel GJ, Choi DW. The changing landscape of ischaemic brain injury mechanisms. *Nature* 1999; **399**: A7–A14.

32. Choi D. Antagonizing excitotoxicity: a therapeutic strategy for stroke? *Mt Sinai J Med* 1998; **65**: 133–138.

33. Narayanan U, Chi OZ, Liu X, Weiss HR. Effect of AMPA on cerebral cortical oxygen balance of ischemic rat brain. *Neurochem Res* 2000; **25**: 405–411.

34. Shimizu Sasamata M, Kano T, Rogowska J, Wolf GL, Moskowitz MA, Lo EH. YM872, a highly water-soluble AMPA receptor antagonist, preserves the hemodynamic penumbra and reduces brain injury after permanent focal ischemia in rats. *Stroke* 1998; **29**: 2141–2148.

35. Schielke GP, Kupina NC, Boxer PA, Bigge CF, Welty DF, Iadecola C. The neuroprotective effect of the novel AMPA receptor antagonist PD152247 (PNQX) in temporary focal ischemia in the rat. *Stroke* 1999; **30**: 1472–1477.

36. Michenfelder JD, Lanier WL, Scheithauer BW, Perkins WJ, Shearman GT, Milde JH. Evaluation of the glutamate antagonist dizocilipine maleate (MK-801) on neurologic outcome in a canine model of complete cerebral ischemia: correlation with hippocampal histopathology. *Brain Res* 1989; **481**: 228–234.

37. Foster AC, Gill R, Woodruff GN. Neuroprotective effects of MK-801 in vivo: selectivity and evidence for delayed degeneration mediated by NMDA receptor activation. *J Neurosci* 1988; **8**: 4745–4754.

38. Bowes MP, Swanson S, Zivin JA. The AMPA antagonist LY293558 improves functional neurological outcome following reversible spinal cord ischemia in rabbits. *J Cereb Blood Flow Metab* 1996; **16**: 967–972.

39. Arias RL, Tasse JR, Bowlby MR. Neuroprotective interaction effects of NMDA and AMPA receptor antagonists in an in vitro model of cerebral ischemia. *Brain Res* 1999; **816**: 299–308.

40. Forstermann U, Closs EI, Pollock JS et al. Nitric oxide synthase isozymes. Characterization, purification, molecular cloning, and functions. *Hypertension* 1994; **23**: 1121–1131.

41. Forstermann U, Boissel JP, Kleinert H. Expressional control of the 'constitutive' isoforms of nitric oxide synthase (NOS I and NOS III). *FASEB J* 1998; **12**: 773–790.

42. Ashwal S, Tone B, Tian HR, Cole DJ, Pearce WJ. Core and penumbral nitric oxide synthase activity during cerebral ischemia and reperfusion. *Stroke* 1998; **29**: 1037–1046.

43. Iadecola C. Bright and dark sides of nitric oxide in ischemic brain injury. *Trends Neurosci* 1997; **20**: 132–139.

44. Samdani AF, Dawson TM, Dawson VL. Nitric oxide synthase in models of focal ischemia. *Stroke* 1997; **28**: 1283–1288.

45. Stagliano NE, Dietrich WD, Prado R, Green EJ, Busto R. The role of nitric oxide in the pathophysiology of thromboembolic stroke in the rat. *Brain Res* 1997; **759**: 32–40.

46. Dalkara T, Moskowitz MA. The complex role of nitric oxide in the pathophysiology of focal cerebral ischemia. *Brain Pathol* 1994; **4**: 49–57.

47. Faraci FM, Heistad DD. Regulation of the cerebral circulation: role of endothelium and potassium channels. *Physiol Rev* 1998; **78**: 53–97.

48. Yamamoto S, Golanov EV, Berger SB, Reis DJ. Inhibition of nitric oxide synthesis increases focal ischemic infarction in rat. *J Cereb Blood Flow Metab* 1992; **12**: 717–726.

49. Zhang ZG, Reif D, Macdonald J et al. ARL 17477, a potent and selective neuronal NOS inhibitor decreases infarct volume after transient middle cerebral artery occlusion in rats. *J Cereb Blood Flow Metab* 1996; **16**: 599–604.

50. Huang Z, Huang PL, Panahian N, Dalkara T, Fishman MC, Moskowitz MA. Effects of cerebral ischemia in mice deficient in neuronal nitric oxide synthase. *Science* 1994; **265**: 1883–1885.

51. Huang Z, Huang PL, Ma J et al. Enlarged infarcts in endothelial nitric oxide synthase knockout mice are attenuated by nitro-L-arginine. *J Cereb Blood Flow Metab* 1996; **16**: 981–987.

52. Lo EH, Hara H, Rogowska J et al. Temporal correlation mapping analysis of the hemodynamic penum-

bra in mutant mice deficient in endothelial nitric oxide synthase gene expression. *Stroke* 1996; **27**: 1381–1385.

53. Dawson TM, Dawson VL, Snyder SH. A novel neuronal messenger molecule in brain: the free radical, nitric oxide. *Ann Neurol* 1992; **32**: 297–311.

54. Moncada S, Palmer RM, Higgs EA. Nitric oxide: physiology, pathophysiology, and pharmacology. *Pharmacol Rev* 1991; **43**: 109–142.

55. Radomski MW, Palmer RM, Moncada S. The anti-aggregating properties of vascular endothelium: interactions between prostacyclin and nitric oxide. *Br J Pharmacol* 1987; **92**: 639–646.

56. Radomski MW, Palmer RM, Moncada S. An L-arginine/nitric oxide pathway present in human platelets regulates aggregation. *Proc Natl Acad Sci USA* 1990; **87**: 5193–5197.

57. Iadecola C, Pelligrmno DA, Moskowitz MA, Lassen NA. Nitric oxide synthase inhibition and cerebrovascular regulation. *J Cereb Blood Flow Metab* 1994; **14**: 175–192.

58. Kubes P, Suzuki M, Granger DN. Nitric oxide: an endogenous modulator of leukocyte adhesion. *Proc Natl Acad Sci USA* 1991; **88**: 4651–4655.

59. Papapetropoulos A, Garcia Cardena G, Madri JA, Sessa WC. Nitric oxide production contributes to the angiogenic properties of vascular endothelial growth factor in human endothelial cells. *J Clin Invest* 1997; **100**: 3131–3139.

60. Ziche M, Morbidelli L, Choudhuri R et al. Nitric oxide synthase lies downstream from vascular endothelial growth factor-induced but not basic fibroblast growth factor-induced angiogenesis. *J Clin Invest* 1997; **99**: 2625–2634.

61. Shweiki D, Itin A, Soffer D, Keshet E. Vascular endothelial growth factor induced by hypoxia may mediate hypoxia-initiated angiogenesis. *Nature* 1992; **359**: 843–845.

62. Kano T, Shimizu Sasamata M, Huang PL, Moskowitz MA, Lo EH. Effects of nitric oxide synthase gene knockout on neurotransmitter release in vivo. *Neuroscience* 1998; **86**: 695–699.

63. Dinerman JL, Dawson TM, Schell MJ, Snowman A, Snyder SH. Endothelial nitric oxide synthase localized to hippocampal pyramidal cells: implications for synaptic plasticity. *Proc Natl Acad Sci USA* 1994; **91**: 4214–4218.

64. Kantor DB, Lanzrein M, Stary SJ et al. A role for endothelial NO synthase in LTP revealed by adenovirus-mediated inhibition and rescue. *Science* 1996; **274**: 1744–1748.

65. O'Dell TJ, Huang PL, Dawson TM et al. Endothelial NOS and the blockade of LTP by NOS inhibitors in mice lacking neuronal NOS. *Science* 1994; **265**: 542–546.

66. Estevez AG, Spear N, Thompson JA. Nitric oxide-dependent production of cGMP supports the survival of rat embryonic motor neurons cultured with brain-derived neurotrophic factor. *J Neurosci* 1998; **18**: 3708–3714.

67. DeGraba TJ. The role of inflammation after acute stroke: utility of pursuing anti-adhesion molecule therapy. *Neurology* 1998; **51**: S62–S68.

68. del Zoppo GJ. Microvascular responses to cerebral ischemia/inflammation. *Ann NY Acad Sci* 1997; **823**: 132–147.

69. Arvin B, Neville LF, Barone FC, Feuerstein GZ. The role of inflammation and cytokines in brain injury. *Neurosci Biobehav Rev* 1996; **20**: 445–452.

70. Barone FC, Feuerstein GZ. Inflammatory mediators and stroke: new opportunities for novel therapeutics. *J Cereb Blood Flow Metab* 1999; **19**: 819–834.

71. Feuerstein GZ, Liu T, Barone FC. Cytokines, inflammation, and brain injury: role of tumor necrosis factor-alpha. *Cerebrovasc Brain Metab Rev* 1994; **6**: 341–360.

72. Feuerstein GZ, Wang X, Barone FC. Inflammatory gene expression in cerebral ischemia and trauma. Potential new therapeutic targets. *Ann NY Acad Sci* 1997; **825**: 179–193.

73. Pantoni L, Sarti C, Inzitari D. Cytokines and cell adhesion molecules in cerebral ischemia: experimental bases and therapeutic perspectives. *Arterioscler Thromb Vasc Biol* 1998; **18**: 503–513.

74. Bian LG, Zhang TX, Zhao WG, Shen JK, Yang GY. Increased endothelin-1 in the rabbit model of middle cerebral artery occlusion. *Neurosci Lett* 1994; **174**: 47–50.

75. Nikolov R, Rami A, Krieglstein J. Endothelin-1 exacerbates focal cerebral ischemia without exerting neurotoxic action in vitro. *Eur J Pharmacol* 1993; **248**: 205–208.

76. Willette RN, Ohlstein EH, Pullen M, Sauermelch CF, Cohen A, Nambi P. Transient forebrain ischemia alters acutely endothelin receptor density and immunoreactivity in gerbil brain. *Life Sci* 1993; **52**: 35–40.

77. Anwaar I, Gottsater A, Lindgarde F, Mattiasson I. Increasing plasma neopterin and persistent plasma endothelin during follow-up after acute cerebral ischemia. *Angiology* 1999; **50**: 1–8.

78. Spera PA, Ellison JA, Feuerstein GZ, Barone FC. IL-10 reduces rat brain injury following focal stroke. *Neurosci Lett* 1998; **251**: 189–192.

79. Choi DW. Ischemia-induced neuronal apoptosis. *Curr Opin Neurobiol* 1996; **6**: 667–672.

80. Clemens JA, Stephenson DT, Smalstig EB, Dixon EP, Little SP. Global ischemia activates nuclear factor-kappa B in forebrain neurons of rats. *Stroke* 1997; **28**: 1073–1080; discussion 1080–1081.

81. Bonfoco E, Krainc D, Ankarcrona M, Nicotera P, Lipton SA. Apoptosis and necrosis: two distinct events induced, respectively, by mild and intense insults with N-methyl-D-aspartate or nitric oxide/superoxide in cortical cell cultures. *Proc Natl Acad Sci USA* 1995; **92**: 7162–7166.

82. Shinoura N, Satou R, Yoshida Y, Asai A, Kirino T, Hamada H. Adenovirus-mediated transfer of Bcl-X(L) protects neuronal cells from Bax-induced apoptosis. *Exp Cell Res* 2000; **254**; 221–231.

83. Matsushita K, Matsuyama T, Kitagawa K, Matsumoto M, Yanagihara T, Sugita M. Alterations of Bcl-2 family proteins precede cytoskeletal proteolysis in the penumbra, but not in infarct centres following focal cerebral ischemia in mice. *Neuroscience* 1998; **83**: 439–448.

84. Chen J, Nagayama T, Jin K et al. Induction of caspase-3-like protease may mediate delayed neuronal death in the hippocampus after transient cerebral ischemia. *J Neurosci* 1998; **18**: 4914–4928.

85. Guegan C, Sola B. Early and sequential recruitment of apoptotic effectors after focal permanent ischemia in mice. *Brain Res* 2000; **856**: 93–100.

86. Schulz JB, Weller M, Moskowitz MA. Caspases as treatment targets in stroke and neurodegenerative diseases. *Ann Neurol* 1999; **45**: 421–429.

87. Velier JJ, Ellison JA, Kikly KK, Spera PA, Barone FC, Feuerstein GZ. Caspase-8 and caspase-3 are expressed by different populations of cortical neurons undergoing delayed cell death after focal stroke in the rat. *J Neurosci* 1999; **19**: 5932–5941.

88. Krajewski S, Krajewska M, Ellerby LM et al. Release of caspase-9 from mitochondria during neuronal apoptosis and cerebral ischemia. *Proc Natl Acad Sci USA* 1999; **96**: 5752–5757.

89. Ouyang YB, Tan Y, Comb M et al. Survival- and death-promoting events after transient cerebral ischemia: phosphorylation of Akt, release of cytochrome C and activation of caspase-like proteases. *J Cereb Blood Flow Metab* 1999; **19**: 1126–1135.

90. Namura S, Zhu J, Fink K et al. Activation and cleavage of caspase-3 in apoptosis induced by experimental cerebral ischemia. *J Neurosci* 1998; **18**: 3659–3668.

91. Snider BJ, Gottron FJ, Choi DW. Apoptosis and necrosis in cerebrovascular disease. *Ann NY Acad Sci* 1999; **893**: 243–253.

92. Abe K, Kawagoe J, Aoki M, Kogure K, Itoyama Y. Stress protein inductions after brain ischemia. *Cell Mol Neurobiol* 1998; **18**: 709–719.

93. Finklestein SP. The potential use of neurotrophic growth factors in the treatment of cerebral ischemia. *Adv Neurol* 1996; **71**: 413–417; discussion 417–418.

94. Kawamata T, Speliotes EK, Finklestein SP. The role of polypeptide growth factors in recovery from stroke. *Adv Neurol* 1997; **73**: 377–382.

95. Krupinski J, Issa R, Bujny T et al. A putative role for platelet-derived growth factor in angiogenesis and neuroprotection after ischemic stroke in humans. *Stroke* 1997; **28**: 564–573.

96. Maiese K. From the bench to the bedside: the molecular management of cerebral ischemia. *Clin Neuropharmacol* 1998; **21**: 1–7.

97. Maiese K, Boniece I, DeMeo D, Wagner JA. Peptide growth factors protect against ischemia in culture by preventing nitric oxide toxicity. *J Neurosci* 1993; **13**: 3034–3040.

98. Mattson MP, Cheng B. Growth factors protect neurons against excitotoxic/ischemic damage by stabilizing calcium homeostasis. *Stroke* 1993; **24**: I136–I140.

99. Tagami M, Yamagata K, Nara Y et al. Insulin-like growth factors prevent apoptosis in cortical neurons isolated from stroke-prone spontaneously hypertensive rats. *Lab Invest* 1997; **76**: 603–612.

100. Grotta J, Clark W, Coull B et al. Safety and tolerability of the glutamate antagonist CGS 19755 (Selfotel) in patients with acute ischemic stroke. Results of a phase IIa randomized trial. *Stroke* 1995; **26**: 602–605.

101. Jiang N, Zhang RL, Baron BM, Chopp M. Administration of a competitive NMDA antagonist MDL-100,453 reduces infarct size after permanent middle cerebral artery occlusion in rat. *J Neurol Sci* 1996; **138**: 36–41.

102. Ozyurt E, Graham DI, Woodruff GN, McCulloch J. Protective effect of the glutamate antagonist, MK-801 in focal cerebral ischemia in the cat. *J Cereb Blood Flow Metab* 1988; **8**: 138–143.

103. Park CK, Nehls DG, Graham DI, Teasdale GM, McCulloch J. The glutamate antagonist MK-801 reduces focal ischemic brain damage in the rat. *Ann Neurol* 1988; **24**: 543–551.

104. Schulz JB, Weller M, Matthews RT et al. Extended therapeutic window for caspase inhibition and synergy with MK-801 in the treatment of cerebral histotoxic hypoxia. *Cell Death Differ* 1998; **5**: 847–857.

105. Tremblay R, Hewitt K, Lesiuk H, Mealing G, Morley P, Durkin JP. Evidence that brain-derived neurotrophic factor neuroprotection is linked to its ability to reverse the NMDA-induced inactivation of protein kinase C in cortical neurons. *J Neurochem* 1999; **72**: 102–111.

106. Yu SP, Yeh C, Strasser U, Tian M, Choi DW. NMDA receptor-mediated K+ efflux and neuronal apoptosis. *Science* 1999; **284**: 336–339.

107. Zivin JA. Neuroprotective therapies in stroke. *Drugs* 1997; **54**(suppl 3); 83–88; discussion 88–89.

108. del Pilar Fernandez Rodriguez M, Belmonte A, Meizoso MJ, Garcia Novio M, Garcia Iglesias E. Effect of tirilazad on brain nitric oxide synthase activity during cerebral ischemia in rats. *Pharmacology* 1997; **54**: 108–112.

109. Taylor BM, Fleming WE, Benjamin CW, Wu Y, Mathews WR, Sun FF. The mechanism of cytoprotective action of lazaroids I: inhibition of reactive oxygen species formation and lethal cell injury during periods of energy depletion. *J Pharmacol Exp Ther* 1996; **276**: 1224–1231.

110. The RANTTAS Investigators. A randomized trial of tirilazad mesylate in patients with acute stroke. *Stroke* 1996; **27**: 1453–1458.

111. Kitagawa K, Matsumoto M, Mabuchi T et al. Deficiency of intercellular adhesion molecule 1 attenuates microcirculatory disturbance and infarction size in focal cerebral ischemia. *J Cereb Blood Flow Metab* 1998; **18**: 1336–1345.

112. Bowes MP, Rothlein R, Fagan SC, Zivin JA. Monoclonal antibodies preventing leukocyte activation reduce experimental neurologic injury and enhance efficacy of thrombolytic therapy. *Neurology* 1995; **45**: 815–819.

113. Chopp M, Li Y, Jiang N, Zhang RL, Prostak J. Antibodies against adhesion molecules reduce apoptosis after transient middle cerebral artery occlusion in rat brain. *J Cereb Blood Flow Metab* 1996; **16**: 578–584.

114. Cheng Y, Deshmukh M, D'Costa A et al. Caspase inhibitor affords neuroprotection with delayed administration in a rat model of neonatal hypoxic–ischemic brain injury. *J Clin Invest* 1998; **101**: 1992–1999.

115. Gillardon F, Kiprianova I, Sandkuhler J, Hossmann KA, Spranger M. Inhibition of caspases prevents cell death of hippocampal CA1 neurons, but not impairment of hippocampal long-term potentiation following global ischemia. *Neuroscience* 1999; **93**: 1219–1222.

116. Wiessner C, Sauer D, Alaimo D, Allegrini PR. Protective effect of a caspase inhibitor in models for cerebral ischemia in vitro and in vivo. *Cell Mol Biol* 2000; **46**: 53–62.

117. Dawson DA, Sugano H, McCarron RM, Hallenbeck JM, Spatz M. Endothelin receptor antagonist preserves microvascular perfusion and reduces ischemic brain damage following permanent focal ischemia. *Neurochem Res* 1999; **24**: 1499–1505.

118. Tatlisumak T, Carano RA, Takano K, Opgenorth TJ, Sotak CH, Fisher M. A novel endothelin antagonist, A-127722, attenuates ischemic lesion size in rats with

temporary middle cerebral artery occlusion: a diffusion and perfusion MRI study. *Stroke* 1998; **29**: 850–857.

119. Grotta J. Rodent models of stroke limitations. What can we learn from recent clinical trials of thrombolysis? *Arch Neurol* 1996; **53**: 1067–1070.

120. del Zoppo GJ. Clinical trials in acute stroke: why have they not been successful? *Neurology* 1998; **51**: S59–S61.

121. Muir KW, Grosset DG. Neuroprotection for acute stroke: making clinical trials work. *Stroke* 1999; **30**: 180–182.

122. Oktem IS, Menku A, Akdemir H, Kontas O, Kurtsoy A, Koc RK. Therapeutic effect of tirilazad mesylate (U-74006F), mannitol, and their combination on experimental ischemia. *Res Exp Med Berl* 2000; **199**: 231–242.

123. Schabitz WR, Li F, Irie K, Sandage BW Jr, Locke KW, Fisher M. Synergistic effects of a combination of low-dose basic fibroblast growth factor and citicoline after temporary experimental focal ischemia. *Stroke* 1999; **30**: 427–431.

124. Aronowski J, Strong R, Grotta JC. Combined neuroprotection and reperfusion therapy for stroke. Effect of lubeluzole and diaspirin cross-linked hemoglobin in experimental focal ischemia. *Stroke* 1996; **27**: 1571–1576.

125. Leker RR, Shohami E, Abramsky O, Ovadia H. Dexanabinol; a novel neuroprotective drug in experimental focal cerebral ischemia. *J Neurol Sci* 1999; **162**: 114–119.

126. Barone FC, Feuerstein GZ, White RF. Brain cooling during transient focal ischemia provides complete neuroprotection. *Neurosci Biobehav Rev* 1997; **21**: 31–44.

127. Nurse S, Corbett D. Neuroprotection after several days of mild, drug-induced hypothermia. *J Cereb Blood Flow Metab* 1996; **16**: 474–480.

128. Sick TJ, Xu G, Perez Pinzon MA. Mild hypothermia improves recovery of cortical extracellular potassium ion activity and excitability after middle cerebral artery occlusion in the rat. *Stroke* 1999; **30**: 2416–2421.

129. Maier CM, Ahern K, Cheng ML, Lee JE, Yenari MA, Steinberg GK. Optimal depth and duration of mild hypothermia in a focal model of transient cerebral ischemia: effects on neurologic outcome, infarct size, apoptosis, and inflammation. *Stroke* 1998; **29**: 2171–2180.

130. Dietrich WD, Lin B, Globus MY, Green EJ, Ginsberg MID, Busto R. Effect of delayed MK-801 (dizocilpine) treatment with or without immediate postischemic hypothermia on chronic neuronal survival after global forebrain ischemia in rats. *J Cereb Blood Flow Metab* 1995; **15**: 960–968.

131. Busto R, Globus MY, Dietrich WD, Martinez E, Valdes I, Ginsberg MD. Effect of mild hypothermia on ischemia-induced release of neurotransmitters and free fatty acids in rat brain. *Stroke* 1989; **20**: 904–910.

132. Li PA, He QP, Miyashita H, Howllet W, Siesjo BK, Shuaib A. Hypothermia ameliorates ischemic brain damage and suppresses the release of extracellular amino acids in both normo- and hyperglycemic subjects. *Exp Neurol* 1999; **158**: 242–253.

133. Karibe H, Chen SF, Zarow GJ et al. Mild intraischemic hypothermia suppresses consumption of endogenous antioxidants after temporary focal ischemia in rats. *Brain Res* 1994; **649**: 12–18.

134. Kader A, Frazzini VI, Baker CJ, Solomon RA, Trifiletti RR. Effect of mild hypothermia on nitric oxide synthesis during focal cerebral ischemia. *Neurosurgery* 1994; **35**: 272–277; discussion 277.

135. Ishikawa M, Sekizuka E, Sato S et al. Effects of moderate hypothermia on leukocyte–endothelium interaction in the rat pial microvasculature after transient middle cerebral artery occlusion. *Stroke* 1999; **30**: 1679–1686.

136. Toyoda T, Suzuki S, Kassell NF, Lee KS. Intraischemic hypothermia attenuates neutrophil infiltration in the rat neocortex after focal ischemia–reperfusion injury. *Neurosurgery* 1996; **39**: 1200–1205.

137. Williams GD, Dardzinski BJ, Buckalew AR, Smith MB. Modest hypothermia preserves cerebral energy metabolism during hypoxia–ischemia and correlates with brain damage: a 31P nuclear magnetic resonance study in unanesthetized neonatal rats. *Pediatr Res* 1997; **42**: 700–708.

138. Verhaegen MJ, Todd MM, Hindman BJ, Warner DS. Cerebral autoregulation during moderate hypothermia in rats. *Stroke* 1993; **24**: 407–414.

139. Burdon RH. Temperature and animal cell protein synthesis. *Symp Soc Exp Biol* 1987; **41**: 113–133.

140. Yenari MA, Fink SL, Sun GH et al. Gene therapy with HSP72 is neuroprotective in rat models of stroke and epilepsy. *Ann Neurol* 1998; **44**: 548–591.

141. Fisher M, Meadows ME, Do T et al. Delayed treatment with intravenous basic fibroblast growth factor reduces infarct size following permanent focal cerebral ischemia in rats. *J Cereb Blood Flow Metab* 1995; **15**: 953–959.

142. Forsberg Nilsson K, Behar TN, Afrakhte M, Barker JL, McKay RD. Platelet-derived growth factor induces chemotaxis of neuroepithelial stem cells. *J Neurosci Res* 1998; **53**: 521–530.

143. Huang Z, Chen K, Huang PL, Finklestein SP, Moskowitz MA. bFGF ameliorates focal ischemic injury by blood flow-independent mechanisms in eNOS mutant mice. *Am J Physiol* 1997; **272**: H1401–H1405.

144. Jiang N, Finklestein SP, Do T, Caday CG, Charette M, Chopp M. Delayed intravenous administration of basic fibroblast growth factor (bFGF) reduces infarct volume in a model of focal cerebral ischemia/reperfusion in the rat. *J Neurol Sci* 1996; **139**: 173–179.

145. Johnston BM, Mallard EC, Williams CE, Gluckman PD. Insulin-like growth factor-1 is a potent neuronal rescue agent after hypoxic–ischemic injury in fetal lambs. *J Clin Invest* 1996; **97**: 300–308.

146. Kent TA, Quast M, Taglialatela G et al. Effect of NGF treatment on outcome measures in a rat model of middle cerebral artery occlusion. *J Neurosci Res* 1999; **55**: 357–369.

147. Lee TH, Kato H, Chen ST, Kogure K, Itoyama Y. Expression of nerve growth factor and trkA after transient focal cerebral ischemia in rats. *Stroke* 1998; **29**: 1687–1696.

148. Lin TN, Te J, Lee M, Sun GY, Hsu CY. Induction of basic fibroblast growth factor (bFGF) expression following focal cerebral ischemia. *Brain Res Mol Brain Res* 1997; **49**: 255–265.

149. Liu X, Zhu XZ. Basic fibroblast growth factor protected forebrain against ischemia–reperfusion damage in rats. *Chung Kuo Yao Li Hsueh Pao* 1998; **19**: 527–530.

150. Nakata N, Kato H, Kogure K. Protective effects of basic fibroblast growth factor against hippocampal neuronal damage following cerebral ischemia in the gerbil. *Brain Res* 1993; **605**: 354–356.

151. Tagami M, Ikeda K, Nara Y et al. Insulin-like growth factor-1 attenuates apoptosis in hippocampal neurons caused by cerebral ischemia and reperfusion in stroke-prone spontaneously hypertensive rats. *Lab Invest* 1997; **76**: 613–617.

152. Ren JM, Finklestein SP. Time window of infarct reduction by intravenous basic fibroblast growth factor in focal cerebral ischemia. *Eur J Pharmacol* 1997; **327**: 11–16.

153. Kawamata T, Alexis NE, Dietrich WD, Finklestein SP. Intracisternal basic fibroblast growth factor (bFGF) enhances behavioral recovery following focal cerebral infarction in the rat. *J Cereb Blood Flow Metab* 1996; **16**: 542–547.

154. Semkova I, Krieglstein J. Neuroprotection mediated via neurotrophic factors and induction of neurotrophic factors. *Brain Res Brain Res Rev* 1999; **30**: 176–188.

155. Yamamoto K, Yoshikawa R, Okuyama S et al. Neuroprotective effect of 4'-(4-methylphenyl)-2,2':6',2-terpyridine trihydrochloride, a novel inducer of nerve growth factor. *Life Sci* 1996; **59**: 2139–2146.

156. Endres M, Scott G, Namura S et al. Role of peroxynitrite and neuronal nitric oxide synthase in the activation of poly(ADP-ribose) synthetase in a murine model of cerebral ischemia–reperfusion. *Neurosci Lett* 1998; **248**: 41–44.

157. Zhang RL, Zhang ZG, Chopp M. Increased therapeutic efficacy with rt-PA and anti-CD18 antibody treatment of stroke in the rat. *Neurology* 1999; **52**: 273–279.

23

Immunomodulation—new therapeutic opportunities for stroke

Giora Z Feuerstein and Xinkang Wang

INTRODUCTION

Ischemic stroke is commonly the outcome of obstruction of bloodflow in a major cerebral vessel (usually the middle cerebral artery), which, if not resolved within a short period of time, will lead to a core of severely ischemic brain tissue that may not be salvageable. The dynamic changes of brain tissue following ischemic stroke are illustrated in Fig. 23.1. Ischemic stroke leads to depletion of energy (ATP, phosphocreatine (PCr)) and hence to membrane voltage reduction, leading to ionic fluxes across the cell membrane. Extracellular potassium can reach levels sufficient to release neurotransmitters such as glutamate and aspartate and stimulate sodium/calcium channels coupled to glutamate

receptors, leading to cytotoxic edema. The calcium overload causes further mitochondrial damage and impairment in ATP production as well as extensive breakdown of cellular phospholipids, proteins and nucleic acids due to activation of phospholipases, proteases, and endonucleases. Free radicals are also produced during ischemia and contribute to membrane lipid peroxidation, protein and nuclear DNA toxic changes, and cellular injury (i.e. necrosis and apoptosis).

The inflammatory response to brain ischemia has been extensively studied. The early accumulation of neutrophils in ischemic brain damage has been demonstrated by histopathological,[1,2] biochemical,[3] and ^{111}In-labeled leukocyte studies.[4] The initiation of cellular inflammation in the brain by ischemic

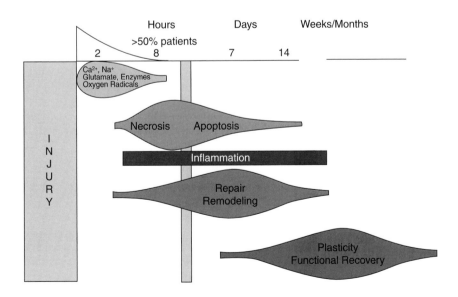

Figure 23.1 The dynamic changes following ischemic stroke.

injury takes place within the microvasculature. Cerebral microvessels are the interface at which polymorphonuclear (PMN) leukocytes adhere and pass into the underlying neuropil.[5,6] Accumulating evidence suggests that this inflammatory response after ischemic brain injury is mediated by a sequence of gene expression, including inflammatory cytokines, chemokines, cellular adhesion molecules, and other proinflammatory genes. The blockade of the expression of these genes or their functions may provide novel therapeutic opportunities in stroke.

CHANGES OF GENE EXPRESSION IN ISCHEMIC BRAIN INJURY

Differential gene expression plays a critical role in the initiation, propagation and maturation of ischemic brain injury. Several waves of new gene expression have been characterized after focal brain ischemia (Fig. 23.2). Transcription factors such as c-fos, c-jun and egr-1 (zif-268) are the first wave induced within minutes after ischemic insult. The second wave consists of heat shock proteins, the mRNA of which is usually expressed at 1–24 h. Of great interest is the third wave, which is largely composed of cytokines, chemokines and adhesion molecules; their mRNA expression usually starts 1–3 h post-injury and reaches its peak at 12 h, and then decreases to a basal level 24 h after focal ischemia.[7] The late wave of new gene expression consists largely of tissue remodeling proteins such as transforming growth factor-β (TNF-β), osteopontin and metalloproteinases.[8–10]

EXPRESSION OF INFLAMMATORY CYTOKINES AFTER ISCHEMIC BRAIN INJURY

Several cell types within the brain are able to secrete cytokines, including microglia, astrocytes, endothelial cells and neurons; in addition, there is also evidence to support the involvement of peripherally derived cytokines in brain inflammation. Peripherally derived mononuclear phagocytes, T-lymphocytes, natural killer (NK) cells and PMNs, which produce and secrete cytokines, can all contribute to central nervous system (CNS) inflammation and gliosis. Brain injury is associated with the expression of inflammatory mediators, e.g. inflammatory cytokines (interleukin-1 (IL-1) and tumor necrosis factor alpha (TNF-α)), chemokines (IL-8, MCP-1 and IP-10) and adhesion molecules (ICAM-1 and selectins).

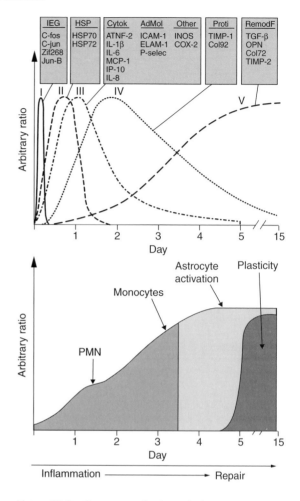

Figure 23.2 Gene expression in rat ischemic cortex after middle cerebral artery occlusion. Five waves of ischemic gene expression include early response genes/transcription factors (wave 1), heat shock proteins (wave 2), proinflammatory mediators (wave 3), proteinases and proteinase inhibitors (wave 4) and delayed remodeling proteins (wave 5). The leukocyte wave, including early polymorphonuclear (PMN) neutrophils and later monocyte/macrophage infiltration, is illustrated in the lower panel. Astrocyte activation (gliosis) occurs following leukocyte infiltration into the ischemic brain tissue.

TNF-α is a proinflammatory cytokine with a diverse array of biological activities. Elevated TNF-α has been repeatedly demonstrated in various experimental models of brain injury. Systemic kainic acid administration induces TNF-α mRNA within 2–4 h in cerebral cortex, hippocampus and hypothalamus. Systemic or intracerebroventricular administration of lipopolysaccharide (LPS) endotoxin has also been shown to increase brain TNF-α levels as determined by bioassay.[11] In a model of non-penetrating head injury, Shohami et al. reported an early increase in TNF-α peptide at the site of the focal insult.[12] Also, in rat traumatic head injury, TNF-α mRNA and protein levels are rapidly elevated.[13] Furthermore, in mice challenged with particles of charcoal injected into the hippocampus, an increase in striatal levels of TNF-α mRNA was observed.[12] Elevated serum TNF-α was also observed following severe head injury in humans.[14]

Elevated expression of TNF-α mRNA and protein occurs shortly (1–3 h) following middle cerebral artery occlusion (MCAO) in rats.[15,16] In ischemic cortex, TNF-α mRNA levels are elevated as early as 1 h post-occlusion (i.e. prior to significant influx of PMN), peak at 12 h and persist for about 5 days. The early expression of TNF-α mRNA preceding leukocyte infiltration suggests that TNF-α may be involved in this response. Double-labeling immunofluorescence studies localized the de novo synthesized TNF-α to neurons but not astroglia. At 5 days following the ischemic insult, neuronally associated TNF-α was diminished, and TNF-α immunoreactivity was localized in the inflammatory cells. The significance of TNF-α expression in the brain was studied by microinjection of TNF-α into the rat cortex; TNF-α induced leukocyte adhesion to the capillary endothelium, but no evidence for neurotoxicity at the site of injection was found. Buttini et al[17] identified a rapid upregulation of TNF-α mRNA and protein in activated microglia and macrophages following focal stroke, again suggesting that TNF-α is part of an intrinsic inflammatory reaction of the brain following ischemia. TNF-α may exert a primary effect on the microvascular inflammatory response as reflected by TNF-α-induced neutrophil adhesion to brain capillary endothelium.[15] Furthermore, intracerebroventricular injection of TNF-α 24 h prior to MCAO exacerbates the ischemia-induced tissue injury.[18] This effect was reversed by ventricular administration of anti-TNF-α monoclonal antibodies (mAb). Further evidence for the involvement of TNF-α in stroke-induced injury is provided by finding that spontaneously hypertensive rats that are stroke-prone have higher levels of TNF-α production in the brain as compared to normotensive rats.[11] These data suggest that TNF-α may prime the brain for subsequent damage by activating capillary endothelium to a pro-adhesive state.

IL-1β is produced in the CNS by various cellular elements, including microglia, astrocytes, neurons and endothelium.[19] Like TNF-α, IL-1β has many pro-inflammatory properties. Increases in IL-1β mRNA

expression have been shown to occur following several types of injury to the brain, including excitotoxicity[20] and LPS.[21] Furthermore, mechanical damage following implantation of a microdialysis probe has been shown to induce expression of IL-1β. Following fluid percussion brain trauma in the rat, a rapid increase in IL-1β mRNA expression has been reported. Microglial IL-1α expression has also been observed in human head injury. IL-β mRNA expression has been shown to increase following transient brain ischemia in the rat.[22] The exacerbation of ischemic brain injury due to exogenous IL-1β administered into the brain has been observed.[23] A rapid (3–6 h post-ischemia) increase in IL-1β mRNA following MCAO peaked at 12 h but returned to basal values at 5 days.[16,24] Early IL-1β expression following focal stroke has also been demonstrated using in situ hybridization. The recent development of tools such as specific antibodies to rat IL-1β has permitted the identification (by immunohistochemistry) of IL-1β peptide in cerebral vessels, microglia and macrophages following focal stroke.

Interleukin-1 receptor antagonist (IL-1ra) is a naturally occurring inhibitor of IL-1 activity, acting by competing with IL-1 for occupancy of the type 1 interleukin-1 receptor (IL-1RI) without inducing a signal of its own. IL-1ra is produced by many different cellular sources including monocytes/macrophages, endothelial cells, fibroblasts, neurons and glial cells. The expression of IL-1ra and interleukin-1 receptor (IL-1R) mRNA following focal stroke has also been reported.[25] The level of IL-1a mRNA was markedly increased in the ischemic cortex at 6 h, and then reached a significantly elevated level from 12 h to 5 days following MCAO. The presence of IL-1ra in the normal brain and the upregulation of IL-1ra mRNA after ischemic injury suggest that IL-1ra may serve as a defense system to attenuate the IL-1-mediated brain injury. It is interesting to observe that the temporal induction profile of IL-1ra following MCAO virtually parallels that of IL-1β,[24] except that IL-1ra mRNA exhibited prolonged elevation beyond that of IL-1β. Thus, the balance between the levels of IL-1β and its antagonist, IL-1ra expressed post-ischemia, may be more critical to the degree of tissue injury than IL-1 levels per se.

ROLE OF INFLAMMATORY CYTOKINES IN ISCHEMIC BRAIN INJURY

Inhibitors of IL-1 or TNF-α have now been shown repeatedly to result in reduced deficits in focal stroke and head trauma models. The detrimental effects of TNF-α and its role as a mediator of focal ischemia may involve several mechanisms. For example,

TNF-α increases blood–brain barrier permeability and produces pial artery constriction that can contribute to focal ischemic brain injury; TNF-α has also been shown to augment pulmonary arterial transendothelial albumin flux in vitro.[26] Furthermore, by stimulating the production of matrix-degradating metalloproteinase (gelatinase B),[27,28] TNF-α may further damage capillary integrity. TNF-α also causes damage to myelin and oligodendrocytes,[29] and increases astrocytic proliferation, thus potentially contributing to demyelination and reactive gliosis. In addition, TNF-α activates the endothelium for leukocyte adherence and procoagulation activity (i.e. increased tissue factor, von Willebrand factor and platelet-activating factor) that can exacerbate ischemic damage. Indeed, increased TNF-α in the brain and blood in response to LPS appears to contribute to increased stroke sensitivity/risk in hypertensive rats.[11] TNF-α activates neutrophils and increases leukocyte–endothelial cell adhesion molecule expression, leukocyte adherence to blood vessels, and subsequent infiltration into the brain.[7]

Several studies have shown that blocking TNF-α results in improved outcome in brain trauma and stroke. Pentoxifyline (a methylxanthine that reduces TNF-α production at the transcriptional level) or soluble TNF receptor I (which acts by competing with TNF-α at the receptor) improve neurological outcome, reduce the disruption of the blood–brain barrier and protect hippocampal cells from delayed cell death following closed head injury in the rat.[30] In rat focal ischemia, an anti-TNF-α mAb and the soluble TNF receptor I were neuroprotective.[18] In the latter studies, TNF-α was blocked by repeated intracerebroventricular (i.c.v.) administrations before and during focal stroke which significantly reduced infarct size. In murine focal stroke, topical application of soluble TNF receptor I on the brain surface significantly reduced ischemic brain injury.[31,32] In addition, in another study evaluating TNF blockade on focal stroke in hypertensive rats, soluble TNF receptor I administered intravenously pre- or post-MCAO significantly reduced the impairment in ischemic cortex microvascular perfusion and the degree of cortical infarction, strongly suggesting an inflammatory/vascular mechanism for TNF-α in focal stroke.[33]

Many studies have demonstrated the protective effects of IL-1ra in brain injury. Thus, administration of recombinant IL-1ra produced a marked reduction in brain damage induced by focal stroke,[34,35] or brain hypoxia.[36] This neuronal protective effect of IL-1ra in focal stroke was further supported by the use of an adenoviral vector that overexpressed IL-1ra in the brain.[37] The excess of IL-1ra significantly reduced infarct size following focal stroke. In addition, IL-1ra expression increases following ischemic preconditioning in a manner that parallels the development of brain ischemic tolerance.[38] Of interest are data showing that peripheral administration of IL-1ra reduces brain injury,[34] suggesting a potential use of IL-1ra as a neuroprotective agent in human stroke and/or neurotrauma.

ROLE OF ADHESION MOLECULES IN ISCHEMIC BRAIN INJURY

Leukocyte adhesion receptors, P-selectin, ICAM-1 and E-selectin are expressed in sequence by microvascular endothelium within the ischemic territory.[39–42] P-selectin is seen within 60–90 min following MCAO,[39] indicating the rapid reactivity of microvascular endothelium to the ischemic insult. P-selectin and E-selectin receptors are continually expressed within the ischemic territory.[42]

The significance of these adhesion molecules in stroke is demonstrated by studies with selective inhibitors to these molecules. For example, rats treated with an antibody against MAC-1 (the leukocyte counterpart to ICAM-1) had smaller lesions (reduction in infarct size by 45–50%) following transient MCAO.[43] Similarly, administration of an anti-ICAM-1 antibody produced a 40% reduction of infarct size in a focal stroke model.[44] Blocking adhesion molecules can also reduce apoptosis induced by focal ischemia.[45] Other studies verified these effects but also illustrated that these antibodies could not reduce infarct size when the ischemia was permanent.[46,47] However, this strategy may only work when both leukocyte and endothelial cell adhesion proteins are blocked. The combination of tissue plasminogen activator (t-PA) and anti-CD18 provides significantly improved outcome, and may increase the therapeutic time window in stroke.[48] In a rabbit embolic model of stroke, anti-ICAM-1 antibody was shown to increase the amount of clot necessary to produce permanent damage.[49] In addition, in a baboon model of transient focal ischemia, anti-CD18 mAb administered 25 min prior to reperfusion led to increase in reflow in microvessels of various sizes.[50] However, in contrast to the demonstrated anti-ischemic effect of antiadhesion molecules in animal models, the recent failure of the murine anti-ICAM mAb (enlimomab) in human stroke[51] and its ability to activate human neutrophils[52] demonstrate the difficulties in extrapolating encouraging data obtained in some animal models to clinical reality.

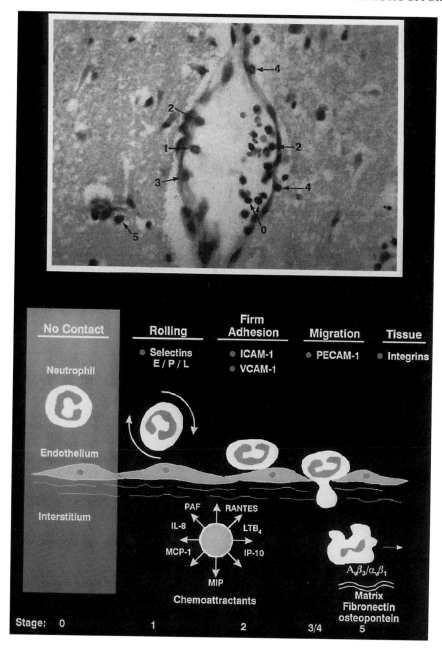

Figure 23.3 Histological (top) and schematic (bottom) representations of changes in the brain microvessels after focal ischemia. Shortly (1–6 h) after middle cerebral artery occlusion, leukocytes (primarily neutrophils) in the ischemic tissue vessels are adherent to the post-capillary venule and capillary walls. This can modify and exacerbate the decreased blowflow occurring in the already ischemic brain. Then, these neutrophils can find their way outside the vessel walls into the focal ischemic cortex over the next 6–24 h. Macrophages move into the brain at 1–5 days and significantly accumulate in the infarct tissue.

ANTI-LEUKOCYTE STRATEGIES FOR NEUROPROTECTION

The infiltration and accumulation of leukocytes in the ischemic brain tissue (Fig. 23.3) has been repeatedly demonstrated. Unlike normal brain microvessels, which are clear of inflammatory cells, brain microvessels from ischemic zones contain leukocytes along with significant perivascular edema. Many of the leukocytes, primarily neutrophils, found in vessels within ischemic tissue are adherent to the endothelium, a situation not normally observed in intact brain microvessels. Some of these neutrophils migrate outside the vascular walls into the focal ischemic cortex.

To explore a role of leukocytes in ischemic brain tissue, anti-leukocyte strategies were applied by using an RP-3 mAb that selectively depletes leukocytes in the rat (about 90–95%).[53] The administration of the RP-3 mAb produced a dramatic reduction in both neutrophil accumulation in focal ischemic brain tissue and infarct size (decreased by 45–50%). However, other reports have failed to reproduce such observations.[54]

THE ROLE OF NITRIC OXIDE IN ISCHEMIC BRAIN INJURY

NO is a mediator involved in a wide variety of physiological and pathological processes. NO is synthesized by the enzyme NO synthase (NOS) by the oxidation of the guanidino nitrogen of L-arginine.[55] Immediately after induction of ischemia, the vasodilator effect of NO, produced mainly by endothelial nitric oxide synthase (eNOS), is believed to protect the brain by limiting the degree of flow reduction produced by the arterial occlusion.[56] However, following ischemia, NO produced by neuronal NOS (nNOS) and, later, by inducible NOS (iNOS), may contribute to the evolution of brain injury.[57] Expression of iNOS occurs in the setting of such inflammatory reactions. Following permanent or transient MCAO in rodents, iNOS mRNA, protein and enzymatic activity are expressed in the post-ischemic brain.[58,59] The expression peaks 12–48 h after ischemia and occurs in inflammatory cells infiltrating the injured brain and in cerebral blood vessels.[60] iNOS expression was also found in neutrophils and vascular cells in human brain after stroke.[61] The role of iNOS in ischemic stroke has been explored by systemic administration of relatively selective iNOS inhibitors, aminoguanidine and 1400GW.[62,63] iNOS inhibition reduced infarct volume by 30–40% in the rat model of transient brain ischemia.[59,62,63] Importantly, the reduction in histological damage was associated with improvement of the neurological deficits produced by the infarct.[64] Other studies have demonstrated that iNOS null mutation mice have smaller infarcts (–30%) and superior neurological outcome to wild-type littermates after focal brain ischemia.[65] The reduction in infarct volume was more pronounced in homozygous than in heterozygous iNOS mice.[66]

ROLE OF MITOGEN-ACTIVATED PROTEIN KINASE IN STROKE AND CNS INJURY

Recent evidence suggests that mitogen-activated protein kinases (MAPK) play an important role in neuronal cell growth, differentiation and death. The MAP kinase/extracellular-signal-response (ERK) kinase signaling pathway was demonstrated to be activated after ischemic injury, and the MEK1-specific antagonist, PD98059, significantly protected from focal cerebral ischemic injury.[67] Stress-activated protein kinases (e.g. SAPKs and p38 MAPK) play an essential role in cells' responses to cytokines and various environmental stimuli. Recently, a new class of compounds, cytokine-suppressive anti-inflammatory drugs (CSAIDs), potent inhibitors of TNF-α and IL-1β production, have been developed.[68] Targeting p38 MAPK may provide an opportunity not only for intervention in early cytokine production but also to block delayed neuronal death by apoptosis after ischemic injury. Very recently, the selective p38 MAPK inhibitor was demonstrated to reduce ischemic infarct (up to 40%) and neurological deficits (35%) in a rat model of focal brain ischemia, supporting the importance of p38 MAPK in focal ischemia-induced brain injury.[69]

CONCLUSION

Inflammation is a well-established phenomenon in brain injury and may serve as a valid target for pharmacological interventions. It has been clearly demonstrated that the brain is capable of producing cytokines, chemokines and adhesion molecules de novo, which may support infiltration and accumulation of leukocytes in brain tissue after injury. A detrimental role of circulating leukocytes in brain injury has been suggested, based on studies with neutrophil depletion, inhibition of cytokines (TNF-α and IL-1β), blockade of adhesion molecules, as well as the inhibition of iNOS and the mitogen-activated protein kinase (e.g. MEK1 and p38 MAPK). Thus, immunomodulation could provide new therapeutic strategies in the management of stroke, head and spinal cord injuries.

REFERENCES

1. Garcia JH, Kamijyo Y. Cerebral infarction: evolution of histopathological changes after occlusion of a middle cerebral artery in primates. *J Neuropathol Exp Neurol* 1974; **33**: 409–421.
2. Hallenbeck JM, Dutka AJ, Tanishima T et al. Polymorphonuclear leukocyte accumulation in brain regions with low blood flow during the early postischemic period. *Stroke* 1986; **17**: 246–253.
3. Barone FC, Hillegass LM, Price WJ et al. Polymorphonuclear leukocyte infiltration into cerebral focal ischemic tissue: myeloperoxidase activity assay and histologic verification. *J Neurosci Res* 1991; **29**: 336–345.
4. Dutka AJ, Kochanek PM, Hallenbeck JM. Influence of granulocytopenia on canine cerebral ischemia induced by an embolism. *Stroke* 1989; **20**: 390–395.
5. del Zoppo GJ. Microvascular changes during cerebral ischaemia and reperfusion. *Cerebrovasc Brain Metab Rev* 1994; **6**: 47–96.

6. Garcia JH, Liu KF, Yoshida Y, Lian J, Chen S, del Zoppo GJ. Influx of leukocytes and platelets in an evolving brain infarct (Wistar rat). *Am J Pathol* 1994; **144**: 188–199.

7. Feuerstein GZ, Wang XK, Barone FC. Inflammatory mediators of ischemic injury: cytokine gene regulation in stroke. In: Ginsberg MD, Bogousslavsky J, eds. *Cerebrovascular Disease: Pathophysiology, Diagnosis and Management.* Blackwell Science Inc., Boston MA, USA 1998: 507–531.

8. Wang XK, Yue TL, White RF, Barone FC, Feuerstein GZ. Transforming growth factor-beta 1 exhibits delayed gene expression following focal cerebral ischemia. *Brain Res Bull* 1995; **36**: 607–609.

9. Wang XK, Louden C, Yue TL et al. Delayed expression of osteopontin after focal stroke in the rat. *J Neurosci* 1998; **18**: 2075–2083.

10. Rosenberg GA, Navratil M, Barone FC, Feuerstein G. Proteolytic cascade enzymes increase in focal cerebral ischemia in rat. *J Cereb Blood Flow Metab* 1996; **16**: 360–366.

11. Siren AL, Heldman E, Doron D et al. Release of pro-inflammatory and prothrombotic mediators in the brain and peripheral circulation in spontaneously hypertensive and normotensive Wistar-Kyoto rats. *Stroke* 1992; **23**: 1643–1651.

12. Shohami E, Novikov M, Bass R, Yamin A, Gallily R. Closed head injury triggers early production of TNF-α and IL-6 by brain tissue. *J Cereb Blood Flow Metab* 1994; **14**: 615–619.

13. Fan K, Young PR, Barone FC, Feuerstein GZ, Smith DH, Mcintosh TK. Experimental traumatic brain injury induces differential expression of TNF-α mRNA in the CNS. *Mol Brain Res* 1996; **36**: 287–291.

14. Goodman JC, Robertson CS, Grossman RG, Narayan RK. Elevation of tumour necrosis factor in head injury. *J Neuroimmunol* 1990; **30**: 2–3.

15. Liu T, Clark RK, Mcdonnell PC et al. Tumour necrosis factor α expression in ischemic neurons. *Stroke* 1994; **25**: 1481–1488.

16. Wang XK, Yue TL, Barone FC, White R, Young PR, Feuerstein GZ, Concomitant cortical expression of TNF-α and IL-1β mRNA following transient focal ischemia. *Mol Chem Neuropathol* 1994; **23**: 103–114.

17. Buttini M, Appel K, Sauater A, Gebicke-Haerter P-J, Boddeke HWGM. Expression of tumour necrosis factor alpha after focal cerebral ischemia in the rat. *Neuroscience* 1996; **71**: 1–16.

18. Barone FC, Arvin B, White RF, Tumour necrosis factor α. A mediator of focal ischemic brain injury. *Stroke* 1997; **28**: 1233–1244.

19. Rothwell NJ. Functions and mechanism of interleukin-1 in the brain. *Trends Pharmacol Sci* 1991; **12**: 430–435.

20. Minami M, Kuraishi Y, Satoh M. Effects of kainic acid on messenger RNA levels of IL-1β, IL-6, TNF-α and LIF in the rat brain. *Biochem Biophys Res Commun* 1991; **176**: 593–598.

21. Buttini M, Boddeki H. Peripheral lipopolysaccharide stimulation induces interleukin-1β mRNA in rat brain microglial cells. *Neuroscience* 1995; **65**: 523–550.

22. Minami M, Kuraishi Y, Yabuuchi K, Yamazaki A, Satoh M. Induction of interleukin-1 beta mRNA in rat brain after transient forebrain ischemia. *J Neurochem* 1992; **58**: 390–392.

23. Yamasaki Y, Matsuura N, Shozuhara H, Onodera H, Itoyama Y, Kogure K. Interleukin-1 as a pathogenetic mediator of ischemic brain damage in the rat. *Stroke* 1995; **26**: 676–681.

24. Liu T, McDonnel PC, Young PR et al. Interleukin-1β mRNA expression in ischemic rat cortex. *Stroke* 1993; **24**: 1746–1751.

25. Wang XK, Barone FC, Aiyar NV, Feuerstein GZ. Increased interleukin-1 receptor and interleukin-1 receptor antagonist gene expression after focal stroke. *Stroke* 1997; **28**: 155–162.

26. Goldblum SE, Sun WL, Tumour necrosis factor-alpha augments pulmonary arterial transendothelial albumen flux in vitro. *Am J Physiol* 1990; **285**: L57–L67.

27. Romanic AM, White RF, Arleth AJ, Ohlstein EH, Barone FC. Matrix metalloproteinase expression increases following cerebral focal ischemia: inhibition of MMP-9 reduces infarct size. *Stroke* 1998; **29**: 1020–1030.

28. Rosenberg GA, Estrada EY, Dencoff JE, Stetler-Stevenson WG. Tumour necrosis factor-α-induced gelatinase B causes delayed opening of the blood brain barrier: an expanded therapeutic window. *Brain Res* 1995; **703**: 151–155.

29. Robbins DS, Shirazi Y, Drydale BE, Lieberman A, Shin HS, Shin ML. Production of cytotoxic factor for oligodendrocytes by stimulated astrocytes. *J Immunol* 1987; **139**: 2593–2597.

30. Shohami E, Bass E, Wallach D, Yamin A, Gallily R. Inhibition of tumour necrosis factor alpha (TNF-α) activity in rat brain is associated with cerebroprotection after closed head injury. *J Cereb Blood Flow Metab* 1996; **16**: 378–384.

31. Nawashiro H, Martin D, Hallenbeck JM. Inhibition of tumour necrosis factor and amelioration of brain infarction in mice. *J Cereb Blood Flow Metab* 1997; **17**: 229–232.

32. Nawashiro H, Tasaki K, Ruetzler CA, Hallenbeck JM, TNF-alpha pre-treatment induces protective effects against focal cerebral ischemia in mice. *J Cereb Blood Flow Metab* 1997; **17**: 483–490.

33. Dawson DA, Martin D, Hallenbeck JM. Inhibition of tumour necrosis factor-alpha reduces focal cerebral ischemic injury in the spontaneously hypertensive rat. *Neurosci Lett* 1996; **218**: 41–44.

34. Relton JK, Martin D, Thompson RC, Russell DA. Peripheral administration of interleukin-1 receptor antagonist inhibits brain damage after focal cerebral ischemia in the rat. *Exp Neurol* 1996; **138**: 206–213.

35. Loddick SA, Rothwell NJ. Neuroprotective effects of human recombinant interleukin-1 receptor antagonist in focal ischemia in the rat. *J Cereb Blood Flow Metab* 1996; **16**: 932–940.

36. Martin D, Chinookoswong N, Miller G. The interleukin-1 receptor antagonist (rhIL-1ra) protects against cerebral infarction in a rat model of hypoxia–ischemia. *Exp Neurol* 1995; **130**: 362–367.

37. Betz AL, Yang GY, Davidson BL. Attenuation of stroke in rats using an adenoviral vector to induce overexpression of interleukin-1 receptor antagonist in brain. *J Cereb Blood Flow Metab* 1995; **15**: 547–551.

38. Barone FC, White RF, Spera PA, Currie RW, Wang XK, Feuerstein GZ. Ischemic preconditioning and brain tolerance: temporal histologic and functional outcomes, protein synthesis requirement, and IL-1ra and early gene expression. *Stroke* 1998; **29**: 1937–1951.

39. Okada Y, Copeland BR, Mori E, Tung MM, Thomas WS, del Zoppa GJ. P-selectin and intercellular adhesion molecule-1 expression after focal brain ischemia and reperfusion. *Stroke* 1994; **25**: 202–211.

40. Wang XK, Siren A-L, Yue T-L, Barone FC, Feuerstein GZ. Upregulation of intracellular adhesion molecule-1

(ICAM1) on brain microvascular endothelial cells in rat ischemic cortex. *Mol Brain Res* 1994; **26**: 61–68.

41. Wang XK, Yue T-L, Barone FC, Feuerstein GZ. Demonstration of increased endothelial–leukocyte adhesion molecule 1 mRNA expression in rat ischemic cortex. *Stroke* 1995; **26**: 1665–1669.

42. Haring H-P, Akamine P, Habermann R, Koziol JA, del Zoppo GJ. Distribution of the integrin-like immunoreactivity on primate brain microvasculature. *J Neuropathol Exp Neurol* 1996; **55**: 236–245.

43. Chen H, Chopp M, Zhang RL et al. Anti-CD11b monoclonal antibody reduces ischemic cell damage after transient focal cerebral ischemia in rat. *Ann Neurol* 1994; **35**: 458–463.

44. Zhang RL, Chopp M, Li Y et al. Anti-ICAM-1 antibody reduces ischemic cell damage after transient middle cerebral artery occlusion in the rat. *Neurology* 1994; **44**: 1747–1751.

45. Chopp M, Li Y, Jiang N, Zhang RL, Prostak J. Antibodies against adhesion molecules reduce apoptosis after transient middle cerebral artery occlusion in rat brain. *J Cereb Blood Flow Metab* 1996; **16**: 578–584.

46. Chopp M, Zhang RI, Chen H, Li Y, Jiang N, Rusche RJ. Post ischemic administration of an anti-MAC-1 antibody reduces ischemic cell damage after transient middle cerebral artery occlusion in the rat. *Stroke* 1994; **25**: 869–876.

47. Zhang RL, Chopp M, Jaing N et al. Anti-intercellular adhesion molecule-1 antibody reduces ischemic cell damage after transient but not permanent middle cerebral artery occlusion in the Wistar rat. *Stroke* 1995; **26**: 1438–1443.

48. Zhang RL, Zhang ZG, Chopp M. Increased therapeutic efficacy with rt-PA and anti-CD18 antibody treatment of stroke in the rat. *Neurology* 1999; **52**: 273–279.

49. Bowes MP, Ziviin JA, Rothlein R. Monoclonal antibody to ICAM-1 adhesion site reduces neurological damage in a rabbit cerebral embolism stroke model. *Exp Neurol* 1993; **119**: 215–219.

50. Mori E, Zoppo M, Chambers GL, Copeland JD, Arfors KE. Inhibition of polymorphonuclear leukocyte adherence suppresses no-reflow after focal cerebral ischemia in baboons. *Stroke* 1992; **23**: 712–718.

51. Degraba TJ. The role of acute inflammation after acute stroke—utility of pursuing anti-adhesion molecule therapy. *Neurology* 1998; **51**: S62–S68.

52. Vourte J, Linsberg PJ, Kaste M et al. Anti-ICAM-1 monoclonal antibody R65 (Enlimomab) promotes activation of neutrophils in whole blood. *J Immunol* 1999; **162**: 2353–2357.

53. Matsuo Y, Onodera H, Shiga Y et al. Correlation between myeloperoxidose-quantified neutrophil accumulation and ischemic brain injury in the rat: effects of neutrophil depletion. *Stroke* 1994; **25**: 1469–1475.

54. Hayward NJ, Elliot PJ, Sawyer SD, Bronson RJ, Bartus RT. Lack of evidence for neutrophil participation during infarct formation following focal cerebral ischemia in the rat. *Exp Neurol* 1996; **139**: 188–202.

55. Griffith OW, Stuehr DJ. Nitric oxide synthases: properties and catalytic mechanism. *Annu Rev Physiol* 1995; **57**: 707–736.

56. Huang Z, Huang PL, Ma J et al. Enlarged infarcts in endothelial nitric oxide synthase knockout mice are attenuated by nitro-L-arginine. *J Cereb Blood Flow Metab* 1996; **16**: 981–987.

57. Iadecola C. Bright and dark sides of nitric oxide in ischemic brain damage. *Trends Neurosci* 1997; **20**: 132–138.

58. Iadecola C, Xu X, Zhang F, El-Fakahany EE, Ross ME. Marked induction of calcium-independent nitric oxide synthase activity after focal cerebral ischemia. *J Cereb Blood Flow Metab* 1995; **14**: 52–59.

59. Iadecola C, Zhang F, Casey R, Clark HB, Ross ME. Inducible nitric oxide synthase gene expression in vascular cells after transient focal cerebral ischemia. *Stroke* 1996; **27**: 1373–1380.

60. Nogawa S, Zhang F, Ross ME, Iadecola C. Cyclooxygenase-2 gene expression in neurons contributes to ischemic brain damage. *J Neurosci* 1997; **17**: 2746–2755.

61. Forster C, Clark HB, Ross ME, Iadecola C. Inducible nitric oxide synthase expression in human cerebral infarcts. *Acta Neuropathol* 1999; **97**: 215–220.

62. Iadecola C, Zhang F, Xu X. Inhibition of inducible nitric oxide synthase ameliorates cerebral ischemic damage. *Am J Physiol* 1995; **268**: R286–R292.

63. Parmentier S, Bohme GA, Lerouet D et al. Selective inhibition of inducible nitric oxide synthase prevents ischaemic brain injury. *Br J Pharmacol* 1999; **127**: 546–552.

64. Nagayama M, Zhang F, Iadecola C. Delayed treatment with aminoguanidine decreases focal cerebral ischemic damage and enhances neurologic recovery in rats. *J Cereb Blood Flow Metab* 1998; **18**: 1107–1113.

65. Iadecola C, Zhang F, Casey R, Nagayama M, Ross ME. Delayed reduction in ischemic brain injury and neurological deficits in mice lacking the inducible nitric oxide synthase gene. *J Neurosci* 1997; **17**: 9157–9164.

66. Zhao X, Haensel C, Ross ME, Iadecola C. Gene-dosing effect of reduction of ischemic brain injury in mice lacking the inducible nitric oxide synthase gene. *Soc Neurosci Abstr* 1999; **25**: 793.

67. Alessandrini A, Namura S, Moskowitz MA, Bonventre JV. MEK1 protein kinase inhibition protects against damage resulting from focal cerebral ischemia. *Proc Natl Acad Sci USA* 1999; **96**: 12866–12869.

68. Lee JC, Laydon JT, McDonnell PC et al. A protein kinase involved in the regulation of inflammatory cytokine biosynthesis. *Nature* 1994; **372**: 739–746.

69. Barone FC, Irving EA, Ohlstein EH et al. p38 MAPK in focal stroke: selective inhibitor reduces brain injury and neurological deficits. *Soc Neurosci Abstr* 1999; **25**: 1060.

24

Toxicity of tumor necrosis factor is enhanced by reactive oxygen species after brain trauma

Esther Shohami

INTRODUCTION

Traumatic brain injury is the major cause of mortality and morbidity in the young age group.[1] It induces acute transient edema and disruption of the blood–brain barrier, and persistent neurological deficits which include motor and memory impairments.[2] The mechanisms underlying the production of these deficits are still unclear, and various mediators have been suggested to contribute to the secondary damage.[3] The complex network of pathways that are triggered by the primary injury and are involved in both damage and recovery include the inflammatory response with the accumulation of cytokines and reactive oxygen species (ROS), excitatory amino acids, eicosanoids, hormones and neurotransmitters. All these mediators are triggered by the injury and have a role in its pathophysiology. In recent years, the concept of opposing responses of injury and healing has emerged, and the role of inflammatory mediators in both processes is emphasized.[4–8] After the initiation of injury, various neurodestructive and neuroprotective genes are expressed. The neurodestructive mediators, such as the inflammatory cytokines and adhesion molecules, or enzymes like metalloproteases, phospholipases, inducible nitric oxide synthase (iNOS) and caspases, can drive brain inflammation to induce cell death either by necrosis or apoptosis. Neuroprotective genes include the neurotrophic and growth factors and anti-inflammatory cytokines that are either brain-derived or infiltrate from the blood. A balance between the anti- and proinflammatory cytokines has been proposed as one of the key factors which controls the life and death of neurons.[9] A shift of balance towards the death signals, e.g. by inhibition of survival signals,

may explain how a cytokine can exert both types of effect. The context of mediators and the interaction between the intracellular signals form the basis for the concept of the intracellular regulation which controls the dual role of cytokines in health and disease.[10]

The proinflammatory cytokine tumor necrosis factor alpha (TNF-α) is produced upon stimulation by monocytes, macrophages, T- and B-lymphocytes, neutrophils and mast cells. Elevated levels of TNF-α (30–40-fold higher than control) were reported in the serum and in the cerebrospinal fluid (CSF) of head-injured patients.[11,12] In the central nervous system, after ischemic or traumatic brain injury TNF-α mRNA is transiently upregulated at the site of injury by neurons, glia, and endothelial cells, and this is followed by induction of TNF-α synthesis.[4,5,13] The cytokine interacts with two high-affinity receptors, R1 (p55) and R2 (p75), and there is conflicting evidence regarding its role in the injured brain. A recent study proposes that regulation between pro- and anti-inflammatory cytokines in the brain occurs at the level of intracellular signaling between heterologous receptors on a single cell.[10]

ACTIVATION OF INFLAMMATORY CYTOKINES AFTER TRAUMATIC BRAIN INJURY

Elevation in rat brain inflammatory cytokines was recorded within 24–48 h after insertion of a microdialysis probe,[14] 3–8 h after fluid percussion,[15–17] or within 1–4 h after closed head injury.[18] The temporal and spatial changes in both TNF-α mRNA and bioactivity indicated that within 1 h of trauma, mRNA expression was markedly enhanced in the contused hemisphere, with only slight alterations contralaterally. The dynamics of the inflammatory response in rat brain were studied following mild contusion, and only delayed (4–6 days), rather than early (4–6 h) expression of TNF-α was observed.[19] Thus, the difference between mild and severe head injury may account for the differences in the temporal profile of TNF-α stimulation. Possibly, the early phase of the post-traumatic inflammatory response is elicited only after severe but not mild trauma. This notion is supported by the findings of Mathiesen et al, who reported that high cytokine levels in the CSF correlated with poor outcome and brain damage in patients suffering subarachnoid hemorrhage.[20]

PHARMACOLOGICAL INHIBITION OF CYTOKINES IS PROTECTIVE IN BRAIN INJURY

TNF-α production is regulated at both transcriptional and translational levels, so a TNF-α mRNA inhibitor such as rolipram (a phosphodiesterase inhibitor) or tyrphostins, which inhibit protein tyrosine kinases, could be used to treat TNF-α-mediated diseases.[21,22] CNI-1493, a tetravalent guanylhydrazone compound that inhibits phosphorylation of p38 mitogen-activated protein (MAP) kinase, has been shown to selectively inhibit TNF-α synthesis.[23,24] This drug, used in cerebral ischemia[25] and trauma (unpublished observations from our laboratory), gave significant cerebroprotection. In our model of closed head injury, we inhibited TNF-α translation (dexanabinol),[18] expression (pentoxyphylline), and activity (TNF-α-binding protein)[26] and demonstrated neuroprotection. Namely, less edema formation and blood–brain barrier disruption were found, along with faster and greater clinical recovery. In addition, the anti-inflammatory cytokine interleukin-10 (IL-10) was used in a model of traumatic brain injury[27] and spinal cord injury.[28] IL-10, when given early (within hours) after injury, inhibited TNF-α production, and improved the clinical outcome.

TNF DEFICIENCY IS DELETERIOUS IN BRAIN INJURY

In contrast to the reports on the beneficial effects of TNF-α inhibition after trauma or ischemia, there are reports showing the opposite effects. TNFR–/– mice were subjected to middle cerebral artery occlusion (MCAO)[29] or to traumatic brain injury[30] and were reported to have greater infarct area at 24 h after the insult. Moreover, these mice were under greater oxidative stress, probably due to their inability to upregulate the antioxidant and neuroprotective enzyme, manganese superoxide dismutase (Mn-SOD). In line with these findings, Stahel et al have also shown in our model of closed head injury (CHI) that TNF/lymphotoxin-α double-knockout mice also suffered higher mortality than their matched wild-type controls during 7 days of recovery after CHI.[31] These authors have analyzed C5aR mRNA and protein expression after CHI, and observed upregulation of both components, mainly on neurons.[32] Whereas intracerebral C5aR expression in the knockout mice remained at low constitutive levels after sham operation, it strongly increased in response to trauma between 24 and 72 h. Interestingly, by 7 days after CHI, the intrathecal C5aR expression was still high in the wild-type animals but was attenuated in the knockout animals. These data show that post-traumatic neuronal expression of C5aR is, at least in part, regulated by TNF and lymphotoxin-α for 7 days after trauma. These findings suggest that C5a-mediated processes are required for brain repair. While the role of C5aR-mediated response after brain injury is not yet fully elucidated, a recent study on C5a-mediated protection from apoptotic neuronal death in a model of intraventricular kainic acid injection in mice supports the present proposed role of C5a in brain recovery.[33]

In a study on the recovery of TNF(–/–) mice after traumatic injury, Scherbel et al proposed a solution to the apparent conflict concerning the role of TNF-α after trauma.[34] They showed that during the first post-trauma days (up to 4 days), the clinical status of the TNF(–/–) mice was better than that of their matched controls, as expected from the pharmacological studies. However, their motor function did not improve from day 1 on, whereas the wild-type mice, who failed in most clinical tests on days 1–4, started to regain function and, by day 7, they performed better in the motor testing, with further improvement up to day 14. A similar biphasic effect was also found when histological changes were analyzed. Support for this notion of the dual, time-dependent role of TNF-α after trauma came from Bethea et al, who studied the effect of TNF-α inhibition on recovery after spinal cord injury. As mentioned above, they treated rats after spinal cord injury with IL-10, an anti-inflammatory cytokine that inhibits the production of TNF-α. When the drug was given within hours after injury, at a single dose, facilitated clinical recovery was evident even at 8 weeks. However, when a second dose of this anti-inflammatory cytokine was given on day 3 after spinal cord injury, the beneficial effect of the first dose at day 1 was completely abolished.[27]

Taken together, the dual effect of TNF-α after brain injury includes the toxic phase, which may last between 1 and 24 h post-injury and can be blocked by inhibitors, and the protective phase, which begins within 2–3 days and lasts for the rest of the recovery period.

SYNERGISM BETWEEN TNF-α AND ROS IN THE EARLY POST-TRAUMATIC PERIOD

The brain is particularly vulnerable to oxidative damage and has efficient antioxidant activity, which includes the antioxidant enzymes (superoxide dismutase (SOD), catalase and peroxidase) and low molecular weight antioxidants (LMWAs). The latter are either synthesized by the cell (glutathione, NAD(P)H, carnosine) or derived from the diet, (ascorbic acid, α-tocopherol, lipoic acid, polyphenols and carotenoids).[35] Following CHI, we have reported dynamic changes in the levels of the endogenous LMWAs, and suggested that they are rapidly consumed, probably due to overproduction of ROS.[36] In addition, we have demonstrated that rats which have been heat-acclimated by exposure to high ambient temperature (30 days at 34°C) respond to CHI with an elevation, rather than a reduction, of brain endogenous LMWAs. Namely, the acclimated rats were able to recruit higher levels of LMWAs after CHI. Heat-acclimated rats were earlier shown to have faster and better recovery from CHI, and to develop less edema and blood–brain barrier disruption, after brain injury.[37] Moreover, we have demonstrated that Tempol, a radical neutralizing agent of the nitroxide family (4-hydroxy-2,2,6,6-tetramethyl-piperidine-1-N-oxyl), has significant beneficial effects on the outcome of CHI. It reduced edema, protected the blood–brain barrier and facilitated functional recovery.[38,39] When the levels of TNF-α were measured after CHI in either the heat-acclimated or the Tempol-treated rats, they were found to be as high as in control, non-treated traumatized rats. However, they displayed better outcome.[40] This observation led us to speculate that high levels of antioxidants, whether of endogenous (as in the acclimated rats) or exogenous (as in Tempol-treated) origin, were able to neutralize the toxic effect of TNF-α. This speculation was supported by our finding that Tempol could attenuate the disruption of the blood–brain barrier which occurred after intracerebral injection of TNF-α.[39]

To try and reconcile the apparent conflicting evidence on the role of TNF-α after brain trauma, and based on our finding on the interaction between antioxidants and TNF-α, we propose that TNF-α activates a 'toxic' signal. This signal probably acts in concert with other mediators[41] such as ROS which accumulate in the brain within minutes after injury. However, at later time points, when the initial TNF-α surge declines and ROS are eliminated, a delayed response, by which low levels of TNF-α activate an 'anti-death' pathway, may contribute to recovery of the injured tissue. At these later time points, the effects of drugs, antibodies or soluble receptors subside and TNF-α can be synthesized, activate its receptors and elicit the cellular response. Thus, the protective mechanisms involved in repair, such as induction of Mn-SOD, regulation of Ca^{2+} influx by actin filaments, expression of Ca^{2+}-binding protein and other actions,[42–44] can be stimulated. Therefore, late inhibition of TNF-α or permanent deletion of TNF-α receptors (as in the knockout mice) are detrimental, and the missing repair phase is expressed as higher rate of mortality, lower rate of recovery and greater area of damage.

To further demonstrate the synergism between TNF and ROS, we studied their combined effect using in vitro models. We have shown that low doses of H_2O_2, which are not capable of causing cell death on their own, synergize with low, non-toxic doses of TNF-α to induce cell death[45] and activation of cellular stress response (unpublished data). We have demonstrated that the mechanism by which this synergism occurs involves inhibition of the nuclear translocation of the p65 subunit of the activated nuclear factor kappa B (NF-κB).[45]

Transcription of many proinflammatory, immune and apoptotic genes, which are induced by TNF-α, is dependent on activation of NF-κB. Kaltschmidt et al proposed that each step of NF-κB activation and DNA binding is redox sensitive,[46] and the final nuclear response to TNF-α and/or ROS depends upon their levels. Taken together, these observations suggest that the point of intersection of TNF-α and ROS after brain insults could be NF-κB, so the nuclear response will be decisive in determining whether the cell will die or survive.

CONCLUSION

The acute inflammatory response of the brain after injury includes the activation of many toxic mediators, among which TNF-α and ROS may cross-talk at the intracellular signaling pathways. A candidate point of convergence is the transcription factor NF-κB, which may signal to induce either pro- or anti-apoptotic genes. Fig. 24.1 summarizes the concept that within the early post-injury period, massive accumulation of ROS and TNF-α

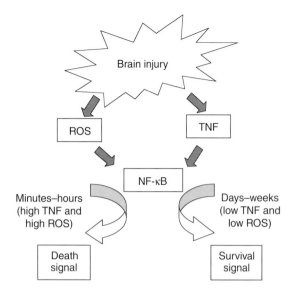

Figure 24.1 A scheme showing the possible checkpoint of cooperation between TNF and ROS. Within the first minutes to hours, interaction of high levels of ROS and high levels of TNF-α with the transcription factor NF-κB shifts the balance of the intracellular signaling towards 'death signals'. At later times, days to weeks, levels of TNF-α and ROS return to normal, and the intracellular signaling is shifted towards 'survival signal'.

lead to their interaction at the death-signaling arm of the TNF-α signal transduction. Therefore, pharmacological inhibition of TNF-α production or activity is protective. However, at later times, ROS are spontaneously neutralized by the endogenous antioxidant system, which includes antioxidant enzymes and low molecular weight compounds. At that time, TNF-α levels return to normal, and this cytokine, acting as a growth factor, is essential for processes of neuronal repair. The intersection of these two mediators could therefore be targeted as a novel therapeutic approach to the treatment of traumatic or ischemic brain injury.

ACKNOWLEDGEMENT

This study was supported by the David R. Bloom Center for Pharmacy, The Hebrew University School of Pharmacy, Jerusalem, Israel.

REFERENCES

1. Waxweiler RJ, Thurman D, Sniezek J, Sosin D, O'Neil J. Monitoring the impact of traumatic brain injury: a review and update. *J Neurotrauma* 1995; **12**: 509–516.

2. McIntosh TK, Smith DH, Meaney DF, Kotapka MJ, Gennarelli TA, Graham DI. Neuropathological sequelae of traumatic brain injury: relationship to neurochemical and biomechanical mechanisms. *Lab Invest* 1966; **74**: 315–342.

3. Siesjo BK, Kristian T, Katsura KI. Overview of bioenergetic failure and metabolic cascades in brain ischemia. In: Ginsberg M, Bogousslavsky J, eds. *Cerebrovascular Disease: Pathophysiology, Diagnosis, and Management*. Malden, MA: Blackwell Science, 1998: 3–13.

4. Rothwell NJ, Hopkins SJ. Cytokines and the nervous system II: action and mechanisms of action. *Trends Neurosci* 1995; **18**: 130–136.

5. Merril JE, Benveniste EN. Cytokines in inflammatory brain lesions: helpful and harmful. *Trends Neurosci* 1996; **19**: 331–338.

6. Barger S. Tumor necrosis factor, the good, the bad and the umbra. In: Mattson MP, ed. *Neuroprotective Signal Transduction*. Totowa, NJ: Humana Press, 1998: 163–183.

7. Munoz-Fernandez M, Fresno M. The role of tumor necrosis factor, interleukin-6, interferon-γ and inducible nitric oxide synthase in the development and pathology of the nervous system. *Prog Neurobiol* 1998; **56**: 307–340.

8. Barone FC, Feuerstein GZ. Inflammatory mediators and stroke: new opportunities for novel therapeutics. *J Cereb Blood Flow Metab* 1999; **19**: 819–834.

9. Venters HD, Tang O, Liu O et al. A new mechanism of neurodegeneration: a proinflammatory cytokine inhibits receptor signaling by a survival peptide. *Proc Natl Acad Sci USA* 1999; **96**: 9879–9884.

10. Venters HD, Dantzer R, Kelley KW. A new concept in neurodegeneration: TNF-α is a silencer of survival signals. *Trends Neurosci* 2000; **23**: 175–183.

11. Goodman JC, Robertson CS, Grossman RG, Narayan RK. Elevation of tumor necrosis factor in head injury. *J Neuroimmunol* 1990; **30**: 213–217.

12. Ross SA, Halliday MI, Campbell GC, Byrnes DP, Rowlands BJ. The presence of tumor necrosis factor in CSF and plasma after severe head injury. *Br J Neurosurg* 1994; **8**: 419–425.

13. Shohami E, Novikov M, Bass R, Yamin A, Gallily R. Closed head injury triggers early production of TNF and IL-6 by brain tissue. *J Cereb Blood Flow Metab* 1994; **14**: 615–619.

14. Woodroofe MN, Sarna GS, Wadhwa M et al. Detection of interleukin-1 and interleukin-6 in adult rat brain, following mechanical injury, by in vivo microdialysis: evidence of a role for microglia in cytokine production. *J Neuroimmunol* 1991; **33**: 227–236.

15. Taupin V, Toulmond S, Serrano A, Benavides J, Zavala F. Increase in IL-6, IL-1 and TNF levels in rat brain following traumatic lesion. Influence of pre- and post-traumatic treatment with Ro5 4864, a peripheral-type (p site) benzodiazepine ligand. *J Neuroimmunol* 1993; **42**: 177–185.

16. Fan L, Young PR, Barone FC, Feuerstein GZ, Smith DH, McIntosh TK. Experimental brain injury induces differential expression of tumor necrosis factor-α mRNA in the CNS. *Mol Brain Res* 1996; **36**: 287–291.

17. Kita T, Liu L, Tanaka N, Kinoshita Y. The expression of tumor necrosis factor-alpha in the rat brain after fluid percussive injury. *Int J Legal Med* 1997; **110**: 305–311.

18. Shohami E, Gallily R, Mechoulam R, Bass R, Ben-Hur T. Cytokine production in the brain following closed head injury: dexanabinol (HU-211) is a novel TNF-α inhibitor

and an effective neuroprotectant. *J Neuroimmunol* 1997; **72**: 169–177.

19. Holmin S, Schalling M, Hojeberg B, Sandberg Nordqvist A-C, Skeftruna A-K, Mathiesen T. Delayed cytokine expression in rat brain following experimental contusion. *J Neurosurg* 1997; **86**: 493–504.

20. Mathiesen T, Edner G, Ulfarsson E, Andersson B. Cerebrospinal fluid interleukin-1 receptor antagonist and tumor necrosis factor-alpha following subarachnoid hemorrhage. *J Neurosurg* 1997; **87**: 215–220.

21. Buttini M, Mir A, Appel K et al. Lipopolysaccharide induces expression of tumour necrosis factor alpha in rat brain: inhibition by methylprednisolone and by rolipram. *Br J Pharmacol* 1997; **122**: 1483–1489.

22. Novogrodsky A, Vanichkin A, Patya M, Gazit A, Osherov N, Levitzki A. Prevention of lipopolysaccharide-induced lethal toxicity by tyrosine kinase inhibitors. *Science* 1994; **264**: 1319–1322.

23. Bianchi M, Bloom O, Raabe T et al. Suppression of proinflammatory cytokines in monocytes by a tetravalent guanylhydrazone. *J Exp Med* 1996; **183**: 927–936.

24. Cohen PM, Nakshatri H, Dennis J et al. CNI-1493 inhibits monocyte/macrophage tumor necrosis factor by suppression of translation efficiency. *Proc Natl Acad Sci USA* 1996; **93**: 3967–3971.

25. Meirstrell 3rd ME, Botchkina GI, Wang H et al. Tumor necrosis factor is a brain damaging cytokine in cerebral ischemia. *Shock* 1997; **8**: 341–348.

26. Shohami E, Bass R, Wallach D, Yamin A, Gallily R. Inhibition of tumor necrosis factor (TNF) activity in rat brain is associated with cerebroprotection after closed head injury. *J Cereb Blood Flow Metab* 1996; **16**: 378–384.

27. Knoblach SM, Faden AI. Interleukin-10 improves outcome and alters proinflammatory cytokine expression after experimental traumatic brain injury. *Exp Neurol* 1998; **153**: 143–151.

28. Bethea JR, Nagashima H, Acosta MC et al. Systemically administered interleukin-10 rescues tumor necrosis factor-alpha production and significantly improves functional recovery following traumatic spinal cord injury in rats. *J Neurotrauma* 1999; **16**: 851–863.

29. Bruce AJ, Boling W, Kindy MS et al. Altered neuronal and microglial responses to excitotoxic and ischemic brain injury in mice lacking TNF receptors. *Nature Med* 1996; **2**: 788–794.

30. Sullivan PG, Bruce-Keller AJ, Rabchevsky AG et al. Exacerbation of damage and altered NF-kappaB activation in mice lacking tumor necrosis factor receptors after traumatic brain injury. *J Neurosci* 1999; **19**: 6248–6256.

31. Stahel PF, Shohami E, Younis FM et al. Experimental closed head injury: analysis of neurological outcome, blood brain barrier dysfunction, intracranial neutrophil infiltration and neuronal cell death in mice deficient in genes for pro-inflammatory cytokines. *J Cereb Blood Flood Metab* 2000; **20**: 369–380.

32. Stahel PF, Kariya K, Shohami E et al. Intracerebral complement C5a receptor (CD88) expression is regulated by TNF and lymphotoxin-α following closed head injury in mice. *J Neuroimmunol* 2000; **109**: 164–172.

33. Osaka H, Mukherjee P, Aisen P, Pasinetti GM. Complement-derived anaphylatoxin C5a protects against glutamate-mediated neurotoxicity. *J Cell Biochem* 1999; **73**: 303–311.

34. Scherbel U, Raghupathi R, Nakamura M et al. Differential acute and chronic responses of tumor necrosis factor-deficient mice to experimental brain injury. *Proc Natl Acad Sci USA* 1999; **96**: 8721–8726.

35. Evans PH. Free radicals in brain metabolism and pathology. *Br Med Bull* 1993; **49**: 577–587

36. Beit-Yannai E, Kohen R, Horowitz M, Trembovler V, Shohami E. Changes in biological reducing activity in rat brain following closed head injury: a cyclic voltammetry study in normal and acclimated rats. *J Cereb Blood Flow Metab* 1997; **17**: 273–279.

37. Shohami E, Novikov M, Horowitz M. Long term exposure to heat protects against brain damage induced by closed head injury in the rat. *Restor Neurol Neurosci* 1994; **6**: 107–112.

38. Zhang R, Shohami E, Beit-Yannai E, Bass R, Trembovler V, Samuni A. Mechanism of brain protection by nitroxide radicals in experimental model of closed head injury. *Free Rad Biol Med* 1998; **24**: 332–340.

39. Beit-Yannai E, Zhang R, Trembovler V, Samuni A, Shohami E. Cerebroprotective effect of stable nitroxide radicals in closed head injury in the rat. *Brain Res* 1996; **717**: 22–28.

40. Trembovler V, Beit-Yannai E, Younis F, Gallily R, Horowitz M, Shohami E. Antioxidants attenuate acute toxicity of tumor necrosis factor α induced by brain injury in rat. *J Interferon Cytokine Res* 1999; **19**: 791–795.

41. Schmidt KN, Amstad P, Cerutti P, Baeuerle PA. The roles of hydrogen peroxide and superoxide as messengers in the activation of transcription factor NF-kappa B. *Chem Biol* 1995; **2**: 13–22.

42. Mattson MP, Barger SW, Furukawa K et al. Cellular signaling role of TGF beta, TNF alpha and beta APP in brain injury responses and Alzheimer's disease. *Brain Res Rev* 1997; **23**: 47–61.

43. Mattson MP. Neuroprotective signal transduction: relevance to stroke. *Neurosci Biobehav Rev* 1997; **21**: 193–206.

44. Wong GH, Elwell JH, Oberlet LW, Goeddel DV. Manganous superoxide dismutase is essential for cellular resistance to cytotoxicity of tumor necrosis factor. *Cell* 1989; **58**: 923–931.

45. Ginis I, Hallenbeck JM, Liu J et al. Tumor necrosis factor and reactive oxygen species cooperative cytotoxicity is mediated via inhibition of NF-kB. *Mol Med* 2000; **6**: 1028–41.

46. Kaltschmidt B, Sparna T, Kaltschmidt C. Activation of NF-κB by reactive oxygen intermediates in nervous system. *Antiox Red Signal* 1999; **1**: 129–144.

25

Protective autoimmunity: is vaccination for neurodegenerative disorders feasible?

Michal Schwartz

INTRODUCTION

Recent work from our laboratory has shown that the spread of damage after a traumatic injury to the central nervous system (CNS) can be slowed down by a controlled adaptive immune response. The immune response is mediated by T-cells directed against a CNS-associated self-antigen, such as myelin basic protein (MBP),[1–3] myelin oligodendrocyte protein (MOG), or proteolipid protein (PLP), or against peptides (with or without encephalitogenic activity) derived from these proteins.[4] T-cells directed against encephalitogenic epitopes were as effective as those directed against cryptic epitopes in displaying neuroprotection,[2,4] indicating that the observed neuroprotection was not related to the virulence of the autoimmune response. The response could be achieved either by active immunization with the relevant proteins or peptides or by passive transfer of T-cells activated by them.[5] On the basis of these findings, we suggested that autoimmune T-cells can protect CNS neurons from the post-injury spread of damage. We further showed that the neuroprotective autoimmunity is not only the result of an experimental manipulation, but is an endogenous response that is stimulated by the damaged neurons, though apparently not strongly enough to be effective (Yoles et al, unpublished results). It thus appears that protective autoimmunity is a physiological mechanism whereby the body attempts to cope with trauma-related nerve damage to the nervous system, but—presumably because of an evolutionary trade-off—the recruited autoimmune response, in its natural state, is neither timely nor effective.[6–8]

The beneficial autoimmunity can, in principle, gain access to the damaged tissue at any time, as even the healthy CNS is permissive to surveillance by T-cells, which (unlike immunoglobulins or macrophages) are not restricted by the blood–brain barrier. We found that T-cells which patrol the CNS accumulate preferentially at sites of injury.[2,9]

NEURODEGENERATIVE DISEASES AND THE IMMUNE SYSTEM

In individuals suffering from a neurodegenerative disease, it is conceivable that at any given time some neurons have already degenerated and died, some are actively undergoing degeneration, and some are still healthy or only marginally damaged but, in the absence of therapeutic intervention, will inevitably succumb to secondary degeneration.[10–13] This progressive spread of damage occurs not only in chronic degenerative diseases, but also after acute traumatic injuries to the CNS, where the functional outcome is often more severe than might be expected from the severity of the injury. Intensive research has therefore been devoted to the problem of progressive degeneration, in an attempt to understand the underlying mechanisms and develop therapies to arrest or retard the spread of damage. Many of these studies employ animal models of acute injury to the optic nerve or spinal cord. Since the spread of damage in neurodegenerative diseases may be viewed as the outcome of a continuous series of acute mini-injuries, findings in the acute injury model are expected to be applicable to chronic syndromes.[14,15]

DEGENERATION IN THE CNS INVOLVES COMMON MEDIATORS OF TOXICITY

One of the compounds responsible for neuronal losses after CNS injury is glutamate, an amino acid which normally serves as a ubiquitous neurotransmitter in brain functions such as learning and memory.[16] When its concentration increases, however, it can become cytotoxic.[17–20] Extracellular glutamate is normally buffered via uptake by astrocytes, and is recycled after being converted to glutamine.[21–23] Under abnormal conditions, caused for example by acute or chronic CNS insults, the local buffering capacity in the CNS is apparently unable to control the inevitable increase in glutamate. Studies in our laboratory have shown that glutamate, when injected intravitreally at different concentrations into rats, exerts a dose-dependent effect on the recruitment of the immune system to counteract the cytotoxicity. This was demonstrated by comparing retinal ganglion cell (RGC) death in normal mice and mice devoid of T-cells (nude mice) from a strain capable of producing a protective T-cell-mediated response (Kipnis et al, unpublished results; Schori et al, unpublished results; Yoles et al, unpublished results). Interestingly, absence of T-cells was correlated with greater neuronal loss.

On the basis of our findings, we suggest that immune neuroprotection may be viewed as a mechanism for the recruitment of a second line of protective activity when the local CNS control mechanism is inadequate. This additional adaptive mechanism might not be specifically evoked by a single potentially toxic compound, but may be a general feature of any compound that has an essential physiological function yet is cytotoxic when present in excessive amounts.

Taken together, our findings in connection with neuroprotective autoimmunity thus appear to ascribe a hitherto unrecognized function to the immune system. Up to now, the adaptive immune response has been viewed as a defensive mechanism that evolved to provide a versatile backup when the innate immune response (involving macrophages) is unequal to the task. Our studies provide evidence that stressful conditions, caused by a pathological increase in potentially toxic compounds (e.g. glutamate), might prove too overwhelming for the nervous system to cope with, and thus alert the adaptive immune system (expressed here by the response to self-antigens) to provide neuroprotective immunity. An inadequate autoimmune response will lead to loss of beneficial autoimmunity and therefore accelerated degeneration, and perhaps also to destructive autoimmunity and hence a predisposition to autoimmune disease.

As all of the above studies were conducted in Lewis rats, a strain susceptible to the development of the paralytic syndrome experimental autoimmune encephalomyelitis (EAE), the results were puzzling in view of our recent finding that beneficial autoimmunity in Lewis rats does not develop spontaneously. First, how can rats that fail to develop a spontaneous beneficial autoimmunity be capable of deriving benefit from immunization that depends on evoking or augmenting such autoimmunity? Second, can we boost the spontaneous beneficial autoimmunity that exists in resistant strains?

It is possible that the autoimmune response evoked by passive transfer or active immunization with myelin-associated antigens requires the participation of multiple cell types, including anti-MBP T-cells and CD4+ regulatory cells. It is also possible that the same T-cell population displays different activities depending on the tissue context, and that in the presence of damaged neuronal tissue (as in the above case of the Lewis rats) such T-cells might exert neuroprotection. This latter possibility obtains some support from the recent finding that neurons can derive benefit from protective substances originating in T-cells, even if the T-cells are encephalitogenic.[24–26] With regard to resistant strains, our data showed, for example, that RAG-1-positive transgenic mice whose genetic background (B10.PL) confers susceptibility to autoimmune disease development, and which overexpress a T-cell receptor to MBP, not only do not develop EAE but also recover better from optic nerve injury than the wild type (Yoles et al, unpublished results). Moreover, recovery from optic nerve injury in rats is better if the insult is preceded about 7–17 days earlier by a spinal cord injury (as mentioned earlier), or if splenocytes withdrawn from spinally injured rats are passively transferred into rats with a newly inflicted spinal contusive injury (caused by dropping a weight onto the laminectomized cord) (Yoles et al, unpublished results). More recently, as discussed below, we found that the outcome of CNS injury was better in SPD rats (an EAE-resistant strain) immunized with MBP, or with spinal cord homogenate emulsified in adjuvant, than in their matched non-immunized controls. Both the antigenic specificity of the evoked physiological response and the phenotype of the cells have yet to be determined.

VACCINATION—A WAY TO EXPLOIT T-CELL-MEDIATED AUTOIMMUNITY FOR THE TREATMENT OF DEGENERATIVE DISEASE

The finding of autoimmune neuroprotection of nerve cell bodies and fibers in the rat optic nerve or spinal cord after mechanical (crush) or biochemical (glutamate) insult leads us to believe that such neuroprotection will prove to be a feature of other degenerative events as well.[27]

We were all taught that vaccination places the immune system on call for action, thus shortening the lag period between invasion of a particular microorganism and recruitment of the specific immune cells needed to fight it. Vaccination is not a preventative measure, in the sense that it does not stop the microorganism from invading, but it endows the individual with protection by making it possible for the immune system to cope promptly and appropriately with the consequences of the invasion. An analogous situation arises when the insult is caused by non-invaders. Just as conventional vaccinations cannot repulse microorganisms or alter the environment which they inhabit, there is no vaccination that will prevent a motor accident or a head trauma from happening—yet here, too, vaccination can ensure speedy recruitment of the immune system by preparing it in advance to protect the individual against the pathological consequences of the trauma. Both types of vaccination are based on eliciting a response by the immune system to the offending stimulus or antigen. When the vaccination is designed to protect the body from invaders, the antigen targeted by the immune response is the invading microorganism itself. When the vaccination is designed to protect the individual from insult-induced endogenous toxicity, the antigen is a self-protein and the reaction elicited is therefore an autoimmune response.

We can thus view the immune system in general as the body's defense mechanism against specific self-antigens. The question is: how can this mechanism be safely exploited? Is there a way to immunize with self-antigens without the risk of introducing an autoimmune disease? And is the therapeutic window wide enough to enable the individual to benefit from immunization performed after the insult?[28] In view of the versatility of the human HLA, it seems unlikely that a self-antigen selected for therapeutic neuroprotection in human patients will be universally safe. One feasible approach might therefore be to use a non-encephalitogenic epitope. Such epitopes exist in any self-antigen. However, since the encephalitogenic property is a function of the specific presentation of the epitope by the antigen-presenting cells, and this presentation is genetically determined by the individual's major histocompatibility complex, selection of a cryptic epitope in one individual does not ensure that it will be cryptic—or even effective—in another individual. An alternative approach, analogous to conventional vaccination using attenuated microorganisms, is to modify the pathogenic self-peptide in a way that renders it non-pathogenic. Another option is to select an antigen that can cross-react with a relevant self-antigen but is known to be completely safe. Peptides of the above two types have been tested for their therapeutic efficacy (via immune deviation or immune suppression) against autoimmune disease. For protective autoimmunity, it is necessary to activate T-cells that will recognize self-epitopes in the damaged CNS, and we therefore tested both types of peptides for their use, not as drugs, but as antigens for vaccination. Each peptide (emulsified in a suitable adjuvant) was administered to the experimental animals, not in repeated doses after the event as in the case of drug treatment, but only once, to evoke an immune response for protective purposes.[29]

Our studies have indicated that autoimmune neuroprotective treatment has a therapeutic window of at least 1 week in the case of spinal cord injury.[5] This window makes it possible to use not only passive T-cell transfer but also vaccination as a therapeutic protocol.[5] In screening the CNS injury-associated proteins for a safe (non-pathogenic) antigen to boost the endogenous response to spinal cord injury, we also examined the post-traumatic effect of peptides which, though originally encephalitogenic, were modified by the replacement of a single amino acid in their T-cell receptor-binding site, a manipulation which attenuated the pathogenic effect. These 'altered peptide ligands' were reported not to cause EAE in susceptible strains even when injected after emulsification in a potent adjuvant such as complete Freund's adjuvant (CFA).[30–33] A single vaccination with such peptides, immediately after spinal cord contusion, exerted a neuroprotective effect, with significant reduction of the injury-induced paralysis in spinally contused rats. It thus appears that it is possible to design a beneficial autoimmunity which, even in susceptible strains, is not accompanied by the risk of autoimmune disease. Recent studies have warned that the therapeutic use of modified peptides for patients with multiple sclerosis may not be safe, as these peptides may, when administered at high dosage to patients predisposed to pathogenic autoimmunity, aggravate the disease as a result of their cross-reactivity with MBP.[32,33] A single injection, however, does not seem to carry any risk. In any case, the ongoing search for a safer peptide may ultimately lead to the development of a safe neuroprotective vaccination for all individuals. Our present results show that both susceptible and resistant strains can benefit from immunization, and that the beneficial effect on neuroprotection is influenced by the choice of both the antigen and the adjuvant.

One non-pathogenic (i.e. safe) peptide that cross-reacts with MBP is copolymer-1 (Cop-1), an FDA-approved drug used as an immunosuppressant in multiple sclerosis. The suppression of disease induction and development by Cop-1 is thought to be the result of Cop-1-mediated suppression of pathogenic T-cells (immune suppression).[34,35] However, recent studies have suggested that immune modulation by bystander suppression rather than by immune suppression might underlie the Cop-1 effect.[34] If the immune response to trauma needs to be modulated in order to achieve immune neuroprotection, such modulation might be mediated by Cop-1-reactive T-cells through bystander suppression, causing a switch in the phenotype of endogenous T-cells towards a protective phenotype.

Passive or active immunization with Cop-1 was shown in our laboratory to lead to significant protection from mechanical insults in the rat optic nerve.[36] We suggest that T-cells reactive to Cop-1 may be activated by cross-recognition with myelin proteins at the site of the injury and consequently act like T-cells reactive to myelin proteins. Alternatively, it is possible that the observed survival of neurons results from Cop-1–mediated modulation of the endogenous immune response. It should be noted that immune neuroprotection with Cop-1 was achieved in both EAE-resistant and EAE-susceptible strains of mice and rats, suggesting that Cop-1 may both boost the beneficial endogenous neuroprotective response that exists in resistant strains and stimulate this response in susceptible strains. Studies in our laboratory have shown that the beneficial autoimmune response to biochemically induced trauma (such as that induced by glutamate insult), like the response evoked by mechanical trauma, is mediated by T-cells and is present in resistant but not in susceptible strains. Accordingly, it should be possible to achieve immune neuroprotection from glutamate insults by boosting or stimulating an endogenous beneficial autoimmune response. Immunization with myelin proteins, however, had no effect on RGC survival when the insult was caused by glutamate toxicity. Thus, even though an adaptive immune response is evoked by both kinds of injuries, it appears that different epitopes might be involved in each case. Since both active and passive immunization with Cop-1 provided efficient neuroprotection in animal models of mechanical and biochemical insults, it might be possible to overcome the problem of antigen specificity among various CNS degenerative disorders by using Cop-1 in order to achieve immune neuroprotection.

Our recent studies have demonstrated that active immunization with Cop-1 immediately after an increase in intraocular pressure in rats results in significant protection from the otherwise inevitable death of RGCs.[29] These findings strongly suggest that it is worth examining the neuroprotective efficacy of Cop-1 vaccination as a therapeutic strategy for different neurodegenerative disorders of the CNS.[37]

SUMMARY

Attempts to halt the spread of damage in cases of traumatic injuries or degenerative diseases of the CNS have not included recruitment of the immune system, on the assumption that immune activity in the CNS, and particularly autoimmune activity, is harmful. Using rat models of injured optic nerve or spinal cord or intraocular glutamate toxicity, we recently showed, however, that neuronal degeneration is affected, at least to some extent, by an insult-induced endogenous protective immunity mediated by autoimmune T-cells. We further showed that this beneficial autoimmunity is genetically controlled and is amenable to boosting. Therapeutic boosting of immunity against self, using suitably modified forms of self-antigens, may be viewed as analogous to conventional vaccination against the invasion of harmful microorganisms using suitably attenuated microbes. Such boosting provides maximal immune-mediated protection with minimal risk of causing an autoimmune disease in the former case, and a microbe-induced disease in the latter. Synthetic peptides that resemble self-antigens but are non-pathogenic may be a useful starting point for the development of neuroprotective anti-self-immunity against acute or chronic degenerative disorders.

REFERENCES

1. Hauben E, Nevo U, Yoles E et al. Autoimmune T-cells as potential neuroprotective therapy for spinal cord injury. *Lancet* 2000; **355**: 286–287.
2. Moalem G, Leibowitz-Amit R, Yoles E, Mor F, Cohen IR, Schwartz M. Autoimmune T-cells protect neurons from secondary degeneration after central nervous system axotomy. *Nature Med* 1999; **5**: 49–55.
3. Moalem G, Yoles E, Leibowitz-Amit R et al. Auto-immune T-cells retard the loss of function in injured rat optic nerves. *J Neuroimmunol* 2000; **106**: 189–197.
4. Fisher J, Yoles E, Levkovitch-Verbin H, Kay JF, Ben-Nun A, Schwartz M. Vaccination for neuroprotection in the mouse optic nerve: implications for optic neuropathies. *J Neurosci* 2000; **21**: 136–142.
5. Hauben E, Butovsky O, Nevo U et al. Passive or active immunization with myelin basic protein promotes recovery from spinal cord contusion. *J Neurosci* 2000; **20**: 6421–6430.

6. Cohen IR, Schwartz M. Autoimmune maintenance and neuroprotection of the central nervous system. *J Neuroimmunol* 1999; **100**: 111–114.

7. Schwartz M, Cohen IR, Lazarov-Spiegler O, Moalem G, Yoles E. The remedy may lie in ourselves: prospects for immune cell therapy in central nervous system protection and repair. *J Mol Med* 1999; **77**: 713–717.

8. Schwartz M, Moalem G, Leibowitz-Amit R, Cohen IR. Innate and adaptive immune responses can be beneficial for CNS repair. *Trends Neurosci* 1999; **22**: 295–299.

9. Schwartz M, Cohen IR. Autoimmunity can benefit self-maintenance. *Immunol Today* 2000; **21**: 265–268.

10. Faden AI, Ivanova SA, Yakovlev AG, Muhkin AG. Neuroprotective effects of group III mGluR in traumatic neuronal injury. *J Neurotrauma* 1997; **14**: 8885–8895.

11. McIntosh TK. Novel pharmacologic therapies in the treatment of experimental traumatic brain injury: a review. *J Neurotrauma* 1993; **10**: 215–261.

12. Povlishock JT, Christman CW. The pathobiology of traumatically induced axonal injury in animals and humans: a review of current thoughts. *J Neurotrauma* 1995; **12**: 555–564.

13. Yoles E, Schwartz M. Degeneration of spared axons following partial white matter lesion: implications for optic nerve neuropathies. *Exp Neurol* 1998; **153**: 1–7.

14. Schwartz M, Belkin M, Yoles E, Solomon A. Potential treatment modalities for glaucomatous neuropathy: neuroprotection and neuroregeneration. *J Glaucoma* 1996; **5**: 427–432.

15. Schwartz M, Yoles E. Neuroprotection: a new treatment modality for glaucoma? *Curr Opin Ophthalmol* 2000; **11**: 107–111.

16. Rose CR, Konnerth A. Self-regulating synapses. *Nature* 2000; **405**: 413–415.

17. Gennarelli TA. Mechanisms of brain injury. *J Emerg Med* 1993; **1**(suppl 1): 5–11.

18. Yoles E, Schwartz M. Elevation of intraocular glutamate levels in rats with partial lesion of the optic nerve. *Arch Ophthalmol* 1998; **116**: 906–910.

19. Mukhin AG, Ivanova SA, Knoblach SM, Faden AI. New in vitro model of traumatic neuronal injury: evaluation of secondary injury and glutamate receptor-mediated neurotoxicity. *J Neurotrauma* 1997; **14**: 651–663.

20. Ikonomidou C, Qin Qin Y, Labruyere J, Olney JW. Motor neuron degeneration induced by excitotoxin agonists has features in common with those seen in the SOD-1 transgenic mouse model of amyotrophic lateral sclerosis. *J Neuropathol Exp Neurol* 1996; **55**: 211–224.

21. Yudkoff M, Daikhin Y, Grunstein L et al. Astrocyte leucine metabolism: significance of branched-chain amino acid transamination. *J Neurochem* 1996; **66**: 378–385.

22. Yudkoff M, Daikhin Y, Nissim I, Grunstein R, Nissim I. Effects of ketone bodies on astrocyte amino acid metabolism. *J Neurochem* 1997; **69**: 682–692.

23. Gritti A, Rosati B, Lecchi M, Vescovi AL, Wanke E. Excitable properties in astrocytes derived from human embryonic CNS stem cells. *Eur J Neurosci* 2000; **12**: 3549–3459.

24. Hammarberg H, Lidman O, Lundberg C et al. Neuroprotection by encephalomyelitis: rescue of mechanically injured neurons and neurotrophin production by CNS-infiltrating T and natural killer cells. *J Neurosci* 2000; **20**: 5283–5291.

25. Hohlfeld R, Toyka KV. Strategies for the modulation of neuroimmunological disease at the level of autoreactive T-lymphocytes. *J Neuroimmunol* 1985; **9**: 193–204.

26. Kerschensteiner M, Gallmeier E, Behrens L et al. Activated human T-cells, B cells, and monocytes produce brain-derived neurotrophic factor in vitro and in inflammatory brain lesions: a neuroprotective role of inflammation? *J Exp Med* 1999; **189**: 865–870.

27. Schwartz M. Autoimmune involvement in CNS trauma is beneficial if well controlled. *Prog Brain Res* 2000; **128**: 259–263.

28. Schwartz M, Kipnis J, Hauben E, Yoles E. Response to trauma is controlled by the immune system: Genetic aspects and prospects for vaccination. *Trends Mol Med* 2001; in press.

29. Schori H, Kipnis J, Yoles E et al. Vaccination for protection of neurons against glutamate cytotoxicity. *Proc Natl Acad Sci USA* 2001; **98**: 3398–403.

30. Vergelli M, Hemmer B, Utz U et al. Differential activation of human autoreactive T-cell clones by altered peptide ligands derived from myelin basic protein peptide (87–99). *Eur J Immunol* 1996; **26**: 2624–2634.

31. Gaur A, Boehme SA, Chalmers D et al. Amelioration of relapsing experimental autoimmune encephalomyelitis with altered myelin basic protein peptides involves different cellular mechanisms. *J Neuroimmunol* 1997; **74**: 149–158.

32. Bielekova B, Goodwin B, Richert N et al. Encephalitogenic potential of the myelin basic protein peptide (amino acids 83–99) in multiple sclerosis: results of a phase II clinical trial with altered peptide ligand. *Nature Med* 2000; **6**: 1167–1175.

33. Kappos L, Comi G, Panitch H et al. Induction of a non-encephalitogenic type 2 T helper-cell autoimmune response in multiple sclerosis after administration of an altered peptide ligand in a placebo-controlled, randomized phase II trial. *Nature Med* 2000; **6**: 1176–1182.

34. Aharoni R, Teitelbaum D, Sela M, Arnon R. Bystander suppression of experimental autoimmune encephalomyelitis by T-cell lines and clones of the Th2 type induced by copolymer 1. *J Neuroimmunol* 1998; **91**: 135–146.

35. Aharoni R, Teitelbaum D, Arnon R, Sela M. Copolymer 1 acts against the immunodominant epitope 82–100 of myelin basic protein by T-cell receptor antagonism in addition to major histocompatibility complex blocking. *Proc Natl Acad Sci USA* 1999; **96**: 634–639.

36. Kipnis J, Yoles E, Porat Z et al. T-cell immunity to copolymer-1 confers neuroprotection on the damaged optic nerve: possible therapy for optic neuropathies. *Proc Natl Acad Sci USA* 2000; **97**: 7446–7451.

37. Schwartz M. Vaccination for T-cell-mediated neuroprotection: dream or reality? *Drug Dev Res* 2000; **50**: 223–225.

26

The molecular biology of blood–brain barrier disruption under stress; the potential involvement of acetylcholinesterase

Hermona Soreq, Daniela Kaufer, Ilan Shelef, Haim Golan, Oren Tomkins, David Glick, Eli Reichenthal and Alon Friedman

INTRODUCTION

The blood–brain barrier (BBB) isolates the brain from the general circulation of the body and thus protects it from harmful xenobiotics. This isolation, however, renders the pharmacological treatment of the brain most difficult, as most drugs cannot enter the brain owing to the existence of the BBB. BBB research addresses multiple clinical questions (Table 26.1), which together utilize powerful techniques for the evaluation of BBB functions in patients (Table 26.2). Answering these questions will have practical clinical benefits that justify these efforts (Table 26.3).

Numerous diseases have been reported to involve perturbations in BBB integrity (Table 26.4). Based on this information, it appears that both carriers of mutations that induce BBB disruption and individuals exposed to BBB-disrupting insults may be at risk for malfunctions of the BBB (Table 26.5).

Table 26.1 Leading questions, research approaches and practical applications related to BBB control

(1) What is the scope of pathological conditions under which BBB integrity is compromised?
(2) What is the space and time resolution for disruption of the BBB in specific brain subregions?
(3) Does the extent of BBB disruption vary with the disease?
(4) Which clinical conditions predict BBB disruption?

Table 26.2 Methods for evaluation of BBB function in humans

(1) Computerized tomography[14]
(2) Avoidance of undesired brain penetrance by a drug
(3) Single photon emission CT[16]
(4) Cerebrospinal fluid analyses[17]

Table 26.3 Potential applications of BBB control

(1) Rationalized drug delivery to the brain
(2) Avoidance of brain penetrance by a drug when undesired
(3) Adaptation of drug dosage according to BBB permeability

Table 26.4 Examples of reported perturbations in BBB integrity

Seizures, status epilepticus[18]
Cerebrovascular disorders[19]
Multiple sclerosis[20]
Brain tumors[21]
Alzheimer's disease[10]
Vascular dementia[5]
Acute psychological stress[5]
Hypoxia/glycemia[22]
Infectious diseases of the meninges and brain[23]
Head trauma[24]

Table 26.5   Who may be at risk?
Carriers of mutations that induce BBB disruption
Hyperactive NO synthase[23]
Malfunctioning mdr1a[25]
'Atypical' butyrylcholinesterase[26]
abnormal glutathione transferase[27]
Individuals exposed to BBB-disrupting insults
Lead batteries[28]
Organophosphate insecticides[29]
Acute psychological stress[1]

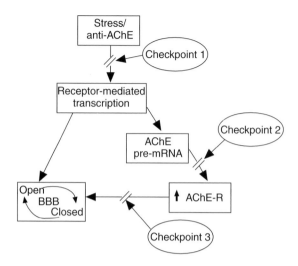

Figure 26.1   Sites of interaction of the cholinergic system with the BBB. Stress or anticholinesterases induce muscarinic receptor-mediated transcriptional responses, which are subject to interruption at checkpoint 1 by muscarinic blockers.[18,38] The transcriptional response involves a shift in pre-mRNA splicing (checkpoint 2) which leads to AChE-R accumulation.[14,15] The BBB is hypothesized to exist in two states, open and closed, i.e. permeable and impermeable. The balance between these states is tilted by AChE-R, the stress-related variant of acetylcholinesterase[1] (checkpoint 3).

Using various imaging techniques, we have recently observed that the cerebral cortex is particularly vulnerable to BBB disruption (Friedman et al, unpublished). This may be due to the physiological properties unique to cerebral cortex microvasculature (Table 26.6), and can lead to deleterious consequences, including changes in neuronal excitability, epileptic synchronized activity, consequent neuronal toxicity and even neurodegenerative disease (Table 26.7).

A dynamic balance of 'open' and 'closed' states of the BBB, affected by stress,[1] exposure to environmental anticholinesterases[2] and changes in acetylcholinesterase (AChE) gene expression, is a useful

Table 26.6   Properties unique to cerebral cortex microvasculature
(1) Mechanism(s) that control bloodflow[30]
(2) Astrocyte endfoot muscarinic receptors[3,31]
(3) Afferent cholinergic innervation[32,33]

Table 26.7   Possible deleterious consequences of cortical BBB disruption
(1) Hyperexcitation of cortical neurons due to extracellular ionic changes[34]
(2) Development of synchronous epileptic activity[35]
(3) Neuronal/excitotoxic damage[36]
(4) Consequent neuronal death[37]
(5) Neurodegeneration[27]

working model for understanding its control and for proposing central nervous system (CNS) therapeutic interventions. Shortly after stress or exposure to anticholinesterases, there is a drastic upregulation of the expression of the 'readthrough' variant, AChE-R; and both acute psychological stress and anticholinesterase exposure cause BBB disruption. Moreover, AChE shares sequence homology and morphogenic functions with *Drosophila* proteins that are essential for the integrity of the hemolymph–neuron barrier, the insect homolog of the BBB. Therefore, we suggest that AChE-R is causally involved in maintenance of non-catalytic function(s), associated with the dynamic equilibrium of BBB integrity. Fig. 26.1 presents this hypothesis in a flow-chart scheme, highlighting three specific checkpoints in AChE regulation: transcriptional enhancement, alternative splicing and protein activity.

THE PHYSICAL ELEMENTS OF THE BBB

Separation of the brain from the peripheral blood serves to protect this most sensitive and crucial organ from various insidious agents that circulate in the blood. Conversely, this separation must allow for the nutrition of the brain and the removal from it of waste products and/or xenobiotics. The existence of a physical barrier that separates the brain tissue from the general circulation was first proposed 100 years ago by Ehrlich. This study was based on injection of a series of dyes into laboratory animals that resulted in uncolored brains, as opposed to highly stained visceral organs (review: Pardridge[3]). The BBB develops during the late embryonic and early postnatal period. Physically, the BBB is an endothelial barrier present in the capillaries throughout the brain. BBB properties are contact-influenced by neighboring astrocytes (review: Rubin and Staddon[4]). Electron microscopic studies reveal two major properties that distinguish brain endothelial cells from their peripheral relatives. First, they contain lower amounts of endocytic vesicles; this implies limited transport by endocytosis. Second, the space between adjacent cells is sealed by tight junctions. Added to the ubiquitously present gap junctions, these structures restrict intercellular flux. These features enable the formation of a barrier that hinders the entry of most xenobiotics into the brain. Moreover, it is actively involved in exporting such substances from the brain when they do enter it. The diffusion-based brain penetration of different substances is determined by their chemical properties: small lipophilic molecules enter the brain fairly freely, but hydrophilic molecules are mostly restricted and can enter only via active transport. Specific transporters exist, therefore, for required nutrients such as glucose, L-DOPA, and certain amino acids (reviewed: Pardridge[3]). We have shown that acute psychological stress causes disruption of the BBB[5] and induces accumulation of AChE-R, a normally rare variant (R) of the AChE.[1] The role of AChE-R as an instrument of BBB integrity may imply that its regulation can assist in the control of BBB functioning. Fig. 26.2 presents a schematic drawing of a section through a brain microvessel that is part of the BBB with AChE-R as its potential modulator.

DROSOPHILA GENETICS SUGGESTS AN INVOLVEMENT OF AChE IN BBB FUNCTIONING

For nearly a century, the fruit fly *Drosophila melanogaster* has served as a model for genetic studies. With the introduction of genetic engineering and genomic databases, this has also become a powerful tool for the discovery of genes and gene products that participate in physiological functions.

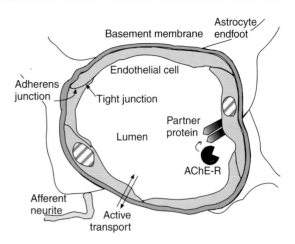

Figure 26.2 The physical components of the BBB. Throughout the mammalian brain, blood vessels and microvessels transverse the brain tissue, bringing in essential compounds from the periphery and removing metabolic end-products and xenobiotics. The three layers surrounding the microvessel lumen comprise the BBB. These include endothelial cells lining the blood vessels as the innermost layer. A basement membrane surrounding them comprises the second layer, and astrocyte endfeet separating these structures create the third. Certain neurons interact with astrocytes through contacting neurites. Two types of intercellular junction cement endothelial cells to each other. These are the tight and adherens junctions.[39] Trans-cellular active transport (parallel arrows) allows the movement of molecules across the BBB. Under stress, AChE-R is produced by depolarized neurons,[1] and it is secreted from cultured endothelial cells (H. Perry, personal communication), where it presumably interacts with as yet unidentified partner protein(s). This potentially affects BBB integrity.

The identification of a physiological defect in the insect can be quickly traced to a specific gene, and the homologous sequence in the mammalian genome can then be identified. There it can serve as a candidate gene for the similar function in the mammal. For instance, a defect in the hemolymph–neuron barrier, which has a function analogous to the BBB in mammals, was shown to depend on the structural and functional integrity of the special septate junctions which seal this barrier in insect larva.[6–8] Disruption of these structures by genomic destruction of either of three different genes, neurexin IV, gliotactin and the multi-PDZ domain protein, disk lost (*dlt*), causes severe neuronal toxicity due to exposure to the high concentrations of K[+] in the hemolymph. This leads to paralysis and death of the developing insect larva.

Such genomic disruption also impaired the subcellular targeting of coracle, a band 4.1 homolog that transduces signals from the cell membrane to the cytoskeleton. Therefore, one may assume that gene homologs sharing sequence with gliotactin, neuroexin, *dlt* and band 4.1 may be involved with the development and/or maintenance of BBB functions.

Gliotactin is one of several structural homologs of the acetylcholine-hydrolyzing enzyme, AChE, that were discovered in the last decade. Like the other AChE homologs, it has no capacity for acetylcholine hydrolysis. However, gliotactin has the capacity to signal into the intracellular space through its interaction with PDZ domain proteins, which serve as intracellular anchors linking membrane proteins to the cytoskeleton. In the extracellular milieu, gliotactin interacts with a homolog of neurexins, neuronal membrane proteins, which also transduce signals into the cytoplasm through PDZ domain proteins.[9]

AChE has been shown to substitute for its structural homologs and complement their action, or compete with them in cell–cell interactions.[5,10] Transgenic mice overexpressing AChE display altered

regulation of neurexin gene expression, suggesting a compensation mechanism and functional linkage for this protein, too.[11]. Finally, the expression of a band 4.1 homolog, designated nitzin, was elevated in cultured pheochromocytoma cells deprived of AChE by antisense transfection.[12] Therefore, all of the insect genes involved in barrier maintenance may do so also in mammals.

The potential involvement of AChE has raised the question which of the three AChE variants, formed by alternative splicing of the human *ACHE* pre-mRNA, is in fact involved in regulating BBB functioning. These variants include AChE-S, the synaptic form, AChE-E, the erythrocyte form, and AChE-R, a soluble monomeric form.[13] Perhaps significantly for BBB physiology, AChE-R has been shown to be overexpressed under stress and anticholinesterase exposure,[14,15] both of which also induce BBB disruption. Fig. 26.3 demonstrates accumulation of catalytically active AChE around a microvessel of a mouse brain, following confined swim stress. This analysis places active AChE in close proximity to BBB elements and supports our hypothesis of AChE's involvement with BBB functioning. Disruption of the BBB under both

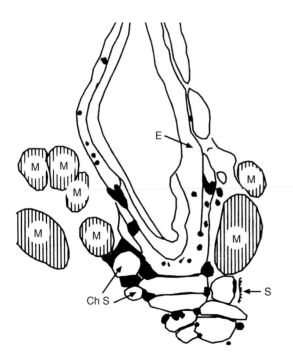
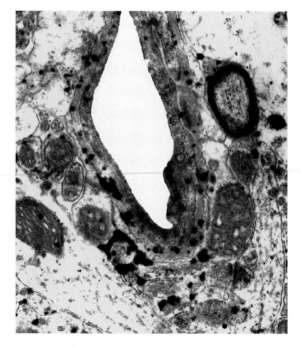

Figure 26.3 Electronmicrograph of a mouse brain microvessel stained for AChE catalytic activity following confined swim. Methodology was as in ref 11. Important features are endothelial cells (E), mitochondria (M), apparently non-cholinergic synapse (S) and cholinergic synapses (Ch S) surrounded by electron-dense regions that have been stained by the Karnovsky method[40] for the product of AChE activity.

anticholinesterase exposure and acute psychological stress may, therefore, reflect this functional involvement.

ACKNOWLEDGEMENTS

This work was supported by the Israel Science Foundation (590/97, to H.S.), the US Army Medical Research and Materiel Command (DAMD17-99-1-9483, to H.S. and A.F.) and Ester Neuroscience, Ltd.

REFERENCES

1. Kaufer D, Friedman A, Seidman S, Soreq H. Acute stress facilitates long-lasting changes in cholinergic gene expression. *Nature* 1998; **393**: 373–377.
2. Kaufer D, Friedman A, Seidman S, Soreq H. Anticholinesterases induce multigenic transcriptional feedback response suppressing cholinergic neurotransmission. *Chem Biol Interact* 1999; **119–120**: 349–360.
3. Pardridge WM. CNS drug design based on principles of blood–brain barrier transport. *J Neurochem* 1998; **70**: 1781–1792.
4. Rubin LL, Staddon JM. The cell biology of the blood–brain barrier. *Annu Rev Neurosci* 1999; **22**: 11–28.
5. Friedman A, Kaufer D, Shemer J, Hendler I, Soreq H, Tur-Kaspa I. Pyridostigmine brain penetration under stress enhances neuronal excitability and induces early immediate transcriptional response. *Nature Med* 1996; **2**: 1382–1385.
6. Auld VJ, Fetter RD, Broadie K, Goodman CS. Gliotactin, a novel transmembrane protein on peripheral glia, is required to form the blood–nerve barrier in Drosophila. *Cell* 1995; **81**: 757–767.
7. Baumgartner S, Littleton JT, Broadie K et al. A Drosophila neurexin is required for septate junction and blood–nerve barrier formation and function. *Cell* 1996; **87**: 1059–1068.
8. Bhat MA, Izaddoost S, Lu Y, Cho KO, Choi KW, Bellen HJ. Discs Lost, a novel multi-PDZ domain protein, establishes and maintains epithelial polarity. *Cell* 1999; **96**: 833–845.
9. Ichtchenko K, Nguyen T, Sudhof TC. Structures, alternative splicing, and neurexin binding of multiple neuroligins. *J Biol Chem* 1996; **271**: 2676–2682.
10. Skoog I, Wallin A, Fredman P et al. A population study on blood–brain barrier function in 85-year-olds: relation to Alzheimer's disease and vascular dementia. *Neurology* 1998; **50**: 966–971.
11. Andres C, Beeri R, Friedman A et al. Acetylcholinesterase-transgenic mice display embryonic modulations in spinal cord choline acetyltransferase and neurexin Ibeta gene expression followed by late-onset neuromotor deterioration. *Proc Natl Acad Sci USA* 1997; **94**: 8173–8178.
12. Grifman M, Galyam N, Seidman S, Soreq H. Functional redundancy of acetylcholinesterase and neuroligin in mammalian neuritogenesis. *Proc Natl Acad Sci USA* 1998; **95**: 13935–13940.
13. Grisaru D, Sternfeld M, Eldor A, Glick D, Soreq H. Structural roles of acetylcholinesterase variants in biology and pathology. *Eur J Biochem* 1999; **264**: 672–686.
14. Roman-Goldstein S, Clunie DA, Stevens J et al. Osmotic blood–brain barrier disruption: CT and radionuclide imaging. *AJNR Am J Neuroradiol* 1994; **15**: 581–590.
15. Merten CL, Knitelius HO, Assheuer J, Bergmann-Kurz B, Hedde JP, Bewermeyer H. MRI of acute cerebral infarcts, increased contrast enhancement with continuous infusion of gadolinium. *Neuroradiology* 1999; **41**: 242–248.
16. Ostergaard L, Hochberg FH, Rabinov JD et al. Early changes measured by magnetic resonance imaging in cerebral blood flow, blood volume, and blood–brain barrier permeability following dexamethasone treatment in patients with brain tumors. *J Neurosurg* 1999; **90**: 300–305.
17. Correale J, Rabinowicz AL, Heck CN, Smith TD, Loskota WJ, DeGiorgio CM. Status epilepticus increases CSF levels of neuron-specific enolase and alters the blood–brain barrier. *Neurology* 1998; **50**: 1388–1391.
18. Cornford EM, Oldendorf WH. Epilepsy and the blood–brain barrier. *Adv Neurol* 1986; **44**: 787–812.
19. Klatzo I. Disturbances of the blood–brain barrier in cerebrovascular disorders. *Acta Neuropathol Suppl* 1983; **8**: 81–88.
20. Larsson HB, Stubgaard M, Frederiksen JL, Jensen M, Henriksen O, Paulson OB. Quantitation of blood–brain barrier defect by magnetic resonance imaging and gadolinium-DTPA in patients with multiple sclerosis and brain tumors. *Magn Reson Med* 1990; **16**: 117–131.
21. Akeson P, Larsson EM, Kristoffersen DT, Jonsson E, Holtas S. Brain metastases—comparison of gadodiamide injection-enhanced MR imaging at standard and high dose, contrast-enhanced CT and non-contrast-enhanced MR imaging. *Acta Radiol* 1995; **36**: 300–306.
22. Abbruscato TJ, Davis TP. Protein expression of brain endothelial cell E-cadherin after hypoxia/aglycemia: influence of astrocyte contact. *Brain Res* 1999; **842**: 277–286.
23. Boje KM. Inhibition of nitric oxide synthase attenuates blood–brain barrier disruption during experimental meningitis. *Brain Res* 1996; **720**: 75–83.
24. Shohami E, Kaufer D, Chen Y et al. Antisense prevention of neuronal damages following head injury in mice. *J Mol Med* 2000; **78**: 228–236.
25. Meijer OC, de Lange EC, Breimer DD, de Boer AG, Workel JO, de Kloet ER. Penetration of dexamethasone into brain glucocorticoid targets is enhanced in mdr1A P-glycoprotein knockout mice. *Endocrinology* 1998; **139**: 1789–1793.
26. Loewenstein Lichtenstein Y, Schwarz M, Glick D, Norgaard Pedersen B, Zakut H, Soreq H. Genetic predisposition to adverse consequences of anticholinesterases in 'atypical' BCHE carriers. *Nat Med* 1995; **1**: 1082–1085.
27. Menegon A, Board PG, Blackburn AC, Mellick GD, Le Couteur DG. Parkinson's disease, pesticides, and glutathione transferase polymorphisms. *Lancet* 1998; **352**: 1344–1346.
28. Kuhn W, Winkel R, Woitalla D, Meves S, Przuntek H, Muller T. High prevalence of parkinsonism after occupational exposure to lead-sulfate batteries. *Neurology* 1998; **50**: 1885–1886.
29. Senanayake N, Sanmuganathan PS. Extrapyramidal manifestations complicating organophosphorus insecticide poisoning. *Hum Exp Toxicol* 1995; **14**: 600–604.
30. Inanami O, Ohno K, Sato A. Responses of regional cerebral blood flow to intravenous administration of

thyrotropin releasing hormone in aged rats. *Neurosci Lett* 1992; **143**: 151–154.

31. Friedman A, Kaufer D, Pavlovsky L, Soreq H. Cholinergic excitation induces activity-dependent electrophysiological and transcriptional responses in hippocampal slices. *J Physiol Paris* 1998; **92**: 329–335.

32. Estrada C, Hamel E, Krause DN. Biochemical evidence for cholinergic innervation of intracerebral blood vessels. *Brain Res* 1983; **266**: 261–270.

33. Triguero D, Lopez de Pablo AL, Gomez B, Estrada C. Regional differences in cerebrovascular cholinergic innervation in goats. *Stroke* 1988; **19**: 736–740.

34. Schwartzkroin PA, Baraban SC, Hochman DW. Osmolarity, ionic flux, and changes in brain excitability. *Epilepsy Res* 1998; **32**: 275–285.

35. Jefferys JG. Mechanisms and experimental models of seizure generation. *Curr Opin Neurol* 1998; **11**: 123–127.

36. Kadota E, Nonaka K, Karasuno M, Nishi K, Teramura K, Hashimoto S. Neurotoxicity of serum components, comparison between CA1 and striatum. *Acta Neurochir Suppl* 1997; **70**: 141–143.

37. Charriaut-Marlangue C, Aggoun-Zouaoui D, Represa A, Ben-Ari Y. Apoptotic features of selective neuronal death in ischemia, epilepsy and gp 120 toxicity. *Trends Neurosci* 1996; **19**: 109–114.

38. Darboux I, Barthalay Y, Piovant M, Hipeau Jacquotte R. The structure–function relationships in Drosophila neurotactin show that cholinesterasic domains may have adhesive properties. *EMBO J* 1996; **15**: 4835–4843.

39. Soreq H, Glick D. Novel roles for cholinesterases in stress and inhibitor responses. In: Giacobini E, ed. *Cholinesterases and Cholinesterase Inhibitors: Basic, Preclinical and Clinical Aspects*. London: Martin Dunitz, 2000: 47–61.

40. Karnovsky MJ, Roots L. 'Direct coloring' thiocholine method for cholinesterase. *J Histochem Cytochem* 1964; **12**: 219–221.

Part 4

Treatment of epilepsy and paroxysmal syndromes

27

Clinically important interactions involving new antiepileptic drugs

Yitzhak Schiller

Epilepsy is a common disease with a prevalence of about 1%, and a lifetime incidence of 2–3%.[1–2] Patients with epilepsy experience recurrent unprovoked seizures. There are multiple subtypes of epileptic seizures, which vary substantially in their clinical manifestations.[3,4] The common feature unifying epileptic seizures is their underlying pathophysiological basis. All epileptic seizures result from hypersynchronized increased electrical activity in cortical neurons.[5]

The treatment of choice for epilepsy is antiepileptic drugs. Patients with epilepsy are found in one of two states. Patients spend the vast majority of their time in the interictal state, in which no or almost no symptoms are experienced. For a small minority of their time (usually less than 0.01% of the total timespan), they are in the symptomatic ictal state of epileptic seizures. All drugs exert their antiepileptic effect by eliminating the transition from the asymptomatic interictal state to the symptomatic ictal state (and hence eliminate seizure initiation). In addition, once seizures are initiated, antiepileptic drugs can shorten their duration, and restrict the propagation of seizure activity from the epileptogenic zone. Presently, we have no drugs at our disposal that influence the underlying pathological processes causing seizures.

Antiepileptic drugs are subdivided into old and new drugs. The old antiepileptic drugs, which include phenobarbital and primidone, phenytoin, ethosuxamide, carbamazepine, valproate and benzodiazepines, had been progressively introduced for clinical use during the first seven decades of the 20th century, and revolutionized the treatment of epilepsy. However, approximately 50% of patients treated with old antiepileptic drugs did not achieve adequate control, because of either recurrent seizures or significant drug-related side-effects.

During the last decade, about 10 new antiepileptic drugs have been developed and introduced for clinical use. The new antiepileptic drugs have improved the treatment of epilepsy in several respects. First, they improve seizure control in patients, who continue to experience seizures despite treatment with old antiepileptic drugs.[6,8] Second, new antiepileptic drugs have an improved side-effect profile. Several double-blind controlled studies have shown that patients receiving new antiepileptic drugs experience fewer side-effects than patients treated with old antiepileptic drugs.[9–10] Third, new antiepileptic drugs have significantly less interactions with other drugs. In contrast, old antiepileptic drugs are notorious for their drug interactions, including significant interactions with other antiepileptic drugs. For example, phenytoin decreases the levels of carbamazepine, oral contraceptives, valproate, warfarin and many other medications that are metabolized in the liver.[11]

In the following section, I will briefly describe each of the new antiepileptic drugs, and discuss clinically significant interactions of each of these drugs with other medications in general and other antiepileptic drugs in particular.

VIGABATRIN

Vigabatrin was the first new antiepileptic drug introduced for use in the late 1980s. The use of vigabatrin has dramatically declined in recent years, following the detection of vigabatrin-induced visual field defects in 30–40% of patients. Vigabatrin exerts its antiepileptic action by inhibiting the enzyme gamma-aminobutyric acid (GABA) transaminase, which is the rate-limiting enzyme in the catabolism of GABA. Vigabatrin is rapidly and almost completely absorbed from the gastrointestinal tract, and is only minimally bound to plasma proteins (5%). The drug is cleared through the kidneys without being metabolized. The plasma half-life of vigabatrin is approximately 6 h. However, as vigabatrin binds to the enzyme GABA transaminase irreversibly, it has a much longer biological life. Regarding the clinical spectrum of vigabatrin, it is used as an add-on drug for intractable partial epilepsy. In addition, it has a special role in treating children with infantile spasm. The dose of vigabatrin used in clinical practice is 1000–3000 mg/day in two divided doses.[12–16]

Drug interactions

Vigabatrin is excreted through the urine unmetabolized, and is only minimally bound to plasma proteins. As such, vigabatrin has to date no known interactions with other drugs, including other antiepileptic drugs. The only known exception is a possible small (up to 20%) reduction of the phenytoin plasma levels reported to occur in some patients.[15,17,18]

FELBAMATE

Felbamate was the first new antiepileptic drug to be approved in the USA in 1993. Felbamate is an effective add-on drug for the treatment of intractable partial epilepsy, and was the first drug to show effectiveness in treating children with Lennox–Gastaut syndrome. Since 1994, the use of felbamate has been limited because of the appearance of potentially fatal adverse events of aplastic anemia and severe hepatotoxicity. The mechanism underlying the antiepileptic effect of felbamate probably combines enhancement of the GABA inhibitory response and partial blockade of the N-methyl-D-aspartate (NMDA) glutamate receptors. Felbamate has a high bioavailability (> 90%), and low plasma protein binding (25%). The drug is metabolized in the liver, in part via the cytochrome P450 pathway. Its plasma half-life is about 14–24 h. Felbamate is usually administered in doses of 2400–3600 mg/day in three or four divided doses.[13,16,19,20]

Drug interactions

Felbamate has relatively numerous drug interactions. Drugs that induce hepatic cytochrome P450 enzymes, such as carbamazepine, phenytoin and phenobarbital, increase the clearance of felbamate, and reduce its plasma concentration. In turn, felbamate can induce the enzymes of the hepatic cytochrome P450 system. Hence felbamate increases the clearance of oral contraceptives, and reduces their plasma levels. In addition, it elevates the plasma concentrations of carbamazepine, phenytoin and valproate, probably by inhibiting their hepatic metabolism. To date, no significant interactions between felbamate and lamotrigine, clonazepam, vigabatrin and oxcarbazepine have been described.[17,19,21,22]

GABAPENTIN

Gabapentin is a new antiepileptic drug with an unknown mechanism of action. It is absorbed in the gastrointestinal tract through an active transport system. Thus, the bioavailability of the drug decreases with increasing doses. As a result, there is no additional benefit in increasing the daily dose of gabapentin above 4800–6400 mg. Once in the blood, only a small fraction of the drug is bound to plasma proteins (< 5%). Gabapentin is cleared through the kidneys without being metabolized. Its plasma half-life is approximately 6 h. Gabapentin has been shown to be effective in partial epilepsy as add-on therapy or monotherapy. The usual dose of gabapentin is 900–3600 mg/day in three or four divided doses.[13,16,22–23]

Drug interactions

Gabapentin has no known clinically significant interactions with other medications, including other antiepileptic drugs.[16–18,24] Gabapentin has a special role in the treatment of epilepsy in the elderly population, and in patients receiving multiple medications, owing to its benign side-effect profile and lack of drug interactions.

LAMOTRIGINE

Lamotrigine is a new antiepileptic drug that probably exerts its antiepileptic effect via use-dependent blockade of voltage-gated sodium channels. Lamotrigine is almost completely absorbed from the gastrointestinal tract (bioavailibility of 98%). Once in the blood, 55% of the drug is bound to plasma proteins. Lamotrigine is cleared by hepatic metabolism, and its half-life is approximately 24–35 h. Lamotrigine has a wide clinical spectrum of efficacy. It is effective in the treatment of partial and generalized epilepsy, including children with Lennox–Gastaut syndrome. In addition, it is used in both adults and children, and can be administered as either add-on therapy or monotherapy. The usual doses of lamotrigine are 100–600 mg/day in two divided doses.[5,9,10,13,15,16,25–27]

Drug interactions

Compared to most other new antiepileptic drugs, lamotrigine has relatively more interactions with other drugs. The most noticeable interaction is with the old antiepileptic drug valproate. Co-administration of valproate approximately doubles the half-life of lamotrigine from 24–35 h to 48–60 h; hence if valproate and lamotrigine are co-administered, dose modifications of the latter are required. Hepatic enzyme-inducing drugs such as phenytoin, phenobarbital and carbamazepine speed the clearance of lamotrigine and reduce its plasma half-life to approximately half of its original value (12 h). Lamotrigine has only minimal effects on other drugs. The exception to the rule is valproate. Lamotrigine slightly reduces valproate plasma levels (up to a 25% reduction). Lamotrigine does not alter the plasma levels of oral contraceptives or other antiepileptic drugs, except valproate.[15,16,22,25–29]

In addition to pharmacokinetic interactions, there are pharmacodynamic interactions between lamotrigine and other antiepileptic drugs. Addition of lamotrigine to carbamazepine results in increased toxicity, probably due to pharmacodynamic interactions between the two antiepileptic drugs.[30]

TOPIRAMATE

Topiramate is a sulfate-substituted monosaccharide. Its antiepileptic mechanism is mediated by multiple mechanisms, including enhancement of GABA-mediated inhibition, interference with the activity of voltage-gated sodium channels, and partial blockade of AMPA glutamate receptors. Topiramate has a high bioavailability, and low plasma protein binding (10–15%). The drug is cleared mostly (50–80%) via the kidneys without being metabolized. However, some topiramate is cleared via hepatic metabolism as well. In the presence of other hepatic enzyme inducer drugs, the relative contributions of the renal and hepatic clearance routes change, and a larger fraction of topiramate is cleared via the liver. The half-life of the drug given in isolation is 20–25 h. Clearance of topiramate is age-dependent, being higher in children than in adults. Topiramate has a wide clinical spectrum of efficacy. It is efficient in the treatment of partial and generalized epilepsy, including Lennox–Gastaut syndrome. Topiramate has been shown to be effective in the adult and pediatric population, and is proven for add-on drug therapy in intractable epilepsy. In addition, recent studies indicate that topiramate is probably effective as first-line monotherapy for newly diagnosed epilepsy as well. The doses used in clinical practice range from 100–600 mg/day in two divided doses.[8,13,15,22,32–34]

Drug interactions

Topiramate has several interactions with other drugs. Hepatic enzyme-inducing drugs such as phenytoin, phenobarbital and carbamazepine increase the hepatic clearance of topiramate, and hence shorten its half-life by up to 50%. Topiramate can slightly increase phenytoin and haloperidol levels owing to inhibition of their hepatic metabolism. In addition topiramate decreases the plasma levels of oral contraceptives.[15,16,18,22,24,32–35]

TIAGABINE

Tiagabine is a new antiepileptic drug that increases the GABA concentration in the central nervous system by inhibiting GABA reuptake. Tiagabine is rapidly absorbed in the gastrointestinal tract, and has a high bioavailability (90%). In contrast to other new antiepileptic drugs, a large fraction of tiagabine in the blood is bound to plasma proteins (approximately 95%). Tiagabine is eliminated in the liver by oxidative metabolism, and has a plasma half-life of 6–9 h.[15–16,36] However, for unknown reasons, the clinical effect of tiagabine lasts much longer than expected solely from its plasma half-life. Tiagabine is used as add-on therapy for intractable partial epilepsy. In addition, it is probably effective as monotherapy for partial epilepsy and in the pediatric population as well.[13,16,36] The commonly used dosage of tiagabine is 15–56 mg/day divided into three or four doses.[37]

Drug interactions

Tiagabine is not known to affect the levels of any other drugs, including other antiepileptic drugs, warfarin, digoxin, cimetidine and oral contraceptives. In addition, despite its high protein binding, it does not significantly displace other antiepileptic drugs from the plasma proteins. In contrast, hepatic enzyme-inducing drugs such as carbamazepine, phenytoin and phenobarbital increase the clearance of tiagabine, and hence reduce its plasma half-life by 40–50%.[15,16,18,22,36]

OXCARBAZEPINE

Oxcarbazepine is a new antiepileptic drug structurally related to the old antiepileptic drug carbamazepine. The antiepileptic effect of oxcarbazepine is probably mediated by blockade of voltage-gated sodium channels. Oxcarbazepine is rapidly absorbed into the bloodstream, and is converted to the active metabolite 10-monohydroxy metabolite (MHD) in the liver. Thirty to forty percent of both active substances are bound to plasma protein. The half-life of oxcarbazepine and its active metabolite MHD is 10–14 h. Oxcarbazepine and MHD are metabolized in the liver. In contrast to carbamazepine, cytochrome P450 is not involved in the process. In addition, a smaller proportion of the MHD is cleared via the kidneys. The metabolism of oxcarbazepine does not produce an epoxide derivative, which is responsible for many of the side-effects of carbamazepine. As a result, oxcarbazepine is much better tolerated than the structurally related old antiepileptic drug carbamazepine. Oxcarbazepine has been shown to be effective as add-on therapy and monotherapy in partial epilepsy. The commonly used dose of oxcarbazepine is 600–2400 mg/day divided into two doses.[15,16,38,39]

Drug interaction

Oxcarbazepine and MHD are not metabolized via the hepatic cytochrome P450 system, and thus they have many fewer interactions with other drugs than carbamazepine. In addition, in contrast to carbamazepine, autoinduction has not been described for oxcarbazepine. Oxcarbazepine can moderately elevate the blood levels of phenytoin and phenobarbital by inhibiting their hepatic clearance, and reduce the blood concentration of oral contraceptives and calcium channel blockers by inducing a subset of cytochrome P450 isoenzymes.[13,16–18,22,38]

LEVETIRACETAM

Levetiracetam is a new antiepileptic drug with unknown mechanisms of action. The drug is almost fully absorbed after oral administration (high bioavailability), and is only minimally bound to plasma proteins (< 10%). Levertiracetam is eliminated via two routes. Most of it is excreted unmetabolized through the urine. The remaining portion is metabolized in the liver via a cytochrome P450-independent enzymatic system.[16,41] The plasma half-life of the drug is 6–8 h. However, the biological action of levetiracetam lasts much longer (about 24 h), and hence the drug can be administered twice daily.[16] The common dose range of levetiracetam is 1000–3000 mg/day. Presently, levetiracetam is approved as add-on therapy for partial epilepsy. Additional studies are required to test its efficacy in generalized epilepsy, and as first-line monotherapy. Moreover, additional data are required regarding the safety and efficacy of levetiracetam treatment in the pediatric population.[16,41]

Drug interactions

Levetiracetam has an ideal interaction profile. Studies have failed to show interactions with any other drugs, including other antiepileptic drugs, oral contraceptives, digoxin and oral anticoagulants. In addition, no antiepileptic drugs or other medications interfere with levetiracetam.[16,42]

ZONISAMIDE

Zonisamide is the latest antiepileptic drug approved for use in the USA. In Japan, however, zonisamide has been approved for use for the past several years. The antiepileptic effect of zonisamide is probably mediated by partial blockade of voltage gated sodium channel and T-type calcium channels. Zonisamide has a high bioavailability (more than 95%), and about 50% of the drug in the blood is bound to plasma proteins. Zonisamide is eliminated via both renal and hepatic routes. The half-life of the drug given as monotherapy is 40–60 h. Zonisamide is a broad-spectrum antiepileptic drug. It is effective for both generalized and partial epilepsy. It has also been shown to be effective in progressive myoclonic epilepsy and infantile spasm. Zonisamide is usually used as add-on therapy for intractable epilepsy. However, in Japan this drug is used as monotherapy as well. The dose of zonisamide used in clinical practice is 200–600 mg/day divided into one or two doses.[16,43–47]

Drug interactions

Zonisamide does not alter the blood levels of other antiepileptic drugs, including carbamazepine, phenytoin, valproate or barbiturates. In contrast, enzyme-inducing antiepileptic drugs such as phenytoin, carbamazepine and phenobarbital increase the hepatic elimination of zonisamide, and hence shorten its half-life by approximately 50% (25–35 h). Similarly, ketoconazole, cyclosporin A and miconazole also increase the liver clearance of zonisamide.[45–49] The effect of zonisamide on oral contraceptives is as yet unknown.[24]

CONCLUSIONS

In the past decade, approximately 10 new antiepileptic drugs have been introduced for clinical use. Moreover, several additional drugs are in the last stages of clinical testing, and will probably join this enlarging list in the next few years. New antiepileptic drugs have several uses in clinical practice. They improve seizure control in some patients with intractable epilepsy, and on average cause less side-effects than the old antiepileptic drugs. In this chapter, I highlight one additional advantage of new antiepileptic drugs. They have many fewer interactions with other medications, as compared to the old antiepileptic drugs. This is especially important for patients receiving polytherapy with several antiepileptic drugs or other medications such as warfarin and digoxin.

REFERENCES

1. Hausser WA, Annegers JF, Kurland LT. The prevalence of epilepsy in Rochester, Minnesota, 1940–1980. *Epilepsia* 1991; **32**: 429–445.
2. Hausser WA, Annegers JF, Kurland LT. Incidence of epilepsy and unprovoked seizures in Rochester, Minnesota, 1935–1984. *Epilepsia* 1994; **34**: 453–468.
3. Commission on Classification and Terminology of the International League Against Epilepsy. Proposal for revised clinical and electroencephalographic classification of epileptic seizures. *Epilepsia* 1981; **22**: 489–501.
4. Commission on Classification and Terminology of the International League Against Epilepsy. Proposal for revised classification of epilepsies and epileptic syndromes. *Epilepsia* 1989; **30**: 389–399.
5. Clark S, Wilson W. Mechanisms of epileptogenesis and the expression of epileptiform activity. In: Eillie E, ed. *The Treatment of Epilepsy: Principles and Practice*, 2nd edn. Baltimore: Williams & Wilkins, 1997: 53–81.
6. Matsuo F, Bergen D, Faught E et al. Placebo-controlled study of the efficacy and safety of lamotrigine in patients with partial seizures. US Lamotrigine Protocol 0.5 Clinical Trial Group. *Neurology* 1993; **43**: 2284–2291.
7. Shorvon SD, Lowenthal A, Janz D, Bielen E, Loiseau P. Multi-center double-blind, randomized, placebo-controlled trial of levetiracetam as add-on therapy in patients with refractory partial seizures. European Levetiracetam Study Group. *Epilepsia* 2000; **41**: 1179–1186.
8. Reife R, Pledger G, Wu SC. Topiramate as add-on therapy: pooled analysis of randomized controlled trials in adults. *Epilepsia* 2000; **41**(suppl 1): S66–S71.
9. Brodie MJ, Richens A, Yuen AW. Double-blind comparison of lamotrigine and carbamazepine in newly diagnosed epilepsy. UK Lamotrigine/Carbamazepine Monotherapy Trial Group. *Lancet* 1995; **345**: 476–479.
10. Steiner TJ, Dellaportas CI, Findley LJ et al. Lamotrigine monotherapy in newly diagnosed untreated epilepsy: a double-blind comparison with phenytoin. *Epilepsia* 1999; **40**: 601–607.
11. Graves NM, Ramsay RE. Phenytoin and fosphenytoin. In: Eillie E, ed. *The Treatment of Epilepsy: Principles and Practice*, 2nd edn. Baltimore: Williams & Wilkins, 1997: 833–844.
12. Ben-Menachem E. Vigabatrin. *Epilepsia* 1995; **36**(suppl 2): S95–S104.
13. Bazil CW, Pedley TA. Advances in the medical treatment of epilepsy. *Annu Rev Med* 1998; **49**: 135–162.
14. French JA, Vigabatrin. *Epilepsia* 1999; **40**(suppl 5): S11–S16.
15. Bialer M, Johannessen SI, Kupferberg HJ, Levy RH, Loiseau P, Perucca E. Progress report on new antiepileptic drugs: a summary of the fourth Eilat conference (EILAT IV). *Epilepsy Res* 1999; **34**: 1–41.
16. Bialer M, Johannessen SI, Kupferberg HJ, Levy RH, Loiseau P, Perucca E. Progress report on new antiepileptic drugs: a summary of the fourth Eilat conference (EILAT V). *Epilepsy Res* 2001; **53**: 11–58.
17. Benedetti MS. Enzyme induction and inhibition by new antiepileptic drugs: a review of human studies. *Fundam Clin Pharmacol* 2000; **14**: 301–319.
18. Sabers A, Gram L. Newer anticonvulsants: comparative review of drug interactions and adverse effects. *Drugs* 2000; **60**: 23–33.
19. Wagner ML. Felbamate: a new antiepileptic drug. *Am J Hosp Pharm* 1994; **51**: 1657–1666.
20. Leppik IE, Felbamate. *Epilepsia* 1995; **36**(suppl 2): S66–S72.
21. Glue P, Banfield CR, Perhach JL, Mather GG, Racha JK, Levy RH. Pharmacokinetic interactions with felbamate. In vitro–in vivo correlation. *Clin Pharmacokinet* 1997; **33**: 214–224.
22. Perucca E. The clinical pharmacokinetics of the new antiepileptic drugs. *Epilepsia* 1999; **40**(suppl 9): S7–S13.
23. McLean MJ. Gabapentin. *Epilepsia* 1995; **36**(suppl 2): S73–S86.
24. Wilbur K, Ensom MH. Pharmacokinetic drug interactions between oral contraceptives and second-generation anticonvulsants. *Clin Pharmacokinet* 2000; **38**: 355–365.
25. Matsuo F. Lamotrigine. *Epilepsia* 1999; **40**(suppl 5): S30–S36.
26. Dulac O, Kaminska A. Use of lamotrigine in Lennox–Gastaut and related epilepsy syndromes. *J Child Neurol* 1997; **12**(suppl 1): S23–S28.
27. Garnett WR. Lamotrigine: pharmacokinetics. *J Child Neurol* 1997; **12**(suppl 1): S10–S15.
28. Kanner AM, Frey M. Adding valproate to lamotrigine: a study of their pharmacokinetic interaction. *Neurology* 2000; **55**: 588–591.
29. Fattore C, Cipolla G, Gatti G et al. Induction of ethinylestradiol and levonorgestrel metabolism by oxcarbazepine in healthy women. *Epilepsia* 1999; **40**: 783–787.
30. Besag FM, Berry DJ, Pool F, Newbery JE, Subel B, Carbamazepine toxicity with lamotrigine: pharmacokinetic or pharmacodynamic interaction? *Epilepsia* 1998; **39**: 183–187.
31. Pisani F, Oteri G, Russo MF, Di Perri R, Perucca E, Richens A. The efficacy of valproate–lamotrigine comedication in refractory complex partial seizures: evidence for a pharmacodynamic interaction. *Epilepsia* 1999; **40**: 1141–1146.
32. Garnett WR. Clinical pharmacology of topiramate: a review. *Epilepsia* 2000; **41**(suppl 1): S61–S65.
33. Perucca E. Pharmacokinetic profile of topiramate in comparison with other new antiepileptic drugs. *Epilepsia* 1996; **37**(suppl 2): S8–S13.
34. Glauser TA. Topiramate. *Epilepsia* 1999; **40**(suppl 5): S71–S80.

35. Sachdeo RC. Topiramate. Clinical profile in epilepsy. *Clin Pharmacokinet* 1998; **34**: 335–346.
36. Schmidt D, Gram L, Brodie M et al. Tiagabine in the treatment of epilepsy—a clinical review with a guide for the prescribing physician. *Epilepsy Res* 2000; **41**: 245–251.
37. Schachter SC. Tiagabine. *Epilepsia* 1999; **40**(suppl 5): S17–S22.
38. Tecoma ES. Oxcarbazepine. *Epilepsia* 1999; **40**(suppl 5): S37–S46.
39. Shorvon S. Oxcarbazepine: a review. *Seizure* 2000; **9**: 75–79.
40. Jain KK. An assessment of rufinamide as an antiepileptic in comparison with other drugs in clinical development. *Expert Opin Invest Drugs* 2000; **9**: 829–840.
41. Willmore LJ. Clinical pharmacology of new antiepileptic drugs. *Neurology* 2000; **55**(suppl 3): S17–S24.
42. Patsalos PN. Pharmacokinetic profile of levetiracetam: toward ideal characteristics. *Pharmacol Ther* 2000; **85**: 77–85.
43. Perucca E, Bialer M. The clinical pharmacokinetics of the newer antiepileptic drugs. Focus on topiramate, zonisamide and tiagabine. *Clin Pharmacokinet* 1996; **31**: 29–46.
44. Kyllerman M, Ben-Menachem E. Zonisamide for progressive myoclonus epilepsy: long-term observations in seven patients. *Epilepsy Res* 1998; **29**: 109–114.
45. Mimaki T. Clinical pharmacology and therapeutic drug monitoring of Zonisamide. *Ther Drug Monit* 1998; **20**: 593–597.
46. Leppik IE. Zonisamide. *Epilepsia* 1999; **40**(suppl 5): S23–S29.
47. Oommen KJ, Mathews S. Zonisamide: a new antiepileptic drug. *Clin Neuropharmacol* 1999; **22**: 192–200.
48. Yanai S, Hanai T, Narazaki O. Treatment of infantile spasms with Zonisamide. *Brain Dev* 1999; **21**: 157–161.
49. Nakasa H, Nakamura H, Ono S et al. Prediction of drug–drug interactions of zonisamide metabolism in humans from in vitro data. *Eur J Clin Pharmacol* 1998; **54**: 177–183.

28

Challenges in monitoring the new antiepileptic drugs*

Svein I Johannessen and Torbjörn Tomson

INTRODUCTION

The treatment of epilepsy is one of the areas where therapeutic drug monitoring (TDM) has made the most significant contributions. Determination of serum concentrations of the antiepileptic drugs phenobarbital and phenytoin came into routine use soon after the development of sensitive and reliable analytical methods in the 1960s. Monitoring of antiepileptic drugs such as carbamazepine, valproate, and ethosuximide has since then also become widely accepted in clinical practice. However, due to indiscriminate overuse, TDM as such has attracted criticism.[1,2] To promote more appropriate use, the International League Against Epilepsy has issued guidelines for monitoring of antiepileptic drugs,[3] and many independent experts have also published reviews and position papers on the topic in recent years.[4–9] Several new antiepileptic drugs have, however, been licensed during the last decade, and the value of monitoring the new antiepileptic drugs is presently under debate.

This chapter will focus on gabapentin, lamotrigine, oxcarbazepine, tiagabine, topiramate, vigabatrin, and zonisamide.

RATIONALE FOR THERAPEUTIC DRUG MONITORING IN EPILEPSY

Drug treatment is ideally monitored by direct observation of therapeutic response and adverse effects in the patient. Sometimes, the interpretation of the clinical response is not so clear-cut, and intermediate physiological markers of clinical effects may serve as surrogates. TDM may be an option if such measurable markers are unavailable. The goal of TDM is to

optimize a patient's clinical outcome by managing their medication regimen with the assistance of measured drug concentrations.[10] TDM will be relevant mainly when there is a need for individualized dosing owing to large inter-individual differences in drug response and when such differences are accounted for by variation in pharmacokinetics. The value of TDM will, however, depend on a number of factors.

It may be useful to distinguish between disease-related and drug-related reasons for TDM. Evidently, measurement of drug plasma concentrations is more likely to be worthwhile in the treatment of disorders where the clinical evidence of therapeutic or toxic effects is difficult to interpret and where therapeutic failures may have serious consequences. This is often the case in the treatment of epilepsy. The clinical manifestations of the disorder, the seizures, occur intermittently, often with long and variable intervals. The drug treatment is prophylactic with the aim of preventing the occurrence of seizures in patients with epilepsy, as even a few unnecessary seizures may have considerable consequences for an individual patient. It may thus be difficult to assess the efficacy of the therapy, and problematic to tailor the treatment on clinical grounds alone. Also, intermediary physiological indices of therapeutic response are lacking in epilepsy. The long treatment duration, often life, reinforces the importance of monitoring the therapy in order to avoid overexposure to potentially toxic drugs and thereby possibly reduce the risks for chronic side-effects. Clinical symptoms and signs of toxicity may sometimes be insidious and difficult to detect and interpret, particularly among the many epilepsy patients with additional neurological handicaps such as mental retardation or cerebral palsy.

Thus, there are many reasons, related to the nature of the disorder, for using TDM as a guide to an individually tailored treatment of patients with

*This review is based on: Tomson T, Johannessen SI. Therapeutic monitoring of the new antiepileptic drugs. *Europ J Clin Pharmacol* 2000; **55**: 697–705

epilepsy. This rationale for TDM in epilepsy will be valid whether new or old antiepileptic drugs are used. However, the value and applicability of TDM will also depend on the pharmacological properties of the drug to be monitored.

Pharmacological properties that would make therapeutic monitoring of a specific drug potentially valuable are as follows:

- pronounced inter-individual variability in pharmacokinetics
- intra-individual variation in kinetics (due to pharmacokinetic drug interactions, concurrent disease or age-related)
- established correlation between the concentration of the drug and its therapeutic or toxic effects
- narrow therapeutic range

The TDM concept rests on the assumption that the drug concentration correlates better with clinical effects than the dose. For most of the established antiepileptic drugs, more or less well-defined therapeutic plasma level ranges, or target ranges, have been determined.[4,5] These are steady-state drug concentrations known to be associated with a high probability of seizure control and low risk of toxicity. Although target ranges have been established for most of the older antiepileptic drugs, one should be aware that there are pharmacological requirements that need to be fulfilled in part or in full in order to obtain a meaningful relationship between serum concentration of a drug and its effect. The drug should act per se and not through active metabolites, it should have a reversible action, and development of tolerance should not occur at receptor sites. In addition, the level of unbound drug at the site of sampling (normally plasma) should ideally equal the unbound drug concentrations at receptor sites. Indeed, some of the traditional antiepileptic drugs have properties that may obscure such a correlation (active metabolites of carbamazepine and primidone are examples) and one cannot presuppose that a target range can be identified for every antiepileptic drug. TDM may, however, under certain circumstances, be meaningful also in the absence of a defined target range. Provided that there is a distinct concentration–effect relationship within the individual patient, TDM may be justifiable to control for intra-individual changes in drug levels due to, for instance, pharmacokinetic drug interactions.

Phenytoin, with its dose-dependent kinetics, was a perfect candidate for TDM, fulfilling most of the criteria and requirements discussed above.[6] Studies in the 1960s and 1970s demonstrated a good correlation between drug plasma concentrations and therapeutic and toxic effects, and TDM was soon considered necessary for the safe use of phenytoin.[11] The fact that this particular drug was the first choice for most types of epilepsy when the concept of TDM was introduced in the 1960s probably contributed to the rapid establishment of TDM in epilepsy.

As for the new antiepileptic drugs, studies of the relationship between plasma drug concentrations and effects are often lacking when the drugs are introduced on to the market, and very few systematic studies have been carried out after licensing. In contrast, extensive information is generally available on the pharmacokinetics and the pharmacokinetic drug interaction potential.

GABAPENTIN

Gabapentin is devoid of enzyme-inducing properties. Since the drug is not protein bound and almost completely eliminated by renal excretion, gabapentin does not appear to be involved in significant pharmacokinetic interactions with other drugs.[12]

The short half-life and the resulting marked inter-dosage fluctuations in gabapentin plasma concentrations are likely to complicate the establishment of a target range. Furthermore, since the mode of action remains elusive, it cannot be excluded that mechanisms are involved that will lead to a dissociation between plasma concentration and effect. Finally, no linear relationship was found between plasma and cerebrospinal fluid concentrations of gabapentin in treated patients.[13] These are circumstances that make the establishment of a meaningful concentration-effect relationship less likely.

The lack of pharmacokinetic drug interactions is a further argument against therapeutic monitoring of gabapentin. However, although gabapentin is excreted unchanged in urine, substantial variation in plasma concentrations at the same daily dose has been found among different patients, and the dose-dependency of the absorption may also vary substantially between patients.[14] Hence, TDM may be used to clarify whether a poor response to dose increments in the individual case is caused by impaired absorption.

A wide range of gabapentin plasma concentrations have been reported to be associated with seizure control. Therapeutic effects of gabapentin were evident in refractory patients with partial seizures only at plasma concentrations above 2 mg/l in a study by Sivenius et al.[15] In another study,[14] using high-dose gabapentin in patients with refractory partial seizures, plasma concentrations among responders ranged from 5.9 to 2 mg/l, but one particular patient responded well to, and tolerated,

61.2 mg/l (at a dose of 6000 mg/day). Although the blood samples in this study were obtained at a standardized time after dosing, they were not necessarily trough levels.

As with other new antiepileptic drugs, systematic studies designed primarily to investigate drug level–effect correlations are lacking, and thus no target range has been established.

LAMOTRIGINE

Phenytoin, carbamazepine and barbiturates induce the metabolism of lamotrigine,[16,17] and the half-life of lamotrigine is considerably shorter, with an average of 15 h, ranging from 8 to 33 h.[18] Conversely, lamotrigine metabolism is inhibited by valproate, prolonging the half-life of lamotrigine to an average of 60 h, with a range of 30–90 h.[19] The clearance is to some extent age-dependent, being higher in children than in adults[20] and further decreased in the elderly.[21]

The pronounced inter-individual variation in pharmacokinetics[22] indicates that lamotrigine is a suitable candidate for TDM. The fact that the kinetics in the individual patient may be altered by concurrent drug therapy and other conditions also suggests that TDM of lamotrigine will be of value in certain situations.

Of all the new antiepileptic drugs, lamotrigine is probably the most extensively studied with respect to concentration–effect correlations. Nevertheless, the information is scarce. A target range of 1–4 mg/l was suggested initially, partly based on preclinical data, and this range has been used in clinical trials.[23] Some investigators have claimed this to be too low, since many patients will benefit from and tolerate considerably higher lamotrigine concentrations. Morris et al[24] proposed a target range of 3–14 mg/l, based on their own experience and on an open trial where lamotrigine and vigabatrin were combined in patients with intractable seizures.[25] The median lamotrigine plasma concentration in the responders in this study was 7.9 mg/l (range 2.1–15.4 mg/l) compared with 16.0 mg/l (range 7.9–19.4 mg/l) in patients reporting dose-related side-effects. Most studies, however, have shown a wide range in plasma concentrations associated with seizure control, and a considerable overlap in plasma concentrations of responders and non-responders, as well as between patients with and without side-effects.[20,26,27] This was also the case in the only prospective study of the relationship between lamotrigine plasma concentrations and effects and toxicity, in which no useful relationship could be demonstrated.[26] The methodology in this study has, however, been criticized and the conclusions questioned.[28]

Clearly, more systematic studies are needed to explore the value of TDM in lamotrigine therapy. Nevertheless, despite the absence of a target range for populations of patients, TDM is likely to be of value in the control of pharmacokinetic changes within an individual patient.

OXCARBAZEPINE

Induction or inhibition of the cytochrome P-450 system, as is often encountered in antiepileptic drug therapy, will have little effect on the kinetics of oxcarbazepine and its active metabolite. In contrast to carbamazepine, oxcarbazepine does not influence its own metabolism after repeated administration.[29,30]

The target range of serum levels for the active metabolite is as yet not well defined. Serum concentrations of 10-hydroxycarbazepine have been reported in a few studies that summarize the post-marketing experience of oxcarbazepine use in some epilepsy centres. Friis et al[31] found a mean trough level of approximately 20 mg/l in their retrospective analysis of 947 patients, but the range in serum concentrations was wide (3–40 mg/l), and the relation to effects and toxicity was not analysed in detail. Similarly, Van Parys and Meinardi[32] reported 10-hydroxycarbazepine concentrations ranging from 3 to 32 mg/l (mean 17.4) in 19 seizure-free adult patients. Neither the mean concentration nor the range differed from what was found in non-responders. In another retrospective analysis, Borusiak et al[33] reported somewhat higher concentrations in children, 15–55 mg/l (mean 30). Side-effects were more frequent at plasma concentrations of 35–40 mg/l. A population pharmacokinetic–pharmacodynamic assessment was recently made, based on more than 1800 blood samples from 513 patients participating in three separate double-blind, placebo-controlled or dose-controlled trials of oxcarbazepine.[34] Generally, safety and efficacy responses could adequately be explained by oxcarbazepine dose alone, and plasma concentrations of the metabolite provided limited additional information according to a preliminary report.

Clearly, also for oxcarbazepine, there is a need for more systematic studies exploring the concentration–effect relationships.

TIAGABINE

Tiagabine serum levels are decreased in patients also treated with enzyme-inducing drugs.[35,36] The marked variability in kinetics and the fact that tiagabine elimination is affected by other antiepileptic drugs suggest that there may be a need for therapeutic monitoring of tiagabine. However, the establishment of a target range is complicated by the pronounced fluctuations in tiagabine plasma concentrations due to the short half-life. In addition, the need to monitor free rather than total levels needs to be explored, considering the high protein binding of tiagabine. A more pronounced reduction in seizures was observed at trough plasma concentrations >40 µg/l in a preliminary analysis of data from a clinical trial of patients with complex partial seizures given three different dosages of tiagabine.[37] The authors are not aware of any other systematic study exploring the relationship between tiagabine concentration in plasma and effects, and no target concentration has been proposed.

The available data are clearly not sufficient to recommend routine monitoring of tiagabine concentrations, and more studies are needed.

TOPIRAMATE

Phenytoin and carbamazepine induce the metabolism of topiramate and decrease the serum levels of topiramate markedly.[38,39] Valproate may also lower topiramate concentrations but to a much lesser extent.[40]

Although topiramate is eliminated mainly unchanged by the renal route in patients on monotherapy, the proportion metabolized will increase in patients on inducing antiepileptic drugs. The magnitude of this pharmacokinetic interaction indicates that TDM might be of value in selected patients. However, systematic studies exploring concentration–effect correlations are lacking, and no target range has been established. Plasma topiramate concentrations have normally ranged from 2 to 5 mg/l[41] in clinical trials, and seizure control has been associated with topiramate levels between 3.4 and 5.2 mg/l.[42,43] A preliminary report based on topiramate as add-on to other antiepileptic drugs in refractory patients suggests that levels over 4 mg/l are necessary for effectiveness[44] but also that there is a greater incidence of improvement in seizure control at concentrations of 10 mg/l or greater (Penovich et al, personal communication).

Further studies are needed to determine the possible role of topiramate plasma level monitoring.

VIGABATRIN

Owing to the irreversible mode of action of the drug, the serum half-life bears practically no relationship to the duration of pharmacological effect, which will depend on resynthesis of new GABA transaminase.[45] Hence, the antiepileptic effect of vigabatrin long outlasts its presence in serum.

The irreversible action of vigabatrin, and the following dissociation between serum concentration and clinical effects, complicates the interpretation of concentration–effect relationships and limits the potential value of monitoring vigabatrin. The fact that vigabatrin is a racemate and that only the S-enantiomer is active adds further to the complexity, in particular since the kinetics of the enantiomers differ. Consequently, Arteaga et al[46] found no correlation between vigabatrin plasma levels and seizure control in a study of 16 children with refractory epilepsy treated with vigabatrin as add-on, and nor did platelet GABA transaminase inhibition correlate with effect.

It has been suggested that monitoring plasma GABA levels may be a better alternative. In a cross-sectional study, patients with complex partial seizures who responded to vigabatrin had significantly higher plasma GABA levels than non-responders.[47] The results indicate that plasma GABA levels might reflect central nervous system GABA concentrations and could serve as an intermediate physiological marker of effect. However, according to a recent prospective study from the same group, plasma GABA does not seem to be a reliable marker of clinical response to viagatrin.[48] Although responders showed a significant increase in plasma GABA concentrations, a similar increase was found also among a subgroup of non-responders.

TDM of vigabatrin has been advocated for checking compliance.[7]

ZONISAMIDE

In patients also receiving carbamazepine or phenytoin, zonisamide serum levels are decreased, suggesting that the metabolism of zonisamide is induced by other antiepileptic drugs.[49,50]

The pronounced inter-individual variation in kinetics, together with the drug interaction potential, indicate that monitoring of zonisamide may be useful.[51] Favourable clinical responses have been observed at plasma levels of 20–30 mg/l[52] and 7–40 mg/l in children with refractory seizures given zonisamide as add-on.[53] There was, however, a considerable overlap between serum concentrations of responders and non-responders, as well as between serum levels associated with seizure control and side-effects.[51]

Again, more systematic studies designed to explore the concentration–effect relationship are needed.

CONCLUSIONS

There are no generally accepted target plasma concentration ranges for any of the new antiepileptic drugs, and in general the available information on the relationship between plasma concentrations and effects is scarce. For most drugs, wide ranges in concentrations associated with seizure control are reported, and a considerable overlap with drug levels among non-responders and also with concentrations associated with toxicity is often noted. However, most observations of concentration–effect correlations come from clinical trials with the primary objective of demonstrating efficacy of the new drug, and there is a remarkable paucity of systematic studies designed primarily to explore the relationship between drug plasma concentrations and effects.

This is true not only for new antiepileptic drugs but also for some of the more established antiepileptic drugs that are frequently monitored in everyday practice. Although the available documentation is clearly insufficient and routine monitoring of the new antiepileptic drugs cannot be recommended at this stage, the pharmacological properties of some of the drugs, in particular lamotrigine, zonisamide, and possibly oxcarbazepine, topiramate and tiagabine, suggest that they may be candidates for TDM. Monitoring some of these new drugs may be of value also in the absence of established target ranges, since concomitant therapy or concurrent disease may affect the kinetics in an individual patient. The case of vigabatrin is special, and the irreversible action of this drug makes TDM irrelevant in most cases.

Owing to the nature of epilepsy, it remains problematic to monitor antiepileptic drug treatment by direct observations of clinical response in the individual patient. Further systematic studies designed specifically to investigate concentration–effect relationships of the new antiepileptic drugs are therefore urgently needed. In such studies, patients with well-defined seizure disorders should ideally be randomized to different drug plasma level ranges and the clinical effects be evaluated with appropriate methods. Alternatively, a more pragmatic study design may be used in which the individual patients are titrated to stepwise increasing predefined drug plasma levels depending on their response. The interpretation of such trials will be facilitated if patients are treated with the new drug in monotherapy, although this will in most cases be possible only rather late in the clinical development programme.

REFERENCES

1. Chadwick D. Overuse of monitoring of blood concentrations of antiepileptic drugs. *BMJ* 1987; **294**: 723–724.
2. Schoenenberger RA, Tanasijevic MJ, Jha A, Bates DW. Appropriateness of antiepileptic drug level monitoring. *JAMA* 1995; **274**: 1622–1626.
3. Commission on Antiepileptic Drugs. Guidelines for therapeutic monitoring on antiepileptic drugs. *Epilepsia* 1993; **34**: 585–587.
4. Johannessen SI. Plasma drug concentration monitoring of anticonvulsants. Practical guidelines. *CNS Drugs* 1997; **7**: 349–365.
5. Eadie MJ. Therapeutic drug monitoring—antiepileptic drugs. *Br J Clin Pharmacol* 1998; **46**: 185–193.
6. Brodie MJ. Routine measurement of new antiepileptic drug concentrations: a critique and a prediction. *Adv Neurol* 1998; **76**(22): 223.
7. Patsalos PN. New antiepileptic drugs. *Ann Clin Biochem* 1999; **36**: 10–19.
8. Tomson T, Johannessen SI. Therapeutic monitoring of the new antiepileptic drugs. *Eur J Clin Pharmacol* 2000; **55**: 60–705.
9. Perruca E. Monitoring the new antiepileptic drugs. *Clin Pharmacokinet* 2000; **38**: 191–204.
10. Gross AS. Best practice in therapeutic drug monitoring. *Br J Clin Pharmacol* 1998; **46**: 95–99.
11. Lund L. Anticonvulsant effect of diphenylhydantoin relative to plasma levels. *Arch Neurol* 1974; **31**: 289–294.
12. Goa KL, Sorkin EM. Gabapentin. A review of its pharmacological properties and clinical potential in epilepsy. *Drugs* 1993; **46**: 409–427.
13. Ben-Menachem B, Söderfelt B, Hamberger T, Hedner T, Persson LI. Seizure frequency and CSF parameters, a double-blind, placebo-controlled trial of gabapentin patients with intractable complex partial seizures. *Epilepsy Res* 1995; **21**: 231–236.
14. Wilson EA, Sills GJ, Forrest G, Brodie MJ. High dose gabapentin in refractory partial epilepsy: clinical observations in 50 patients. *Epilepsy Res* 1998; **29**: 161–166.
15. Sivenius J, Kälviäinen R, Ylinen A, Riekkinen P. Double blind study of gabapentin in the treatment of partial seizures. *Epilepsia* 1991; **32**: 539–542.
16. Eriksson A-S, Hoppu L, Nergårdh A, Boréus L. Pharmacokinetic interactions between lamotrigine and other antiepileptic drugs in children with intractable epilepsy. *Epilepsia* 1996; **37**: 769–773.
17. May TW, Rambeck B, Jürgens U. Serum concentrations of lamotrigine in epileptic patients: the influence of dose and comedication. *Ther Drug Monit* 1996; **18**: 523–531.
18. Jawad S, Yuen AWC, Peck AW, Hamilton MJ, Oxley JR, Richens A. Lamotrigine: single-dose pharmacokinetics and initial one-week experience in refractory epilepsy. *Epilepsy Res* 1987; **1**: 194–210.
19. Yau MK, Wargin WA, Wolf KB et al. Effect of valproate on the pharmacokinetics of lamotrigine (Lamictal) at steady state. *Epilepsia* 1992; **33**(suppl 3): 82.
20. Bartoli A, Guerrini R, Belmonte A, Alessandri MG, Gatti G, Perruca E. The influence of dosage, age and comedication on steady-state plasma lamotrigine concentrations in epileptic children: a prospective study with

preliminary assessment of correlations with clinical response. *Ther Drug Monit* 1997; **19**: 252–260.

21. Posner J, Holdich T, Crome P. Comparison of lamotrigine pharmacokinetics in young and elderly healthy volunteers. *J Pharm Med* 1991; **1**: 121–128.

22. George S, Wood AJ, Braithwaite RA. Routine therapeutic monitoring of lamotrigine in epileptic patients using a simple and rapid high performance liquid chromatographic technique. *Ann Clin Biochem* 1995; **32**: 584–588.

23. Brodie MJ, Richens A, Yuen AWC. Double-blind comparison of lamotrigine and carbamazepine in newly diagnosed epilepsy. *Lancet* 1995; **345**: 476–479.

24. Morris RG, Black AB, Harris AL, Batty AB, Sallustio BC. Lamotrigine and therapeutic drug monitoring: retrospective survey following the introduction of a routine service. *Br J Clin Pharmacol* 1998; **46**: 547–551.

25. Schapel G, Black A, Lam E, Robinson M, Dollman W. Combination vigabatrin and lamotrigine therapy for intractable epilepsy. *Seizure* 1996; **5**: 51–56.

26. Kilpatric ES, Forrest G, Brodie M. Concentration–effect and concentration–toxicity relations with lamotrigine: a prospective study. *Epilepsia* 1996; **37**: 534–538.

27. Eriksson A-S, Nergårdh A, Hoppu K. The efficacy of lamotrigine in children and adolescents with refractory generalized epilepsy: a randomized, double-blind, cross-over study. *Epilepsia* 1998; **39**: 495–450.

28. Gidal BE, Welty TE. The concentration–effect relationship with lamotrigine (LE). *Epilepsia* 1997; **38**: 260.

29. Lloyd P, Flesch G, Dieterle W. Clinical pharmacology and pharmacokinetics of oxcarbazepine. *Epilepsia* 1994; **35**(suppl 3): S10–S13.

30. Baruzzi A, Albani F, Riva R. Oxcarbazepine: pharmacokinetic interactions and their clinical relevance. *Epilepsia* 1994; **35**(Suppl 3): S14–S19.

31. Friis ML, Kristensen O, Boas J et al. Therapeutic experiences with 947 epileptic out-patients in oxcarbazepine treatment. *Acta Neurol Scand* 1993; **87**: 224–227.

32. Van Parys JAP, Meinardi H. Survey of 260 patients treated with oxcarbazepine (Trileptal) on a named-patient basis. *Epilepsy Res* 1994; **19**: 79–85.

33. Borusiak P, Korn-Merker B, Holert N, Boenigk HE. Oxcarbazepine in treatment of childhood epilepsy: a survey of 46 children and adolescents. *J Epilepsy* 1998; **11**: 355–360.

34. Nedelman JR, Gasparini M, Hossain M et al. Oxcarbazepine: analysis of concentration–efficacy/safety relationships. *Neurology* 1999; **52**(suppl 2): A524–A525.

35. Adkins JC, Noble S. Tiagabine. A review of its pharmacodynamic and pharmacokinetic properties and therapeutic potential in the management of epilepsy. *Drugs* 1998; **55**: 437–460.

36. So EL, Wolff D, Graves NM et al. Pharmacokinetics of tiagabine as add-on therapy in patients taking enzyme-inducing antiepileptic drugs. *Epilepsy Res* 1995; **22**: 221–226.

37. Rowan AJ, Gustavson L, Shu V, Sommerville KW. Dose concentration relationship in a multicentre tiagabine (Gabitril) trial. *Epilepsia* 1997; **38**(suppl 3): 40.

38. Johannessen SI. Pharmacokinetics and interactions of topiramate. *Epilepsia* 1997; **38**(suppl 1); S18–S23.

39. Sachdeo RC, Sachdeo SK, Walker SA, Kramer LD, Nayak RK, Doose DR. Steady-state pharmacokinetics of topiramate and carbamazepine in patients with epilepsy during monotherapy and concomitant therapy. *Epilepsia* 1996; **37**: 774–778.

40. Rosenfeld WE, Liao S, Kramer LD et al. Comparison of the steady-state pharmacokinetics of topiramate and valproate in patients with epilepsy during monotherapy and concomitant therapy. *Epilepsia* 1997; **38**: 24–33.

41. Reife RA. Topiramate. In: Shorvon S, Dreifuss F, Fish D, Thomas D, eds. *The Treatment of Epilepsy*. Oxford: Blackwell Science, 1996: 471–481.

42. Reife RA, Pledger G, Doose D, Lim P, Ward C. Topiramate PK/PD analysis. *Epilepsia* 1995; **36**(suppl 3): S152.

43. Perruca E, Bialer M. The clinical pharmacokinetics of the newer antiepileptic drugs. Focus on topiramate, zonisamide and tiagabine. *Clin Pharmcokinet* 1996; **31**: 29–46.

44. Penovich PE, Schroeder-Gustafson M, Gates JR, Moriarty GL. Clinical experience with topiramate: correlation of serum levels with efficacy and adverse events. *Epilepsia* 1997; **38**(suppl 8): 181.

45. Schechter PJ. Clinical pharmacology of vigabatrin. *Br J Clin Pharmacol* 1989; **27**(suppl 1); 19S–22S.

46. Arteaga R, Herranz JL, Valdizán EM, Armijo JA. Vinyl GABA (Vigabatrin): relationship between dosage, plasma concentrations, platelet GABA-transaminase inhibition, and seizure reduction in epileptic children. *Epilepsia* 1992; **33**(5): 923–931.

47. Löscher W, Fassbender CP, Gram L. Determination of GABA and vigabatrin in human plasma by a rapid and simple HPLC method: correlation between clinical response to vigabatrin and increase in plasma GABA. *Epilepsy Res* 1993; **14**: 245–255.

48. Erdal J, Gram L, Alving J, Löscher W. Changes in plasma GABA concentration during Vigabatrin treatment of epilepsy: a prospective study. *Epilepsy Res* 1999; **34**: 145–150.

49. Ojemann, LM, Shastri RA, Wilensky AJ et al. Comparative pharmacokinetics of zonisamide (CI-912) in epileptic patients on carbamazepine or phenytoin monotherapy. *Ther Drug Monit* 1986; **8**: 293–296.

50. Seino M, Miyazaki H, Ito T. Zonisamide. *Epilepsy Res* 1991; **3**: 169–174.

51. Mimaki T. Clinical pharmacology and therapeutic drug monitoring of zonisamide. *Ther Drug Monit* 1998; **20**: 593–597.

52. Wilensky AJ, Friel PN, Ojemann LM, Dodrill CB, McCormick KB, Levy RH. Zonisamide in epilepsy: a pilot study. *Epilepsia* 1985; **26**: 212–220.

53. Mimaki T, Mino M, Sugimoto T, Murata R. Antiepileptic effect and serum levels of zonisamide in epileptic patients with refractory seizures. In: Sunshine I, ed. *Recent Developments in Therapeutic Drug Monitoring and Clinical Toxicology*. New York: Marcel Dekker, 1992: 437–442.

29

Aggravation of seizures by antiepileptic drugs: pathophysiology and clinical implications

Miri Y Neufeld

INTRODUCTION

The medications prescribed by physicians for the treatment of a specific disease or condition may occasionally cause an effect opposite to the expected one. For instance, benzodiazepines, which are given for sedation, can paradoxically induce reactions of anxiety, hostility or rage.[1] Antipsychotic agents have been reported to induce dose-related sudden and dramatic exacerbations of psychosis, albeit rarely.[2] Such paradoxical effects are not limited to the central nervous system (CNS). Virtually any arrhythmia can be induced by antiarrhythmic drugs.[3] Antiepileptic drugs (AEDs) are administered to treat seizures; however, as is the case with the above-mentioned drugs, there are reports of anticonvulsants either exacerbating seizures or inducing new ones.[4–30] The mechanisms that are involved are not always clearly defined, and there is little certainty concerning the true extent of the problem, since authors frequently report interesting anecdotal cases, and reports of AED efficacy studies rarely mention aggravation of seizures in response to therapy.

ENCEPHALOPATHY CAUSING AN INCREASE OF SEIZURES WITH ADDITIONAL SIGNS OF CNS TOXICITY

Excessive doses of most drugs acting on the CNS may cause intoxication encephalopathy, a condition which may be characterized by specific signs. AEDs, in particular, have low therapeutic indices. Certain patients can use and benefit from higher blood levels of these drugs, while others will experience signs of intoxication. Levy and Fenichel were the first to describe a syndrome of phenytoin encephalopathy in their presentation of three patients in whom the frequency of generalized tonic–clonic seizures increased with high levels of the anticonvulsant medication.[7] All three patients had additional manifestations of drug toxicity to the CNS that included nystagmus, ataxia, mental clouding and EEG slowing.

An increased seizure frequency has also been observed (very rarely) during treatment with valproic acid[8] and carbamazepine,[9] with elevated drug levels being associated with coma and seizures.

EXACERBATION OF SEIZURES RELATED TO INTOXICATION, WITHOUT ADDITIONAL SIGNS OF CNS TOXICITY

It is rare for toxic levels of the anticonvulsant medications not to be accompanied by other toxic signs, but the frequency of seizures nevertheless increases in their absence. This so-called 'paradoxical intoxication'[10] probably reflects the fact that some patients can tolerate increasing doses of anticonvulsants with minimal side-effects. Biological variation apparently causes some individuals to develop seizures prior to developing other side-effects involving CNS function. Troupin and Ojemann described nine patients with poorly controlled focal as well as generalized seizures who experienced increased seizure frequency (the seizure type that was increased was not specified) following high levels of phenytoin (eight patients) or carbamazepine (one patient).[10] Neufeld described one patient with increased complex partial seizures during carbamazepine treatment.[11] Both Troupin and Ojemann's and Neufeld's patients' seizures were exacerbated by high levels of carbamazepine with no evidence of encephalopathy.

EXACERBATION OR INDUCTION OF NEW TYPES OF SEIZURES ASSOCIATED WITH THERAPEUTIC DRUG LEVELS

There is increasing evidence that AEDs may provoke aggravation of seizures by a pharmacodynamic mechanism: whether this is due to an inappropriate choice of the AED or to paradoxical activity is not clear. A paradoxical phenomenon of unexpected exacerbation or induction of seizures in patients while they were under AED treatment and whose blood levels were being maintained within accepted therapeutic limits was described mainly with carbamazepine, particularly in children and often in the children with generalized epilepsies. Shields and Saslow described five children aged 3–11 years who were being treated with carbamazepine for epilepsy, all with serum levels within the therapeutic range, who experienced the onset of myoclonic, atonic and atypical absences after the institution of carbamazepine therapy.[12] Snead and Hosey reported a series of 15 children who mainly had increased minor motor seizures or experienced the onset of minor motor seizures, but who also had more frequent and severe generalized seizures following carbamazepine administration: they, too, had carbamazepine levels within the therapeutic range.[13] The use of video-EEG monitoring allowed precise examination of ictal electrical events during their patients' seizures. They suggested that the pattern of 2.5–3-Hz spike- and wave-generalized activity represented a risk factor for carbamazepine-induced seizures. Talwar et al found that the EEG obtained after the initiation of carbamazepine in young children could predict the ones at increased risk of exacerbation: the tracings became significantly more abnormal, highlighted by the new appearance of generalized spike and wave discharges following drug intoxication.[14] Although these phenomena were mainly observed in children, carbamazepine was associated with an increase of absence seizures in older patients who had absence and generalized tonic–clonic seizures, in cases when carbamazepine was given to adults for generalized tonic–clonic seizures, and with an increase of myoclonic seizures in adolescents and young adults with juvenile myoclonic epilepsy.[15] Only rarely were increased focal seizures reported with normal carbamazepine levels: Dhuna et al described a patient with generalized tonic–clonic seizures who had an onset of complex partial seizures when carbamazepine was added: the serum levels of carbamazepine were within the therapeutic range, but there were toxic levels of carbamazepine epoxide which were speculated to contribute to the neurotoxicity.[16] So et al

reported on six adults with focal and generalized seizures who unexpectedly developed partial seizure status epilepticus and daily multiple partial and generalized seizures which the authors attributed to high serum levels of carbamazepine epoxide.[17]

Phenytoin was reported to aggravate absence seizures[18] as well as myoclonic seizures in patients with juvenile myoclonic epilepsy.[19] It was also believed to be responsible for exacerbating complex partial seizures induced by photic stimulation in a child.[20]

In add-on studies and also in monotherapy, vigabatrin was reported to increase seizures in 10–20% of patients.[21,22] The seizures that were increased with this drug were mainly generalized, and only rarely were they partial. The onset of new seizure types was also described with vigabatrin:[21,22] the occurrence was clearly related to specific epileptic syndromes, particularly symptomatic infantile spasms, symptomatic partial seizures and nonprogressive myoclonic epilepsy. The new types were either generalized or partial, with the former being myoclonic and the latter often replacing generalized tonic–clonic seizures.

The reoccurrence of myoclonic, absence and generalized tonic–clonic seizures was reported after the adjunctive use of gabapentin in a child with Lennox–Gastaut syndrome, as was an increased frequency of seizures in patients with partial epilepsy treated with gabapentin.[23,24]

Tiagabine was associated with the precipitation of non-convulsive status epilepticus.[25]

While benzodiazepines and phenobarbital are effective against several types of seizures, they were occasionally reported to have an opposite effect. Tonic status epilepticus was reported to have been precipitated following treatment with diazepam in children with Lennox–Gastaut sydrome[26] or with absence status.[27] Phenobarbital was reported to increase the frequency of generalized tonic–clonic seizures, and was implicated in the worsening of absence seizures.[28]

Exacerbation of generalized non-convulsive seizures was described with ethosuximide therapy,[29] and exacerbation of myoclonic seizures was reported in an add-on trial of lamotrigine in patients with severe epilepsy.[30]

POSSIBLE EXPLANATIONS FOR THE PARADOXICAL EFFECTS OF ANTIEPILEPTIC DRUGS

Several facts are known about the paradoxical effects of AEDs. To begin with, they are not frequent in occurrence. Most information comes from case reports or small numbers of patients. Second, this phenomenon appears to occur more often in children with certain types of refractory epilepsy and with specific drugs.

There are several possible and speculatory explanations for this phenomenon. An increase in seizures can occur with toxic levels of AEDs, such as that encountered in other types of drug encephalopathy. This can unmask certain pharmacodynamic effects of high concentrations on other cell populations. Carbamazepine can also have non-direct effects, such as drug-induced drowsiness, or pharmacological action outside the brain, such as hyponatremia.

It must be remembered that if carbamazepine is introduced to a large number of patients and only a few of them develop increased seizure frequency, it must be considered that the chances are that this increase reflects the natural fluctuation of seizure frequency. It must also be borne in mind that the new drug was introduced in many cases because seizures were uncontrolled in the first place. To add to the confusion, in some instances a previously administered drug may be simultaneously withdrawn, and this, rather than the newly introduced drug, could be responsible for the increased frequency of seizures. Moreover, most of the patients described in the literature were on multiple drugs; therefore, one further explanation would necessarily involve the drop in the blood level of AEDs following an interaction with the new drug, which will then be implicated as being responsible. These considerations relate primarily to situations in which the incriminated drug was within the therapeutic range and the seizure type was not new.

Switching from a brand name to a generic drug must also be considered, since this was shown to cause reduced serum concentrations and seizures or, alternatively, increased concentrations and clinical toxicity with seizures, in spite of an unaltered daily drug dosage.[31]

Carbamazepine deserves special attention, since the paradoxical effect was most often seen with this drug. An active metabolite, carbamazepine epoxide, is speculated to increase seizure frequency in certain situations.[17] When drugs that are known to increase carbamazepine epoxide levels, such as valproic acid,[32] are added to carbamazepine therapy, determination of carbamazepine epoxide levels or reduction of the carbamazepine dose should be considered. Another possibility is that this paradoxical situation may stem from the use of inappropriate anticonvulsants for a specific seizure type, such as what happens when carbamazepine is used for absence seizures. In idiopathic generalized epilepsies, many patients have multiple seizure types that appear to have different underlying pathophysiological mechanisms. The mechanism of aggravation in these epilepsies is largely unknown. AEDs that elevate GABA levels, e.g. vigabatrin, do not appear to be effective in generalized epilepsies. Blockade of voltage-gated sodium channels, such as that which occurs with carbamazepine, may be counterproductive in patients with absence or myoclonus. Still another possibility is the activation of epileptiform discharges by the carbamazepine itself. Wilkus et al have shown that adult patients with seizures who are treated with carbamazepine have a higher incidence of generalized epileptiform discharges in their EEGs.[33] The reason that this action of carbamazepine on the EEG results in an increase in clinical seizures mainly in children but rarely in adults may relate to the greater susceptibility of the developing brain to the types of seizures induced by carbamazepine, such as absence seizures, and to the fact that adults rarely have the constellation of mixed seizures and EEG abnormalities seen in children.

The GABA system that is involved in the mechanism of action of drugs such as vigabatrin, tiagabine and gabapentin was investigated with regard to the mechanism of seizure precipitation. While GABA-mediated inhibition is usually considered as being protective against seizures, enhancement of GABA ergic transmission has actually been shown to prevent or to facilitate seizures, depending on the primary site at which the action of the transmitters is exerted.[34]

Some cases are even more intriguing because exacerbation of seizures occurs at therapeutic dosages in the patients with the types of epilepsy which normally respond favorably to the offending drug.

As for the paradoxical effect associated with benzodiazepines and barbiturates, sleep activates epileptic discharges to a degree which amounts to a subclinical status in certain cases. Since benzodiazepines cause drowsiness or sleep, the question arises of whether sleep thus induced could precipitate that status.

Seizure exacerbation as a paradoxical phenomenon has to be differentiated from non-epileptic seizures such as movement disorders and psychogenic seizures. Dystonic movements and choreoathetoid dyskinesias were described with carbamazepine[35,36] felbamate[37] and phenytoin.[38] Myoclonic movements deserve special consideration, because of their differential diagnosis from myoclonic epilepsy. Multifocal myoclonus was occasionally described with toxic but also with therapeutic doses of carbamazepine,[39] as well as with vigabatrin[40] and gabapentin.[41]

Psychogenic seizures can occur in isolation or be associated with epileptic seizures, and a correct diagnosis may often be a difficult and challenging task.[42]

CONCLUSION—SALIENT POINTS

The phenomena described above underscore the possibility that increased seizure frequency can occur as a drug effect rather than as an exacerbation of the underlying disease, the risk depending both on the type of the drug and the specific epileptic syndrome.

Whenever a paradoxical reaction to AEDs is suspected, it is important to verify the diagnosis of epilepsy. It should also be ascertained whether the provoked abnormality under investigation is a non-epileptic one, i.e. a physiological or psychological event such as a movement disorder or a pseudo-seizure. It is important to make certain that the increased frequency is not related to identifiable conditions such as a progressive brain lesion, recent withdrawal of another AED, or interaction between several AEDs resulting in subtherapeutic or toxic blood levels, or due to tolerance or non-compliance. It is necessary to verify whether the diagnosis of epilepsy, the type of seizure and the epileptic syndrome are correct. Risk factors often associated with the development of paradoxical effects of AEDs include childhood, multiple types of seizures, mental retardation, AED polytherapy, and prominent epileptiform activity in the EEG.

More light on the paradoxical effects of AEDs could be shed by future prospective monotherapy drug studies and documentation of the phenomenon by video-EEG monitoring.

SUMMARY

Although they generally produce the expected results, various antiepileptic drugs have been reported to increase seizure frequency or even provoke new types of seizures. This effect can occur under several conditions: (1) when the drug levels in the blood are excessively high and there are concomitant clinical signs of drug intoxication; (2) in 'paradoxical intoxication', wherein an increase in seizure frequency is the only manifestation of high blood levels of the antiepileptic drugs; and (3) when there is unexpected exacerbation or induction of seizures with no apparent relationship to drug levels in the blood. The mechanisms associated with exacerbation of seizures are poorly understood. They may include spontaneous fluctuations of the epileptic disorder, changes in the drug levels due to polytherapy, and adverse interactions between the mode of action of the drug and the nature of the pathogenic mechanism underlying specific seizure types or syndromes. The real prevalence of the above-mentioned phenomena can be evaluated accurately only in prospective studies.

REFERENCES

1. Hall RCW, Zisook S. Paradoxical reactions to benzodiazepines. *Br J Clin Pharmacol* 1981; **11**: 995–1045.
2. Putten TV, Mutalipassi LR, Malkin MD. Phenothiazine induced decompensation. *Arch Gen Psychiatry* 1974; **30**: 102–105.
3. Horowitz LN. Proarrhythmia—taking the bad with the good. *N Engl J Med* 1988; **319**: 304–305.
4. Bauer J. Seizure-inducing effects of antiepileptic drugs: a review. *Acta Neurol Scand* 1996; **94**: 367–377.
5. Genton P, McMnemin J. Can antiepileptic drugs aggravate epilepsy? Proceedings of a symposium held at the 22nd International Epilepsy Congress, June 1997, Dublin, Ireland. *Epilepsia* 1998; **39**(suppl 3): S26–S29.
6. Perucca E, Gram L, Avanzini G, Dulac O. Antiepileptic drugs as a cause of worsening of seizures. *Epilepsia* 1998; **39**: 5–17.
7. Levy LL, Fenichel GM. Diphenylhydantoin activated seizures. *Neurology* 1965; **15**: 716–722.
8. Eeg-Olofsonn O, Lindskog U. Acute intoxication with valproate. *Lancet* 1982; **i**: 2306.
9. Weaver DF, Camfield P, Fraser A. Massive carbamazepine overdose: clinical and pharmacological observations. *Neurology* 1988; **38**: 755–759.
10. Troupin AS, Ojemann LM. Paradoxical intoxication—a complication of anticonvulsant administration. *Epilepsia* 1975; **16**: 753–758.
11. Neufeld MY. Exacerbation of focal seizures due to carbamazepine treatment in an adult patient. *Clin Neuropharmacol* 1993; **16**: 359–361.
12. Shields WD, Saslow E. Myoclonic, atonic and absence seizures following institution of carbamazepine therapy in children. *Neurology* 1983; **33**: 1487–1489.
13. Snead OC III, Hosey LC. Exacerbation of seizures in children by carbamazepine. *N Engl J Med* 1985; **313**: 916–921.
14. Talwar D, Maninder SA, Sher PK. EEG changes and seizure exacerbation in young children treated with carbamazepine. *Epilepsia* 1994; **34**: 1154–1159.
15. Horn CS, Ater SB, Hurst DL. Carbamazepine-exacerbated epilepsy in children and adolescents. *Pediatr Neurol* 1986; **2**: 340–345.
16. Dhuna A, Pascual-Leone A, Talwar D. Exacerbation of partial seizures and onset of non-epileptic myoclonus with carbamazepine. *Epilepsia* 1991; **32**: 275–278.
17. So EL, Ruggles KH, Cassino GD, Ahmann PA, Weatherlord KW. Seizure exacerbation and status epilepticus related to carbamazepine-10,11-epoxide. *Ann Neurol* 1994; **35**: 743–746.
18. Lerman P. Seizures induced or aggravated by anticonvulsants. *Epilepsia* 1986; **276**: 706–710.

19. Kivity S, Rechtman E. Juvenile myoclonic epilepsy: Serious consequences due to pitfalls in diagnosis and management. *Epilepsia* 1995; **36**(suppl 3): S66.

20. Shufer A, Vining EPG. Photosensitive complex partial seizures aggravated by phenytoin. *Pediatr Neurol* 1991; **7**: 471–472.

21. Lortie A, Chiron C, Mumford J, Dulac O. The potential for increasing seizure frequency, relapse, and appearance of new seizure types with vigabatrin. *Neurology* 1993; **43**(suppl 5): S24–S27.

22. Luna D, Dulac O, Pajot N, Beaumont D. Vigabatrin in the treatment of childhood epilepsies: a single-blind placebo-controlled study. *Epilepsia* 1989; **30**: 430–437.

23. Vossler DG. Exacerbation of seizures in Lennox–Gastaut syndrome by gabapentin. *Neurology* 1996; **46**: 852–853.

24. Ojemann LM, Wilensky AJ, Temkin NR, Chmelir T, Ricker BA, Wallace J. Long-term treatment with gabapentin for partial seizures. *Epilepsy Res* 1992; **13**: 159–165.

25. Ettinger AB, Bernal OG, Andriola MR et al. Two cases of non-convulsive status epilepticus in association with tiagabine therapy. *Epilepsia* 1999; **40**: 1159–1162.

26. Tassinari CA, Dravet C, Roger J, Cano JP, Gastaut H. Tonic status epilepticus precipitated by intravenous benzodiazepine in five patients with Lennox–Gastaut syndrome. *Epilepsia* 1972; **13**: 421–435.

27. Prior PF, Maclaine GN, Scott DF, Laurance BM. Tonic status epilepticus precipitated by intravenous diazepam in a child with petit mal status. *Epilepsia* 1972; **13**: 467–472.

28. Hominer D, Tverskoy M, Zakut H. Paradoxical convulsions following barbiturate as an anticonvulsant. *Harefuah* 1980; **98**: 67–69.

29. Todorov AB, Lenn NJ, Gabor AJ. Exacerbation of generalized non-convulsive seizures with ethosuximide therapy. *Arch Neurol* 1978; **35**: 389–391.

30. Sander JWAS, Patsalos PN, Oxley JR, Hamilton MJ, Yuen WC. A randomized double blind placebo controlled add-on trial of lamotrigine in patients with severe epilepsy. *Epilepsy Res* 1990; **6**: 221–226.

31. Gilman JT, Alvarez LA, Duchovny M. Carbamazepine toxicity resulting from generic substitution. *Neurology* 1993; **43**: 2696–2697.

32. Robbins DK, Wedlund PJ, Kuhn R, Baumann RJ, Levy RH, Chang SL. Inhibition of epoxide hydrolase by valproic acid in epileptic patients receiving carbamazepine. *Br J Clin Pharmacol* 1990; **29**: 759–762.

33. Wilkus RJ, Dodrill CB, Troupin AS. Carbamazepine in the electroencephalogram of epileptics: a double blind study in comparison to phenytoin. *Epilepsia* 1978; **19**: 291–293.

34. Gale K. GABA and epilepsy: basic concepts from preclinical research. *Epilepsia* 1992; **33**(suppl 5): S3–S15.

35. Joccome D. Carbamazepine induced dystonia. *JAMA* 1979; **25**: 263.

36. Bimpong-Buta K, Froescher W. Carbamazepine induced choreoathetoid dyskinesias. *J Neurol Neurosurg Psychiatry* 1982; **45**: 560–567.

37. Kerrick JM, Kelley BJ, Maister BH, Graves NM, Leppik IE. Involuntary movement disorder associated with felbamate. *Neurology* 1995; **45**: 185–187.

38. Klawans HL, Weiner WJ. Phenytoin and choreic movements. *N Engl J Med* 1978; **298**: 1093–1094.

39. Agulia V, Zappia M, Quattrone A. Carbamazepine induced non-epileptic myoclonus in a child with benign epilepsy. *Epilepsia* 1987; **28**: 515–518.

40. Neufeld MY, Vishnevska S. Vigabatrin and multifocal myoclonus in adults with partial seizures. *Clin Neuropharmacol* 1995; **18**: 280–283.

41. Reeves AL, So EL, Sharbrough FW, Krahn LE. Movement disorders associated with the use of gabapentin. *Epilepsia* 1996; **37**: 988–990.

42. Lesser RP. Psychogenic seizures. *Neurology* 1996; **46**: 1499–1506.

30

Management of paroxysmal symptoms in multiple sclerosis

Christian Confavreux, Françoise Bouhour and Sandra Vukusic

The first anecdotal reports on paroxysmal symptoms or signs in multiple sclerosis date back to the last century. The first comprehensive review was made by McAlpine in 1972 in his classical monograph[1] devoted to multiple sclerosis with the collaboration of Lumsden and Acheson. Several other authors should also be mentioned for their pioneer work in the field. The description of tonic seizures is due to Matthews,[2] paroxysmal dysarthria and ataxia to Andermann et al,[3] paroxysmal akinesia to Zeldowicz,[4] paroxysmal paraesthesias and pain to Espir and Millac,[5] and paroxysmal hemitaxia and crossed paraesthesias, paroxysmal diplopia and paroxysmal itching to Osterman and Westerberg.[6] Owing to quite similar physiopathology and response to antiepileptic drugs, the current trend is to include Lhermitte sign and trigeminal neuralgia in the list of paroxysmal symptoms and signs in multiple sclerosis. It may also be argued that epileptic manifestations, which are a classic feature in multiple sclerosis, should be included.

THE COMMON CLINICAL PATTERN

Paroxysmal manifestations in multiple sclerosis share several clinical characteristics. They correspond to positive symptoms or signs related to hyperactivity of the central nervous system. They occur suddenly, at any time or place. Their duration is short, a few seconds to 1 or 2 min. They often recur from a few times per day to several times an hour. Their semiological expression may vary considerably from one patient to another, but, as shown on the occasion of the frequent recurrences, remains stereotyped for a given patient. Paroxysmal manifestations may either occur spontaneously or be triggered by external stimuli. Typical examples are neck flexion for Lhermitte sign, tactile stimuli for trigeminal neuralgia, and limb movements for kinesigenic choreoathetosis. Eye movements have also been described at the origin of phosphenes in optic neuritis. Paroxysmal manifestations may recur in a given patient for several days, weeks or months until remission appears. This time-scale of the cluster is similar to that of exacerbations of the disease. A dramatic response to carbamazepine is another characteristic of paroxysmal manifestations.

Considering these definitions, paroxysmal manifestations are quite similar to epileptic attacks: positive signs, possible triggering, duration of a few seconds. Conversely, they are clearly different from the Uhthoff phenomenon and the exacerbations of the disease. In both of these instances, clinical manifestations are negative. The Uhthoff phenomenon is particular for being triggered by an increase in body temperature or warm atmosphere (hot bath test), or by muscular effort, and by having few minutes' duration, since the phenomenon disappears when physiological temperature returns to normal or physical effort stops. As for the exacerbations, they are spontaneous in most cases and their time-scale varies from a few days to a few weeks (Fig. 30.1).

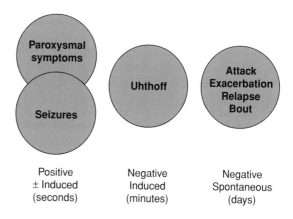

Figure 30.1 Comparison of the clinical characteristics of paroxysmal manifestations, epileptic seizures, Uhthoff phenomenon and exacerbations in multiple sclerosis.

CLINICAL DIVERSITY

The clinical range of paroxysmal manifestations is incredibly large.[7] Some syndromes may nonetheless be highlighted with respect to their frequency or particular clinical expression. Paroxysmal dysarthria and ataxia[3] is the most famous of them. It is characterized by slurred speech and gait ataxia. In some cases, the syndrome is associated with incoordination of one or both upper limbs, some sensory disturbances in one limb, and even, sometimes, diplopia.

Another classical syndrome is that of paroxysmal hemiataxia and crossed paraesthesias.[6] The first symptom is unpleasant prickling, with painful sensations in some cases, these manifestations affecting one side of the face and ipsilateral arm. This is followed by ataxia of the contralateral arm and leg and, in some cases, dysarthria. From a clinical point of view, one should rather speak of paroxysmal paraesthesias and crossed hemiataxia.

The paroxysmal tonic seizures correspond to a tonic spasm without clonic movements or loss of consciousness. They affect the upper limb and are often manifested by adduction of the shoulder, flexion of the elbow, wrist and metacarpophalangeal joints, and extension of the interphalangeal joints. In some cases, the lower limb is also affected, causing flexion of hip and knee and extension of the feet and toes. The tonic spasms may sometimes be bilateral. The syndrome may be purely motor or, conversely, painful with sensory disturbances. When the latter affect the involved limb, one speaks of 'spinal sensorimotor seizure'.[8] When they affect the contralateral limb, one speaks of the 'Brown–Sequard syndrome in reverse'.[6] Finally, the tonic seizures may also be associated with dysarthria.

The paroxysmal manifestations may take the form of paraesthesia or pain.[5] In most cases, such manifestations affect a single limb. Paraesthesias are usually unpleasant. When painful, they are often intense and severe. Paroxysmal itching is another variety of sensory manifestation.[6] This phenomenon may affect different parts of the body, usually one upper limb or the trunk. It may be extremely intense and is not relieved by scratching or pinching.

Among the motor manifestations, one should note paroxysmal akinesia.[4] When it affects the lower limbs, which is most often the case, the patient complains that 'knees are locking', 'legs are collapsing', or 'legs do not go'. These manifestations may lead to unexpected falls. They may also affect the upper limbs. There are some dramatic descriptions, notably in a piano player.[9]

Manifestations in the brainstem have also been reported. This is the case with paroxysmal diplopia[6]

and, more recently, paroxysmal vertigo, which has been diagnosed as 'benign paroxysmal positional vertigo'.[10]

The list of possible paroxysmal manifestations does not end here. Tremor, kinesigenic choreoathetosis, focal dystonia of the jaw and cataplexy have also been described. In the area of the eyes, superior rectus and levator palpebrae spasm, ocular convergence spasm, chromatopsia and umbropsia, and movement phosphenes in optic neuritis should also be mentioned. At the sensory level, attacks of epigastric or pelvic pain and paraesthesias in the form of girdle sensation have been reported. Vegetative manifestations have also been reported, such as visually induced nausea and vomiting, and urinary incontinence, attacks of hyperventilation and atrial fibrillation. This diversity of paroxysmal manifestations is made more complex by the frequency of combinations. Indeed, it is not unusual to see a patient affected with several of the elementary manifestations described above.

It is not easy to give an estimate of the precise incidence of paroxysmal manifestations in multiple sclerosis. Indeed, the literature often deals with one or a few particular types of paroxysmal manifestations described by authors trying to collect as many representative cases as possible but without the aim of listing all the multiple sclerosis cases in the corresponding geographical area. Conversely, in some cohorts of patients with multiple sclerosis who are representative of the disease, one may wonder whether the number of cases with paroxysmal manifestations has not been underestimated, as a specific review of all the patients' case records is necessary to report these paroxysmal manifestations. The latter remark applies to the Lyon Multiple Sclerosis Cohort.[11] The available data allow us to estimate the incidence of the paroxysmal manifestations in multiple sclerosis as being between 4% and 9% for the population of the western countries[5,6,11] and around 15% for the eastern countries[12] (Table 30.1).

We would like to underline our experience of the Lyon MS Cohort, in which the most frequent paroxysmal manifestation could be called 'paroxysmal contraction of the resting lower limb(s)'. It seems that this kind of manifestation has not been described in the literature, whereas our experience proves it to be the most frequent one by far. Typically, these manifestations occur late in the afternoon or in the evening, while the patient is resting with the legs stretched out on a sofa or in bed. The patient feels the lower limb retract under a flexion of the hip and knee in response to a phasic muscular contraction, usually isolated. The limb returns to normal afterwards, until the next

Table 30.1   Incidence of paroxysmal manifestations in multiple sclerosis

	N	%
Espir and Millac[5]	23/600	4
Osterman and Westerberg[6]	22/235	9
Shibasaki and Kuroiwa[12]	N/A	17
Lyon MS Cohort[11]*	133/2926	5

* Including paroxysmal contractions of the resting lower limb(s); NA, not available

Table 30.2   Relative frequency of paroxysmal manifestations in multiple sclerosis[11]

Paroxysmal manifestation	Total number	Number of inaugural manifestations
Dysarthria/ataxia	51	11
Hemiataxia/paraesthesias	2	0
Tonic seizures	64	7
Paraesthesias	9	4
Pain	15	3
Itching	3	1
Akinesia	18	13
Diplopia	5	4
Vertigo	0	0
Total	167	43

contraction occurs 5–10 s later. The phenomenon may recur for several hours. The syndrome is often purely motor and unilateral. There are scarcely any sensory symptoms. The phenomenon may recur every day under the same conditions and, like the other paroxysmal manifestations, responds readily to carbamazepine.

Another issue is the relative incidence of the various paroxysmal manifestations. As far as we know, only one study has provided an answer, that of Twomey and Espir[13] (Table 30.2). Table 30.2 shows that for the 167 cases of multiple sclerosis with paroxysmal manifestations, the two most frequent types are tonic seizures and dysarthria/ataxia. In about 20% of the cases, the manifestations mark the onset of multiple sclerosis.

In fact, this description of the clinical range of paroxysmal manifestations of multiple sclerosis would not be exhaustive if we did not mention the trigeminal neuralgia and the Lhermitte sign. The first case of trigeminal neuralgia in multiple sclerosis was described by Oppenheim.[14] A review of the literature allows to conclude that about 1% of multiple sclerosis patients are affected on one day or another with trigeminal neuralgia, and that 1% of the patients affected with trigeminal neuralgia also suffer from multiple sclerosis. In the Lyon MS Cohort, we have traced 41 cases of trigeminal neuralgia among 2926 multiple sclerosis cases (1.4%). The clinical presentation usually mimicks perfectly idiopathic trigeminal neuralgia. Pain is distributed in the area covered by the trigeminal nerve. Its nature is frankly paroxystic with stabbing sensations. There is often a trigger zone corresponding to the part of the face affected, which is well defined in a given patient. The pain is short in duration. There is no persisting pain between the paroxystic bouts. Neurological examination does not reveal any sign in the trigeminal area. Some cases are less typical, with long-lasting pain or even persisting pain between the paroxystic attacks, paraesthesias or even sensory deficits in the trigeminal area. Trigeminal neuralgia in multiple sclerosis differs from idiopathic trigeminal neuralgia in two ways: onset is 5 years earlier; and it is more often bilateral. Trigeminal neuralgia in multiple sclerosis is unusual but possible at the onset of the disease.

The Lhermitte sign may be spontaneously reported by the patients or revealed through systematic examination. It was described by Lhermitte et al in 1924.[15] It is defined as an electric feeling passing down (the arms and) the back to the legs on flexing the neck. The younger the patient is, the more suggestive of multiple sclerosis the symptom is. It is not specific for the disease, however, as it is not infrequently observed in cervical compression, cervical spondylotic myelopathy, and subacute combined degeneration of the spinal cord. Its rate of occurrence is between 1% and 38% according to different series in the literature. In the Lyon MS Cohort, the Lhermitte sign has been reported in 329 out of the 2926 cases (11%). It is useful to remember that the Lhermitte sign may be an isolated manifestation, if not the inaugural manifestation, of multiple sclerosis.

THE LOCALIZATIONAL VALUE

Like the classic negative signs of multiple sclerosis, the paroxysmal manifestations may have localizational value. This is how trigeminal neuralgia, dysarthria ataxia and diplopia lead to the diagnosis of a brain-stem lesion. The Lhermitte sign, the tonic seizures, and even more the Brown–Sequard reverse syndrome suggest an affection of the spinal cord. Other manifestations are suggestive of a motor pathway lesion, without allowing more precision in the absence of other signs. This is the case for dyskinesia and dystonia. This is also valid for the paraesthesias and pains suggestive of a sensory pathway lesion. It is only when these manifestations concern a very well-defined dermatome that the localizational value can be more precise. Itching suggests a spinal cord lesion in the corresponding metamere. Some motor, sensory or dysarthric manifestations may correspond to subcortical lesions revealed by MRI, thus overlapping epileptic manifestations. Oculomotor movement-induced phosphenes suggest a lesion of the optic nerves.

THE DIAGNOSIS

The main risk is of underestimating these manifestations. They are indeed transient, and often have an original, if not odd, expression; also, many patients are reluctant to report them spontaneously, as they are afraid to describe disorders that could seem too extraordinary to be true. The clinician himself may be tempted to consider these manifestations as the expression of fatigue, which is often present in multiple sclerosis. He may find it difficult to individualize these paroxysmal manifestations when they develop within a chronic neurological deficit syndrome.

The diagnosis itself may be discussed with regard to three main syndromes. This is notably the case when the paroxysmal manifestations correspond to the onset of multiple sclerosis. This may also be the case in overt multiple sclerosis, as an intercurrent disease may always appear. A first alternative diagnosis is migrainous aura. The aura is visual in most cases, which is exceptional in multiple sclerosis-related paroxysmal manifestations. It may also be sensory, hemicorporeal or facial, which often leads to misdiagnosis. It may be dysphasic, which is also exceptional for a paroxysmal manifestation of multiple sclerosis, the latter being usually limited in that case to dysarthria. The motor manifestations, so frequent in the paroxysmal manifestations of multiple sclerosis, are not present in migrainous aura. Positive signs and subacute development over a few minutes until a plateau is reached and maintained for about 10 min are other characteristics of migrainous aura. Remission is also subacute on a few minutes' scale. The overall duration of migrainous aura is much greater than that of the paroxysmal manifestations of multiple sclerosis. It is usually followed by a typical headache.

Transient ischaemic attacks (TIAs) may cause many difficulties with their sudden occurrence and short duration. In fact, they differ from the paroxysmal manifestations of multiple sclerosis in several respects. They involve negative signs instead of positive ones. The episode may last several minutes to several hours. It rarely recurs with such a high frequency and symptomatic stereotypy as is the case with paroxysmal manifestations of multiple sclerosis.

Epileptic attacks are usually even more misleading. Generalized epilepsy is perfectly well documented in multiple sclerosis, with a frequency similar to that observed in the general population (0.5–1%). More specifically, focal epileptic attacks in multiple sclerosis may correspond to a cortical or subcortical plaque. Neurological symptoms may then be similar to those of a paroxysmal manifestation. It is the localization of the concerned plaque which makes the difference: cortical or subcortical in epilepsy, subcortical or clearly distant from the cortex in paroxysmal manifestations. This being said, there is obviously a clear continuum between epileptic attacks and paroxysmal manifestations in multiple sclerosis. In some cases, electroencephalography may allow us to see the difference. According to the available literature, the overall rate of epilepsy may reach 4% of the patients with multiple sclerosis. In the Lyon MS Cohort, 46 cases with epilepsy out of 2926 patients with multiple sclerosis have been traced (1.5%).

None of the paroxysmal manifestations which have been reported in multiple sclerosis has a specific diagnostic value. This is obvious for trigeminal neuralgia. Clinically, nothing may distinguish the multiple sclerosis-related and the idiopathic trigeminal neuralgia. As explained above, the Lhermitte sign has been reported in cases of radiation myelopathy, cord compression, acute combined degeneration of the cord, and other conditions. Tonic seizures have been described in neuro-Behçet, systemic lupus erythematosus and many other collagene diseases.

PATHOPHYSIOLOGY

We are indebted to the Uppsala Group[6,8] for the current interpretation of the pathogenesis of the paroxysmal manifestations of multiple sclerosis. This interpretation is based on several lines of evidence. The common clinical pattern described above is one of these. It is very close to that of epilepsy. The second line of evidence is the common pathology, the plaques of multiple sclerosis being characterized by the original combination of demyelination and axonal preservation. As multiple sclerosis primarily affects myelin, focal lesions are subcortical or located within the central white matter. The common mechanism of these paroxysmal manifestations is, similarly to epileptic attacks, paroxysmal hyperactivity of a group of neurons but, in contrast to epilepsy, from a subcortical or deep area, i.e. axonal and not neuronal. This is the basis for the theory of ephaptic transmission. Considering the plaque of demyelination with axonal preservation, transmission of the nerve influx in one of the axons tends to spread transversely from one axon to the other. One may speak of transversely spreading activation of axons in the damaged fibre tracts at the affected level. Obviously, this transverse activation is observed in the circumstances likely to activate the fibres of the affected plaque. This is the likely explanation for the frequency of triggering factors of these paroxysmal manifestations (Fig. 30.2).

This theory of ephaptic transmission allows us to interpret, though in a simplistic way, the Lhermitte sign. It corresponds to a plaque of the posterior columns of the cervical spinal cord. As it is a sensory centripetous pathway, fibres from the lower limbs enter the cord first. They arrange themselves deeply in the posterior columns of Goll and Burdach, close to the grey matter. The sensory fibres penetrating higher in the spinal cord place themselves at the surfaces of the previous fibres. Consequently, there is a somatotopy in the posterior columns of the spinal cord, with the fibres related to the arms, the trunk and the legs distributed from the surface to the interior. In the case of plaques in that area at the cervical level, neck flexion causes mechanical stimulation at the surface of the cord which spreads to the interior inducing this particular subjective sensation going down along the back from the neck to the feet (Fig. 30.3).

TREATMENTS

The paroxysmal manifestations in multiple sclerosis are among the most satisfactory symptoms to treat in multiple sclerosis. The treatment must first of all be symptomatic. It is based on the antiepileptic drugs, among which carbamazepine holds the first place. Its outstanding efficiency was first reported by Espir and Walker.[16] Low doses may be effective. In some cases, one must resort to higher doses like

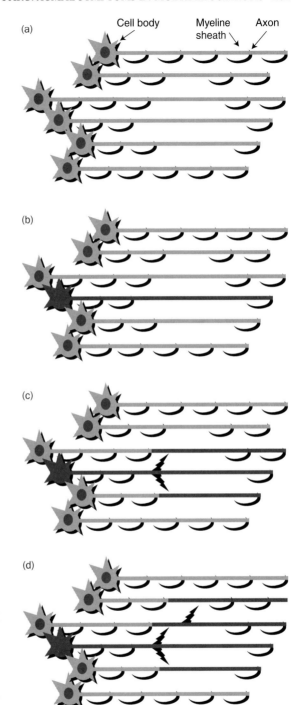

Figure 30.2 Schematic representation of ephaptic transmission: (a) resting state; (b) activation of one neuron; (c) propagation of the nerve impulse from the first activated axon to the adjacent axons; (d) propagation of the nerve impulse from the secondarily activated axons to the adjacent axons.

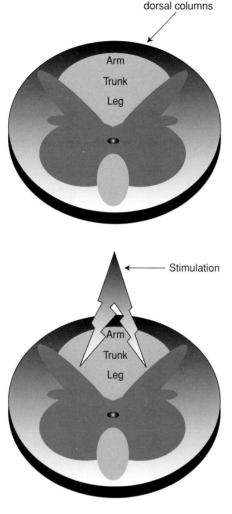

Plaque in the dorsal columns

Arm
Trunk
Leg

Stimulation

Arm
Trunk
Leg

Figure 30.3 Schematic representation of the mechanism underlying the Lhermitte sign.

those used in epilepsy, i.e. 10 mg/kg per day. Usually, this treatment brings about a dramatic response. Tolerance is not always perfect. It is preferable to start with the slowly escalating doses before reaching the efficient dose. Once the efficient, well-tolerated treatment has been established, it is possible after a few days or weeks to try to taper the posology. Indeed, as mentioned earlier, most of these paroxysmal manifestations evolve in the same way as a relapse of the disease, which implies a spontaneous remission after some time. This being said, in some cases the paroxysmal manifestations do persist, thus requiring continuous treatment.

For obscure reasons, the other traditional antiepileptic drugs are less effective than carbamazepine. This is the case with phenytoin and phenobarbital. In contrast, among the new antiepileptic therapies, some drugs such as gabapentin and lamotrigine seem to be as effective as carbamazepine. Interestingly, these are often much better tolerated than carbamazepine, notably regarding wakefulness.

However, there is another consideration when using antiepileptic drugs in multiple sclerosis. Though their efficacy has been proven for paroxysmal manifestations and epileptic seizures, i.e. for positive manifestations that involve axonal or neuronal hyperactivity, these drugs have a worsening effect on negative manifestations, whether related to Uhthoff's phenomenon or to relapses, neurological sequelae or progression of the disease. These neurological deficits result from blocked nerve conduction. Interestingly, they are improved with certain molecules such as aminopyridine. These are potassium channel blockers that improve nerve conduction in experimentally demyelinated nerves, decrease epileptic threshold, and induce bursting of nerve impulses. Here again they act as a two-edged sword; that is, they improve the negative signs of multiple sclerosis while triggering paraesthesia, pain and, most of all, convulsions at the same time (Fig. 30.4).

Quite a number of other drugs or techniques have been described as symptomatic treatment of the paroxysmal manifestations of multiple sclerosis. Benzodiazepines are among these, notably clonazepam. They are often effective but poorly tolerated, causing drowsiness and worsening of the

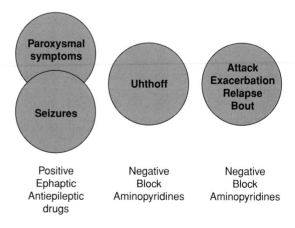

Figure 30.4 Comparison of the pathophysiology and the treatments of the positive and negative manifestations in multiple sclerosis

negative signs, for instance worsening of the balance disorders and reduction of the muscular tonus in the lower limbs. Sodium channel blockers such as lidocaine and mexiletine have also been described as useful. This is also true for acetazolamide, which inhibits carbonic anhydrase. Bromocriptine has shown some efficacy according to some authors. Weak electromagnetic fields and, more recently, smoked cannabis have also been proposed.

Trigeminal neuralgia is often well controlled by antiepileptic drugs, especially carbamazepine. It may evolve like a relapse of multiple sclerosis, and antiepileptic drugs may then be reduced or even stopped. In fact, the signs recur afterwards and become chronic so that the drugs are necessary. Under these conditions, one has to prescribe quite a high dose of carbamazepine, which unfortunately implies an adverse effect on the deficits. Surgical treatment has then to be considered. As the trigeminal neuralgia corresponds to a plaque in the area of the nerve entry zone in the protuberance, the most appropriate surgery is a rhizotomy performed, either a radiofrequency rhizotomy (mechanical) or a glycerol injection (chemical). The results are often positive, with complete disappearance of pain, thus allowing us to stop the symptomatic drugs. The results are nonetheless obtained at the expense of thermoalgic hypo-aesthesia in the area of the initial pain. After several months or years, the pain may also reappear and require further treatment. This is also true for idiopathic trigeminal neuralgia. This is why the surgery technique of microvascular decompression is recommended in that setting. This kind of technique should be discarded in theory in multiple sclerosis, since the physiopathological mechanism of neuralgia is presumably related to a plaque and not to vascular–nerve compression. However, microvascular decompression has recently been proposed,[17] with results which, though preliminary, are considered as satisfactory for 50% of the cases.

The majority of the paroxysmal manifestations of multiple sclerosis are associated with relapse of the disease. It is always possible to add steroids to the symptomatic treatment to accelerate the remission.

Many factors and circumstances may trigger paroxysmal manifestations of multiple sclerosis. Overbreathing is so characteristic that the 20 deep breaths test has long been suggested to establish the diagnosis. Likewise, coffee, tea and alcohol absorption may also be at the origin of these manifestations. Hypocalcaemia is another triggering factor. Cold baths are likely to be such factors too. As far as we know, this has never been reported, whereas the worsening effect of hot baths on the neurological deficits in multiple sclerosis is well known. The worsening effect of aminopyridines has been mentioned above. In the context of this wide range of triggering factors, there are quite a number of preventive measures with respect to these paroxysmal manifestations.

To conclude, the paroxysmal manifestations of multiple sclerosis are much more frequent than initially seemed to be the case. They are easily identifiable by the attentive clinician. They share a characteristic common pattern, even if their clinical and semiological diversity are amazing, owing to the fact that the plaques may be located anywhere in the central nervous system. It is essential to identify them clearly. They may indeed cause great handicap in some patients, but can easily be controlled with antiepileptic drugs. The latter are often highly effective for the paroxystic ephaptic transmission which is the assumed mechanism of these manifestations within the demyelinated plaques with axon preservation.

REFERENCES

1. McAlpine D. In: McAlpine D, Lumsden CE, Acheson ED, eds. *Multiple Sclerosis: A Reappraisal*. Edinburgh: Churchill Lvingstone, 1972: 185–190.
2. Matthews WB. Tonic seizures in disseminated sclerosis. *Brain* 1958; **81**: 193–206.
3. Andermann F, Cosgrove JBR, Lloyd-Smith D, Walters AM. Paroxysmal dysarthria and ataxia in multiple sclerosis. *Neurology (Minneap)* 1959; **9**: 211–215.
4. Zeldowicz L. Paroxysmal motor episodes as early manifestations of multiple sclerosis. *Can Med Assoc* 1961; **84**: 937–941.
5. Espir MLE, Millac P. Treatment of paroxysmal disorders in multiple sclerosis with carbamazepine (Tegretol). *J Neurol Neurosurg Psychiatry* 1970; **33**: 528–531.
6. Osterman PO, Westerberg CE. Paroxysmal attacks in multiple sclerosis. *Brain* 1975; **98**: 189–202.
7. Matthews WB. Clinical aspects: symptoms and signs. In: Matthews WB, Compston A, Allen IV, Martyn CN, eds. *McAlpine's Multiple Sclerosis*, 2nd edn. London: Churchill Livingstone, 1991: 43–77.
8. Ekbom KA, Westerberg CE, Osterman PO. Focal sensory-motor seizures of spinal origin. *Lancet* 1968; **1**: 67.
9. Castaigne P, Cambier J, Masson M et al. Les manifestations motrices paroxystiques de la sclérose en plaques. *Presse Med* 1970; **78**: 1921–1924.
10. Dumas G, Charachon R, Ghozali S. Benign paroxysmal positional vertigo. *Ann Otolaryngol Chir Cervicofac* 1994; **111**: 301–313.
11. Confavreux C, Vukusic S, Moreau T and Adeleine P. Relapses and progression of disability in multiple sclerosis. *New Engl J Med* 2000; **343**: 1430–38.
12. Shibasaki H, Kuroiwa Y. Painful tonic seizure in multiple sclerosis. *Arch Neurol* 1974; **30**: 47–51.
13. Twomey JA, Espir MLE. Paroxysmal symptoms as the first manifestations of multiple sclerosis. *J Neurol Neurosurg Psychiatry* 1980; **43**: 296–304.

14. Oppenheim H. *Textbook of the Nervous Diseases,* Vol. 1, 5th edn. London, 1911: 337.

15. Lhermitte J, Bollak J, Nicolas M. Les douleurs à type de décharge électriqued consécutives à la flexion céphalique dans la sclérose en plaques: un cas de forme sensitive de la sclérose multiple. *Rev Neurol* 1924; **31**: 56–62.

16. Espir MLE, Walker ME. Carbamazepine in multiple sclerosis. *Lancet* 1967; **1**: 280.

17. Broggi G, Ferroli P, Franzini A, Servello D, Dones I. Microvascular decompression for trigeminal neuralgia: comments on a series of 250 cases, including 10 patients with multiple sclerosis. *J Neurol Neurosurg Psychiatry* 2000; **68**: 59–64.

Part 5

Degenerative diseases

31

An update on therapy for Parkinson's disease

Sharon Hassin-Baer and Nir Giladi

INTRODUCTION

Parkinsonism results from hypofunction of the dopaminergic system originating at the substantia nigra. Its severity correlates with the neurodegenerative process. Pharmacological restoration of dopaminergic input to the striatum ameliorates the motor symptoms associated with parkinsonism and is the mainstay for effective symptomatic therapy for Parkinson's disease (PD). Over the last decade, there have been significant achievements in this field. New drugs have been introduced and neurosurgical interventions have been renovated and reintroduced as potential treatment for selected patients. The combination of effective symptomatic drugs, modern functional intervention and careful use of the two gives patients the opportunity to function reasonably well with good quality of life for 10–20 years after the diagnosis is made.

Thirty years of experience with effective dopaminergic treatment for PD have raised several therapeutic dilemmas and modified the modern therapeutic strategies. This chapter will review the current achievements and future developments.

GENERAL GUIDELINES

Several issues should be considered before prescribing a medication for a recently diagnosed PD patient, as follows.

Does a recently diagnosed patient need medications and, if so, what should be the goal of treatment?

Since no definite neuroprotective agent is yet available, there is no rush to begin pharmacotherapy. Physical exercises should be encouraged if the patient does not experience significant functional disability. The therapeutic strategy should be discussed with the patient as well as the expectations from treatment in terms of benefit or adverse events. The major goal of treating PD remains symptomatic treatment tailored individually in order to maintain maximal function, with minimal short-term and long-term complications.

Which agents should be prescribed for which symptoms?

Most antiparkinsonian agents have a similar effect on the parkinsonian symptoms. Bradykinesia and rigidity respond better than tremor or postural disturbances. Age, cognitive function and degree of disability are the three major factors taken into consideration while choosing a drug. Other clinical characteristics, such as compliance, comorbid disorders and the presence of autonomic symptoms, affect the choice as well.

Which agents should be taken first?

In younger patients (those below 70), it is common practice to initially withhold levodopa therapy, and start with amantadine, selegiline or anticholinergics. Patients may enjoy symptomatic improvement with these drugs for several months. Only when disability becomes significant should one consider adding dopamine agonists (DAs) or levodopa. For elderly patients, levodopa may be the first choice for maximizing rapid benefit and minimizing side-effects.

When and how to escalate with therapy?

Since a chronic progressive illness is dealt with, one should consider milder medications and lowest doses early in the course of the disease and escalate slowly, trying to prescribe minimal dosages with maximal benefit. 'Using up' all the 'ammunition' at early stages is not advisable.

SPECIFIC AGENTS

Anticholinergics

Drugs that block the muscarinic receptor have a modest place in PD pharmacotherapy. They are mildly beneficial mostly for rest tremor and rigidity, with little effect on other cardinal symptoms.

Their use in PD has been limited because of the common occurrence of both peripheral (dry mouth, constipation, urinary hesitancy and visual blurring) and central (memory loss and confusion) side-effects. The latter are especially problematic in the elderly, and anticholinergics should therefore be avoided in elderly patients.

Medications such as trihexyphenidyl (Artane), procyclidine (Kemadrin), biperiden (Dekinet) and benztropine (Cogentin) can be used, starting at a low dose and increasing slowly.

Anticholinergics may be the initial therapy for early stages when rest tremor is a dominant symptom.

Amantadine

The mechanism of action of amantadine is not completely clear. There is evidence for various mechanisms, such as enhancing dopamine release, blockage of dopamine reuptake, anticholinergic effect and glutamate-N-methyl-D-aspartate (NMDA) receptor blockage.[2,3] Many patients have some symptomatic benefit, especially in the early stages, but also in the late stages of PD.

Apart from its effect on the cardinal features of parkinsonism, amantadine has been shown to decrease drug-induced dyskinesias (DID), and was suggested to have a positive effect on longevity and to improve lethargy.[4,5] Side-effects of amantadine are common and include leg edema, livedo reticularis (mottled skin on the legs), urinary retention and hallucinations.

The possible neuroprotective effect of amantadine through its NMDA antagonistic properties have made it a commonly used drug throughout the course of the disease. Memantine is another NMDA receptor antagonist related to amantadine, and which shows antiparkinsonian activity in animal models and in Parkinson's patients. Its role as a symptomatic or neuroprotective agent for PD has not yet been established.

MAO-B inhibitors

Selegiline (Eldepryl) is the only agent from this group which has been approved for PD. It is an irreversible inhibitor of monoamine oxidase B (MAO-B), is known to prevent 1-methyl-4-phenyl-1,2,3,6-tetrahydropyridine (MPTP)-induced parkinsonism in animal models, and has been shown in vitro to possess unique anti-apoptotic properties that could have neuroprotective implications.[6] Unfortunately, the evidence for slowing of PD progression is sparse, and, in addition, selegiline does not delay the development of dyskinesias or fluctuations associated with chronic levodopa therapy.[7]

Selegiline has a mild symptomatic effect in the early stages and is also beneficial for the later stages in fluctuating patients as a dopa-sparing drug, which allows a reduction of about 20% of levodopa dose.[8] The side-effects of selegiline when given in combination with other antiparkinsonian agents are those of increased dopaminergic stimulation and insomnia, which have also been seen with monotherapy. The insomnia may be attributed to the metabolism of selegiline to amphetamine. For this reason, it is recommended to take selegiline no later than at noon. The recommended dose is 5 mg twice-daily (morning and noon).

Other MAO-B inhibitors are being developed (see later).

Levodopa

Levodopa in combination with a peripheral dopa-decarboxylase inhibitor (DDI) is the most effective symptomatic medication for PD. In the brain, levodopa is converted to dopamine and both act to stimulate the monoaminergic system. The peripheral DDIs, carbidopa and benserazide, are combined with levodopa in order to increase its bioavailability in the brain and to reduce peripheral side-effects.

Despite an excellent response, most PD patients will develop levodopa-induced side-effects within 5 years of levodopa treatment.[9] These include motor fluctuations (wearing off) and/or dyskinesias (choreiform movements) as well as psychiatric or autonomic disturbances. It has become common practice to delay the use of levodopa, especially in young-onset patients, who are more prone to develop response fluctuations.

The possibility that levodopa may be toxic to dopaminergic neurons through enhancement of oxidative stress[10] raises some concern, but currently there is no convincing evidence in animal models or in humans that levodopa is toxic. When mild disability persists despite the initial antiparkinsonian treatment (anticholinergics, amantadine and selegiline), and certainly when disability increases, more potent dopaminergic therapy should be initiated. For older patients it is safer to begin levodopa. At a younger age, DAs should be introduced first, since they may result in less motor complications (see section on DAs). An alternative is to begin with low-dose levodopa combined with a low-dose DA, while further augmentation of the antiparkinsonian effect is achieved by increasing the dosage of the agonist. When the patient develops occupational or social disability despite other dopaminergic therapy, levodopa therapy should be installed or increased.

Levodopa should be given at the lowest effective dose. The maximal carbidopa or benserazide blockage effect is reached at or above 75 mg/day. If nausea is bothersome, higher doses of carbidopa can be given, or domperidone (a peripheral dopamine receptor antagonist) can be supplemented.

If the response to levodopa is unclear, the dosage should be gradually escalated until benefit or side-effects are reached. A patient that does not respond to 500 mg levodopa in a single dose is unlikely to have primary PD.

Some recommend commencing therapy with the controlled-release formulations of levodopa and a DDI, in order to provide more stable concentrations of levodopa in the brain and, as a result, to cause less long-term side-effects.[11] However, a long-term prospective study, comparing standard versus controlled-release formulations of levodopa, could not confirm this hypothesis.[12]

When motor response fluctuations develop, it becomes a real art to keep the patient in a good functional state for most of the waking hours. Manipulation of the levodopa dose and type of levodopa given is usually the first step in treating 'wearing-off' fluctuations. Increasing the number of levodopa dosages may be necessary to provide continuous coverage throughout the waking day. Changing from immediate-release to sustained-release levodopa (e.g. Sinemet CR) is another option. These formulations enable slower and more sustained levodopa absorption. Levodopa bioavailability is lower (about 70%), so the actual total dose of levodopa must be increased by about one-third. Since the peak effect is also delayed, in order to get a 'kick-in' effect patients add a small dose of the regular levodopa formulation, especially in the morning. Another approach is to add amantadine, selegiline and/or DAs.

It has been suggested that delayed gastric emptying and competition with dietary amino acids over the amino acid transporters in the small intestine and the blood–brain barrier may contribute to the development of a delayed effect to levodopa (delayed 'on') or its absence (dose failure). Therefore, in patients with motor fluctuations, levodopa should be taken on an empty stomach at least 60 min prior to meals. Dietary protein should be minimized during the day and eaten predominantly in the evening.

One may form a 'liquid levodopa' formulation, by crushing 1000 mg levodopa and 100 mg of a DDI with 1 l of water and 2 g ascorbic acid (creating a solution that contains 1 mg levodopa = 1 ml solution). This may be a solution for patients with long delayed 'on' and others who need fast absorption or very small adjustments in dosage that cannot be achieved by breaking the pills. Nocturnal akinesia can be eased by a bedtime dose of a controlled-release formulation of levodopa.

Drug-induced choreiform dyskinesias may resolve with a reduction in the daily levodopa dose. As the disease progresses, the levodopa dosage needed to produce an adequate motor response approaches the dosage that causes dyskinesia, and eventually any 'on' is accompanied by dyskinesia. Other alternatives for treating drug-induced dyskinesias are mentioned later.

Dopamine agonists

The DAs are a group of antiparkinsonian agents acting directly on the dopamine receptors. There are currently six commercially available DAs: bromocriptine (Parlodel), lisuride (Dopergin), pergolide (Permax), pramipexole (Mirapex), ropinirole (Requip) and cabergoline (Cabaser).

The DAs have a longer half-life than levodopa, and are thought to cause less response fluctuations. In addition, they do not increase oxidative stress, and may have neuroprotective effects on dopaminergic neurons. As a result of all the above and their established efficacy in parkinsonism, they are being used increasingly in the treatment of PD. DAs are given as monotherapy early in the course of disease, in order to delay the introduction of levodopa. It has recently been shown that early PD can be managed successfully for up to 5 years with a reduced risk of dyskinesia by initiating treatment with ropinirole alone and supplementing it with levodopa if necessary.[13]

DAs work in concert with levodopa at all stages, ameliorating the symptoms and enabling lower levodopa dosage. DAs are commonly given to PD patients with levodopa-induced motor fluctuations in order to smoothen the fluctuations by decreasing the patient's 'off' periods.

One of the disadvantages of DA therapy is the long and complex titration period needed to reach effective doses. In addition, their side-effect profile is more complex and frequent. The most frequent adverse effects of DAs are nausea and vomiting, postural hypotension, drowsiness, constipation and mental disturbances (hallucinations and confusion). The latter are more common in elderly and demented patients. Serious but rare adverse events associated with the ergoline DAs (bromocriptine, pergolide, lisuride and cabergoline) include pulmonary and retroperitoneal fibrosis as well as erythromelalgia, which are unlikely with the newer non-ergot DAs (pramipexole and ropinirole). Recently, it has been reported that DAs may cause in addition to somnolence sudden bouts of sleep that are often unpredictable.[14] Therefore, DAs should be taken with caution when driving.

DAs are much more expensive than levodopa, and at a time when pharmacoeconomics have an important place in healthcare strategies this is a serious disadvantage.

The various DAs differ in receptor affinity and activity (Tables 31.1 and 31.2). Stimulation of the D2 dopamine receptor is primarily responsible for their antiparkinsonian effect. How the other pharmacological profiles translate into clinical events is uncertain. The drugs differ also in their half-life, formulations and, to a lesser extent, in their adverse events.

One important advantage of DAs is the possibility of their parenteral administration. Lisuride and apomorphine are DAs that can be given parenterally. Subcutaneous injections of apomorphine display an immediate effect and thus are frequently used as rescue therapy during 'off' periods. Continuous subcutaneous infusions of apomorphine are another effective approach for patients with severe motor fluctuations.

Clinical comparisons between the DAs have been done only by comparing pergolide and some of the new DAs to the oldest drug in this group, bromocriptine. Some of these studies did indeed show superiority over bromocriptine in some aspects, i.e. motor improvement, 'off' time reduction and side-effects, whereas some of them did not. In spite of this there is no convincing evidence unequivocally demonstrating the superiority of the newer drugs.[15–19]

COMT inhibitors

There are two agents belonging to another class of antiparkinsonian medications that work by inhibiting the enzyme catechol-*O*-methyltransferase

Table 31.1   In vitro receptor binding affinities of dopamine agonists

DA	D2 Family	D1 Family	5-HT$_{1/2}$	α_1	α_2
Ropinirole	++	–	–	–	–
Pramipexole	++	–	–	+	–
Bromocriptine[a]	++	+[a]	++	++	++
Pergolide	+++	++	++	+	++
Cabergoline	++	+	–	–	–
Apomorphine	++	+++	–		

+, ++, +++, increasing agonist affinity; –, negligible affinity.
[a] Bromocriptine is a mild D1 antagonist.

Table 31.2   Characteristics of dopamine receptor agonists

Drug	Formulations (mg)	$T_{1/2}$ (h)	Starting daily dose (mg)	Usual maintenance dose (mg)	Maximal dose (mg)
Bromocriptine (Parlodel)	2.5, 5	3–8	1.25	5–10 t.i.d.	60–100
Pergolide (Permax)	0.05, 0.25, 1.0	27	0.05 b.i.d.	0.5–1.0 t.i.d.	12
Lisuride (Dopergin)	0.2		0.1 b.i.d	0.2–0.6 t.i.d. or q.i.d.	3
Pramipexole (Mirapex)	0.125, 0.25, 0.5, 1.0, 1.5	8–12	0.125 t.i.d.	1.0–1.5 t.i.d.	6
Ropinirole (Requip)	0.25, 0.5, 1.0, 2.0, 5.0	6	0.25 t.i.d.	1.0–6 t.i.d.	27
Cabergoline (Cabaser)	1, 2, 4	65	0.5 once	2–6 mg once-daily	6
Apomorphine	10 mg/ml	0.5	1.5–3 mg, single injection	As needed	

(COMT), an enzyme involved in levodopa and dopamine metabolism in the periphery and centrally. COMT metabolizes levodopa into 3-O-methyldopa (3-OMD), whose half-life is about 15 h, compared to about 1 h for levodopa, and which is suggested to compete with levodopa for uptake into the brain.

The COMT inhibitors tolcapone (Tasmar) and entacapone (Comtan) have been proven to improve 'on' time and reduce motor fluctuations in advanced PD patients treated with levodopa.[20–22] Tolcapone inhibits COMT peripherally and possibly centrally, and entacapone works only at the periphery. Their action augments levodopa bioavailability and its entrance into the central nervous system by increasing its plasma concentration–time curve. Introducing one of these agents was shown to reduce the necessary levodopa dose by about 30%.

Long-term exposure to the oscillations in levodopa-derived dopamine is suggested to cause postsynaptic changes within the dopaminergic system, leading to further reductions in the drug's efficacy and development of DID. Early COMT inhibition along with levodopa therapy even in stable responders might decrease the pulsatile stimulation and lessen the development of long-term complications, but this hypothesis needs further confirmation.

The major side-effects of both drugs are dopaminergic (dyskinesias, hallucinations, nausea) and these usually respond to reductions in levodopa dose. Tolcapone causes diarrhea in up to 20% of the patients, commonly leading to treatment withdrawal. Abnormalities in liver function tests have been observed in up to 4% of the patients participating in clinical studies with tolcapone. There have also been a few cases of hepatic failure and death while taking tolcapone, leading to restrictions on its use.[23]

Future developments

There is a continuous effort being made to improve symptomatic therapy for PD. Levodopa ethyl ester (LDEE), a new highly soluble prodrug of levodopa, is one such development, enabling faster absorption of levodopa from the gastrointestinal tract and shortening the time to 'on'.[24] LDEE can be given as a soluble oral preparation and also by subcutaneous and intramuscular injections. Oral LDEE is under investigation in phase III studies in advanced PD. Other methods of levodopa administration are under development, such as transdermal patches. Combining DDIs, MAO-B inhibitors and COMT inhibitors in one 'magic' levodopa preparation is another proposal.

Currently, no treatment has been proven to slow the progression of PD. The past decade has seen major advances in deciphering genetic and molecular causes of parkinsonism as well as mapping some of the events involved in nigral cell death. The present efforts towards developing disease-modifying neuroprotective strategies concern mechanisms of oxidative stress, excitotoxicity and apoptosis. Since the largest part of nigral cell loss occurs before PD symptoms appear, neuroprotection relies on early presymptomatic diagnosis and therapy.

The potential of DAs to provide neuroprotection in PD by mechanisms other than a levodopa-sparing effect, e.g. stimulation of dopamine autoreceptors resulting in decreased dopamine synthesis, release, and turnover or direct antioxidant effects, is under investigation, and several clinical trials have been initiated to test their effect on clinical and neuroimaging markers of disease progression.

Evidence for mitochondrial dysfunction in PD has been published, rendering the dopaminergic neurons vulnerable to oxidative injury. Levodopa has been claimed to have a toxic effect on the nigral cells through oxidative mechanisms. This issue is now being prospectively studied in a clinical study. MAO-B inhibition, high doses of vitamin E and other antioxidants as well as agents that enhance mitochondrial function (coenzyme Q10, idebenone, nicotinamide, sodium dichloroacetate and creatine) have never been shown to have any significant protective effect.

In addition, antiexcitatory agents are under investigation. Glutamate NMDA receptor antagonists, such as amantadine and memantine, have been shown to be associated with increased survival in PD. Remacemide, a glutamate NMDA receptor antagonist,[25] and riluzole, a drug which inhibits glutamate release and has been proven to slow progression of amyotrophic lateral sclerosis, are being investigated as possible neuroprotective agents for PD.

Other strategies, such as treatment with neurotrophic factors, immunophilin ligands, antiapoptotic agents and caspase inhibitors, are in various stages of research.

NEUROSURGICAL INTERVENTIONS FOR PD

Selected patients who suffer severe disability despite optimal medical therapy may be candidates for neurosurgical interventions

Currently, three types of surgery are performed:

Table 31.3 Neurosurgical interventions in Parkinson's disease[26]

Type of operation	Site of intervention	Best candidate	Effect on drug therapy	Effect on parkinsonian symptoms			Disadvantages
				Tremor	'Off' symptoms	Dyskinesia	
Lesioning procedures	Thalamus Vim (unilateral)	Unilateral tremor-predominant PD	Can replace drug therapy for tremor	++	0	+	speech disturbances when done bilaterally
	Pallidum GPi/GPe (unilateral)	Advanced PD with unilateral dyskinesias	Minor changes of medications	++	++ (30%)	+++	Cognitive changes when done bilaterallly
Deep brain stimulation	Thalamus Vim	Tremor-predominant PD	Decrease anti-tremor treatment	+++	0	0	Improves only tremor
	Pallidum GPi (bilateral)	Advanced PD with dyskinesias	Minor changes of medications	+	++	+++	Mild effect on tremor
	Subthalamic nucleus (bilateral)	Advanced PD, on/off, dyskinesia, and good response to levodopa	60–80% decrease in total levodopa dose-day	+++	+++	0	Needs fine tuning Dyskinesia as side-effect

Vim, ventral intermediate; GPi, internal globus pallidus, GPe, internal globus pallidus; PD, Parkinson's disease; +, mild effect; ++, moderate effect; +++, marked effect; 0, no effect.

(1) ablative or destructive surgery (lesioning procedures)
(2) stimulation surgery or deep brain stimulation
(3) transplantation or restorative surgery.

The first two are in common practice, while the third is still experimental and will not be discussed here. Recent advances in neurosurgical techniques and in understanding the pathophysiology of motor disturbances in PD have made functional neurosurgery safer and more effective. The various indications are shown in Table 3.3.[26]

REFERENCES

1. Wasielewski PG, Burns JM, Koller WC. Pharmacologic treatment of tremor. *Mov Disord* 1998; **13**: 90–100.

2. Stoof JC, Booij J, Drukarch B. Amantadine as N-methyl-D-aspartic acid receptor antagonist: new possibilities for therapeutic applications? *Clin Neurol Neurosurg* 1992; **94**: S4–S6.

3. Lang AE, Blair RDG, Anticholinergic drugs and amantadine in the treatment of Parkinson's disease. In: Calne DB, ed. *Handbook of Experimental Pharmacology.* Berlin: Springer-Verlag, 1989: 307–323.

4. Verhagen Metman L-P, Del Dotto P, van den Munckhof P et al. Amantadine as treatment for dyskinesias and motor fluctuations in Parkinson's disease. *Neurology* 1998; **50**: 1323–1326.

5. Snow, BJ, Macdonald L, McAuley D et al. The effect of amantadine on levodopa-induced dyskinesias in Parkinson's disease: a double-blind, placebo-controlled study. *Clin Neuropharmacol* 2000; **23**: 82–85.

6. Snyder SH, D'Amato RJ. MPTP: a neurotoxin relevant to the pathophysiology of Parkinson's disease. The 1985 George C. Cotzias lecture. *Neurology* 1986; **36**: 250–258.

7. Parkinson Study Group. Impact of deprenyl and tocopherol treatment on Parkinson's disease in DATATOP patients requiring levodopa. *Ann Neurol* 1996; **39**: 37–45.

8. The Parkinson Study Group. Effect of deprenyl on the progression of disability in early Parkinson's disease. *N Engl J Med* 1989; **321**: 1364–1371.

9. Miyawaki E, Lyons K, Pahwa R et al. Motor complications of chronic levodopa therapy in Parkinson's disease. *Clin Neuropharmacol* 1997; **20**: 523–530.

10. Jenner PG, Brin MF. Levodopa neurotoxicity: experimental studies versus clinical relevance. *Neurology* 1998; **50**: S39–S43; discussion S44–S48.

11. Chase TN. The significance of continuous dopaminergic stimulation in the treatment of Parkinson's disease. *Drugs* 1998; **55**: 1–9.

12. Yeh KC, August TF, Bush DF et al. Pharmacokinetics and bioavailability of Sinemet CR: a summary of human studies. *Neurology* 1989; **39**: 25–38.

13. Rascol O, Brooks DJ, Korczyn AD et al. A five-year study of the incidence of dyskinesia in patients with early Parkinson's disease who were treated with ropinirole or levodopa. 056 Study Group. *N Engl J Med* 2000; **342**: 1484–1491.

14. Frucht S, Rogers JD, Greene PE et al. Falling asleep at the wheel: motor vehicle mishaps in persons taking pramipexole and ropinirole. *Neurology* 1999; **52**: 1908–1910.

15. Inzelberg R, Nisipeanu P, Rabey JM et al. Double-blind comparison of cabergoline and bromocriptine in Parkinson's disease patients with motor fluctuations. *Neurology* 1996; **47**: 785–788.

16. Guttman M. Double-blind comparison of pramipexole and bromocriptine treatment with placebo in advanced Parkinson's disease. International Pramipexole–Bromocriptine Study Group. *Neurology* 1997; **49**: 1060–1065.

17. Lambert D, Waters CH. Comparative tolerability of the newer generation antiparkinsonian agents. *Drugs Aging* 2000; **16**: 55–65.

18. Pezzoli G, Martignoni E, Pacchetti C et al. A crossover, controlled study comparing pergolide with bromocriptine as an adjunct to levodopa for the treatment of Parkinson's disease. *Neurology* 1995; **45**: S22–S27.

19. Korczyn AD, Brunt ER, Larsen JP et al. A 3-year randomized trial of ropinirole and bromocriptine in early Parkinson's disease. The 053 Study Group [published erratum appears in *Neurology* 1999; **53**(5); 1162] *Neurology* 1999; **53**: 364–370.

20. Rajput AH, Martin W, Saint-Hilaire MH et al. Tolcapone improves motor function in parkinsonian patients with the 'wearing-off' phenomenon: a double-blind, placebo-controlled, multicenter trial. *Neurology* 1998; **50**: S54–S59.

21. Rinne UK, Larsen JP, Siden A et al. Entacapone enhances the response to levodopa in parkinsonian patients with motor fluctuations. Nomecomt Study Group. *Neurology* 1998; **51**: 1309–1314.

22. Kurth MC, Adler CH. COMT inhibition: a new treatment strategy for Parkinson's disease. *Neurology* 1998; **50**: S3–S14.

23. Olanow CW. Tolcapone and hepatotoxic effects. Tasmar Advisory Panel. *Arch Neurol* 2000; **57**: 263–267.

24. Djaldetti R, Melamed E. Levodopa ethylester: a novel rescue therapy for response fluctuations in Parkinson's disease. *Ann Neurol* 1999; **39**: 400–404.

25. Parkinson Study Group. A multicenter randomized controlled trial of remacemide hydrochloride as monotherapy for PD. *Neurology* 2000; **54**: 1583–1588.

26. Giladi N, Melamed E. The role of functional neurosurgery in Parkinson's disease. *Isr Med Assoc J* 2000; **2**: 455–461.

32

Restoring structure and function of the nigrostriatal system in Parkinson's disease

Olle Lindvall and Peter Hagell

INTRODUCTION

Intracerebral transplantation of various types of cells, including primary neurons from fetal central nervous system (CNS) tissues, genetically modified cells, adrenal medulla cells, sympathetic ganglia and stem cells, has over the past two decades been proposed as a novel therapeutic approach to repair the diseased or damaged brain. Clinical trials have been started, e.g. in Parkinson's disease (PD), Huntington's disease, stroke, and epilepsy. However, convincing experimental data must be available before any clinical trials should be undertaken, i.e. animal data demonstrating not only functional efficacy in relevant animal models, but also a defined biological mechanism for the proposed therapeutic effect. The cell replacement strategy in PD is based on such a well-defined biological mechanism, namely the recovery of function by restoration of dopamine (DA) neurotransmission in the striatum. It was demonstrated over 20 years ago that fetal mesencephalic DA-rich tissue implanted in an animal model of PD reinnervated the denervated striatum and ameliorated some functional deficits. Extensive animal studies have subsequently shown that the grafted DA neurons display many of the morphological and functional characteristics of intrinsic DA neurons: they reinnervate the denervated striatum and form synaptic contacts with host neurons, are spontaneously active and release DA, and receive afferent inputs from the host.[1] The reinnervation by the grafts is accompanied by significant amelioration of several aspects of the DA deficiency syndrome, both in rodents and monkeys.[1,2] Based on these animal experimental data, the first trials with transplantation of human fetal mesencephalic tissue to the striatum in patients with PD were started in 1987. From the clinical point of view, there is definitely a need for new therapeutic approaches in this disorder. The cell replacement strategy is also particularly suitable to explore in PD because the main pathology is a rather selective degeneration of the nigrostriatal DA system, i.e. of a specific neuronal population within a restricted area of the brain. The dopaminergic deficit in PD should, therefore, be easier to correct by transplantation as compared to, for example, the more widespread loss of many different cell types in Alzheimer's disease.

SHORT- AND LONG-TERM GRAFT SURVIVAL AND GROWTH

So far, about 300 patients with PD have been grafted with fetal tissue of human or porcine origin. It is now well established that the fetal mesencephalic DA neurons can survive transplantation into the human parkinsonian brain. Significant increase of fluorodopa uptake in the grafted striatum has been shown using positron emission tomography (PET) in 24 PD patients.[3–13] In one patient, the fluorodopa uptake in the putamen was normalized after transplantation.[9,14] Histopathological studies have confirmed the survival of dopaminergic grafts and demonstrated reinnervation of the striatum in two parkinsonian patients who died after transplantation.[15–17] Between 80 000 and 135 000 dopaminergic neurons had survived on each side. The neuritic outgrowth from the grafted neurons extended up to approximately 7 mm within the putamen. With six tracts, placed 5 mm apart, confluent reinnervation of 24–78% of the designated target area in the postcommissural putamen could be obtained, although in the patient with the densest reinnervation, the putamen was shrunken.[16] The dopaminergic innervation occurred in a patch-matrix pattern and electron microscopy revealed synaptic connections between graft and host. There was no evidence that sprouting had occurred from the patient's own DA neurons.

Fetal mesencephalic grafts can exhibit long-term survival despite an ongoing disease process and continuous antiparkinsonian drug treatment. In two patients, who were transplanted unilaterally in the putamen, the fluorodopa uptake in the grafted structure was still high at 6 and 10 years after surgery.[9,14] In contrast, there had been a progressive fall of tracer uptake in non-grafted striatal regions, indicating degeneration of the patient's own DA neurons. Immunological rejection of the grafts has not been reported in any PD patient, even several years after withdrawal of immunosuppression.

MAGNITUDE OF CLINICAL IMPROVEMENT

Several clinical research groups have demonstrated therapeutic improvement associated with graft survival.[3–13,18,19] In the most successful cases, patients have been able to cease L-dopa treatment after transplantation.[9,10,13] In our own series, three patients have managed without L-dopa for 3.5–5 years. About two-thirds of grafted patients have shown clinically useful, partial recovery of motor function, mainly characterized by decreased time spent in the 'off'

phase and reduced rigidity and bradykinesia during remaining 'off' phases. Both improvement and worsening of dyskinesias and gait have been observed after transplantation. Posture, postural function, swallowing and speech have been unchanged or only modestly improved in single patients.

Table 32.1 summarizes the magnitude of the overall clinical benefit at 10–24 months postoperatively in three series of patients who were grafted bilaterally with human fetal mesencephalic tissue.[10,11,13] These patients received tissue from about 3–5 donors into each putamen. In addition, tissue from one or two donors was implanted into the caudate nucleus, bilaterally in the patients of Brundin et al[13] and unilaterally in one patient reported by Hagell et al.[10] According to the Unified Parkinson's Disease Rating Scale (UPDRS)[20] motor score during practically defined 'off' phase (i.e. in the morning, at least 12 h after the last dose of antiparkinsonian medication), the overall symptomatic relief was between 30% and 40%. In addition, there was a decrease (by 43–59%) of the average daily time spent in the 'off' phase. The mean daily L-dopa requirements were reduced by 16–45% (Table 32.1).[10,11,13]

In the study by Brundin et al,[13] the patients received less fetal mesencephalic tissue than in the

Table 32.1   Amount of graft tissue and magnitude of postoperative changes of putaminal fluorodopa uptake and motor function in three series of patients with idiopathic PD at 10–24 months after bilateral intrastriatal implantation of human fetal mesencephalic tissue

	Hauser et al[11] (n = 6)	Hagell et al[10] (n = 4[a])	Brundin et al[13] (n = 5)
Number of VM/putamen	3–4	4.9	2.8[b]
Fluorodopa uptake (putamen):			
Preop[c]	34%	31%	31%
Postop[c]	55%	52%	48%
Δ	+61%	+69%	+55%
UPDRS motor score in 'off' (Δ)[d]	–30%	–30%	–40%
Daily time in 'off' phase (Δ)	–43%	–59%	–43%
Daily L-dopa dose (Δ)	–16%	–37%	–45%

[a]Excluding one patient with possible multiple system atrophy.
[b]The graft tissue was treated with the lazaroid tirilazad mesylate.
[c]Mean percentage fluorodopa uptake compared to the normal mean as measured in healthy volunteers.
[d]As assessed during practically defined 'off'.
VM, ventral mesencephalon; Δ, mean postoperative change (%) from baseline; Preop, preoperatively; Postop, postoperatively; UPDRS, Unified Parkinson's Disease Rating Scale.

other two clinical trials. In order to increase graft survival, the lazaroid tirilazad mesylate was supplied to the tissue before transplantation and given intravenously to the patients for 3 days thereafter. Lazaroids are a group of free radical scavengers that inhibit oxidative stress caused by lipid peroxidation. These compounds increase the survival of rat and human DA neurons in culture and after grafting in the rat PD model about 2-fold.[21–25] Although not providing definite proof, the observations of Brundin et al[13] indicate that exposure of human fetal mesencephalic tissue to tirilazad mesylate prior to implantation into the striatum of PD patients promotes dopaminergic graft survival similarly to what has been found in experimental animals.

MECHANISMS OF GRAFT FUNCTION

The clinical observations discussed above demonstrate that the grafts can survive, store DA, and give rise to symptomatic relief. But can the grafts really restore the specific biological mechanism that is deficient in PD, i.e. dopaminergic neurotransmission in the striatum?

Using PET, we have started to address questions regarding the mechanisms of action of neural grafts in vivo in PD patients. We first wanted to explore whether the grafts release DA, and therefore studied one of our most successful patients, who was grafted unilaterally in the right putamen more than 10 years ago using mesencephalic tissue from four donors.[3–5,9,14,18] 'On–off' fluctuations disappeared

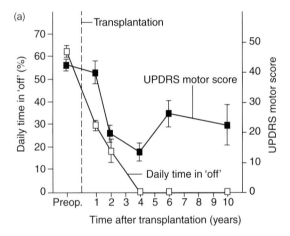

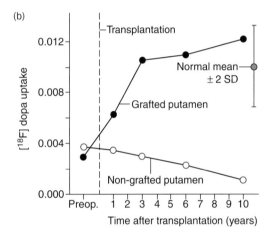

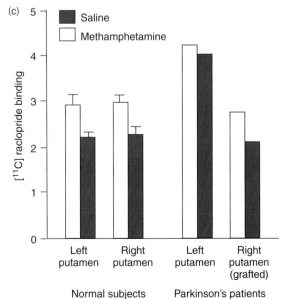

Figure 32.1 Neural grafts can restore DA storage and release in the striatum to normal levels and give major symptomatic relief for more than a decade in patients with PD. (a) Percentage of the day spent in the 'off' phase and UPDRS motor score (maximum score = 108) in the practically defined 'off' phase preoperatively and at various time points after transplantation of human fetal mesencephalic tissue unilaterally into the right putamen. Data are mean ± 95% confidence interval. (b) Fluorodopa uptake in the grafted and non-grafted putamen in the same patient. Comparative data (mean ± 2 SD) are given for a group of 16 healthy volunteers. (c) Basal and drug-induced DA release as assessed using [11C]raclopride PET to measure DA D2 receptor occupancy by the endogenous transmitter. In the baseline condition (saline infusion; open bars), [11C]raclopride binding is increased in the non-grafted putamen in the patient, while it is normal on the grafted side (right putamen). After methamphetamine administration (filled bars), the binding reduction in the grafted putamen is similar to that seen in the putamen of normal subjects, whereas it is negligible in the non-grafted putamen. Data from Piccini et al.[14]

after 3 years (Fig. 32.1a), and L-dopa treatment and immunosuppression were withdrawn. His motor score on the UPDRS was reduced by 50–60%. The patient was without L-dopa treatment for 3.5 years, at which time it was reintroduced (using one-third of his preoperative dose), owing to slight symptom progression axially and on the side of the body ipsilateral to the graft. In agreement with his major clinical improvement, fluorodopa uptake in the grafted putamen was normalized after 3 years and has been stable thereafter (Fig. 32.1b). In contrast, the non-grafted putamen has exhibited a progressive decrease of fluorodopa uptake, which at 10 years after surgery was only about 10% of the normal level.

DA release from the grafts could be visualized in this patient using [^{11}C]raclopride and PET to measure DA D2 receptor occupancy by endogenous DA.[14] Scans were performed twice, giving an intravenous dose of saline in one scan and of methamphetamine in the other scan. Following saline injection, we observed a 30% upregulation of D2 receptor binding in the non-grafted putamen, whereas binding was normal in the grafted putamen (Fig. 32.1c). This indicates that the graft continuously releases DA at a level comparable to that released from the normal nigrostriatal system. Following amphetamine injection, there was only a 5% reduction of raclopride binding in the non-grafted putamen. In contrast, the binding reduction in the grafted putamen was much more pronounced (27%), and similar to the amphetamine-induced decrease observed in normal controls (23%). These observations strongly suggest that efficient restoration of DA release in this patient underlies his major clinical improvement.

In a second study, we wanted to investigate if neural grafts can improve the deficit in movement-related frontal cortical activation in PD. We analyzed the activation of the supplementary motor area (SMA) and the dorsolateral prefrontal cortex (DLPFC) associated with movements in four patients grafted bilaterally in the caudate and putamen, using a motor task (joystick movements with the left hand) and regional cerebral blood flow measurement with PET.[26] The SMA and DLPFC are known to be important in the preparation and selection of voluntary movements, their function is influenced by basal ganglia–thalamo–cortical circuitries, and their impairment is believed to underlie parkinsonian akinesia. Preoperatively, there was only small activation of the SMA and no significant activation of the DLPFC. No significant differences in activation were observed in these patients at 6.5 months after grafting, as compared to preoperatively, while

at 18.3 months there was significantly increased activation of both the SMA and DLPFC (Fig. 32.2). The time course of clinical improvement paralleled that of the increase of cortical activation, with partial recovery after 6.5 months and substantial improvement at 18.3 months. In contrast, striatal fluorodopa

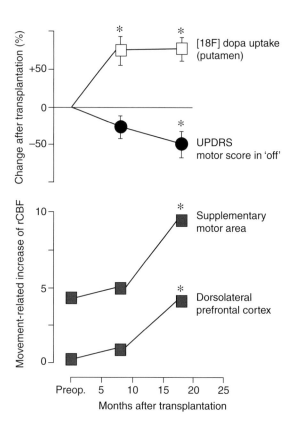

Figure 32.2 Evidence for functional integration of dopaminergic grafts in PD patients. Changes of fluorodopa uptake in the putamen and UPDRS motor score in the 'off' phase (upper panel) and movement-related increases of regional cerebral blood flow (rCBF) compared to resting condition in the supplementary motor area and dorsolateral prefrontal cortex (lower panel), preoperatively and at 6.5 and 18.3 months after bilateral implantation of fetal mesencephalic tissue into the putamen and caudate nucleus in four PD patients. Caudate and putaminal fluorodopa uptake is already significantly elevated at 6.5 months after transplantation, with no further changes thereafter. In contrast, the symptomatic relief is only partial at 6.5 months, and substantial clinical improvement, as measured by the UPDRS motor score, does not occur until the second postoperative year. The gradual and delayed symptomatic relief is paralleled by the recovery of movement-related cortical activation. Data are mean ± SD. *$P < 0.001$, compared to preoperatively, t-test. Modified from Piccini et al.[26]

uptake was already significantly elevated at 6.5 months, with no further change at 18.3 months after grafting (Fig. 32.2). These findings indicate that successful grafts in patients with PD, by improving striatal dopaminergic neurotransmission, can restore movement-related cortical activation, which is probably necessary to induce substantial clinical improvement. They also provide new evidence that the functional effects of the grafted neurons go beyond those of a simple DA delivery system. Restoration of non-regulated DA release, as in the early stages of graft maturation, when fluorodopa uptake is already significantly elevated, seems to be insufficient to improve cortical activation during movement and to induce maximum clinical recovery. In order to increase basal ganglia–thalamo–cortical neurotransmission and movement-related cortical activation, the grafted DA neurons probably need to establish both efferent and afferent synaptic connections with the host.

Taken together, these advances in our understanding of graft function in the human parkinsonian brain make it possible to propose specific neurobiological properties that are required in order for implants of DA-producing cells to be capable of inducing marked clinical improvements in PD patients: (1) at least 100 000 grafted DA neurons should survive in each putamen; (2) graft-derived reinnervation should cover as much as possible of the putaminal volume; (3) grafted cells should restore striatal DA release; and (4) grafts have to become functionally integrated into the host basal ganglia–thalamo–cortical circuitries.

FUTURE DIRECTIONS

The clinical observations after neural transplantation clearly document that cell replacement has the potential to become a novel and effective therapeutic strategy in PD. Presently, however, neural transplantation remains an experimental approach and can only be applied to small groups of patients. The most urgent problem is that new sources of dopaminergic cells have to be developed. These cells should be available in large amounts and suitable for transplantation into humans. Less than 4% of human DA neurons survive grafting into rats,[27] and similar findings (5–10% survival) have been reported after transplantation into patients.[15–17] Using currently available procedures, mesencephalic tissue from at least three or four human fetuses (giving rise to about 100 000–150 000 surviving grafted DA neurons) probably needs to be implanted per side in each patient in order to induce a substantial clinical improvement.

At present, three main research strategies are being pursued in order to solve the problem of the need for large amounts of human fetal mesencephalic tissue. The first strategy is to increase the survival of the human DA neurons after transplantation. In animal experiments, the survival of grafted mesencephalic DA neurons can be increased 2–4-fold by exposure of the graft to growth factors, and compounds that reduce oxidative stress or inhibit caspases (review: Brundin et al[25]). The only compounds that have been tested clinically are the lazaroid, tirilazad mesylate (see above), and glial cell line-derived neurotrophic factor (GDNF).[12,13] These clinical studies provide evidence that both tirilazad mesylate and GDNF (administered to the graft tissue during 6-day pregrafting storage) may improve survival of grafted DA neurons in PD patients. The second strategy is to use xenografts. However, in the initial attempts with porcine xenografts in PD patients, the survival of DA neurons has been poor and the clinical benefits only modest.[28,29] Major concerns with porcine xenografts, apart from immunological rejection and transfer of virus, are, first, that a very large number of porcine donors and many implant sites may be needed to effectively reinnervate the human striatum, and second, that the porcine DA neurons may have a lesser capacity to integrate functionally into the patient's brain as compared to human DA neurons. The third strategy is to generate large numbers of DA neurons from immature progenitor or stem cells. This has been explored using four different approaches, starting from committed mesencephalic DA neuron percursors from rat embryos,[30] in vitro expanded rat mesencephalic progenitors,[31,32] immortalized mouse neural stem cells[33] or mouse embryonic stem cells.[34] All four procedures have been reported to generate large numbers of neurons with a dopaminergic phenotype. However, major problems are that the survival of these predifferentiated DA neurons after grafting, if tested, has been poor, and it is unknown whether these cells display the functional characteristics of fully mature nigral DA neurons. Also, relatively little is known about whether DA neurons can be generated from human progenitors, since most studies have used rodent progenitors. The further progress of stem cell therapies towards clinical application in patients with PD should be made with great care, and the complexity of the biological problems involved should not be underestimated. However, given time and effort, the stem cell technology could become the scientific breakthrough that will turn cell therapy from an experimental procedure into a clinically useful treatment for large numbers of PD patients.

ACKNOWLEDGEMENTS

Our own work was supported by grants from the Swedish Medical Research Council, the Kock Foundation, the Wiberg Foundation, the King Gustav V and Queen Victoria Foundation and the Söderberg Foundation.

REFERENCES

1. Brundin P, Duan WM, Sauer H. Functional effects of mesencephalic dopamine neurons and adrenal chromaffin cells grafted to the rodent striatum. In: Dunnett SB, Björklund A, eds. *Functional Neural Transplantation*. New York: Raven Press, 1994: 9–46.
2. Annett LE. Functional studies of neural grafts in parkinsonian primates. In: Dunnett SB, Björklund A, eds. *Functional Neural Transplantation*. New York: Raven Press, 1994: 71–102.
3. Lindvall O, Brundin P, Widner H et al. Grafts of fetal dopamine neurons survive and improve motor function in Parkinson's disease. *Science* 1990; **247**: 574–577.
4. Lindvall O, Sawle G, Widner H et al. Evidence for long-term survival and function of dopaminergic grafts in progressive Parkinson's disease. *Ann Neurol* 1994; **35**: 172–180.
5. Sawle GV, Bloomfield PM, Björklund A et al. Transplantation of fetal dopamine neurons in Parkinson's disease: PET [^{18}F]6-L-fluorodopa studies in two patients with putaminal implants. *Ann Neurol* 1992; **31**: 166–173.
6. Peschanski M, Defer G, N'Guyen JP et al. Bilateral motor improvement and alteration of L-dopa effect in two patients with Parkinson's disease following intrastriatal transplantation of foetal ventral mesencephalon. *Brain* 1994; **117**: 487–499.
7. Remy P, Samson Y, Hantraye P et al. Clinical correlates of [^{18}F]fluorodopa uptake in five grafted parkinsonian patients. *Ann Neurol* 1995; **38**: 580–588.
8. Freeman TB, Olanow CW, Hauser RA et al. Bilateral fetal nigral transplantation into the postcommissural putamen in Parkinson's disease. *Ann Neurol* 1995; **38**: 379–388.
9. Wenning GK, Odin P, Morrish P et al. Short- and long-term survival and function of unilateral intrastriatal dopaminergic grafts in Parkinson's disease. *Ann Neurol* 1997; **42**: 95–107.
10. Hagell P, Schrag A, Piccini P et al. Sequential bilateral transplantation in Parkinson's disease: effects of the second graft. *Brain* 1999; **122**: 1121–1132.
11. Hauser RA, Freeman TB, Snow BJ et al. Long-term evaluation of bilateral fetal nigral transplantation in Parkinson disease. *Arch Neurol* 1999; **56**: 179–187.
12. Mendez I, Dagher A, Hong M et al. Enhancement of survival of stored dopaminergic cells and promotion of graft survival by exposure of human fetal nigral tissue to glial cell line-derived neurotrophic factor in patients with Parkinson's disease. *J Neurosurg* 2000; **92**: 863–869.
13. Brundin P, Pogarell O, Hagell P et al. Bilateral caudate and putamen grafts of embryonic mesencephalic tissue treated with lazaroids in Parkinson's disease. *Brain* 2000; **123**: 1380–1390.
14. Piccini P, Brooks DJ, Björklund A et al. Dopamine release from nigral transplants visualized *in vivo* in Parkinson's disease. *Nature Neurosci* 1999; **2**: 1137–1140.
15. Kordower JH, Freeman TB, Snow BJ et al. Neuropathological evidence of graft survival and striatal reinnervation after the transplantation of fetal mesencephalic tissue in a patient with Parkinson's disease. *N Engl J Med* 1995; **332**: 1118–1124.
16. Kordower JH, Rosenstein JM, Collier TJ et al. Functional fetal nigral grafts in a patient with Parkinson's disease: chemoanatomic, ultrastructural, and metabolic studies. *J Comp Neurol* 1996; **370**: 203–230.
17. Kordower JH, Freeman TB, Chen EY et al. Fetal nigral grafts survive and mediate clinical benefit in a patient with Parkinson's disease. *Mov Disord* 1998; **13**: 383–393.
18. Lindvall O, Widner H, Rehncrona S et al. Transplantation of fetal dopamine neurons in Parkinson's disease: 1-year clinical and neurophysiological observations in two patients with putaminal implants. *Ann Neurol* 1992; **31**: 155–165.
19. Defer GL, Geny C, Ricolfi F et al. Long-term outcome of unilaterally transplanted parkinsonian patients: I. Clinical approach. *Brain* 1996; **119**: 41–50.
20. Fahn S, Elton RL, members of the UPDRS Development Committee. Unified Parkinson's Disease Rating Scale. In: Fahn S, Marsden CD, Calne DB, Goldstein M, eds. *Recent Developments in Parkinson's Disease*, Vol. 2. New Jersey: Florham Park, MacMillan Healthcare Information, 1987: 153–163.
21. Nakao N, Frodl EM, Duan WM, Widner H, Brundin P. Lazaroids improve the survival of grafted rat embryonic dopamine neurons. *Proc Natl Acad Sci USA* 1994; **91**: 12408–12412.
22. Othberg A, Keep M, Brundin P, Lindvall O. Tirilazad mesylate improves survival of rat and human embryonic mesencephalic neurons *in vitro*. *Exp Neurol* 1997; **147**: 498–502.
23. Björklund L, Spenger C, Strömberg I. Tirilazad mesylate increases dopaminergic neuronal survival in the in oculo grafting model. *Exp Neurol* 1997; **148**: 324–333.
24. Hansson O, Kaminski-Schierle GS, Karlsson J, Brundin P. The lazaroid tirilazad mesylate and the caspase inhibitor Ac-YVAD-cm improve the survival of grafted dopamine neurons. *Soc Neurosci Abstr* 1999; **25**: 745.
25. Brundin P, Karlsson J, Emgård M et al. Improving the survival of grafted dopaminergic neurons: a review over current approaches. *Cell Transplant* 2000; **9**: 179–195.
26. Piccini P, Lindvall O, Björklund A et al. Delayed recovery of movement-related cortical function in Parkinson's disease following striatal dopaminergic grafts. *Ann Neurol* 2000; **48**: 689–695.
27. Frodl EM, Nakao N, Brundin P. Lazaroids improve the survival of cultured rat embryonic mesencephalic neurones. *NeuroReport* 1994; **5**: 2393–2396.
28. Deacon T, Schumacher J, Dinsmore J et al. Histological evidence of fetal pig neural cell survival after transplantation into a patient with Parkinson's disease. *Nature Med* 1997; **3**: 350–353.
29. Schumacher JM, Ellias SA, Palmer EP et al. Transplantation of embryonic porcine mesencephalic tissue in patients with PD. *Neurology* 2000; **14**(54): 1042–1050.
30. Studer L, Tabar V, McKay RDG. Transplantation of expanded mesencephalic precursors leads to recovery in parkinsonian rats. *Nature Neurosci* 1998; **1**: 290–295.

31. Ling Z, Potter ED, Lipton JW, Carvey PM. Differentiation of mesencephalic progenitor cells into dopaminergic neurons by cytokines. *Exp Neurol* 1998; **149**: 411–423.

32. Potter ED, Ling Z, Carvey PM. Cytokine-induced conversion of mesencephalic-derived progenitor cells into dopamine neurons. *Cell Tissue Res* 1999; **296**: 235–246.

33. Wagner J, Åkerud P, Castro DS et al. Induction of a midbrain dopaminergic phenotype in Nurr1-overexpressing neural stem cells by type 1 astrocytes. *Nature Biotchnol* 1999; **17**: 653–659.

34. Lee SA, Lumelsky N, Studer L, Auerbach JM, McKay RD. Efficient generation of midbrain and hindbrain neurons from mouse embryonic stem cells. *Nature Biotechnol* 2000; **18**: 675–679.

33

Therapy of hyperkinetic movement disorders

Jose Martin Rabey

This chapter deals with therapy of hyperkinetic movement disorders. An extensive review of the treatment of movement disorders was published a few years ago (see Table 33.1).[1]

TREMOR

Tremor may be defined as a rhythmic, mechanical oscillation of any functional body region. Although any movement is accompanied by a normal physiological tremor, we are usually concerned with pathological tremors (like the kinetic tremors) that affect the activities of daily living or produce an esthetic problem (like the rest tremor of Parkinson's disease).[2,3]

Resting tremor occurs in a body part that is not voluntarily activated and that is completely supported against gravity. Usually it occurs in a relaxed limb, and is one of the major symptoms observed in Parkinson's disease. Action tremor is any tremor occurring during a voluntary contraction of muscle. This includes postural, isometric and kinetic tremor. Kinetic tremor includes intention tremor. Postural tremor occurs while a subject voluntarily maintains a position against gravity. This type of tremor sometimes occurs also in Parkinson's disease, but has usually been described in essential or familial tremor and in upper midbrain or thalamic lesions. Variants of this type of tremor have been described and are usually position-specific or position-sensitive.

Tremor observed during target-oriented movements is called intentional tremor, and usually represents a disturbance of the cerebellum or its afferent or efferent pathways. Task-specific kinetic tremor may appear or become exacerbated during specific activities, e.g. writing tremor.

Tremor is usually increased in fatigue, weakness, anxiety, hypercapnia, drug and alcohol withdrawal, and some metabolic and endocrine syndrome (uremia, hypoglycemia, hepatic disease, thyrotoxicosis and heavy-metal intoxication). Some medications increase physiological tremor, e.g. amphetamines, valproic acid, theophyllines, lithium,

Table 33.1 Drug responsiveness of various basal ganglia diseases	
Highly responsive	**Poorly responsive**
Parkinson's disease	Cerebellar tremor
Neuroleptic 'persistent' parkinsonism	Rubral tremor
DOPA-responsive dystonia	Writer's cramp
Paroxysmal hypnogenic dystonia	Palatal tremor (myoclonus)
Paroxysmal kinesigenic choreoathetosis/dystonia	Oromandibular dystonia
Neuroleptic-induced, acute dystonic reactions	Spasmodic dysphonia
Postanoxic action myoclonus	Blepharospasm
Restless leg syndrome	Striatonigral degeneration
Hereditary periodic ataxia	

steroids, anti-psychotic drugs and tricyclic antide-pressants.

Essential tremor

Essential tremor (ET) is the most common movement disorder, affecting 0.5% of the population.

It may be of the postural or action type, and is inherited in an autosomal dominant pattern. Senile tremor is considered a variant of ET. It may improve with alcohol. The underlying cause of this tremor is still not clear, although some recent studies suggest a role of cerebellar output pathways related to the Guillain–Mollaret triangle: (1) cerebellar cortex, dentate and globose-emboliform nucleus; (2) contralateral red nucleus; (3) contralateral inferior olive.[4]

Treatment of ET

β-Adrenergic receptor antagonists
These have been used extensively for the treatment of essential tremor. Their effect is due to antagonism of β_2 receptors on muscle spindles peripherally.[5] For this reason, β-antagonists that are not selective (for β_1 receptors) are desirable. Propranolol (Inderal), either as a regular or a long-acting formulation, is usually utilized (40–240 mg daily in divided doses). Propranolol is contraindicated in insulin-dependent diabetes and asthma. For patients with asthma, metoprolol (Lopressor), a cardioselective β-blocker, is preferred (50 mg b.i.d. increasing to 100 mg b.i.d).

Common side-effects which limit the use of this drug are congestive heart failure, aggravation of atrioventricular heart block, bradycardia, worsening of obstructive lung disease, masking signs of hypoglycemia for diabetes, and worsening of perfusion in obstructive peripheral vascular disease. Another problem is that aged males may complain of erection perturbations with β-blockers. Although two-thirds of patients with ET respond to β-adrenergic antagonists, the effect is unpredictable in individual patients.

Primidone (Mysoline)
This is an anticonvulsant that, for unknown reasons, is useful for the treatment of ET. The useful dosage of primidone for ET is lower than that used for its anticonvulsant properties. Treatment is usually started at 25 or 50 mg before sleeping. One of the most common side-effects observed is drowsiness and dizziness. Patients usually develop tolerance, and within a couple of weeks they can receive daily 250 mg or more without side-effects

Nimodipine (Nimotop)
At a dose of 30 mg q.i.d., this has been recently proposed as a useful medication for treating action tremor.

Carbonic anhydrase inhibitors
These include methazolamide (Neptazane) and acetozolamide (Diamox), and have also been shown recently to have some effect in some patients with ET. Some side-effects, like paresthesias and taste alterations, may occur.

Benzodiazepines
These may be used if other medication has failed. However, they produce only partial improvement. Long-acting agents such as clonazepam (Klonopin) can be used, but many patients prefer to use shorter-acting agents such as alprazolam. Sedation, tolerance and ataxia are common side-effects.

Alcohol
A small amount of alcohol can also be useful for 3–4 h for the treatment of ET.

Botulinum toxin A (Botox, Dysport)
Focal injections have been used when oral medication of tremors has failed.[6] Even head ET has been treated in this way, although with only partial success.[7]

Clozapine
This has been found useful for the treatment of ET as well as for the alleviation of parkinsonian tremor when other drugs have failed.[8] No tolerance has been observed within 6 months. The dosage is 18–75 mg/day. Major side-effects are sedation and leukopenia. It is mandatory with its use to take blood tests every week during the first 18 weeks, and later once a month.

Dystonic voice tremor (isolated)

This can often be very successfully treated with local injections of botulinum toxin into the vocal cords.[9]

Orthostatic tremor (a variant of essential tremor)

This may respond to clonazepam and primidone. Valproate and propranolol have been utilized with poor results.

Dystonic tremors

Propranolol is useful in this type of tremor. Botulinum toxin is also well documented.[6]

Surgical treatment of tremor

Stereotactic ventrolateral thalamotomy has been used with success in severe action tremor and in cerebellar action tremor of the limbs, such as in ET combined with parkinsonian tremor.[10] The use of deep-brain high-frequency stimulation (DBHS) constitutes a new therapeutic advance. The results reported apply to tremor in Parkinson's disease and ET. In patients with bilateral stimulation, dysarthria is not as common as with bilateral lesions.[11] In one controlled study in patients with cerebellar and Holmes' tremor (upper midbrain, red nucleus), good results were reported in almost 40% of the patients.[12] The major advantages of DBHS are the reversibility of the procedure and the fact that stimulation parameters can be changed over time. Some studies are dealing with the question of a possible antitremor effect of DBHS applied in the subthalamic nucleus.

Cerebellar tremors

These are usually difficult to treat. Studies with cholinergic substances (lecithin, physostigmine) have shown benefit in some patients but not in most of them. Isoniazid was reported to be effective in some isolated cases, but failed in a double-blind study.[13] Single reports have been reported with propranolol, clonazepam, carbamezapine, tetrahydrocannabinol, and trihexyphenidil.[14] A recent double-blind study supported the use of ondansetron.[15] A surgical approach with DBHS may result in an improvement, although the information gathered is still insufficient.

Holmes' tremor (rubral, midbrain)

Some patients respond to levodopa or anticholinergics.[16,17] Clonazepam and clozapine have been tried, but with limited results. Surgery may provide some success. However, we still lack a good convincing therapy for this type of tremor.

DYSTONIA

The term dystonia refers to sustained contractions of agonist and antagonist muscles, causing twistings and repetitive movements or abnormal postures. The twisting nature of dystonic movements and postures is distinctive and has led to the use of the term torsion dystonia. Dystonia can be idiopathic or secondary to several causes. Structural lesions may involve the putamen but may be found in other parts of the basal ganglia. The segmental dystonias include torticollis, retrocollis writer's cramp and other craft-associated dystonias, Meige facial dystonia and blepharospasm. Hemifacial spasms are a form of focal dystonia.

Several inherited disorders with known metabolic defects have been identified as causes of dystonia. Wilson's disease and dopa-responsive dystonia (DRD) (or dystonia with diurnal variation or Segawa's variant) are examples of this group. Idiopathic dystonia may be generalized, or limited to a particular muscle group. In idiopathic dystonia the basal ganglia show no gross or microscopic abnormalities, and no specific biochemical abnormality that explains the motor symptoms. As could be expected, given the lack of understanding of the relevant neurochemistry involved, a wide variety of medications have been reported to be effective for some patients.

Most cases of childhood-onset dystonia are inherited, usually in an autosomal dominant pattern. In 1989,[18] a DNA marker in the q32–34 region of chromosome 9 in a large non-Jewish kindred was identified. About a third of those carrying the gene express it clinically (30–40% penetrance). After the recent identification of a 3-base-pair deletion in a gene coding for a novel ATP-binding protein in the 9q34 locus, termed torsin A (resulting in the loss of a pair of glutamic acid residues), gene testing for this abnormal DYT1 gene can be carried out on individuals with dystonia.[19]

The gene for DRD was mapped to a locus on chromosome 14.[20] The use of botulinum toxin A (Botox, Dysport) injections for focal and segmental dystonia has greatly improved the therapeutic possibilities in this type of disorder.[21,22]

Unfortunately, botulinum toxin injections cannot be used to treat segmental and generalized dystonias, because of the greater number of muscles involved and the larger doses that would be needed. Very large doses may stimulate antibody formation or even induce generalized weakness. Even doses used to treat cervical dystonia have been found to produce blocking antibodies in some patients. A list of medications used for the treatment of this disorder is presented in Table 33.2.

Since 5–10% of children respond to small doses of levodopa, this drug in small doses is the drug of first choice for the treatment of dystonia in children and

Table 33.2   Medications used in the treatment of dystonia

Class	Example	Dosage (mg/day)
Dopaminergics	Levodopa	≤ 300
	Bromocriptine	7.5–40
Anticholinergics	Trihexyphenidyl	6–100
Antidopaminergics	Haloperidol	2–20
Benzodiazepines	Diazepam	5–100
GABA agonists	Baclofen	15–100
Antidepressants	Amitriptyline	25–150
Anticonvulsants	Carbamezapine	100–1000

adults (levodopa with a decarboxylase inhibitor). The second choice in patients unresponsive to levodopa are anticholinergic agents. High-dosage anticholinergics have become the main palliative treatment in dystonia.[23]

Approximately 50% of children and 40% of adults with idiopathic dystonia obtain moderate to dramatic benefit from their use. The main dose-limiting factors are the peripheral and central adverse effects of anticholinergics. Peripheral effects, such as dry mouth and blurred vision, are common but can be neutralized by co-administration of a peripherally acting anticholinesterase drug, such as pyridostigmine bromide (Mestinon) and pilocarpine eyedrops, muscarinic agonists. Central effects (hallucinations, confusion, memory decline) can be overcome by reducing the dose. High-dose baclofen appears to be the most effective medication after the anticholinergics.[24]

CHOREA

The term chorea refers to involuntary, irregular, purposeless, abrupt, rapid movements that flow randomly from one body part to another. Chorea is usually accompanied by motor impersistence, the inability to maintain a sustained contraction, manifested by drooping of objects, an inability to keep the tongue protruded ('serpentine tongue') and the presence of a 'milk-maid grip', reflecting an inability to maintain a tight hand grip.

Chorea can be caused by a variety of disorders of the basal ganglia. The treatment of the choreiform movements themselves is identical regardless of the cause.

Treatment of choreas

Neuroleptics

Choreiform movements can be controlled by neuroleptics that have prominent extrapyramidal side-effects. Most commonly, haloperidol (Haldol) (1–4 mg q.i.d.) is prescribed, but others, like pimozide (1–10 mg/day) and thioridazine (Mellaril), can be used. However, these drugs can also induce extrapyramidal and tardive syndromes (tardive dyskinesia and tardive dystonia) and should be used only if absolutely needed to control troublesome symptoms.

Clozapine, an atypical antipsychotic drug that does not seem to cause tardive dyskinesia, may be a useful alternative to the typical neuroleptics; however, the risk of agranulocytosis and its high cost limit its use.

Tetrabenazine (TBZ) (Nitoman) (25 mg tablets)

This depletes central biogenic monoamine stores. Treatment is started with half a tablet (12.5 mg), and then the dose can be increased to 200 mg/day. Drowsiness, parkinsonism and depression may be seen while using TBZ. Anxiety, insomnia and akathisia have also been described. TBZ is not available in the USA and some other countries.[25]

Reserpine (Seropasil)

This depletes central biogenic monoamine stores, like TBZ. A dose of 0.5 mg PO q.i.d. has been used in Sydenham's chorea and increased slowly to 2–4 mg/day. Orthostatic hypotension is a major problem during treatment. Tolerance usually develops in 1–2 weeks.

There are other potential adverse effects with the use of reserpine, including parkinsonism, depression and peptic ulcer disease.

Benzodiazepines

These can also have some effectiveness in the treatment of choreas. Clonazepam (0.5–6 mg/day) has been used with some benefit.

Corticosteroids

These have been used in Sydenham's chorea when the laboratory parameters suggest active inflammation.

Other drugs, such as baclofen and valproic acid, have not been proven to be effective.

PAROXYSMAL DYSKINESIAS

These are defined as abnormal dystonic and/or choreoathetotic movements that are only intermittently present.[26] The pathogenesis of paroxysmal dyskinesias is still not known but two main theories have been presented: one considers the features to be an expression of a dysfunction of the basal ganglia, and the other considers that they have an epileptic basis.

Paroxysmal dyskinesias can be distinguished phenomenologically and classified in the following way: diurnal versus nocturnal; brief (<5 min) versus prolonged (>5 min), and kinesigenic (occurring while active movements are produced) versus non-kinesigenic. In addition, we differentiate between primary (either familial or sporadic) and secondary (as a manifestation of another disorder). Four categories have been studied pharmacologically and summarized in a review by Goetz and Bennet.[27]

Prolonged familial paroxysmal dykinesias

Two-thirds of cases reported are males. Most cases suggest an autosomal dominant form of inheritance with variable penetrance. Most cases appear before 5 years of age. The most successful drugs used have been benzodiazepines, especially clonazepam. Anticonvulsants are usually not helpful. Also anticholinergics have sometimes been used.

Brief familial paroxysmal dyskinesias

This disorder is autosomal dominant with variable penetrance. Most cases are males. The majority of attacks are dystonic and brief. In this type of disorder, anticonvulsants such as phenytoin, carbamezapine and phenobarbital have been shown to be very effective.

Brief non-familial paroxysmal dyskinesias

Almost all cases of primary dyskinesias, non-familial and familial, are kinesigenic. Secondary cases are usually non-kinesigenic. The treatment of choice for this type of abnormal movement comprises anticonvulsants: phenytoin, carbamezapine, and phenobarbital. Chlodiazepoxide, imipramine and levodopa have been reported in single cases to be effective.

Nocturnal paroxysal dyskinesias

Nocturnal dyskinesias are usually cases of nocturnal dystonia. Cases are sensitive to carbamezapine and phenobarbital.

MYOCLONUS

This is a sudden, rapid, irregular, lightning-like movement produced by an abrupt and brief muscular contraction (positive myoclonus) or inhibition (negative myoclonus) like asterixis. Myoclonus may be classified as focal, multifocal, segmental or generalized, and, according to the site of origin, as cortical, brain stem (reticular) or spinal. Cortical back-averaging evoked potentials and polyelectromyography have permitted the physiological subclassification of myoclonus into cortical, subcortical, cortical–subcortical, spinal and peripheral.

Cortical myoclonus is usually manifested as focal myoclonus, which may be repetitive (epilepsia partialis continua) or evoked by muscle stretch reflex or abrupt movement of a phalanx. Myoclonus arising in the brainstem is manifested typically as generalized or palatal myoclonus.

Acquired causes of myoclonus include infections, metabolic conditions (hypoxia, uremia, hepatic encephalopathy), drug and poison intoxication (imipramine, levodopa, lithium, monoamine oxidase inhibitors, piperazine, penicillin, chlorambucil, thalium) and tumors (neuroblastoma). Treatment is directed to the underlying condition. Some dementias also present with myoclonus, such as Jakob–Creutzfeld disease (prion-related disease), Lewy body dementia, Alzheimer's disease and subacute sclerosing panencephalitis.

Treatment of myoclonus

The most common drugs used are as follows:

(1) Clonazepam (Rivotril, Clonopil) 7–12 mg daily in divided doses, starting with 1.5 mg and increasing gradually.
(2) Valproic acid in gradually increasing doses up to 2400 mg has been used in post-hypoxic myoclonus.
(3) Piracetam (Notropyl) 18–24 mg daily has been reported to be useful as a coadjuvant.
(4) TBZ been reported to be useful in spinal myoclonus.
(5) 5-Hydroxytryptophan (5-HT) 15–1500 mg PO daily with and without carbidopa has been used

in the treatment of post-hypoxic myoclonus with some success.[28]

TICS

These can be defined as quick repetitive movements (motor tics), abnormal sounds (phonic tics) or a combination of the two. When both types of tic are present for longer than a year, the syndrome is called Gilles de la Tourette. Tics frequently vary in severity over time and may have remissions and exacerbations. Usually, most of the patients admit that most of the motor and vocal tics are purposefully executed in response to an uncontrollable urge. Moreover, tics can be suppressed voluntarily by the patient for some time, but later on there is an urgent necessity to move and then the tics are manifested even more strongly. Motor and vocal tics may be simple or complex.

Treatment of tics

Haloperidol (Haldol)
This is one of the best treatments; however, success is limited by the frequent side-effects of the drug. The starting dose is 0.5 mg t.i.d., and the maximal dose achieved is between 8 and 16 mg t.i.d. Sedation, parkinsonism and hypotension are common side-effects. The development of tardive syndromes is another limiting factor.

Pimozide (Orap)
This is an oral dopamine receptor blocking drug, and may be used when haloperidol fails. The starting dosage is 1–2 mg daily, increasing gradually to 7–14 mg daily.

Risperidone (Risperdal)
This is an antipsychotic, and at a dose of 0.5–9 mg/day has been reported to be helpful in some trials.

Clonidine (Catapres)
This is an α_2-adrenergic agonist, and helps in some patients who fail to respond to haloperidol. This finding suggests that norepinephrine may play a role in the pathophysiology of tics. Clonidine is started at 0.1 mg/day and gradually increased to a maximal dose of 2 mg/day. Improvement may be seen after a couple of months. Sedation, postural hypotension and fatigue are common side-effects. The drug should be withdrawn slowly because of the possibility of rebound hypertension.[29]

TBZ (Nitoman)
This has been reported to be useful in some patients.

Calcium channel blockers
Calcium channel blockers, like nifedipine, flunarizine and verapamil, have been used for this disorder.

Botulinum toxin A (Botox)
This has been used for dystonic tics.

TARDIVE DYSKINESIA (TD)

This is a syndrome of abnormal involuntary stereotypic jerks secondary to long-term exposure to dopamine receptor antagonists such as the neuroleptics, but antiemetics such as metoclopramide and sulpiride (selective D2 receptor antagonists) can also produce the syndrome. TD usually manifests as hyperkinesias involving mainly the orofacial, limb and truncal regions. The pathophysiology of TD is not completely understood. The classical hypothesis claims an upregulation of dopamine receptors in the striatum. As a consequence, there is no specific treatment which completely abates the syndrome.

In order to avoid the occurrence of TD when it is withdrawn, the neuroleptic should be reduced gradually over as much as 2 years. On the other hand, if the offending drug is stopped after the syndrome of TD appears, the symptoms will vanish within approximately 2 years. The eventual rate of remissions is about 60%. In general, anticholinergics usually worsen the symptomatology.

Treatment of TD

(1) Amantadine and dopamine receptor agonists[30] have been claimed to be partially effective as drugs that can 'downregulate' dopamine receptors.

(2) Presynaptic dopamine depletors, such as TBZ and reserpine, have been proven to be effective in the treatment of TD (see section on chorea for drug characteristics and dosage).[31]

(3) Benzodiazepines may also prove useful for patients with mild TD. Long-acting agents such as clonazepam (Rivotril, Klonopin) (1.5–3 mg/day) have been shown to be useful in some patients.[32]

(4) Sodium valproate, g-vinyl GABA and vigabatrin have also shown mild clinical efficacy in small groups of patients.[33]

For years it was advised to restart neuroleptics in very low dosage (haloperidol 0.25 mg t.i.d.) if psychiatric symptoms emerged again and affected the quality of life in patients with TD. However, since the introduction of atypical antipsychotics such as clozapine, olanzapine, quetiapine and risperidone, classical neuroleptics should be completely avoided in patients with TD if the psychotic symptoms worsen.

AKATHISIA

This is a very common and early dose-related side-effect of neuroleptics. It may also occur after prolonged exposure to those drugs (tardive akathisia). It has also been described in patients with unmedicated encephalitic parkinsonism. Patients often complain of a feeling of inner tension in their limbs and body, causing them to shift from one position to another in attempts to relieve it.

Any therapeutic strategy in individuals exposed to neuroleptics should include dose reductions, and changing to atypical antipsychotics if possible (clozapine, ondansetron, quetiapine). In some cases, amantadine and anticholinergics may be useful. Other drugs, such as propranolol, clonidine, benzodiazepines and opioid agonists, e.g. propoxyphene, have been found to be effective in a number of patients.[34]

In refractory cases, buspirone, amitriptyline, piracetam and dopamine depleters (TBZ) can be tried.

RESTLESS LEGS SYNDROME

This is characterized by unusual sensations in the musculoskeletal parts of the lower limbs that occur at rest, mostly at night, and that are improved by movement. The pathogenesis is still unknown. It has been seen in patients with chronic renal failure and patients with iron-deficient anemia. Sometimes the symptoms are seen in subjects who also present with periodic movements during sleep; however, both syndromes can be differentiated. The treatment of both syndromes includes clonazepam, carbamezapine, dopaminergic agents (levodopa, bromocriptine, pergolide, pramipexole, cabergoline), clonidine and opioids.[35]

STIFF-PERSON SYNDROME

This is a chronically progressive condition of stiffness and rigidity in axial and then proximal limb muscles, making voluntary muscles and ambulation difficult. A fixed spinal deformity is common. Episodic spasms are precipitated by sudden movement, emotional upset and unexpected noise. An autoimmune pathogenesis is suspected, and antibodies to the enzyme glutamic acid decarboxylase (GAD) are frequently found in the plasma and cerebrospinal fluid of the patients. Corticosteroids and plasmapheresis have been used with some success.[36]

NEUROLEPTIC MALIGNANT SYNDROME

This is characterized by muscle rigidity, severe hypertremia, autonomic instability, confusion, leukocytosis and elevated creatine phosphokinase (CPK) level. It is a potentially fatal side-effect of neuroleptic drugs, but can also be produced by treatment with presynaptic dopamine depletors (reserpine) and by the sudden interruption of dopaminergic medication in parkinsonian patients. Owing to the rigidity of muscles, patients may also suffer from dyspnea, dysphagia and rhabdomyolisis. Treatment with levodopa, bromocriptine and lisuride has been successful. Also, the muscle relaxant dantrolen has been suggested. I also have good experience with the administration of amantadine intravenously, especially in patients who cannot take any medication orally. Unfortunately intravenous amantadine is not available in all countries.

ATAXIA

Ataxia does not improve with drug therapy. However some disorders with ataxia may respond to treatment.

Ataxia associated with vitamin E deficiency

Vitamin E deficiency can be associated with the development of spinocerebellar degeneration and ataxia. In abetalipoproteinemia and pure vitamin E deficiency, both autosomal recessive disorders, vitamin E can prevent or arrest the progression of the neurological dysfunction.[37]

Hereditary periodic ataxia

Periodic ataxia is an autosomal dominant disorder characterized by attacks of limb and gait ataxia associated with nystagmus, dysarthria and intention tremor. The attacks can be controlled by treatment with the carbonic anhydrase inhibitor acetazolamide.[38]

CHOLESTANOLOSIS

Cholestanolosis of cerebrotendinous xanthomatosis is an autosomal recessive disorder characterized by ataxia and tendon xanthomata. Treatment with chenodeoxycolic acid is reported to improve neurological function in this disorder.[39]

REFERENCES

1. Burns RS, Rabey JM. Drug treatment in movement disorders. In: Munson PL, Mueller RA, Breese GR, eds. *Principles of Pharmacology, Basic Concepts and Clinical Applications*. New York: Chapman & Hall, 1995: 325–362.

2. Hallet M. Classification and treatment of tremor. *JAMA* 1991; **266**: 1115–1117.

3. Deushl G, Krack P. Tremors: differential diagnosis, neurophysiology and pharmacology. In: Jancovic J, Tolosa E, eds. *Parkinson's Disease and Movement Disorders*, 3rd edn. Baltimore: Williams & Wilkins, 1998: 419–452.

4. Elble RJ, Koller WC. *Tremor*. Baltimore: Johns Hopkins University, 1990.

5. Young RR, Growdon JH, Shahani BT. Beta-adrenergic mechanism in action tremor. *N Engl J Med* 1975; **293**: 950–953.

6. Jankovic J, Shwartz K. Botulinum toxin treatment of tremors. *Neurology* 1991; **41**: 1185–1188.

7. Pahwa R, Busenbark K, Swanson-Hyland EF et al. Botulinum toxin treatment of essential head tremor. *Neurology* 1995; **45**(4): 822–824.

8. Packenberg H, Packenberg B. Clozapine in the treatment of tremor. *Acta Neurol Scand* 1986; **73**: 295–297.

9. Findley LG, Gresty MA. Head, facial, and voice tremor. *Adv Neurol* 1988; **49**: 239–253.

10. Narabayashi H. Analysis of intention tremor. *Neurol Neurosurg* 1992; **94**: S130–S132.

11. Pollak P, Benabid AL, Gervason CL et al. Long term effect of chronic stimulation of the ventral intermediate thalamic nucleus in different types of tremor. *Adv Neurol* 1993; **60**: 406–413.

12. Geny C, Nguyen JP, Pollin B et al. Improvement of severe postural cerebellar tremor in multiple sclerosis by chronic thalamic stimulation. *Mov Disord* 1996; **11**: 489–494.

13. Hallet M, Ravits J, Dubinsky RM et al. A double blind trial of isoniazid for essential tremor and other action tremors. *Mov Disord* 1991; **6**: 253–256.

14. Deuschl G, Koester B. Diagnose und Behandlung des Tremors. In: Conrad B, Ceballos-Baumann AO, eds. *Bewegungsstorungen in der Neurologie*. Stuttgart: Thieme, Verlag, 1996: 222–253.

15. Rice GP, Lesaux J, Vandervoort P et al. Ondansetron a 5HT3 antagonist, improves cerebellar tremor. *J Neurol Neurosurg Psychiatry* 1997; **62**: 282–284.

16. Friedman JH. 'Rubral' tremor induced by a neuroleptic drug. *Mov Disord* 1992; **7**: 281–282.

17. Remy P, de Recondo A, Defer G et al. Peduncular 'rubral' tremor and dopaminergic denervation: a PET study. *Neurology* 1995; **45**: 472–477.

18. Ozelius L, Kramer PL, Moskowitz CB et al. Human gene for torsion dystonia located on chromosome 9q32–34. *Neuron* 1989; **2**: 1427–1434.

19. Kramer PL, Deleon D, Ozelius L et al. Dystonia gene in Askenazi Jewish population located on chromosome 9q32–34. *Ann Neurol* 1990; **27**: 114–120.

20. Nygaard TG, Wilhelmsen KC, Risch NJ et al. Linkage mapping of dopa-responsive dystonia (DRD) to chromosome 14q. *Nature Gene* 1993; **5**: 386–391.

21. Brin MF, Fahn S, Moskowitz C et al. Localized injections of botulinum toxin for the treatment of focal dystonia and hemifacial spasm. *Mov Disord* 1987; **2**: 237–254.

22. Jankovic J, Schwartz KS. Longitudinal follow-up of botulinum toxin for treatment of blepharospasm and cervical dystonia. *Neurology* 1993; **43**: 834–836.

23. Burke RE, Fahn S, Marsden CD. Torsion dystonia: a double-blind, prospective trial of high-dosage trihexyphenidyl. *Neurology* 1986; **36**: 160–164.

24. Greene PE, Fahn S. Baclofen in the treatment of idiopathic dystonia in children. *Mov Disord* 1992; **7**: 48–52.

25. Jankovic J, Beach J. Long-term effects of tetrabenazine in hyperkinetic movement disorders. *Neurology* 1997; **48**: 358–362.

26. Bennet DA, Goetz CG. Paroxysmal dyskinesias. In: Chokroverty S, ed. *Movement Disorders*. New York: Spectrum, 1990: 287–307.

27. Goetz CG, Bennet D. Pharmacology of paroxysmal dyskinesias. In: Klawans H, Goetz CG, Tanner CM, eds. *Textbook of Clinical Neuropharmacology and Therapeutics*. New York: Raven Press, 1992: 207–213.

28. Van Woert MH, Rosembaum D. L-5-Hydroxytryptophan therapy in myoclonus. *Adv Neurol* 1979; **144**: 862–863.

29. Cohen DJ, Dettlor J, Young JC, Shaywitz BA. Clonidine ameliorates Gilles de la Tourette's syndrome. *Arch Gen Psychiatry* 1980; **37**: 1350–1357.

30. Tolosa ES. Modification of tardive dyskinesia and spasmodic torticollis by apomorphine: possible role of dopamine autoreceptors. *Arch Neurol (Chicago)* 1978; **35**: 459–462.

31. Jankovic J, Orman J. Tetrabenazine therapy of dystonia, chorea, tics and other dyskinesias. *Neurology* 1988; **38**: 391–394.

32. Thaker GK, Nguyen JA, Straus ME. Clonazepam treatment of tardive dyskinesias: a practical GABA mimetic strategy. *Am J Psychiatry* 1990; **147**: 445–451.

33. Srinivasan J, Richens A. A risk–benefit assessment of vigabatrin treatment of neurological disorders. *Drug Safety* 1994; **10**: 5.

34. Walters A, Hening W, Chokroverty S, Fahn S. Opioid responsiveness in patients with neuroleptic-induced akathisia. *Mov Disord* 1986; **1**: 119–127.

35. Akpinar S. Restless legs syndrome treatment with dopaminergic drugs. *Clin Neuropharmacol* 1987; **10**: 69–79.

36. Blum P, Kankovic J. Stiff-man syndrome: an autoimmune disease. *Mov Disord* 1991; **6**: 12–20.

37. Muller DPR, Lloyd JK, Wolff OH. Vitamin E and neurological functions. *Neurology* 1985; **35**: 969–974.

38. Criggs RC, Moxley RT, Lafrance RA, Mcquillen J. Hereditary paroxysmal ataxia: response to acetazolamide. *Neurology* 1978; **28**: 1259–1264.

39. Berginer VM, Salen G, Shefer S. Long-term treatment of cerebrotendinous xanthomatosis with chenodeoxycholic acid. *N Engl J Med* 1984; **311**: 1649–1651.

34

Molecular events in dopaminergic neurodegeneration and neuroprotection in MPTP model of Parkinson's disease employing cDNA microarray

Silvia Mandel, Edna Grünblatt, Yona Levites, Gila Maor and Moussa BH Youdim

INTRODUCTION

The etiology of Parkinson's disease and mechanism of nigrostriatal dopaminergic neurodegeneration remains elusive. The biochemical studies so far done on the substantia nigra pars compacta (SNPC) of Parkinson's disease (PD) and the striatum from 6-hydroxydopamine-*N*-methyl-4-phenyl-1,2,3,6-tetrahydropyridine (MPTP)-treated mice point to an ongoing biochemical process of abnormal iron metabolism within the reactive microglia and melanin-containing dopamine (DA) neurons, resulting in oxidative stress and inflammation that propagates the degeneration of the DA neurons.[1–3] Both neurotoxins are considered to be relevant models of the disease and are thought to induce neurodegeneration via oxidative stress (OS) since iron chelator (e.g. desferrioxamine and R-apomorphine) and radical scavenger (vitamin E, ebselen, lipoic acid) pretreatment induces neuroprotection against the two neurotoxins.[4,5] However, it is not known whether these are primary or secondary events. It is most likely that a cascade of biochemical events, similar to a domino effect, takes place, resulting eventually in the death of DA neurons. Many of these processes are not established or known.

The advent of cDNA microarrays has provided a potential tool for gene expression analysis. The most attractive application of cDNA microarrays is in the study of differential gene expression in disease and animal models.[6] The opportunity to compare the expression of thousands of genes between disease and normal tissues will allow the identification of multiple potential targets. Furthermore, this technique allows the monitoring of gene expression in response to drug treatments and drug action, namely, how the drug affects the expression of genes. Detailed profiling of gene expression in the MPTP Parkinson model may yield additional insights into cellular, animal and human physiology, which is critical to the discovery and validation of therapeutic targets. Since gene expression reflects biochemical events, they may point out how these reactions interact.

In the present study, we applied a cDNA array including 1200 gene fragments for comparing gene expression in brains of control and MPTP-treated mice. The results were further confirmed by quantitative real-time PCR analysis and in situ hybridization. Furthermore, the neuroprotective actions in this model of R-apomorphine (R-APO) and the tea extract catecine, ECGC (3,3-epigallocatecine-3-gallate), which previously have been shown to have neuroprotective activities in neuronal cell culture and the in vivo MPTP model, have been evaluated.[5,7–9]

METHODS

We have used the Atlas mouse cDNA expression array from Clontech to investigate gene alterations occurring in neurodegeneration induced by MPTP in mice.[10] MPTP specifically destroys the nigrostriatal DA neurons, leading to DA depletion. Male C57-BL mice (weighing 20–30 g) were injected (subcutaneously) with R-APO (10 mg/kg per day) before MPTP (intraperitoneally, 24 mg/kg per day) injection, for 5 days. Control animals received saline or R-APO. The animals were decapitated 3 days after the last injection. Brains were dissected on an ice-chilled glass plate, quickly frozen in liquid nitrogen, and stored at –70°C. The main steps of this method are extraction of total RNA from control and MPTP-treated mouse brains, followed by synthesis of a first-strand cDNA radioactive probe using a gene-specific primer mix specifically designed to retrieve only those genes that are embedded in the membranes. This mix gives better signals with less background noise. Four identical membranes were used in parallel, in order to obtain the expression profiles of four RNA populations (MPTP, R-APO and the combination of MPTP- and R-APO-treated mice compared to controls). The hybridization pattern was quantified by phosphorimaging followed by AtlasImage 1.0 program (Clontech) analysis. The relative expression level of a given cDNA from two different RNA sources was assessed by comparing the signal obtained in each membrane after normalizing to the global value of all the genes provided on the membranes.

The Atlas mouse cDNA expression array contains six functional gene groups. Plasmid and bacteriophage DNAs are included as negative controls to confirm hybridization specificity, along with house-keeping cDNAs as positive controls for normalizing mRNA abundance.

Real-time quantitative PCR was performed using the LightCycler System (Roche Molecular Biochemicals). This technique measures PCR-specific products being synthesized in each cycle by staining the double-strand PCR product with SYBR Green I dye.[10] Fluorescence was measured at the end of the annealing period of each cycle to monitor amplification. Target concentrations were calculated by the parallel construction of a dose curve with increasing concentrations of a given gene as standard. The LightCycler software analyzes all the values that are in the log-linear phase, so the absolute concentration in the unknown sample can be calculated by extrapolation.

RESULTS AND DISCUSSION

MPTP differentially affected the expression of prominent genes: 51 of 1200 genes whose expression was altered by the treatment were divided into eight major functional groups, as shown in Table 34.1. It is now apparent that MPTP-altered gene expression is a time-dependent event. The patterns of gene

---

Table 34.1 Differential gene expression analysis identified by the Atlas mouse cDNA arrays

Inflammation		Oxidative stress	Neurotrophic factors		Iron-related proteins
↑ IL-1β	↑ IL-1βR	↓ NADPH P450	↑ EGF	↑ NGF-α	↓ Transferrin receptor
↑ IL-6	↑ IL-2R	↓ Glutathione reductase	↑ GNDF	↑ NGF-β	protein
↑ IL-7	↑IL-6R	↓ Glutathione transferase-5	↑ VEGF	↑ TGF-β	
↑ IL-10	↑ IL-7R	↑ Oxidative stress-induced	↑ TNF-β		
↑ iNOS	↑IL-9R	protein (A 170)	↑ TNF-α-induced protein		
↓ NF-κB p65	↑ NF-κB p105	↓ Osp94 osmotic stress			
↓ I-kappa alpha subunit		protein			

Transporters and channels	Glutamate receptors	Apoptosis and cell cycle	Others
↓ Glucose transporter 1	↑ NMDA 2AR	↓ cdk inhibitor protein 1	↑ Prolactin R2
↓ Voltage-gated sodium	↑ NMDA 2BR	↓ Cyclin B1	↑ LDL R
channels		↑ G1/S-specific cyclin E1 and D3	↑ 5-Hydroxytryptamine
↓ Golgi 4 transmembrane-		↓ bcl-x, BCL2LI	↑ c-rel proto-oncogene
spanning transporter		↓ G2/M-specific cyclin B2	
		↓ cdk 4 and 6 inhibitors	
		↑ STAM	
		↑BAX	

expression at early times (3, 6, 12 and 24 h after MPTP) differ significantly from those seen 10 days after treatment with MPTP. Thus, early gene changes may have a far more crucial role in dictating future gene expression that leads to neurodegeneration.[11] In addition, we investigated the effect of R-APO and EGCG on genes by themselves and those expression induced by MPTP since we previously showed that R-APO and EGCG are relatively potent neuroprotective drugs against MPTP insult, both in cell culture and in vivo.[5,7-9,11] The initial gene expression changes

obtained from cDNA hybridization studies were further verified by quantitative real-time RT-PCR and in situ hybridization.[11]

MPTP upregulated the expression of several mRNAs related to inflammation, such as interleukin-1β (IL-1β), IL-6, IL-7 and IL-10, as well as of their receptors. The general increase in cytotoxic cytokines and in cytokine receptors induced by MPTP, confirms the concept of inflammation in neurodegeneration.[12-13] Indeed, in PD and the MPTP model there is a proliferation of reactive microglia

Table 34.2   Differential gene expression in chronic R-APO and MPTP-treated mice as measured by quantitative real-time PCR

Name of protein/gene	Control (pg/μg total RNA)	MPTP	R-APO	R-APO + MPTP
Plasma glutathione peroxidase precursor	1.00 ± 0.044 (0.0673 ± 0.014)	0.61 ± 0.108[a]	0.69 ± 0.298	0.60 ± 0.119[a]
Glutathione reductase	1.00 ± 0.167 (0.7028 ± 0.081)	0.97 ± 0.152	0.95 ± 0.141	0.72 ± 0.119
Glutathione S-transferase A	1.00 ± 0.010 (0.1194 ± 0.004)	0.74 ± 0.083[a]	0.63 ± 0.266	0.75 ± 0.044[a]
NADPH–cytochrome P450 reductase	1.00 ± 0.052 (52.57 ± 5.5)	0.61 ± 0.026[b]	0.78 ± 0.0067[a]	0.78 ± 0.340
iNOS	1.00 ± 0.182 (0.2157 ± 0.043)	0.78 ± 0.104	0 90 ± 0.081	0.76 ± 0.203
AMPA 1	1.00 ± 0.110 (66.15 ± 2.25)	0.96 ± 0.120	0.78 ± 0.118	0.86 ± 0.265
NMDAA2A	1.00 ± 0.173 (24.67 ± 1.19)	0.97 ± 0.130	0.85 ± 0.206	0.44 ± 0.123[a]
IL-1β	1.00 ± 0.167 (0.0273 ± 0.003)	1.45 ± 0.358	0.57 ± 0.131	0.59 ± 0.207
IL-1R type II	1.00 ± 0.08	1.43 ± 0.11[a]	0.66 ± 0.06[d]	1.27 ± 0.11
IL10	1.00 ± 0.151 ($3.4 \times 10^{-5} ± 2.7 \times 10^{-6}$)	6.81 ± 2.039[b]	1.83 ± 0.804[d]	2.49 ± 0.622
NFκB P65[e]	1.00 ± 0.07	0.75 ± 0.06	0.73 ± 0.07[a]	0.85 ± 0.08
NFκB P105[e]	1.00 ± 0.12	1.23 ± 0.12	1.05 ± 0.12	1.06 ± 0.12
Oxidative stress-induced protein mRNA (A170)	1.00 ± 0.18	1.25 ± 0.17	1.16 ± 0.17	1.15 ± 0.16
GDNF[e]	1.00 ± 0.09	1.59 ± 0.14[b]	0.70 ± 0.08[d]	1.23 ± 0.14

The amount of each product was normalized to β-actin (138 ± 7.26 pg/μg total RNA in control). Control was set arbitrarily as one. ANOVA: [a] $P < 0.05$, [b] $P < 0.01$, [c] $P < 0.001$ versus control; [d] $P < 0.05$ versus MPTP ($n = 3$–9). [e] Amplified products from regular PCR reaction visualized on ethidium bromide-stained agarose gel and semiquantified by densitometry. iNOS, inducible nitric oxide synthase.

around and on top of dying DA neurons,[14] suggesting an ongoing microglia-induced inflammatory process. In line with these findings, pretreatment with R-APO attenuated the elevation of expression of most of those genes[10,11] and this was further confirmed for IL-1β, IL-1R type II and IL-10 by quantitative real-time PCR analysis (Table 34.2). This protection by R-APO may be related to its potent radical scavenger and iron-chelating properties. It is assumed that the chelatable iron has a pivotal role in the process of neurodegeneration and participates in a Fenton reaction with hydrogen peroxide to generate the most reactive of all reactive oxygen species (ROS), namely hydroxyl radical, leading to OS and inflammation (review: see Youdim et al[15]).

Increased iron in macrophages and microglia, as seen in PD,[15] may lead to iron-dependent activation of NFκB.[16] Indeed, a 70-fold increase in immunoreactive NFκB in the nuclei of melanized DA neurons of PD patients was recently reported.[17] In the present study, the expression of mRNA for the precursor of NFκB p50 subunit, NFκB p105, was increased as a consequence of chronic MPTP treatment, whereas pretreatment of animals with R-APO prevented this effect. Conversely, inhibitor-κB (I-κB), responsible for keeping NFκB inactive in the cytoplasm, was decreased by MPTP and increased upon pretreatment with R-APO,[10,11] indicating a tight regulation of both proteins in neurodegeneration. Antioxidants, and specifically iron chelators, were found to be potent inactivators of NFκB,[16,18] suggesting a pivotal role for iron in NFκB activation. Indeed, in our studies we have shown that EGCG, which protects against 6-hydroxydopamine-induced neuroblastoma

Table 34.3 The comparison of gene expression induced by the neuroprotective drugs R-APO and EGCG in the nigrostriatum of mice

Gene coordinate	Apo	EGCG	Gene/Protein name
Cell surface antigens			
A01d	Up	Up	Gap junction α_1 protein (GJA1); connexin 43 (CXN43; CX43); gap junction 43-kDa heart protein
Transcription factors and DNA-binding protein			
A041	NS	Up	Zinc finger protein of the cerebellum 3 (ZIC3)
B03b	Up	Up	Erf; Ets-related transcription factor
B05j	Down	Up	Nuclear hormone receptor ROR-α_1
B08d	Down	Up	Embryonic ectoderm development protein (EED)
B08e	Down	Up	Ring finger protein 2 (RNF2); polycomb-M33-interacting protein ring 1B (RING1B)
B08e	Down	Up	Ring finger protein 2 (RNF2); polycomb-M33-interacting protein ring 1B (RING1B)
B08m	Down	Up	Activating transcription factor 2 (ATF2); cAMP response element DNA-binding protein 1 (CREBP1)
B09a	Down	Up	Signal transducer and activator of transcription 1 (STAT1)
B09e	Down	Up	D-3-phosphoglycerate dehydrogenase (PGDH); transcription factor A10
Cell adhesion receptors and proteins			
B14m	NS	Down	Semaphorin J
Oncogenes and tumor suppressors			
C04i	NS	Down	junB
C06a	Up	Up	Adenomatous polyposis coli protein (APC)
Ion channels and transport proteins			
C11c	Down	Down	CCHB3; calcium channel (voltage-gated; dihydropyridine-sensitive; L-type) β_3 subunit
C11g	Down	Down	Synaptotagmin III (SYTIII)
C11l	Down	Up	Insulin-like growth factor I receptor α-subunit (IGF-I-Rα)

Table 34.3 Continued

Gene coordinate	Apo	EGCG	Gene/Protein name
Post-translational modification and folding			
C131	Down	Down	ERp72 endoplasmic reticulum stress protein; protein disulfide isomerase-related protein
Apoptosis-associated proteins			
C14a	Down	Up	Survival of motor neuron (hSMN)
C14b	Down	Up	Growth arrest and DNA-damage-inducible protein 45 (GADD45); DNA-damage-inducible transcript 1 (DDIT1)
C14n	Down	Down	Adenosine A2A receptor (ADORA2A)
Receptors			
D05d	NS	Down	Granulocyte–macrophage colony-stimulating factor receptor low-affinity subunit precursor (GM-CSF-R)
D09d	Up	Down	Nociceptin receptor; orphanin FQ receptor; kappa-type 3 opioid receptor (KOR-3)
D10m	NS	Down	Lymphotoxin receptor (TNFR family)
Extracellular cell signaling and communication			
D11g	Up	Up	β-Protachykinin a
D11k	Up	Up	Secretogranin II precursor (SGII); chromogranin C
D12c	Up	Up	Pleotrophin precursor (PTN) (heparin-binding growth-associated molecule) (HB-GAM) (heparin-binding growth factor 8) (HBGF-8) (osteoblast-specific factor 1) (OSF-1) (heparin-binding neurotrophic factor) (HBNF)
E02m	Down	Down	Neurogenic locus notch homolog 1 precursor (notch 1); notch protein
Modulators, effectors and intracellular transducers			
E05g	NS	Up	TGF-β-activated kinase 1 (TAK1); mitogen-activated protein kinase kinase kinase 7 (MAP3K7)
E08g	Down	Down	Interleukin-6 receptor β-chain; membrane glycoprotein gp130
E13m	Up	Down	Transducin β_5-subunit; GTP-binding protein G(i)/G(s)/G(t) β-subunit 3
E14d	Down	Down	Rab GDI-α, Rab GDP-dissociation inhibitor-α; GDI-1; XAP4
F01c	Up	Down	S100 calcium-binding protein A1; S-100 protein α-chain
F02j	NS	Down	Dv12; dishevelled-2 tissue polarity protein
F02k	Up	Down	Zyxin (ZYX)
Cytoskeleton and motility proteins			
F05k	NS	Down	Kinesin motor protein 3C (KIF3C)
F06h	Down	Down	Mena protein; enabled homolog (ENAH)
F06m	NS	Down	Nidogen precursor (NID); entactin (ENT)
F07b	NS	Down	Vitronectin precursor (VTN); serum-spreading factor; S-protein
F07k	NS	Down	Endoglin precursor (EDG; ENG); cell surface MJ7/18 antigen
F08j	NS	Down	Fibronectin 1 precursor (FN1)
DNA synthesis, repair and recombination proteins			
F13l	NS	Down	WSB2 protein
F14d	NS	Down	Four and a half domains 1 (FLH1); skeletal muscle LIM protein 1 (SLIM1)
F14k	Up	Down	Huntingtin, Huntington disease homolog (HDH)
F14l	NS	Down	Frataxin; Friedreich ataxia protein (FRDA)
G31		Down	Ornithine decarboxylase (ODC)

or PC12 cells and in vivo MPTP neurotoxicity, inhibits the nuclear translocation and activity of NFκB in neuroblastoma cells.[8,9] This action has been attributed to the iron-chelating/radical-scavenging action of EGCG, since other iron chelators (desferal and R-APO) or radical scavengers (vitamin E) have the same effects.

MPTP (10 days) increased the mRNA expression of several neurotrophic factors, such as GDNF, EGF and VEGF. This increased expression may reflect a compensatory mechanism, stimulating the sprouting of the surviving neurons. GDNF and EGF have been shown to exert growth-promoting and survival effects on DA neurons.[19,20] Pretreatment with R-APO prevented MPTP-induced EGF and GDNF induction.

Genes corresponding to oxidative stress, stress response protein and OS functional groups were found to be affected by MPTP; plasma glutathione peroxidase precursor and glutathione-S-transferase A mRNAs were decreased by MPTP. The expression of Osp94 osmotic stress protein, a member of a recently described HSP110/SSE subfamily of heat shock and osmotic stress proteins, shown to be downregulated in response to hydrogen peroxide,[21] was reduced by MPTP. The decreased expression of this gene supports the role of hydrogen peroxide-induced OS in the mechanism of MPTP neurotoxicity. Upregulation of this gene by R-APO in control and MPTP-treated mice,[10] confirms the protection provided by this drug against hydrogen peroxide and 6-hydroxydopamine-induced OS in pheochromocytoma cells.[7]

In addition to the protective effects conferred by R-APO and EGCG against MPTP-induced transcriptional gene changes, these drugs display by themselves a specific pattern of gene expression or, in other words, what is termed 'pharmacogenetics' (Table 34.3). Nevertheless, the two neuroprotectants also show similar gene changes that might account for their neuroprotective activity, since both are iron chelators and radical scavengers (Table 34.3). For example, EGCG alters the expression of some 31 genes, such as signal tranducers, transcriptional repressors and growth factors, and this is time-dependent. The alteration in gene expression resulting from their actions becomes an extremely important factor to take into consideration, especially in the process of drug action, development or consumption. R-APO alone was shown to downregulate the expression of OS-induced protein (A 170), NMDA 2A, IL-1β, GDNF and tyrosine hydroxylase mRNAs. Thus, these results point to possible gene targets for R-APO action.

The gene profile displayed by MPTP-induced neurodegeneration and neuroprotection by R-APO indicates that, in addition to OS, glutamate excitotoxicity and inflammatory processes, a cascade of other events (e.g. cell cycle modulators and transduction pathways), as yet undefined, act in parallel to converge finally into a common pathway leading to cell death (Fig. 34.1). We are currently examining the pattern of gene expression in the 6-hydroxy-dopamine model of PD and in SNPC from idiopathic PD to evaluate the homology between animal models and clinical manifestations of the disease.

CONCLUSIONS

This study provides the first global assessment of the gene processes involved in neurodegeneration of DA neurons and the neuroprotection afforded by iron chelator/radical scavenger (R-APO and EGCG) treatment at the molecular level in a well-defined model of PD. For the first time, we have direct evidence for the involvement of OS and inflammatory processes, as well as glutamate excitotoxicity, nitric oxide, iron, neurotrophic factors and a cascade of other as yet undefined gene events in neurodegeneration (Fig. 34.1). The cDNA array-based method represents an attractive and powerful application for studying differential gene expression involved in the cell cycle, death and protection. This method can contribute to the development of new and more effective antiparkinson drugs as well as understanding their mechanism of action. The most important aspect is drug development for neuroprotection. It is well known that there have been many attempts to develop drugs as neuroprotectives for the treatment of neurodegenerative diseases, especially ischemia and neurotrauma. These drugs work very well in the animal models, yet they have all failed in the clinical setting. It is more than possible that the drugs so far developed do not affect the gene expression of the specific biochemical events that are ultimately involved in neurodegeneration. In future, microarrays will also contribute to the identification of induced gene products that can be used as markers to follow the effect and dose of a drug in the clinical setting (review: Debouck and Goodfellow[6]). This approach will be particularly useful in progressive diseases such as PD and Alzheimer's disease, to identify possible early biological markers that might be expressed before the first symptoms of the disease are manifested.

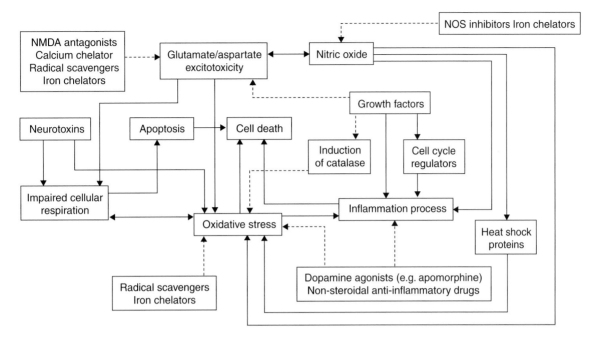

Figure 34.1 Current hypothesis for neurodegeneration cascade of events in the MPTP model of PD. Solid lines indicate those pathways so far identified as participating in the mechanism of cell death. Dotted lines indicate drugs used to induce neuroprotection.[10]

ACKNOWLEDGEMENTS

We wish to thank the NPF (Miami), Golding Parkinson Research Fund (Technion) and the Stein Foundation (Philadelphia) for supporting this work.

REFERENCES

1. Youdim MBH, Ben-Shachar D, Riederer P. The possible role of iron in the etiopathology of Parkinson's disease [published erratum appears in *Mov Disord* 1993; **8**(2): 255]. *Mov Disord* 1993; **8**: 1–12.
2. Gerlach M, Ben-Shachar D, Riederer P, Youdim MB. Altered brain a metabolism of iron as a cause of neurodegenerative diseases? *J Neurochem* 1994; **793**: 793–807.
3. Jenner P, Olanow CW. Oxidative stress and the pathogenesis of Parkinson's disease. *Neurology* 1996; **47**: 161–170.
4. Cadet JL, Katz M, Jackson-Lewis V. Fahn S. Vitamin E attenuates the toxic effects of intrastriatal injection of 6-hydroxydopamine (6-OHDA) in rats: behavioral and biochemical evidence. *Brain Res* 1989; **476**: 10–15.
5. Grünblatt E, Mandel S, Berkuzki T, Youdim MBH. Apomorphine protects against MPTP-induced neurotoxicity in mice. *Mov Disord* 1999; **14**: 612–618.
6. Debouck C, Goodfellow PN. DNA microarrays in drug discovery and development. *Nat Genet* 1999; **21**(1 suppl.): 48–50.
7. Gassen M, Gross A, Youdim MBH. Apomorphine enantiomers protect cultured pheochromocytoma (PCL2) cells from oxidative stress induced by H_2O_2 and 6-hydroxydopamine. *Mov Disord* 1998; **13**: 242–248.
8. Levites Y, Mandel S, Youdim MBH. Protective effect of green tea extract against MPTP-induced neurotoxicity: possible gene changes. *Neurosci* 2000; Suppl 55: S34.
9. Mandel M, Royak-Kebites Y, Maor G, Youdim MBH. Neuroprotection by black and green tea extracts involves inhibition of translocation and activity of NfkappaB in neuronal cells. *Neurosci Lett* 2000; Suppl 55: S35.
10. Grünblatt E, Mandel S, Maor G, Youdim MBH. Alterations of oxidative-stress and inflammatory gene expression in MPTP-induced neurotoxicity and their prevention by R-apomorphine. In: *Sixth International Congress of Parkinson's Disease and Movement Disorders*, Barcelona, Spain, 2000.
11. Grünblatt E, Mandel S, Maor G, Youdim MBH. Gene expression analysis in MPTP model of Parkinson's disease using cDNA microarray. *J Neurochem* (in press).
12. Mogi M, Harada M, Narabayashi H, Inagaki H, Minami M, Nagatsu T. Interleukin (IL)-1β, IL-2, IL-4, IL-6 and transforming growth factor-α levels are elevated in ventricular cerebrospinal fluid in juvenile parkinsonian and Parkinson's disease. *Neurosci Lett* 1996; **211**: 13–16.
13. Bessler H, Djaldetti R, Salman H, Bergman M, Djaldetti M. IL-1β, IL-2, IL-6 and TNF-α production by peripheral blood mononuclear cells from patients with Parkinson's disease. *Biomed Pharmacother* 1999; **53**: 141–145.
14. Jellinger K, Paulus W, Grundke-Iqbal I, Riederer P, Youdim MBH. Brain iron and ferritin in Parkinson's and Alzheimer's disease. *J Neural Transm Park Dis Dement Sect* 1990; **2**: 327–340.

15. Youdim MB, Grünblatt E, Mandel S. The pivotal role of iron in NF-kappaB activation and nigro-striatal dopaminergic neurodegeneration; prospects for neuroprotection in Parkinson's Disease with iron chelators. *Ann NY Acad Sci* 1999; **890**: 7–25.

16. Lin M, Rippe RA, Niemela O, Brittenham G, Tsukamoto H. Role of iron in NFkB activation and cytokine gene expression by rat hepatic macrophages. *Am J Physiol* 1997; **272**: G1355–G1364.

17. Hunot S, Brugg B, Ricard D et al. Nuclear translocation of NF-κB is increased in dopaminergic neurons of patients with Parkinson's disease. *Proc Natl Acad Sci USA* 1997; **94**: 7531–7536.

18. Schreck R, Rieber P, Baeuerle PA. Reactive oxygen intermediates as apparently widely used messengers in the reactivation of the NF-kappa B transcription factor and HIV-1. *EMBO J* 1991; **10**: 2247–2258.

19. Hadjiconstantinou M, Fitkin JG, Dalia A, Neff NH. Epidermal growth factor enhances striatal dopaminergic parameters in the 1-methyl-4-phenyl-1,2,3,6-tetrahydropyridine-treated mouse. *J Neurochem* 1991; **57**: 479–482.

20. Lin LF, Doherty DH, Lile JD, Bektesh S, Collins F. GDNF: a glial cell line-derived neurotrophic factor for midbrain dopaminergic neurons. *Science* 1993; **260**: 1130–1132.

21. Santos BC, Chevaile A, Kojima R, Gullans SR. Characterization of the Hsp110/SSE gene family response to hyperosmolarity and other stresses. *Am J Physiol* 1998; **274**: F1054–F1061.

35

Alzheimer's disease

Abdalla Bowirrat, Robert P Friedland and Amos D Korczyn

INTRODUCTION

Alzheimer's disease (AD) is the major neurological disorder of aging and the most common cause of dementia in the elderly.[1] The disease is characterized as a chronic neurodegenerative process with an unknown etiology. AD is a common process and every old person may become a victim of this disorder.

AD is the most common form of dementia, accounting for two-thirds or more of all dementia cases, while vascular dementia (VaD) has been reported to be the second major subtype of dementia, accounting for 15–30% of all dementias. The two types of dementia have distinct pathological features, but these frequently coexist,[2] and the combination results in more severe symptoms of dementia.[3,4]

Although dementia syndromes, and particularly AD, are not new disorders, Western communities face a huge increase in their frequency, with an immense economic burden to families and societies, above which human suffering must be considered. Much of the available data from developed countries suggest a prevalence of over 10% in elderly subjects, with at least a doubling in frequency every 5 years from age 65 (about 1%) to age 90 (about 50%).

Clinically, AD is slowly progressive with memory complaints as the presenting symptom (Table 35.1). The earliest memory problem can be a defect in delayed verbal recall,[5] although the person should have normal alertness and an insidious onset of symptoms. As the disease advances, problems with language, calculation, visuospatial functions and praxis become increasingly apparent. Behavioral alterations such as depression, agitation, delusions, anxiety and hallucinations may become evident at any time during the course of the illness.[6–9] These progressive events lead to separation from reality and eventually death. The physical neurological examination in AD is usually normal. Commonly

Table 35.1 Clinical features of AD
Slow, insidious onset and progression starting usually in senescence
Memory decline at onset, leading to loss of all cognitive abilities, including insight executive skills
Lack of focal neurological signs (but primitive reflexes are common).

associated features include primitive reflexes (snout, glabellar, grasp), impaired graphesthesia, and an abnormal face–hand test.[10–12]

The laboratory evaluation of patients with dementia is an important adjunct to the neurological and cognitive screening tests in the diagnosis and differential diagnosis of dementia. Using the NINCDS-ADRDA or other criteria, with suitable laboratory and diagnostic studies, at least 80% accuracy in the clinical diagnosis of AD can be achieved.[13–15]

THE PATHOLOGY OF ALZHEIMER'S DISEASE

Pathologically, AD consists of two classical predominant neuropathological lesions. Neuritic (senile) plaques contain extracellular deposits of the amyloid β-proteins (Aβ). A portion of these deposits occur as clumps of insoluble amyloid fibrils,[16] but these are intermixed with an as-yet poorly defined array of non-fibrillar forms of this peptide. After it had been established by protein sequencing that Aβ was the subunit of fibrillar plaque cores, immunohistochemistry with sensitive antibodies to Aβ revealed a large number of deposits in AD brain that appeared to lack the altered microglia and astrocytes and the surrounding dystrophic neurites which characterize the neuritic plaques. Such lesions, referred to as 'diffuse' plaques, represent deposits of Aβ that are mostly in a non-fibrillar, apparently granular form in the neuropil.[17] The compacted fibrillar cores of 'mature' neuritic plaques appear to contain mixtures of the Aβ42 and the Aβ40 peptides. Aβ deposits do not occur simply in these two extreme forms (diffuse and neuritic) but rather as a continuum in which mixtures of fibrillar and non-fibrillar forms of the peptide can be associated with varying degrees of local glial and neuronal alterations.

In regions of the AD brain that are generally not implicated in the clinical manifestations, e.g. the cerebellum and thalamus, Aβ deposits are meager and usually of the diffuse type, with little evidence of local gliosis and neuritic change. Likewise, the brains of aged, cognitively normal humans often contain Aβ deposits, but these are overwhelmingly of the diffuse type, with relatively few neuritic plaques and neurofibrillary tangles present in the cerebral cortex. Perhaps the most frequently voiced criticism of the 'amyloid hypothesis' of AD is that Aβ plaques can be found in moderate or sometimes high density in the cortex of cognitively normal elderly subjects. Again, these are frequently diffuse plaques that appear to represent still cytologically benign precursor lesions not associated with surrounding cytopathology, analogous to the fatty streaks in the vasculature of individuals who have not yet developed frank cardiovascular events. There is significant debate as to what extent the relationship between amyloid plaque burden and the extent of cognitive impairment is significant.[18]

The other classical lesion observed by Alois Alzheimer in his original patient is the neurofibrillary tangle (NFT). Tangles are generally intraneuronal cytoplasmic bundles of paired, helically wound ~10-nm filaments, sometimes interspersed with straight filaments.[19] NFTs usually occur in large numbers in the AD brain, particularly in entorhinal cortex, hippocampus, amygdala, associated cortices of the frontal, temporal and parietal lobes, and certain subcortical nuclei that project to these regions. The subunit protein of the NFT is the microtubule-associated protein, tau. NFTs are not limited to the tangles found in the cell bodies of neurons, but also occur in many of the dystrophic neurites present within and outside the amyloid plaques. Biochemical studies reveal that the tau present in NFTs comprises hyperphosphorylated, insoluble forms of this normally highly soluble cytosolic protein.[20] Tangles composed of tau aggregates that are similar to and sometimes indistinguishable from those that occur in AD have been described in several less common neurodegenerative diseases, usually without accompanying Aβ deposits and neuritic plaques. Conversely, Aβ deposits can be seen in aged 'normal' human brain in the virtual absence of tangles. Infrequently, AD cases are seen which are 'tangle-poor', i.e. with very few NFTs despite abundant Aβ plaques.[21]

EPIDEMIOLOGY

While there is no question that dementia of the Alzheimer type (DAT) occurs all over the world, the exact frequencies are not known for many communities. (We prefer to use the term AD for the pathologically confirmed disease, and the term DAT for those cases where firm diagnosis is not established and can only be assumed, such as in epidemiological surveys.) Few data on DAT have been published for eastern Mediterranean countries, and there is little information available on the occurrence of DAT in Arabs. We have studied an Arab community living in Wadi Ara, which is homogeneous in terms of living conditions (rural), language (Arabic) and religion (Moslem), with low levels of education (illiteracy >70%). Also, this Arab population is notable with regard to the high levels of inbreeding and smoking. The prevalence of DAT in this population appears to be very high.[22] The prevalence of DAT in our population followed the usual pattern, increasing steeply with advancing age, and reaching higher frequencies than seen in previous similar studies. After adjustment for age, gender and schooling, it appeared that DAT was 3.9 times more frequent than among the population of Ashkelon, Israel (where a similar study has been conducted using identical methods),[23,24] even after adjustment for age, gender and schooling. In a study in Tunisia, unspecified dementia was found to be three times less prevalent than in the USA.[25] Two other studies regarding the prevalence of DAT were reported in Arabs: one prevalence study was reported from a University Hospital in Saudi Arabia,[26] and the second was recently reported from Assiut, Upper Egypt.[27]

These results used different methodologies and are difficult to compare to our data. However, it is possible that the high prevalence of DAT in Wadi Ara may not be representative of other communities in the Middle East. The elderly population of Wadi Ara have generally limited activities in their villages and usually no formal occupation. Almost all elderly Arab subjects live within a protective environment of their extended families, are cared for and are not required to be involved actively in daily activities, in accordance with tradition and religion. This stereotypic life may influence the intellectual activity and the mental capacity of the elderly.

The diagnosis of dementia and DAT among elderly illiterate Arab subjects is difficult. The fact that these subjects are living within a protective environment of their extended families and not allowed to participate in strenuous or complex activities outside the house, according to the traditions and the religion, may delay the correct diagnosis and require intensive investigation and new strategies. DAT was considered to be present if the DSM-IV criteria were fulfilled. One potential problem is that the standard diagnostic tool used here (DSM-IV criteria) might not have been appropriate for the Wadi Ara population.

There are no known genes affecting the development of DAT which are recessive, perhaps because there have been few studies of AD in populations with high levels of inbreeding.

GENETICS OF ALZHEIMER'S DISEASE

Etiologically, AD is heterogeneous. About 10% of patients have a strong family history of AD consistent with a mendelian pattern of inheritance that often results in early onset of disease that runs a rapid and malignant clinical course. Less than one-half of these cases are produced by mutations or polymorphisms on chromosomes 1, 14 and 21. The discovery of these gene mutations (Table 35.2) is among the most exciting and illuminating discoveries of the 1990s. However in the majority of cases, the family history is non-contributory and there is no identified mutation. Autosomal dominant AD is uncommon, but provides precise molecular genetic information that helps to decipher the elusive pathways of disease causation, providing valuable insights into the causes of sporadic, non-genetic disease, which characterizes the majority of patients with AD.

The first gene associated with early-onset AD was the amyloid precursor protein (APP) gene[28,29] on chromosome 21, in part because of its role in the formation of amyloid, which is found in the characteristic senile plaques of brain of patients with AD, and in part because of the relationship between Down's syndrome (trisomy 21) and AD. However, this mutation has been found in only about 20 families worldwide. A second gene involved in AD was identified on chromosome 14, coding for a protein called presenilin-1 (PS1).[30–32] PS1 mutations are thought to account for about 75% of early-onset familial AD (FAD). PS1 mutations are therefore much more common than APP mutations. The age of onset in families with PS1 mutations is the earliest observed (28–60 years).[33] The third gene, the PS2 (presenilin-2) gene, occurs on chromosome 1.[34] Mutations in this gene are the least common genetic factor underlying the development of early-onset FAD identified so far. The PS2 gene was identified by studying the Volga Germans (VGs), a group of eight pedigrees in which FAD is a result of a founder effect. These ethnic Germans migrated to Russia in

Table 35.2 Genetic alterations in AD and effects on amyloid precursor protein (APP)

Chromosome	Gene product	Age of onset	Effect
21	APP mutations	Early	Increased production of Aβ (1–42)
Trisomy 21	APP overproduction	Early	Overproduction of Aβ
14	Presenilin-1 mutations	Early	Increased production of Aβ (1–42)
1	Presenilin-2 mutations	Early	Increased production of Aβ (1–42)
19	Apolipoprotein ε4 allele (polymorphism)	Late	Increased deposition of Aβ plaques and vascular deposits; earlier onset of AD

the 1760s and remained distinct from the surrounding population, and many of them later migrated to the USA.

Several independent research groups have examined the frequency distribution of apolipoprotein E (ApoE) ε4 haplotypes in AD patients. ApoE is a polypeptide composed of 299 amino acids found in chylomicrons, very low-density lipoproteins, and high-density lipoproteins. Although many tissues synthesize ApoE, the liver is the primary source.[35] ApoE is one of the constituents of plasma lipoproteins that participate in the transport of cholesterol and specific lipids through an interaction with low-density lipoprotein receptors and hepatic ApoE receptors.[36] In the central nervous system (CNS), ApoE is synthesized in astrocytes[37] and neurons[38] and upregulated in response to neuronal damage and deafferentation.[39]

The three common polymorphisms of ApoE, ε2, ε3 and ε4, differ by single-base substitutions in the coding region of the gene. Among them, the ε4 allele is well established as a major susceptibility gene for AD.[40] ApoE ε4 is present in about 20–30% of the general Caucasian population, but in 45–60% of patients with AD. The frequency of the ApoE ε4 allele was shown to be markedly increased in sporadic[41] as well as in late-onset FAD.[40] Compared to the most common ApoE ε3/ε3 genotype, reported odds ratios (ORs) range from 2.8 to 4.4 for subjects with one ApoE ε4 allele, and from 7.0 to 19.3 for subjects with two ApoE ε4 alleles (ApoE ε4 homozygotes).[42] ApoE ε4/ε4 homozygotes constitute approximately 2–3% of the general population, but 12–15% of patients with AD.[43] Remarkably, many ApoE ε4 carriers, including ε4/ε4 homozygotes),[42] remain cognitively healthy at advanced ages, including those surviving into the 10th decade,[44] and more than one-third of AD patients

do not carry an ApoE ε4 allele.[43] We[45] have examined the frequency of the ApoE ε4 allele among AD patients and controls in Israeli Jews, and found that the ApoE ε4 frequency is 2.5-fold higher among patients compared to controls (27% and 11%, respectively), although the frequency of the ApoE ε4 allele differs among different ethnic Jewish groups in Israel. Ethiopian Jews had a high frequency of ApoE ε4 (0.27), compared to Libyan, Bucharian, Ashkenazi and Sepharadi Jews (0.067, 0.083, 0.095, 0.1, respectively). Interestingly, the ApoE ε4 allele seems to determine not if but when an individual will develop the disease.[46] ApoE ε4 allele copy number was shown to correlate not only with a lower age of onset of DAT,[40] but also with increased senile plaque density,[47] lower choline acetyltransferase activity[48] and cholinergic neuron density,[49] and more cortical NFTs.[50] Moreover, neuroimaging studies have shown greater atrophy in medial temporal structures in AD patients carrying the ApoE ε4 allele.[48] Recent PET studies showed that ApoE ε4 homozygotes have impaired cortical metabolism before they manifest clinical signs of dementia.[51]

There are several hypotheses concerning how ApoE ε4 mediates the increased risk of AD. It has been speculated that ApoE ε4 may serve as a pathological chaperone, facilitating fibrillar amyloid deposition,[52] which might aid conversion of diffuse Aβ into the β-pleated sheet conformation by direct binding of ApoE ε4 protein to amino acids 12–28 of diffuse Aβ.[53]

The high prevalence of dementia described by us recently in Wadi Ara[22] may, of course, be explained by environmental or genetic factors (or both). The most important genetic risk factor for DAT, the ApoE ε4 allele, is of immediate concern. To date, ApoE genotypes have been determined for 441 people from Wadi Ara study, as shown in Table 35.3.

Table 35.3 The frequency of the ApoE ε4 allele in the Wadi Ara study (total number = 441)

	Age Mean ± SD (years)	Number of subjects	ε4	ε4 allele frequency
Healthy subjects	73.5 ± 13	173	10	0.029
DAT patients	81.8 ± 9	92	5	0.027
Age-associated memory impairment (AAMI)	74.4 ± 6	136	9	0.033
Others	74 ± 7	4	4	0.05

Like the Nigerian study[54] and in marked contrast to previous studies, our study found no correlation between the ApoE ε4 allele frequency and the diagnosis of DAT. However, the reasons were completely different in the Wadi Ara and Nigerian population. The ApoE ε4 allele frequencies in our non-demented subjects (0.029) and DAT patients (0.027) were similar. These data suggest that the ε4 allele is uncommon among Arabs in Wadi Ara and not a risk factor for DAT. This may be the lowest ApoE ε4 frequency in the world.

In the light of these results, other genetic risk factors for DAT must be evaluated for this particular community with the high prevalence of DAT, genetic isolation and high rate of intermarriage. We hypothesize that consanguinity has increased the prevalence of homozygosity for autosomal recessive genes, which are responsible, in part, for the increased prevalence of the disease. It is difficult to evaluate recessive models in outbred populations, especially for a condition such as DAT, when parents have died before awareness of the disease existed and prior to the advent of modern diagnostic methods, particularly because a high proportion of siblings are censored at an age before DAT symptoms are expected to occur. Because the Wadi Ara area is actually composed of less than 14 hamulas (extended families), we studied the distribution of DAT among the largest (4) hamulas and among the other 10 small families. We observed that the prevalence of DAT in family (A) was 21%, in family (B) 21%, in family (C) 22.5%, in family (D) 11%, and in the other 10 small hamulas 24.5%.

In our epidemiological study of DAT in Wadi Ara, we found a high prevalence of late-onset DAT, although the ApoE ε4 frequency is low. High consanguinity in this community led us to speculate that recessive genes for AD may be responsible for this high prevalence. Scientists have long suspected that more than one gene may be involved in increasing an individual's risk of developing late-onset AD. Investigators worldwide have searched intensively for other genes, on other chromosomes, that might also play a role. In Wadi Ara we carried out a study to set the groundwork for the possible identification of genes that contribute to the vulnerability to AD. Finding genetic loci associated with a disease can help us further identify the risk factors and describe the biological mechanisms at work in AD, bringing new promise to the search for ways to diagnose, treat or prevent this devastating illness.

Consanguinity increases the expression in a population of autosomal recessive genes, which may have undesirable characteristics. For example, an additional 1/16 of the variation of DNA is made homozygous by the inbreeding of a marriage of first cousins.[52] Conversely, the probability of identifying recessive or quasi-recessive susceptibility factors is enhanced by inbreeding. Childhood mortality is increased in the offspring of first cousin marriages by a factor of 1.4–1.7, and children born to consanguineous unions have poorer health than the offspring of non-consanguineous unions (including malignancies, congenital abnormalities, mental retardation and physical handicap).[55] Curiously, there are few studies of the effects of inbreeding on the health of adults and, to our knowledge, only one involving AD.[56]

De Brackeleer et al reported an association between inbreeding and the development of AD (inbreeding coefficient nine times higher in AD cases than in controls) in a rural population in Quebec, Canada.[56] Studies in the Older Old Amish in the USA have found a low prevalence of AD in this inbred community, which also has a low frequency of the ApoE ε4 allele (0.037).[57]

NON-GENETIC RISK FACTORS FOR ALZHEIMER'S DISEASE

Age is clearly the most important risk factor for AD. Alois Alzheimer originally described this disorder as a form of premature aging.[58] Many studies have implicated low education as a risk factor for cognitive impairment in elderly people.[59,60] Although Filley et al[61] and Beard et al[62] did not find that education provides protection against dementia, it must be recalled that their subjects had relatively high schooling levels. Education may enhance brain reserve by increasing synaptic density in the neocortical association cortex.[63] Individuals with higher levels of education may have greater brain capacity (i.e. more cortical synapses) than individuals with lower levels of education, and thus have more resistance to the deterioration caused by the progressive synaptic and neuronal loss associated with aging than do less educated individuals.[24]

Our study in Wadi Ara confirmed an association between education and dementia. However, these factors could only partly explain the very high rates of dementia observed by us in this Arab population. Most of the elderly Arab population in Wadi Ara received no formal education (illiteracy rate >70%), and therefore we used illiteracy or literacy for analysis in the contingency tables but a continuous variable (number of school years) in the logistic regression model. Thus, it is possible to suggest that the protective effect of education is non-linear, with a marked effect related to low schooling and a minimal additional effect beyond 6–8 years in school.[22]

One confounding factor that should be discussed as being responsible for the correlation between education and dementia is smoking. In most developed countries, smoking is more frequent in lower socio-economic classes. The higher prevalence of dementia among less educated groups is, therefore, the reverse of what would be expected if smoking were protective. In addition, people who had more school years usually belong to higher social classes and are more likely to take better care of their health in general, e.g. blood pressure control and hyperlipidemia. These in turn may affect the development of dementia.

The relationship of smoking to dementia is complex. Epidemiological studies have established a negative association between cigarette smoking and the prevalence of DAT.[64] In these studies, the risk of DAT in non-smokers has generally been about twice that of smokers. This negative association has been interpreted as suggesting that cigarette smoking exerts a biological neuroprotective influence against the development of AD.[65] Before accepting this seemingly counterintuitive interpretation, however, we should remember the golden rule of statistics: association alone, no matter how significant, does not, cannot, and will not ever mean causation.[66,67] Moreover, other epidemiological studies found non-significant negative correlations between DAT and smoking.[68,69] Ford et al[70] also reported that the prevalence of cognitive impairment was lower among smokers than among non-smokers, but logistic regression, adjusted for age, income, and gender, showed this difference to be non-significant (OR = 0.73; 95% CI 0.42–1.29). For several reasons, it is difficult to generalize concerning the studies carried out to date. Case–control studies have often included cases from hospital series and may not represent dementia cases in the general population.

Moreover, prevalence studies are susceptible to survival bias if demented patients who smoked had a relatively higher mortality than non-demented smokers. This would produce an image of a protective effect of smoking against DAT. Cases referred to a memory clinic may be more likely to have other diseases (perhaps due to smoking) and thus poorer survival than healthy controls. Population-based studies on prevalent cases may have similar biases due to shorter survival of smokers. Population-based prospective studies focusing on smoking in relation to cognitive impairment failed to confirm the protective effect of smoking on the occurrence of DAT.[68,71,72]

Thus most previous studies which suggested a protective effect of smoking on AD were case–control studies based on prevalent cases. In contrast, the findings of several incidence studies suggest that smoking is a risk factor for the development of DAT (Tables 35.4 and 35.5).

Several studies suggest an association between head injury and AD,[73,74] but these observations have remained inconsistent because most studies have been cross-sectional. The risk of AD and dementia increased with severity of head injury.[75] The observed dose–response pattern may support a causal effect of head injury in the pathogenesis of AD and dementia.

Epidemiological studies have suggested that female gender is an independent risk factor for AD,[76] even allowing for the increased proportion of women in the older, at-risk population, which is caused by their relative longevity, with a female/male prevalence ratio in DAT of 2 : 1.[76] In our study we also observed a higher prevalence of dementia among females, with a female/male prevalence ratio in DAT of 1.7 : 1 (Table 35.6). Possible explanations for the higher prevalence of DAT among women could include unrecognized environmental influences, hormonal effects such as late effects of the menopause, or the use of estrogens by

Table 35.4   Association between smoking and DAT in prevalence studies in different countries

Prevalence studies	OR (95% CI)
Cleveland, Ohio, USA[70]	OR 0.73 (95% CI = 0.4–1.3), NS
Manhattan, USA[110]	RR 0.7 (95% CI = 0.5–1.1), protective effect
Rotterdam, The Netherlands[64]	OR 0.8 (95% CI = 0.6–1.0), protective effect
Stockholm, Sweden[72]	OR 0.6 (95% CI = 0.4–1.0), protective effect
Wadi Ara (first prevalence study, 1995)	OR 0.7 (95% CI = 0.4–1.2), NS
Wadi Ara (second prevalence study, 2000)	OR 0.88 (95% CI = 0.5–1.5), NS

Table 35.5   Association between smoking and DAT in different incidence studies in different countries

Incidence studies	OR (95% CI)
Cleveland, Ohio, USA[70]	OR 1.03 (95% CI = 0.5–2.0), NS
Boston, USA[68]	OR 0.7 (95% CI = 0.3–1.4), NS
Manhattan, USA[110]	RR 1.9 (95% CI = 1.2–3.0), risk factor
London, UK[71]	RR 2.3 (95% CI = 0.8–6.3), NS
Rotterdan, The Netherlands[69,111]	RR 2.2 (95% CI = 1.3–3.6)
	RR 1.7 (95% CI = 1.2–2.5), risk factor
Stockholm, Sweden[72]	OR 1.1 (95% CI = 0.5–2.4), NS
Wadi Ara study	OR 2.7, $P = 0.01$, risk factor

Table 35.6   Gender effect in the distribution of DAT in different prevalence studies in different countries

Study site	Age	Population sex ratio F/M	AD sex ratio F/M
Hong Kong[112]	70+	1	1.8
Stockholm[15]	75+	4.2	1.3
Denmark[113]	65+	1.25	0.8
Rotterdam[114]	60+	1.6	2
Pamploma[115]	70+	1	1.4
Korea[116]	65+	1	2
Appignano[76]	60+	1.3	2.3
Taiwan[117]	60+	0.9	1
Framingham[118]	60+	1.55	2.6
Shanghai[119]	65+	1.3	2.6
Wadi Ara	60+	1.3	1.7

postmenopausal women,[77] a possible higher prevalence of the ApoE ε4 allele in older women,[42] as well as the presence of protecting genes on the X chromosome.

VASCULAR COMPONENTS IN ALZHEIMER'S DISEASE

Vascular disease appears to be a risk factor for AD[78,79]. Previous myocardial infarction has been reported to increase the risk of probable AD five-fold in older women.[78] Coronary artery disease at autopsy, with or without myocardial infarction, was found to be associated with a six-fold increase in the proportion of older patients with significant Alzheimer amyloid deposits in the brain.[79] Brun and Englund[80] reported that 60% of patients with autopsy-proven DAT also had white matter changes, which are usually attributed to compromised circulation. Thus, vascular disease may contribute to DAT pathogenesis or may accelerate the clinical presentation of DAT. A significant interaction might exist between aging and vascular risk factors such as hypertension. For example, one study found that midlife blood pressure is the strongest predictor of later-life brain volume and the extent of white matter hyperintensities.[81,82] Hypertension in later life may have less influence on brain structure and function than does midlife hypertension.[82]

Further evidence shows that abnormalities of cerebral white matter share stroke risk factors[83,84] and that these abnormalities significantly predict future stroke[81] and mortality.[85] These findings support the notion of a spectrum of vascular-related brain injury[81] that also may impact on the clinical presentation and progression of AD. The presence of concurrent, albeit clinically silent, cerebrovascular disease may therefore be common in patients with AD and may impact on the presentation and progression of the disease, although stroke risk factors may have a differential influence on the incidence of dementia according to ethnic background.[86,87]

HOMOCYSTEINE AND DEMENTIA

The utility of standard laboratory tests in the work-up of dementia and the true prevalence of potentially reversible etiologies has been examined by several authors. Recent evidence suggests an association between several specific nutrient excesses and deficiencies and AD, including alcohol abuse, vitamin B$_{12}$ and folate deficiency and elevated total homocysteine levels. The exact nature and significance of this association remains uncertain. Three possible explanations exist for this association:

(1) 'Low-intake' hypothesis—cobalamin deficiency develops secondarily to impaired nutritional intake due to dementia.
(2) The 'common pathophysiology' hypothesis—there is a related mechanism for development of both AD and cobalamin deficiency.
(3) The 'etiological' hypothesis—the cobalamin deficiency itself contributes to the dementia.

Homocysteine metabolism is absolutely dependent on five B-complex vitamins: B$_1$, B$_2$, B$_6$, B$_{12}$ and folate. Total homocysteine is a useful indicator of a subtle and early cobalamin-deficient state, as tissues cannot utilize this amino acid in the usual manner. Homocysteine has been shown to be associated with cardiovascular disease,[88] such as heart attack and stroke. It is also an important emerging risk factor for AD and cognitive dysfunction in the elderly.[89] Several associations also have been observed for cognitive impairment in the elderly.[90] Whether vitamin B$_{12}$ deficiency can alter the clinical presentation of DAT or contribute to its pathology is not clear.[91] Vitamin B$_{12}$ levels reflect multiple environmental causes, such as diet and reduced access to preventive medicine. In Wadi Ara, high levels of total homocysteine in both the control and demented cases and low levels of folic acid and vitamin B$_{12}$ that were observed also in our study had no associations with DAT. It is well known that high total homocysteine is a risk factor for vascular damage[88,92] and possibly for dementia.[89,93,94] The fact that such a relationship has not been observed by us is of interest. High levels are not considered to be causative for AD by themselves, but rather to be important factors in the pathogenesis of this multifactorial disorder. The high prevalence of elevated total homocysteine levels in the general population of Wadi Ara thus may set the stage for other factors to set in and cause dementia.

The available information on risk factors for DAT (aging, genetic predisposition, lack of education, female gender, head injury and vascular risk factors), and microscopic pathology of DAT (amyloid plaques, NFTs) suggest that DAT is a clinical syndrome which can arise from a variety of causes. The relationship between genes and environmental risk factors in complex disorders (e.g. stroke, Parkinson's disease and DAT) is a subject of great interest to investigators and is responsible for the growth in the discipline of genetic epidemiology. Thus, both genes and environment are important in AD susceptibility.

THERAPY OF ALZHEIMER'S DISEASE

Propelled by remarkable advances in the understanding of AD pathogenesis, novel therapeutic strategies are being developed that hold the promise of preventing the occurrence of AD or even reversing the disease process once it is established. The identification of the cholinergic deficiency in AD has led to an effort to correct the deficiency, with an attempt to reduplicate the success of levodopa and dopamine agonists as replacement therapies. In retrospect, these hopes seem naive, since the neurotransmitter deficiency is much more complex than just acetylcholine. Nevertheless, limited efficacy was seen with several cholinesterase inhibitors, particularly donepezil, rivastigmine and galantamine. At present, drugs are available that treat the core symptoms of AD: memory and other cognitive and functional loss as well as behavioral symptoms. Even though the benefit is modest in magnitude, the growing acceptance of these agents is eroding the formerly pervasive therapeutic nihilism about AD.[95]

These agents improve cognition and independence, although quite frequently their main effect is on attention and concentration, but an impressive effect is seen on behavioral disorders and activities of daily living, delaying institutionalization. They are more similar than different, and the practical importance of butyrylcholinesterase inhibition by rivastigmine or nicotinic receptor interaction with galantamine remains unknown. Although these drugs have a clear symptomatic effect, the claims that they modify the disease process are as yet unsubstantiated.

Based on the hypothesis of a cortical cholinergic deficit in AD that correlates with dementia, the main classes of drugs evaluated to date in AD are cholinomimetic agents, including cholinesterase inhibitors,[93–103] as well as nicotinic and muscarinic[104] agonists. The expected outcome of cholinergic enhancement is palliation (improved symptoms) rather than an effect on the underlying biology of AD. Cholinesterase inhibitors may provide benefit in AD beyond cognitive performance. Behavioral symptoms such as apathy and loss of initiative, agitation, delusions, hallucinations and irritability appear to develop less often in treated patients.[105–107] Evidence for increased oxidative stress and free radical injury in AD provides the rationale for antioxidant strategies. A large-scale trial of the antioxidants selegiline and α-tocopherol (vitamin E) provided some evidence that both drugs alone (but less in combination) resulted in a delay of about 8 months for moderately demented AD patients in reaching clinical milestones such as institutionalization or death, without necessarily improving cognition.[108]

Recent studies have confirmed that different 3-hydroxy-3-methylglutaryl coenzyme A reductase inhibitors (lovastatin and pravastatin), which inhibit the synthesis of cholesterol, decrease the prevalence of AD.[109]

CONCLUSIONS

AD is a common disorder among the elderly, and will attain an ever-increasing importance in the future. Recent years have witnessed an immense expansion in our understanding of disease pathogenesis and its risk factors, with important epidemiological conclusions pertinent to the delay or prevention of the cognitive decline.

The study of Wadi Ara presents a unique opportunity to dissect out recessive factors linked to AD. Given the extraordinarily high prevalence of DAT in this relatively isolated community, it may be speculated that the population is enriched for one or several predisposing genes, other than ApoE, which increase susceptibility to DAT. Several mapping methods which take advantage of identity by descent at the disease locus have previously been used to successfully map disease loci in inbred populations. In particular, this study may shed light on possible gene–environment interactions leading to the development of DAT.

REFERENCES

1. Larson EB, Kukull WA, Katzman RL. Cognitive impairment, dementia and Alzheimer's disease. *Annu Rev Public Health* 1992; **13**: 431–439.
2. Esiri M, Wilcock GK. Cerebral amyloid angiopathy in dementia and in old age. *J Neurol Neurosurg Psychiatry* 1986; **49**: 1221–1226.
3. Nagy ZS, Esiri M, Jobst KA et al. The effects of additional pathology on the cognitive deficit of Alzheimer's disease. *J Neuropathol Exp Neurol* 1997; **56**: 165–170.
4. Snowden DA, Greiner LH, Mortimer JA et al. Brain infarction and the clinical expression of Alzheimer's disease: the Nun study. *JAMA* 1997; **277**: 813–817.
5. Welsh K, Butters N, Hughes J et al. Detection of abnormal memory decline in mild cases of Alzheimer's disease using CERAD neuropsychological measures. *Arch Neurol* 1991; **48**: 278–281.
6. Mega MS. Cummings JL, Fiorello T, Gombein J. The spectrum of behavioral changes in Alzheimer's disease. *Neurology* 1996; **46**: 130–135.
7. Drevets WC, Rubin EH. Psychotic symptoms and longitudinal course of senile dementia of the Alzheimer type. *Biol Psychiatry* 1989; **25**: 39–48.
8. Wragg RE, Jeste DV. Overview of depression and psychosis in Alzheimer's disease. *Am J Psychiatry* 1989; **146**: 577–587.
9. Burns A. Psychiatric phenomena in Alzheimer's disease II. Disorders of perception. *Br J Psychiatry* 1990; **157**: 76–81.
10. Koller WC. Primitive reflexes and cognitive function in the elderly. *Ann Neurol* 1982; **12**: 302–304.
11. Huff FJ, Growdon JH. Neurological abnormalities associated with severity of dementia in Alzheimer's disease. *Can J Neurol Sci* 1986; **13**: 403–405.
12. Bakchine S. Relationship between primitive reflexes, extrapyramidal signs, reflexive apraxia, and severity of cognitive impairment in dementia of the Alzheimer type. *Acta Neurol Scand* 1989; **79**: 38–46.
13. Tierney MC. The NINCDS-ADRDA Work Group criteria for the clinical diagnosis of probable Alzheimer's disease: a clinico-pathological study of 57 cases. *Neurology* 1988; **38**: 359-364.
14. Kukull WA, Larson EB, Reifler BV et al. The validity of 3 clinical diagnostic criteria for Alzheimer's disease. *Neurology* 1990; **40**: 1364–1369.
15. Galasko D. Clinical–neuropathological correlations in Alzheimer's disease and related dementias. *Arch Neurol* 1994; **51**: 888–895.
16. Glenner GG, Wong CW. Alzheimer's disease and Down's syndrome: sharing of a unique cerebrovascular amyloid fibril protein. *Biochem Biophys Res Commun* 1984; **122**: 1131–1135.
17. Tagliavini F. Preamyloid deposits in the cerebral cortex of patients with Alzheimer's disease and nondemented individuals. *Neurosci Lett* 1988; **93**: 191–196.
18. Cummings BJ. β-Amyloid deposition and other measures of neuropathology predict cognitive status in Alzheimer's disease. *Neurobiol Aging* 1996; **17**: 921–933.
19. Goedert M. The neurofibrillary pathology of Alzheimer's disease. In: Rosenberg RN, Prusiner SB, DiMauro S, Barchi RL, eds. *The Molecular and Genetic Basis of Neurological Disease*, 2nd edn. Boston: Butterworth-Heinemann, 1998 613–627.
20. Kosik KS. Microtubule-associated protein, tau, is a major antigenic component of paired helical filaments in Alzheimer's disease. *Proc Natl Acad Sci USA* 1986; **83**: 4044–4048.
21. Terry RD. Senile dementia of the Alzheimer type without neocortical neurofibrillary tangles. *J Neuropathol Exp Neurol* 1987; **46**: 262–268.
22. Bowirrat A, Treves TA, Friedland RP, Korczyn AD. Prevalence of Alzheimer's type: dementia in an elderly Arab population. *Eur J Neurol* 2000; **8**: 119–123.
23. Korczyn AD, Kahana E, Galper Y. Epidemiology of dementia in Ashkelon, Israel. *Neuroepidemiology* 1991; **10**: 100.
24. Korczyn AD, Kahana E, Friedland RP. Education and dementia. In: Lomraz J, ed. *Handbook of Aging and Mental Health: An Integrative Approach.* New York: Plenum Press, 1998: 448–458.

25. Attia Romdhane N, Ben Hamida M, Mrabet A et al. Prevalence study of neurologic disorders in Kelibia (Tunisia). *Neuroepidemiology* 1993; **2**: 285–299.

26. Ogunniyi A, Daif AK, Al-Rajeh S et al. Dementia in Saudi Arabia: experience from a university hospital. *Acta Neurol Scand* 1998; **98**: 116–120.

27 Farrag A, Farwiz HM, Kheder EH et al. Prevalence of Alzheimer's disease and other dementing disorders: the Assiut-Upper Egypt study. *Dement Geriatr Cogn Disord* 1998; **9**: 323–324.

28. Goate AM, Chartier-Harlin MC, Mullan MC et al. Segregation of a missense mutation in the amyloid precursor protein gene with familial Alzheimer's disease. *Nature* 1991; **349**: 704–706.

29. Tanzi RE, Gusella JF, Watkins PC et al. Amyloid β protein gene: cDNA, mRNA distribution and genetic linkage near the Alzheimer's locus. *Science* 1987; **235**: 880–884.

30. Sherrington R, Rogaev EI, Liang Y et al. Cloning of a gene bearing missense mutation in early-onset familial Alzheimer's disease. *Nature* 1995; **375**: 754–760.

31. Reznik-Wolf H, Treves TA, Davidson M et al. A novel mutation of presenilin-1 in familial Alzheimer's disease in Israel detected by denaturing gradient gel electrophoresis. *Hum Genet* 1996; **98**: 700–702.

32. Reznik-Wolf H, Treves TA, Shabtai H et al. Germline mutational analysis of presenilin 1 and APP genes in Jewish-Israeli individuals with familial or early-onset Alzheimer's disease using denaturing gradient gel electrophoresis (DGGE). *Eur J Hum Genet* 1998; **6**: 176–180.

33. Cruts M, Hendriks L, Van Broeckhoven C. The presenilin genes: a new gene family involved in Alzheimer disease pathology. *Hum Mol Genet* 1996; **5**: 1449–1455.

34. Levy-Lehad E, Wasco W, Pookaj P et al. Candidate gene for the chromosome 1 familial Alzheimer's disease locus. *Science* 1995; **269**: 973–977.

35. Zannis VI, Cole FS, Jackson CL et al. Distribution of apolipoprotein A-I, C-Il, C-Ill and E mRNA in fetal human tissues. Time-dependent induction of apolipoprotein E mRNA by cultures of human monocyte–macrophages. *Biochemistry* 1985; **24**: 4450–4455.

36. Mahley AW. Apolipoprotein E: cholesterol transport protein with expanding role in cell biology. *Science* 1988; **240**: 622.

37. Pitas RE, Boyles JK, Lee SH, Foss D, Mahley RW. Astrocytes synthesize apolipoprotein E and metabolize apolipoprotein E-containing lipoproteins. *Biochem Biophys Acta* 1987; **917**: 148–161.

38. Xu PT, Gilbert JR, Qiu HL et al. Specific regional transcription of apolipoprotein E in human brain neurons. *Am J Pathol* 1999; **154**(2): 601–611.

39. Poirier J, Hess M, May PC, Finch CE. Astrocytic apolipoprotein E mRNA and GFAP mRNA in hippocampus after entorhinal cortex lesioning. *Mol Brain Res* 1991; **11**: 97–106.

40. Corder EH, Saunders AM, Strittmatter WJ et al. Gene dose of apolipoprotein E type 4 allele and the risk of Alzheimer's disease in late onset families. *Science* 1993; **261**: 921–923.

41. Payami H, Kaye J, Heston LL et al. Apolipoprotein E and Alzheimer's disease. *Lancet* 1993; **342**: 738.

42. Poirier J, Davignon J, Bouthillier D et al. Apolipoprotein Alzheimer's disease. *Lancet* 1993; **342**: 697–699.

43. Blacker D, Tanzi RE. The genetics of Alzheimer disease: Current status and future prospects. *Arch Neurol* 1998; **55**: 294–296.

44. Martinez M, Campion D, Brice A et al. Apolipoprotein E ∊4 allele and familial aggregation of Alzheimer's disease. *Arch Neurol* 1998; **55**: 810–816.

45. Treves TA, Bornstein NM, Chapman J et al. APOE-∊4 in patients with Alzheimer disease and vascular dementia. *Alzheimer Dis Assoc Disord* 1996; **10**: 189–191.

46. Meyer MR, Tschanz JT, Norton MC et al. ApoE genotype predicts when—not whether—one is predisposed to develop Alzheimer disease. *Nat Genet* 1998; **19**: 321–322.

47. Schmechel D, Saunders AM, Strittmatter WJ et al. Increased amyloid β-peptide deposition in cerebral cortex as a consequence of apolipoprotein E genotype in late-onset Alzheimer's disease. *Proc Natl Acad Sci USA* 1993; **90**: 9649–9653.

48. Soininem H, Kosumen O, Helisami S et al. A severe loss of choline acetyl transferase in the frontal cortex of Alzheimer patients carrying apolipoprotein ∊4. *Neurosci Lett* 1995; **87**: 79–82.

49. Poirier J, Aubert I, Bertrand P et al. Apolipoprotein E4 and cholinergic dysfunction in AD: a role for the amyloid/ApoE4 complex? In: Giacobini E, Becker AE, eds. *Alzheimer's Disease: Therepeutic Strategies*. Boston: Birkhauser, 1994: 72–76.

50. Polvikoski T, Sulkava R, Haltia M et al. Apolipoprotein E, dementia, and cortical deposition of beta-amyloid protein. *N Engl J Med* 1995; **331**: 1242–1247.

51. Reiman EM, Caselli RJ, Yun LS et al. Preclinical evidence of Alzheimer's disease in persons homozygous for the epsilon 4 allele for apolipoprotein. *N Engl J Med* 1996; **21**(334): 752–758.

52. Wisniewski T, Frangione B. Apolipoprotein E: a pathological chaperone protein in patients with cerebral and systemic amyloid. *Neurosci Lett* 1992; **135**: 235–238.

53. Ma J, Yee A, Brewer HBJ et al. Amyloid-associated proteins alpha 1-antichymotrypsin and apolipoprotein E promote assembly of Alzheimer beta protein into filaments. *Nature* 1994; **372**: 92–94.

54. Osuntokun BO, Sahota A, Ogunniyi AO et al. Lack of an association between apolipoprotein E ∊4 and Alzheimer's disease in elderly Nigerians. *Ann Neurol* 1995; **38**: 463–465.

55. Gibbons A. The risks of inbreeding. *Science* 1993; **259**: 1252.

56. De Braekeleer M, Cholette A, Mathieu J et al. Familial factors in Alzheimer's disease (IMAGE project). *Eur Neurol* 1989; **29**: 2–8.

57. Holder J, Warren AC. Prevalence of Alzheimers disease and ApoE allele frequencies in the Old Older Amish. *J Neuropsychiatry Clin Neurosci* 1998; **10**: 100–102.

58. Bick K, Amaducci L, Pepeu G. *The Early Story of Alzheimer's Disease*. Padua: Living Press, 1987.

59. Fratiglioni L, Grut M, Farmer M et al. Prevalence of Alzheimer's disease and other dementias in an elderly urban population: relationship with age, sex and education. *Neurology* 1991; **41**: 1886–1892.

60. Katzman R. Education and the prevalence of dementia and AD. *Neurology* 1993; **43**: 13–20.

61 Filley CM, Brownell HH, Albert ML. Education provides no protection against Alzheimer's disease. *Neurology* 1985; **35**: 1781–1784.

62. Beard CM, Kokmen E, Offord KP et al. Lack of association between Alzheimer's disease and education, occupation, marital state, or living arrangement. *Neurology* 1992; **42**: 2063–2068.

63. Stern Y, Alexander GE, Prohounik I et al. Inverse relationship between education and parietotemporal perfusion deficit in Alzheimer's disease. *Ann Neurol* 1992; **32**: 371–375.

64. Graves AB, Van Duijn CM, Chandra V et al. Alcohol and tobacco consumption as risk factors for Alzheimer's disease: a collaborative re-analysis of case–control studies. *Int J Epidemiol* 1991; **20**: 48–57.

65. Lee PN. Smoking and Alzheimer's disease: a review of the epidemiology evidence. *Neuroepidemiology* 1994; **13**: 131–144.

66. Riggs JE. The 'protective' influence of cigarette smoking on Alzheimer's and Parkinson's diseases: quagmire or opportunity for neuroepidemiology? *Neurol Clin* 1996; **14**: 353–358.

67. Hill AB. The environment and disease: association or causation? *Proc R Soc Med* 1965; **58**: 295–300.

68. Hebert LE, Scherr PA, Beckett LA et al. Relation of smoking and alcohol consumption to incident Alzheimer's disease. *Am J Epidemiol* 1992; **135**: 347–355.

69. Ott A, Slooter AJC, Hofman A et al. Smoking and risk of dementia and Alzheimer's disease in a population-based cohort study: the Rotterdam Study. *Lancet* 1998; **351**: 1840–1843.

70. Ford AB, Mefrouche Z, Friedland RP, Debanne SM. Smoking and cognitive impairment: a population-based study. *J Am Geriat Soc* 1996; **44**: 905–909.

71. Cervilla JA, Prince M, Mann A. Smoking, drinking and incident cognitive impairment: a cohort community based study included in the Gospel Oak project. *J Neurol Neurosurg Psychiatry* 2000; **68**: 622–626.

72. Wang HW, Fratiglioni L, Giovanni B et al. Smoking and the occurrence of Alzheimer's disase: cross-sectional and longitudinal data in a population-based study. *Am J Epidemiol* 1999; **149**: 640–644.

73. Geyde A, Beattie BL, Tuokko H et al. Severe head injury hastens age of Alzheimer's disease. *J Am Geriatr Soc* 1989; **37**: 970–973.

74. O'Meara ES, Kukull WA, Sheppard L et al. Head injury and risk of Alzheimer's disease by apolipoprotein E genotype. *Am J Epidemiol* 1997; **146**: 373–384.

75. Plassman BL, Havlik RJ, Steffens DC et al. Documented head injury in early adulthood and risk of Alzheimer's disease and other dementias. *Neurology* 2000; **55**: 1158–1166.

76. Rocca WA, Banaiuto S, Lippi A et al. Prevalence of clinically diagnosed Alzheimer's disease and other dementing disorders. A door-to-door survey in Appignano, Italy. *Neurology* 1990; **40**: 626–631.

77. Paganini-Hill A, Henderson VW. Estrogen deficiency and risk of Alzheimer's disease in women. *Am J Epidemiol* 1994; **140**: 256–261.

78. Aronson MK, Ooi WL, Morgenstern H et al. Women, myocardial infarction and dementia in the very old. *Neurology* 1990; **40**: 1102–1106.

79. Sparks DL, Hunsaker JC, Scheff SW et al. Cortical senile plaques in coronary artery disease, aging and Alzheimer's disease. *Neurobiol Aging* 1990; **11**: 601–607.

80. Brun A, Englund E. A white matter disorder of dementia of the Alzheimer's type: a pathoanatomical study. *Ann Neurol* 1986; **19**: 253–262.

81. DeCarli C, Miller BL, Swan GE et al. Predictors of brain morphology among the men of the NHLBI Twin Study. *Stroke* 1999; **30**: 529–536.

82. Elias ME, Wolf PA, D'Agostino RB et al. Untreated blood pressure level is inversely related to cognitive functioning: the Framingham study. *Am Epidemiol* 1993; **138**: 353–364.

83. Launer LJ, Andersen K, Dewey ME et al. Rates and risk factors for dementia and Alzheimer's disease. Results from Eurodem pooled analyses. *Neurology* 1999; **52**: 78–84.

84. Woo J, Ho SC, Lau S et al. Prevalence of cognitive impairment and associated factors among elderly Hong Kong Chinese aged 70 years and over. *Neuroepidemiology* 1994; **13**: 50–58.

85. Miyar S Takano A, Teramoto J et al. Leukoaraiosis in relation to prognosis for patients with lacunar infarction. *Stroke* 1992; **23**: 1434–1438.

86. Streifler JY, Eliasziw M, Fox AJ et al. Prognostic importance of leukoaraiosis in patients with ischemic events and carotid artery disease. *Stroke* 1999; **30**: 254.

87. Gorelick PB. Cerebrovascular disease in African Americans. *Stroke* 1998; **29**: 2656–2664.

88. Nygard O, Vollset SE, Refsum H et al. Total homocysteine and cardiovascular disease. *J Intern Med* 1999; **246**: 425–454.

89. Clarke R, Smith AD, Jobst KA et al. Folate, vitamin B12 and serum total homocysteine levels in confirmed Alzheimer disease. *Arch Neurol* 1998; **55**: 1449–1455.

90. Riggs KM. Spiro A, Tucker K et al. Relations of vitamin B12, vitamin B6, folate and homocysteine to cognitive performance in the normative aging study. *Am J Clin Nutr* 1996; **63**: 306–314.

91. Bernard MA, Nakonezny PA, Kashner TM. The effect of vitamin B12 deficiency on older veterans relationship to health. *J Am Geriatr Soc* 1998; **46**: 1199–1206.

92. Carmel R, Jacobsen DW (eds). *Homocysteine in Health and Disease.* New York: Cambridge University Press, 2001.

93. Nilson K, Gustafson L, Faldt R et al. Hyperhomocysteinaemia—a common finding in a psychogeriatric population. *Eur J Clin Invest* 1996; **26**: 853–859.

94. Joosten E, Lesaffre E, Riezler R et al. Is metabolic evidence for vitamin B12 and folate deficiency more frequent in elderly patients with Alzheimer's disease? *J Gerontol A Biol Sci Med Sci* 1997; **52**: 76–79.

95. Gauthier S. Do we have a treatment for Alzheimer disease? Yes. *Arch Neurol* 1999; **56**: 738–739.

96. Selkoe DJ. Translating cell biology into therapeutic advances in Alzheimer's disease. *Nature* 1999; **399**: 23–31.

97. Schenk D, Barbour R, Dunn K et al. Immunization with amyloid-β attenuates Alzheimer-disease-like pathology in the PDAPP mouse. *Nature* 1999; **400**: 173–174.

98. Haass C, Strooper B. The presenilins in Alzheimer's disease—proteolysis holds the key. *Science* 1999; **286**: 916–919.

99. Cummings JL. Cholinesterase inhibitors: a new class of psychotropic compounds. *Am J Psychiatry* 2000; **157**: 4–15.

100. Rogers SL, Doody RS, Mohs RC, Friedhoff LT, Group DS. Donepezil improves cognition and global function in Alzheimer disease: a 15-week, double-blind, placebo-controlled study. *Arch Intern Med* 1998; **158**: 1021–1031.

101. Tariot PN, Solomon PR, Morris JC et al. A 5-month, randomized, placebo-controlled trial of galantamine in AD. *Neurology* 2000; **54**: 2269–2276.

102. Corey-Bloom J, Anand R, Veach J. A randomized trial evaluating the efficacy and safety of ENA 713 (rivastigmine tartrate), a new acetylcholinesterase inhibitor, in patients with mild to moderately severe Alzheimer's disease. *Int J Geriatr Psychopharmacol* 1998; **1**: 55–65.

103. Giacobini E. Cholinesterase inhibitors stabilized Alzheimer's disease. *Neurochem Res* 2000; **25**: 1185–1190.

104. Korczyn AD. Muscarinic M_1 agonists in the treatment of Alzheimer's disease. *Exp Opin Invest Drugs* 2000; **9**: 2259–2267.

105. Morris JC, Cyrus PA, Orazem J et al. Metrifonate benefits cognitive, behavioral and global function in patients with Alzheimer's disease. *Neurology* 1998; **50**: 1222–1230.

106. Mega MS, Masterman DM, O'Connor SM et al. The spectrum of behavioral responses to cholinesterase inhibitor therapy in Alzheimer disease. *Arch Neurol* 1999; **56**: 1388–1393.

107. Mega MS, Cummings JL, Fiorello T, Gornbein J. The spectrum of behavioral changes in Alzheimer's disease. *Neurology* 1996; **46**: 130–135.

108. Sano M, Ernesto C, Thomas RG et al. A controlled trial of selegiline, alpha-tocopherol, or both as treatment for Alzheimer's disease. *N Engl J Med* 1997; **336**: 1216–1222.

109. Wolozin B, Kellman W, Ruosseau P et al. Decreased prevalence of Alzheimer's disease associated with 3-hydroxy-3-methyglutaryl coenzyme A reductase inhibitors. *Arch Neurol* 2000; **57**: 1439–1443.

Part 6

Nerve and muscle

36

Vasculitic neuropathies

Gérard Said

INTRODUCTION

The term vasculitis applies to a heterogeneous group of diseases characterized by damage to blood vessels with infiltration of the vessel wall by inflammatory infiltrate, which leads to occlusion of the blood vessel and subsequent tissue ischemia. The classification of vasculitis still remains mainly based on pathological aspects and on the size of affected blood vessels. Peripheral neuropathy is a common complication of vasculitis, especially of the polyarteritis nodosa (PAN) type, because the size of the blood vessels affected in this type of vasculitis corresponds to that of vasa nervorum. Since histological evidence is needed for the diagnosis of vasculitis, the search for vasculitis is the most common indication for nerve and muscle biopsy.

The clinical spectrum of vasculitis ranges from diseases considered primary vasculitis syndromes to diseases associated with underlying conditions such as collagen vascular diseases, infections, or malignancies. Vasculitis often occurs in the context of a multisystem disorder, but in a substantial proportion of patients the neuropathy is the first and only manifestation of vasculitis. In most cases, necrotizing arteritis of the type observed in PAN is responsible for the lesions, but classification of vasculitis is still uncertain. In contrast, the mechanism of the nerve lesions associated with vasculitis is rather uniform, with nerve ischemia as the common consequence of the occlusion of blood vessels in necrotizing arteritis.

Vasculitides are assumed to have an autoimmune pathogenesis, but little is actually known about the pathogenesis of most patterns of vasculitis encountered in humans, and the treatment of primary vasculitis, in spite of attempts to use innovative treatments based on presumed pathophysiological mechanisms, empirically rests on corticosteroids. Recent reviews on the subject have failed to bring more clarification.[1]

PRIMARY VASCULITIS

Pathophysiological aspects of necrotizing arteritis

Little is actually known of the pathophysiology of primary vasculitis. It is highly likely that a number of factors, some of which may have been identified, play a role in the onset of inflammatory lesions of blood vessels. It is widely accepted that necrotizing arteritis of the type observed in PAN is related to the formation of soluble, circulating immune complexes, which is a logical consequence of the large-scale synthesis of antibodies by plasma cells. The pathophysiological significance of immune complexes contrasts with the contestable usefulness of their demonstration for disease description and therapy.[2] The immune complexes are phagocytosed through the interaction of neutrophil Fc receptors with the Fc portion of the complexed antibody.[3] Proteolytic enzymes, free radicals and various inflammatory peptides may be released by neutrophilic polymorphonuclear cells, which damage the vessel wall.[4,5] The complement attack complex (C5b-9) may also contribute to the vessel wall injury.[4,6] The demonstration of deposits of immunoglobulins and complement in the epineural vessels of nerve biopsies from patients with vasculitic neuropathy supports a role for immune complexes in this setting.[7–9]

Other humoral mechanisms may be involved in the pathogenesis of vasculitis, including anti-endothelial cell antibodies found in several connective tissue and systemic disorders, but the incidence of detection of anti-endothelial cell antibodies is very variable; they are more often found in conditions that are seldom associated with peripheral nervous system involvement, such as scleroderma, Kawasaki's disease or systemic lupus erythematosus. Thus the role played by such antibodies and the usefulness of their detection in sera from patients with vasculitic neuropathy remain to be established.[10,11]

In patients with Wegener's granulomatosis anti-neutrophil cytoplasmic autoantibodies (ANCAs) are commonly detected, and their serum level seems to correlate with disease activity.[12,13] ANCAs are able to induce neutrophil degranulation and inactivate protease inhibitors,[14] and damage endothelial cells through activation of polymorphonuclear cells and release of reactive oxygen species.[15] An important review article on ANCAs summarizes and clarifies both technical and, practical aspects of these markers, with special emphasis on the clinical utility of ANCAs and the role that these antibodies may play in the pathogenesis of small and medium-sized vessel vasculitis.[16] The authors conclude that the ANCAs are quite heterogeneous, and the determination of ANCA status can be a very useful diagnostic adjunct to the evaluation of patients with suspected Wegener's granulomatosis, but cannot substitute for clinical expertise and histopathological data, in the course of providing patient care. In addition, the identification of this important marker of disease activity in Wegener's granulomatosis is not reliable in PAN, which is responsible for the vast majority of vasculitic neuropathy.

The role of endothelial cell adhesion molecule expression has recently been investigated in vessels from patients with PAN.[17] In early lesions they found similar expression of intercellular adhesion molecules (ICAM) ICAM-1, platelet endothelial cell adhesion molecule 1 (PCEAM-1) and P-selectin in vasculitic specimens and in controls. Vascular cell adhesion molecule-1 (VCAM-1) and E-selectin were induced in vascular endothelium. In advanced lesions, immunostaining for adhesion molecules diminished or disappeared in luminal endothelium, whereas these molecules were clearly expressed in microvessels within and surrounding inflamed vessels. A high proportion of infiltrating leukocytes expressed lymphocyte function-associated antigen-1 and very late antigen-4 (VLA-4), and only a minority expressed L-selectin. These results are interesting but it is important to note the high standard deviation found in quantitative assessment of labeled leukocytes, which illustrates both the difficulty of this type of work and the heterogeneity of tissue specimens from patients with vasculitis. The authors found no relationship between the expression pattern of adhesion molecules and clinical features, disease duration, or previous corticosteroid treatment. The authors logically conclude that endothelial adhesion molecule expression in PAN is a dynamic process that varies according to the histopathological stage of vascular lesions.

An interesting review on cell adhesion molecules in vasculitis[18] focused on the use of adhesion molecules as clinical markers of disease activity, and on the use of adhesion molecules as targets for treatment in animal models of vasculitis. The authors report that levels of soluble ICAM-1, VCAM-1 and E-selectin are generally highly elevated in patients with generalized vasculitis. In limited forms of vasculitis, levels of soluble adhesion molecules tend to be lower. Therefore, the value of these markers as predictors of disease activity is limited, because elevated levels are also found in other conditions in which endothelial cells are activated, including infection, atherosclerosis[19] and malignancy.[20]

Another interesting study on mechanisms of tissue injury in vasculitic neuropathies has been performed on nerve biopsy samples.[21] The authors studied the expression of candidate molecules for tissue injury in vasculitic neuropathies and found numerous infiltrating cells positive for perforin, macrophage nitric oxide synthetase (m-NOS), cyclooxygenase-2 (COX-2) or matrix metalloproteinase-1 (MMP-1). The authors suggest that cell-mediated cytotoxicity may be involved in the pathogenesis of small-vessel injury in vasculitic neuropathies. Following axonal degeneration, all endoneural macrophages showed immunostaining for m-NOS and MMP-1. However, only macrophages involved in phagocytosis were COX-2 positive, which suggests a role for prostaglandins in nerve damage. In this study, too, the standard deviation for characterization of infiltrating cells is high. The findings of these two studies on human specimens bring some insight into the pathogenesis of vasculitic lesions but do not increase our ability to diagnose vasculitis other than histologically.

Cellular factors should also be considered in vasculitis. In this respect, macrophages and cytotoxic T-lymphocytes are likely to play a role in vasculitic lesions.[6–8] Cytotoxic lymphocytes specific for class 2 major histocompatibility complex also seem able to lyse endothelial cells in vitro, after action of interferon-γ.[22] Endothelial cells can serve as antigen-presenting cells and can be induced to secrete a number of cytokines, including interleukin-6 (IL-6), IL-1 and intercellular adhesion molecules, which can recruit and activate lymphocytes and increase cell damage.[23]

In summary, the mechanisms which trigger vasculitis are extremely complex. Both humoral and cellular immunological and inflammatory factors seem to play a role in the occurrence of necrotizing arteritis, which will, in turn, when symptomatic, induce ischemic nerve lesions.

Classification of primary vasculitis

Vasculitides are often classified according to the size of vessels predominantly affected,[24] but overlaps are common, and the nomenclature of the systemic vasculitides remains enigmatic.[25] Recent attempts to classify systemic vasculitides have not brought much clarification. Large-vessel vasculitis, which includes giant cell arteritis and Takayasu's arteritis, is seldom associated with peripheral neuropathy. In medium-sized vessel vasculitis, which includes PAN and Kawasaki disease, neuropathy occurs only in patients with PAN. The group of small-vessel vasculitides of this recent classification includes Wegener's granulomatosis, the Churg–Strauss syndrome, and what the group calls microscopic polyangiitis with involvement of capillaries, which also occurs in PAN, and thus does not represent a clear entity, since overlaps with PAN are common (Table 36.1).

In addition, the Churg–Strauss syndrome, which associates asthma and eosinophilia with eosinophil-rich and granulomatous inflammation involving the respiratory tract, and necrotizing vasculitis affecting small to medium-sized vessels, is often difficult to differentiate from classical PAN, in which eosinophilia and asthma are rather common.

Essential cryoglobulinemia vasculitis is ranged in microscopic polyangiitis but cryoglobulinemia may be associated with small-vessel involvement as well as with typical PAN in our experience.

Thus, no classification of systemic vasculitis is fully satisfactory, since overlaps are common and there is no specific biological marker for any of these forms of vasculitis. The classification recommended by Lie[25] (Table 36.1) seems, however, the most practical.

Pathophysiology of nerve lesions associated with vasculitis

From a neurological point of view, the lesions observed in vasculitic neuropathy are ischemic in nature and result from occlusion of the vasa nervorum, which occurs mainly in the course of PAN, in which condition necrotizing arteritis affects blood vessels of the size of those located in the epineurium. Because of that, necrotizing arteritis is commonly associated with symptomatic or subclinical peripheral nerve involvement through a mechanism of nerve ischemia.[27–29] Clinical neuropathy occurs in 50–75% of the patients with systemic vasculitis of the PAN group,[30,31] but subclinical lesions are much more common. The same pattern of lesions of blood vessels occurs in allergic angiitis. Peripheral neuropathy also occurs in the context of Wegener's granulomatosis,[32] but less often as the presenting manifestation of the disease than in PAN.

Necrotizing arteritis
Necrotizing arteritis is the most common primary vasculitis responsible for vasculitic neuropathy. This process, which is related to local or systemic vascular inflammation, involves large or small vessels, and produces vessel and tissue necrosis with typical leukocytic infiltration, leukocytoclasia, hemorrhage and fibrinoid change.[24] This pattern of vasculitis is commonly associated with symptomatic or subclinical peripheral nerve involvement through a mechanism of nerve ischemia.[27–29] The same pattern of lesions of blood vessels occurs in allergic angiitis.

Secondary lymphocytic vasculitis
Lymphocytic vasculitis (LV), which is characterized by infiltration by cells of the lymphomonocytic lineages of the vessel wall, is common in infectious disorders. These include leprosy, Chagas' and Lyme diseases, and infection with the human immunodeficiency virus (HIV). In many instances, inflammatory infiltration around endo- and perineural blood vessels, mainly venules and capillaries, cannot

---

Table 36.1 A revised, practical classification of primary vasculitis[25]

Affecting large, medium, and small-sized blood vessels
Takayasu arteritis
Giant cell (temporal) arteritis
Isolated angiitis of the central nervous system

Affecting predominantly medium and small-sized blood vessels
Polyarteritis nodosa
Churg–Strauss syndrome
Wegener's granulomatosis

Affecting predominantly small-sized blood vessels
Microscopic polyangiitis
Schönlein–Henoch syndrome
Cutaneous leukocytoclastic angiitis

Miscellaneous conditions
Buerger's disease
Cogan syndrome
Kawasaki disease

be termed vasculitis because the vessel wall is not infiltrated with mononuclear cells. In some cases, however, which include some forms of vasculitis associated with the HIV infection, with lymphoproliferative disorders, with reversal leprous neuropathy and even with diabetes mellitus, lymphocytic vasculitis is complicated by necrosis of the arterial wall which leads to ischemic lesions superimposed on those induced by endoneural inflammatory infiltrates.

The neuropathy of necrotizing arteritis

Neuropathy associated with necrotizing arteritis of the PAN type

In the group of vasculitides, comprising necrotizing arteritis (NA) of the PAN type, which represents the most homogeneous entity, occurs de novo in PAN, or as a secondary feature in diseases such as rheumatoid arthritis and, occasionally, in other connective tissue disorders. The diagnostic criteria of necrotizing arteritis of the PAN type, which represents the most common type of primary vasculitis encountered in association with neuropathy, include: transmural infiltration of small arteries with polymorphonuclear cells, often admixed with lymphocytes and eosinophils; leukocytoclasia; fibrinoid necrosis; destruction of the internal elastic lamina; occlusion of the lumen; and the usual sparing of adjacent venules.

The consequences of vascular inflammation and occlusion depend on the size and number of blood vessels affected. Clinical neuropathy occurs in 50–75% of the patients with systemic vasculitis of the PAN group.[30] The ischemic neuropathy induced by NA can be observed in apparent isolation[33–35] or in the context of a multisystemic disorder. We have recently reviewed the clinical and pathological data of 200 patients in whom we found NA in nerve and/or in muscle biopsy specimens in our department at the Hopital de Bicêtre. NA occurred in the context of multisystem disorders in 131 patients (65%), including 116 patients with connective tissue disorders. Patients in this group commonly manifested loss of weight, fever, asthenia, and myalgia, in association with multisystemic involvement such as arthritis, cutaneous vasculitis, and renal lesions in 10%.

CLASSIC PAN

Classic PAN affected 36% of our patients. In these patients, multisystem involvement was present, with cutaneous vasculitis as the most common non-neurological manifestation. Specific skin involvement, including livedo, cutaneous necrosis

and nodules, was present in 22 patients. In 17 patients, non-specific edema, usually affecting one limb extremity, was present. In patients with cutaneous vasculitis and neuropathy, a nerve biopsy should be performed for diagnostic purposes only in those in whom the skin biopsy did not provide specific vasculitic lesions. Renal involvement was observed in 10% of the patients. Asthma was present in 12.6% of the patients of another large series.[31]

The much-debated Churg–Strauss variant of PAN was diagnosed in 11 patients of our series. In 1951, Churg and Strauss reported a study of 14 cases of a form of disseminated necrotizing vasculitis occurring frequently among asthmatic patients, with fever, eosinophilia, and a fulminant multisystem disease with a pathology of NA, eosinophilic infiltration and extravascular granulomas. Fauci et al[36] classify this syndrome with classic PAN, whereas Chumbley et al[37] clearly differentiate their cases from classic PAN. Pulmonary infiltrates can be transient or nodular and chronic; the asthma may be of short or long duration, and peripheral eosinophilia is observed routinely. Neurological involvement, usually mononeuritis multiplex, was found in 19 of 30 cases.[37] In our experience, the vascular and nerve lesions observed in nerve biopsies from patients with this syndrome are similar to those observed in classic PAN, and peripheral eosinophilia and eosinophilic infiltration occurs in classic PAN as well. The response of the so-called Churg–Strauss allergic granulomatosis to corticosteroid therapy is not different from that observed in classic PAN. Although pANCA seem to be commonly found in this syndrome,[38] the series studied are not large enough to make of this syndrome more than a variant of PAN, as far as the peripheral nervous system and the muscle are concerned.

The clinicopathological and immunopathological aspects of the neuropathy associated with Churg–Strauss syndrome have been reviewed by Hattori et al.[39] The diagnosis of Churg–Strauss syndrome was achieved on clinical criteria, after the onset of peripheral nerve involvement. The sural nerve, which was biopsied in all patients, showed necrotizing vasculitis in 54% of the patients. It is not clear whether the sural nerve was clinically affected or not in all cases. In 89% of the patients, electrophysiological abnormalities were present in the sural nerve territory. Simultaneous muscle sampling, which increases the yield of tissue biopsy for vasculitis, was not performed in this series. In their series, Harrati et al found granuloma in only 3 of the 28 patients included in their series. The other pathological features were similar to those of classic PAN. IgG and C3d deposits were seen only occasionally in epineural vessel walls, a feature which underlines the lack of reliability of this diagnostic criterion used in some studies. The perinuclear antineutrophil antibodies were found positive, at low titers, in 42% of the patients, which is less than the incidence observed in some series of Wegener's granulomatosis and more than in classic PAN.[16]

NECROTIZING ARTERITIS AND NEUROPATHY IN PATIENTS WITH RHEUMATOID ARTHRITIS

Vasculitis is a common manifestation of rheumatoid arthritis (RA).[40] Forty-three patients of our series (21.5%) fitted into this group, which represents the second largest group of patients with NA and multisystem connective tissue disorder. The occurrence of NA in the context of RA is classically associated with a poor outcome. Of the 32 patients with RA and neuropathy due to histologically proven necrotizing vasculitis in muscle and/or in nerve biopsy specimens,[41] 15 had a sensory and motor neuropathy, and the others had a sensory neuropathy. Two-thirds of the patients had a multifocal pattern of neurological deficit, and the other third manifested distal symmetrical sensory neuropathy. In this group of patients, a Sjögren's syndrome was present in 22%, rheumatoid factor in 97%, nodules in 31% and articular erosions in all of them. NA, which was demonstrated in nerve and/or muscle biopsy specimens in all patients, was more often found in the muscle (86%) than in the nerve biopsy specimens (64%). The survival rate was 57% at 5 years. Low CH50 and C4 complement levels, which were found in 60% of our patients, versus in 26% of the patients with RA but without neuropathy, were associated with a poorer outcome. C4 levels returned to normal values in patients in whom remission of vasculitis occurred. Cryoglobulinemia was present in 13% of the patients of this series. A search for hepatitis B antigens was negative in all of them.

NECROTIZING ARTERITIS AND NEUROPATHY IN PATIENTS WITH OTHER CONNECTIVE TISSUE DISORDERS

NA was associated with other connective tissue disorders, including isolated Sjögren's syndrome in 4% of our patients, systemic lupus erythematosus in 1%, and systemic sclerosis in 1%. In 16 patients (8%) there was more than one connective tissue disorder associated with NA and neuropathy, including 12 patients with Sjögren's syndrome and RA.

NECROTIZING ARTERITIS AND NON-CONNECTIVE TISSUE DISORDER

NA occurs in retroviral infection, in patients with chronic hepatitis and in association with hepatitis B infection. Infection with hepatitis B virus was found in 19% of our patients, including two with chronic hepatitis. These figures confirm that infection with the hepatitis B virus is more common in patients with NA than in controls and that it may play a role in the onset of NA.[42–45] Hepatitis C virus infection, associated or not with chronic hepatitis, is also occasionally associated with vasculitic neuropathy, and at times with cryoglobulinemia.

NECROTIZING ARTERITIS AND ISOLATED NEUROPATHY

In a large proportion of patients with peripheral neuropathy related to NA seen in neurology, there is no other organ clinically involved than the peripheral nervous system. This group of patients accounted for 35% of the 200 patients seen in our service with NA and neuropathy. In such patients, peripheral neuropathy is the presenting and only manifestation of NA.

There may be such a syndrome as vasculitis restricted to the peripheral nervous system, as suggested by Dyck et al,[34] who consider that these patients have a non-systemic, organ-specific vasculitis affecting only the peripheral nervous system. In fact, silent involvement of other organs is common in such patients, as shown by the frequent finding of NA in muscle biopsy specimens. In our series of patients with isolated vasculitic neuropathy, the muscle biopsy was as often diagnostic for vasculitis as the nerve biopsy, demonstrating that silent lesions of medium-sized muscle arteries were common in this context, and that vasculitis was not restricted to the nervous system. The same problem was raised by the so-called cutaneous vasculitis, in which 52% of the patients supposed to have a cutaneous variety of periarteritis nodosa actually had associated neuromuscular manifestations.[46] It is thus more appropriate to consider that the patients with apparently isolated vasculitic neuropathy are affected by a milder form of vasculitis, symptomatic in nerves only.

In this group, the mean age of the patients was 61 years, with 61% females. General signs or symptoms, usually minor, including fever and loss of weight, were present in half of them. Fifty-nine percent of them complained of spontaneous pains of neurogenic or muscular origin. The erythrocyte sedimentation rate was normal in 33% of the patients of this group. Patients with cryoglobulinemia were not included in this group. From a neurological standpoint, approximately one-fourth of the patients presented with a distal symmetrical sensory or sensorimotor neuropathy, and the diagnosis of NA had seldom been considered before the results of the nerve and muscle biopsies.

We followed 29 patients for an average 6 years (extremes 2–14 years): 37% of them developed systemic manifestations; 37% died after an average of 3.3 years after the onset of the neuropathy, including eight from systemic manifestations and three from infection; and 24% had one or more relapses of neuropathy. The mean interval between the first and the second episodes of neuropathy was 3.5 years versus 6 months to 1 year in patients who had multisystemic signs from the beginning. Thirty-one percent did not relapse. These findings are in keeping with the better prognosis observed in the 'non-systemic' vasculitis than in the polysystemic forms by Dyck et al.[34] In all subgroups of NA, the neuropathies have common clinical, electrophysiological and pathological characteristics, which are those of an ischemic neuropathy.

The peripheral neuropathy of necrotizing arteritis (Table 36.2)

CLINICAL ASPECTS

Focal (mononeuritis) neuropathy affected 16.5% of the patients and multifocal neuropathy (mononeuritis multiplex) 56.5% of them. Distal symmetrical sensory or sensorimotor neuropathy was present in 50 patients (25%), and central nervous system (CNS) involvement in 3 patients (2%). The peroneal nerve was affected unilaterally in 62.5%, and bilaterally in one-third. Unilateral involvement of the popliteal nerve was present in 27.5% of the patients, on both

sides in 5%. The ulnar nerve was affected on one side in 25.5% of the patients and on both sides in 8% of them. The median nerve was affected on one side in 21.5% of the patients, and on both sides in 3%. Unilateral involvement of the radial nerve was present in 8% of the patients, and in 2% on both sides. Unilateral involvement of the femoral nerve was observed in 6% of the patients. Proximal sciatic nerve or sciatic root involvement was observed in 2% of the patients. Involvement of the fifth and seventh cranial nerves was observed once. Clinical signs of CNS involvement were observed in 3% of the patients.

In typical cases, the onset of the neuropathy is abrupt and the deficit severe, but in many cases only partial deficit is observed. Also, the course of the neuropathy may be slowly progressive in some cases, especially in the elderly. The cerebrospinal fluid (CSF) was normal in nearly all our patients, but a mild elevation of the protein content occurs.

Recovery from motor deficit due to ischemic neuropathy takes months, because of the axonal lesions. Residual pains, which are common, may sometimes be difficult to differentiate from relapses of the neuropathy.

ELECTROPHYSIOLOGICAL DATA

The electrophysiological studies show an axonal neuropathy in all cases. Some authors have suggested using electrophysiological data to orientate the site of the nerve biopsy.[47] Occasionally, an early ischemic conduction block has been observed,[48,49] but conduction block is more suggestive of nerve entrapment or of acute focal demyelination, as observed in Guillain–Barré syndrome or in other forms of acquired demyelinative neuropathy, than an ischemic nerve lesion.

MORPHOLOGICAL ASPECTS

Demonstration of NA in biopsy specimens
The diagnosis of NA demands histological confirmation, which can be easily achieved by biopsying a specific skin lesion. If not, nerve and/or muscle biopsies can be advised in the search for characteristic lesions of muscular or epineural arteries.[47,50–52] Biopsy of the kidney is less frequently demonstrative, even in patients with nephropathy. It is impossible to tell how often the diagnosis of NA cannot be achieved histologically, but it must be remembered that a negative biopsy does not rule out the diagnosis of NA; however, repetition of biopsies seldom helps in our experience.

In patients with vasculitic neuropathy due to NA, vasculitis can be demonstrated in muscle biopsy

Table 36.2 Nerves affected in a series of 200 consecutive patients with demonstrated necrotizing arteritis (Service de Neurologie, Hôpital de Bicêtre, Université Paris-Sud)

Nerve affected	Unilaterally	Bilaterally
Peroneal nerve	125 (62.5%)	66 (33%)
Popliteal nerve	55 (27.5%)	9 (5%)
Ulnar nerve	51 (25.5%)	15 (8%)
Median nerve	23 (21.5%)	6 (3%)
Radial nerve	17 (8.5%)	3
Femoral nerve	12 (6%)	1
Sciatic roots	4 (2%)	
Cranial nerves (V, VII)	2 (1%)	

specimens, in the nerve biopsy specimen, or in both of them. In our most recent evaluation, in 27% of our patients with vasculitic neuropathy the vascular lesion was in the muscle specimen only, in 35% in the nerve specimen only, and in 27% both in the nerve and muscle specimens. It is thus wiser to sample both the nerve and the muscle during the same procedure[35] especially when the peroneal nerve is affected. In such cases, we biopsy the superficial peroneal nerve and the peroneus brevis muscle during the same procedure, under local anesthesia.

Biopsy specimens must be studied on serial sections, because arteritis is segmental, and characteristic lesions may be present on segments of the arteries as short as 50 μm in our experience. Total nerve biopsy must be performed instead of fascicular biopsy, because, almost invariably, only the epineural arteries are affected, sometimes in association with inflammatory infiltration of perineural vessels. Epineural and perineural inflammatory infiltrates were common in the vicinity of characteristic arterial lesions, but they are seldom observed in the endoneural space, except in the patients with NA occurring in the context of HIV infection.

Lesions of nerve fibers—the ischemic neuropathy
Nerve ischemia, as observed in vasculitic neuropathy, induces acute axonal degeneration in most cases. In our series, Wallerian degeneration affected an average of $65 \pm 35\%$ (SD) of the isolated fibers, with simultaneous degeneration of fibers in many cases (normal value: less than 1%), a pattern which fits well with an ischemic lesion and may suggest vasculitis when characteristic arterial lesions have not been found. The average incidence of fibers showing segmental abnormalities of the myelin sheath was 1.9% (range 0–15%; normal <1%), often with paranodal and internodal demyelination clustered in individual fibers, in a pattern suggesting that demyelination was secondary to minor axonal involvement. Asymmetry of lesions between and within fascicles is also common in vasculitic neuropathy. Sometimes, axon loss predominates in the centrofascicular area, which suggests an ischemic origin.

Quantitative studies of epon-embedded specimens and teased-fiber preparations showed that: (1) the intensity of axon loss and the incidence of degenerating fibers varied greatly from case to case, and between fascicles of individual nerves; (2) axon loss predominates on myelinated fibers larger than 7 μm in diameter; (3) the unmyelinated fibers are less affected; (4) occasionally, even the Schwann cells degenerated, which may preclude axonal regenera-

tion and clinical recovery; and (5) in most cases, the nerve lesions appeared to result from the summation of lesions of different age of nerve blood vessels.[53]

Neuropathy in the other types of necrotizing vasculitis
Peripheral neuropathy is less common in the other types of necrotizing vasculitis

WEGENER'S GRANULOMATOSIS
In Wegener's granulomatosis, which is characterized by granulomatous vasculitis of upper and lower respiratory tract with or without glomerulonephritis, peripheral neuropathy occurs in 25% of the patients.[32] In this group, smaller vessels are affected and, in our experience, Wegener's granulomatosis is much less frequently the cause of a peripheral neuropathy than in the previous groups.

The neurological manifestations of Wegener's granulomatosis have been reviewed in a large retrospective study of 324 patients at the Mayo Clinic.[55] One hundred and nine patients (33.6%) had neurological manifestations, including 53 with peripheral neuropathy, 42 of whom had multifocal neuropathy, 6 a distal symmetrical polyneuropathy and 5 an unclassified peripheral neuropathy. Neuropathy was one of the major presenting symptoms in 8 of the 22 patients with mononeuropathy multiplex who had detailed evaluation at this institution. The mean interval between the onset of Wegener's granulomatosis and the onset of the neuropathy was 8.4 months. As in patients with PAN,[35] the peroneal nerve, which was affected in 21 patients, was the most commonly involved nerve. In the upper limbs, as also observed in PAN, the ulnar nerve, which was affected in 10 patients with Wegener's granulomatosis, is the most commonly involved in the upper limbs. Biopsy of the sural nerve was performed in 2 patients only, and was diagnostic in 1. Examination of a biopsy specimen of the superficial peroneal nerve, which was clinically affected in nearly all cases, might have been more contributive. Unlike what occurs in PAN, and especially in some patients with isolated neuropathy and NA, in which conditions the peripheral neuropathy often reveals or is even the only manifestation of NA, neuropathy occurred on average 8.4 months after that of the other manifestations of Wegener's granulomatosis. The peripheral neuropathy of Wegener's granulomatosis is very similar to that seen in PAN, with the important exception of the frequent involvement of the cranial nerve in Wegener's granulomatosis. In Wegener's granulomatosis 21 patients of the 109 presented cranial neuropathy, including 16 patients with external ophthalmoparesis. This high frequency of external ophthalmoplegia in Wegener's granulomatosis is attributed to granulomatous infiltration of the orbit or the cavernous sinus.

GIANT CELL ARTERITIS

Giant cell arteritis includes temporal arteritis and Takayasu's arteritis, two distinct disorders that have in common a granulomatous vasculitis of medium-sized and large arteries.

Temporal arteritis

In temporal arteritis, which affects people over 55 years of age, a polyneuropathy has been noted in some patients.[56] In a clinical retrospective study of 166 patients with biopsy-proven giant cell arteritis, 14% of the patients had peripheral neuropathy, 7% mononeuritis and 7% what the authors call peripheral neuropathy,[57] which probably includes neuropathies of different origin. It is unusual to see symptoms of ischemia related to giant cell arteritis below the neck, although the potential involvement of any systemic intermediate-sized or large muscular artery has been established in post-mortem series.[58] We have encountered two patients who developed mononeuritis multiplex a few months after cranial arteritis; both had characteristic PAN in nerve and muscle biopsies. These findings confirm that PAN should be considered when systemic vasculitis develops in patients with cranial arteritis.[59]

Takayasu's disease

Takayasu's disease is characterized by diminished or pulseless signs, inflammatory prodrome with fever, malaise, polymyalgia pains, arthralgias and weight loss. This may be followed by pain in local vessels. The cardiovascular changes depend upon the vessels involved. Coronary insufficiency may cause infarction. The arterial lesions respond well to treatment with steroids. The lesions observed suggest that Takayasu's disease represents a special form of necrotizing angiitis involving large vessels, the size of which is not in the range of that of nerve blood vessels.

THE NEUROPATHIES ASSOCIATED WITH LYMPHOCYTIC VASCULITIS

Perivascular cuffing and lymphocytic vasculitis occur in infectious and parasitic disorders affecting the peripheral nervous system such as leprosy and Chagas' disease, and sometimes in association with malignant disorders, especially with lymphomas.[60]

Angiocentric lymphoproliferative disorders[61]

This group of disorders, which encompasses the previously nosologic entities of lymphomatoid granulomatosis, represents an uncommon type of vasculitis which combines the angiodestructive and granulomatous features of Wegener's granulomatosis with the cellular atypicality of lymphoma.[62–64] Evidence now indicates that lymphomatoid granulomatosis is a T-cell lymphoma.[65] Jaffe has also described a histological grading for angiocentric lymphoproliferative disorders.[66] Grade I is characterized by a predominantly polymorphous lymphocytic infiltrate without cytological atypia; grade II is characterized by the polymorphous infiltrate but with clear cytological atypia; grade III, also termed angiocentric lymphoma, is clearly malignant histologically. This type of vasculitis seems to carry a more severe prognosis than most cases of NA, with frequent involvement of the CNS. Still, this entity associates an angiocentric proliferation of T-lymphocytes with lesions of blood vessels that induce nerve ischemia. Neuropathy associated with angiocentric proliferation of lymphocytes and necrosis of blood vessels, and infiltration predominantly composed of CD8+ lymphocytes, occur in the course of infection with HIV.[67] Occasionally, vasculitis occurs in the context of a malignant monoclonal gammopathy, including multiple myeloma or malignant lymphoma with monoclonal gammopathy.

Vasculitis in the inflammatory neuropathy due to infectious agents

Leprous neuropathy

Non-necrotizing lymphocytic vasculitis is observed in the different patterns of leprous neuropathy, including lepromatous, tuberculoid and type 1 and type 2 reversal reactions. In lepromatous leprosy, vasculitis is associated with infection of endothelial cells by *Mycobacterium leprae*. A role for ischemia is likely in some reverse reactions during treatment of lepromatous leprosy and borderline lepromatous neuropathy.[68]

Vasculitis in HIV infection

In the course of HIV infection, different patterns of lymphocytic vasculitis are observed, in association with the various types of inflammatory neuropathy encountered in this setting.[68] Clinically, the usual pattern of neuropathy associated with prominent vasculitis is that of a subacute, multifocal, often bilateral, mixed, motor and sensory deficit associated with polyclonal hypergammaglobulinemia, and increased protein content and pleocytosis in the CSF. The most common type of lymphocytic vasculitis is just an exaggerated inflammatory infiltrate that invades the vessel wall without causing more damage. In a few instances, the pattern is that of an angiocentric lymphocytic proliferation associated or not with necrosis of the vessel wall. In such cases, axonal degeneration of nerve fibers is ssociated with a large proportion of demyelinated fibers.

NA of the type observed in PAN, with fibrinoid necrosis and leukocytoclasia, is also observed in HIV neuropathy.[67,69] In this setting, however, in contrast with the usual pattern of lesions observed in PAN, mononuclear cells predominate in the inflammatory infiltrate, which is often present in the endoneural space, and affect small endoneural blood vessels. The lesions of nerve fibers observed in this setting often included a higher than usual proportion of demyelinated fibers in a series of patients with necrotizing vasculitis and HIV infection. Additionally, inflammatory myopathy and lesions of muscle arteries are often present. At late stages of the immunosuppression induced by HIV infection, opportunistic infection of nerve blood vessels, especially of endothelial cells of endoneural capillaries by cytomegalovirus, can further damage nerves.

Vasculitis in focal and multifocal diabetic neuropathy

In a recent study on nerve lesions of the intermediate cutaneous nerve of the thigh and of the superficial peroneal nerve in patients with multifocal and proximal diabetic neuropathy, we found occlusion of epineural blood vessels associated with vasculitis and inflammatory in filtration in some patients.[70] These findings come as a surprise in this setting. Clinically, the neuropathy was not accompanied by general signs or symptoms of inflammation. The lesions spared muscle blood vessels of the same size, and the cellular infiltration was made up of mononuclear cells only, without polymorphonuclear cells, leukocytoclasia or recanalization, as observed in PAN, This possibly, however, stresses the need for studying nerve and muscle biopsy specimens in this context. The link between the occurrence of inflammatory infiltrates, vasculitis and diabetes is not clear, but small inflammatory infiltrates have been occasionally encountered in sural nerve biopsy specimens of diabetic patients with neurological deficits,[71] in autonomic nerve bundles and ganglia,[72] and in only detailed autopsy study of a patient with proximal diabetes neuropathy.[73] It is thus suggested

that lesions of nerve fibers and of blood vessels due to diabetes can trigger an inflammatory reaction and vasculitis in some patients, with secondary ischemic nerve lesions due to occlusion of epi- or perineural blood vessels. Patients with inflammatory infiltrate and vasculitis occurring in this context may respond well to treatment with corticosteroids, but they can also improve spontaneously.[74]

Vasculitis and sarcoidosis

Granulomatous vasculitis may complicate the course of chronic sarcoidosis and can be responsible for diffuse encephalopathy with psychiatric presentation and short-term memory deficit. Necrotizing vasculitis occurs in this context and induces ischemic lesions. This angiitic pattern of neurosarcoidosis has been demonstrated histologically in patients with neuro-ophthalmologic manifestations[75] and in patients with sarcoid neuropathy (Said et al, unpublished). These cases pose the problem of their border with Wegener's granulomatosis, with which they share many features, but sarcoidosis, even in the cases with granulomatous angiitis, has a more benign course than Wegener's granulomatosis.[76,77]

TREATMENT

The treatment of vasculitic neuropathy related to primary vasculitis rests mainly on corticosteroids. It is widely admitted that one should start with prednisone at 1 mg/kg per day. High doses of corticosteroids may not be well tolerated in the elderly. Simultaneous treatment with cyclophosphamide, 2 g/kg per day, may help to reduce the doses of corticosteroids. In cases with severe general manifestations, pulses of intravenous prednisolone may help. It is difficult to tell how long this treatment should be maintained at full dose. This depends on the response to treatment, on the course and form of the disease and on the tolerance of the treatment. We usually prescribe a full dose of steroids for approximately 6–8 weeks and then start tapering the dose of steroids very gently. It is necessary to control the erythrocyte sedimentation rate (ESR) periodically and to increase prednisone if the ESR increases, if this increase in ESR is not due to another factor, especially to infection. The patients with HIV infection and NA also responded well to steroids.

In cases without clinical evidence of polysystemic involvement, in cases with normal ESR, and in elder patients, the benefit of prolonged treatment with high doses of steroids is less certain. Indomethacin (100 mg/day) may be associated with steroids when fever persists or when the ESR remains abnormal in spite of large doses of steroids.

The usefulness of treatments like intravenous immunoglobulin[78] and monoclonal antibodies directed against the human CD4 molecules of T-helper cells[79] deserve further investigation. In the evaluation of the efficacy of treatments of vasculitic neuropathies, it must be remembered that there is a wide range of modalities of evolution in NA, with spontaneous remissions of several years of the disease in some cases.

REFERENCES

1. Jeanette JC, Falk RJ. Small vessel vasculitis. *New Eng J Med* 1997; **337**: 1512–23.
2. Nydegger UE. A place for soluble immune complexes in clinical immunology? *Immunol Today* 1985; **6**: 80–82.
3. Hogg N. The structure and function of Fc receptors. *Immunol Today* 1988; **9**: 185–187.
4. Smiley JD, Moore SE. Immune complex vasculitis: role of complement and IgG-Fc receptor functions. *Am J Med Sci* 1989; **298**: 267–297.
5. Moore PM. Immune mechanisms in the primary and secondary vasculitides. *J Neurol Sci* 1989; **93**: 129–145.
6. Kissel JT, Riethman JL, Ormeza J et al. Peripheral nerve vasculitis: immune characterization of the vascular lesions. *Ann Neurol* 1989; **93**: 129–145.
7. Hawke SHB, Davies L, Pamphlett R et al. Vasculitic neuropathy. A clinical and pathological study. *Brain* 1991; **114**: 2175–2190.
8. Panegyres PK, Blumbergs PC, Leong AS-Y, Bourne AJ. Vasculitis of peripheral nerve and skeletal muscle: clinicopathological and immunopathic mechanisms. *J Neurol Sci* 1990; **100**: 193–202.
9. Kissel JT, Mendell JR. Peripheral neuropathy due to vasculitis: immunopathogenesis, clinical features and treatment. In: Hohlfeld R, ed. *Immunology of Neuromuscular Disease*. Dordrecht: Kluwer Academic Press, 1994: 105–121.
10. Brasile L, Kremer JM, Clarke JL, Cerilli J. Identification of an autoantibody to vascular endothelial cell-specific antigens in patients with systemic vasculitis. *Am J Med* 1989; **87**: 74–80.
11. Ferraro G, Meroni PL, Tincani A et al. Anti-endothelial cell antibodies in patients with Wegener's granulomatosis and micropolyarteritis. *Clin Exp Immunol* 1990; **79**: 47–53.
12. Parlevliet KJ, Henzen-Logmans SC, Qe PL et al. Antibodies to components of neutrophil cytoplasm: a new diagnostic tool in patients with Wegener's granulomatosis and systemic vasculitis. *Q J Med* 1988; **66**: 55–63.
13. Goeken JA. Antineutrophil cytoplasmic antibody—a useful serological marker for vasculitis. *J Clin Immunol* 1991; **11**: 161–174.
14. Frampton G, Jayne DRW, Perry GJ et al. Autoantibodies to endothelial cells and neutrophil cytoplasmic antigens in systemic vasculitis. *Clin Exp Immunol* 1990; **79**: 47–53.
15. Ewert BH, Jennette JC, Falk RJ. The pathogenetic role of antineutrophil cytoplasmic antibodies. *Am J Kidney Dis* 1991; **18**: 188–195.
16. Hoffman G, Speck U. Antineutrophil cytoplasmic antibodies. *Arthritis Rheum* 1998; **41**: 1521–1537.
17. Coll-Vinent B, Cebrian M, Cid M. Dynamic pattern of endothelial cell adhesion molecule expression in muscle and perineural vessels from patients with classic polyarteritis nodosa. *Arthritis Rheum* 1998; **41**: 435–444.
18. Cohen-Tervaert J, Kallenberg C. Cell adhesion molecules in vasculitis. *Curr Opin Rheumatol* 1997; **9**: 16–25.
19. Blann A, McCollum C. Circulating endothelial cell/leukocyte adhesion molecules in atherosclerosis. *Thromb Hemost* 1994; **72**: 151–154.
20. Banks R, Gearubg A, Hemingway I, Norfolk D, Perren T, Selby P. Circulating intercellular adhesion molecule-1, E-selectin and vascular cell adhesion molecule-1 in human malignancies. *Br J Cancer* 1993; **68**: 122–124.
21. Satoi H, Oka N, Kawasaki T, Miyamoto K, Akiguchi I, Kimura J. Mechanisms of tissue injury in vasculitic neuropathies. *Neurology* 1998; **50**: 492–496.
22. Pober JS, Cotran RS. Cytokines and endothelial cell biology. *Physiol Rev* 1990; **70**: 427–451.
23. Panegyres PK, Faull RJ, Russ GR et al. Endothelial cell activation in vasculitis of peripheral nerve and skeletal muscles. *J Neurol Neurosurg Psychiatry* 1992; **55**: 4–7.
24. Winkelmann RK. Classification of vasculitis. In: Vasculitis. Wolff K, Winkelmann RK, eds. London: Lloyd-Luke Ltd, 1980: 1–24.
25. Lie JT. Nomenclature and classification of vasculitis: Plus ça change, plus c'est la même chose. *Arthritis Rheumatol* 1994; **2**: 181–186.
26. Jennette JC, Falk RJ, Andrassy K et al. Nomenclature of systemic vasculitides. *Arthritis Rheumatol* 1994; **37**: 187–192.
27. Kussmaul A, Maier R. Uber eine bisher nicht beschrebene eigenthumliche Arterienerkrankung (Periarteritis nodosa), die mit Morbus Brightii un rapid fortschreitender allgemeiner Muskellah-mung einhergeht. *Dtsch Arch Klin Med* 1866; **1**: 484–517.
28. Lovshin LI, Kernohan JW. Peripheral neuritis in periarteritis nodosa. *Arch Intern Med* 1948; **82**: 321–338.
29. Asbury AK, Johnson PC. Vasculitic neuropathy. In: Bennington JL, ed. *Major Problems in Pathology*, Vol 9, *Pathology of Peripheral Nerve*. Philadelphia: Saunders, 1978: 110–119.
30. Moore PM, Cupps TR. Neurologic complications of vasculitis. *Ann Neurol* 1983; **14**: 155–167.
31. Godeau P, Guillevin L. Périartérite noueuse systémique. In: Kahn M-F, Peltier AP, eds. *Maladies dites systémiques*. Paris: Flammarion, 1982: 414–445.
32. Stern GM, Hoffbrand AV, Urich H. The peripheral nerves and skeletal muscles in Wegener's granulomatosis: clinicopathological study of four cases. *Brain* 1965; **88**: 151–164.
33. Kissel JT, Slivka AP, Warmolts JR, Mendell JR. The clinical spectrum of necrotizing angiopathy of the peripheral nervous system. *Ann Neural* 1985; **18**: 251–257.
34. Dycke PJ, Benstead TJ, Conn DL et al. Nonsystemic vasculitic neuropathy. *Brain* 1987; **110**: 843–854.
35. Said G, Lacroix C, Fujimura H et al. The peripheral neuropathy of necrotizing arteritis: a clinicopathologic study. *Ann Neurol* 1988; **23**: 461–465.
36. Fauci AS, Haynes BF, Katz P. The spectrum of vasculitis. *Ann Intern Med* 1978; **89**: 660–676.
37. Chumbley LC, Harrison EG Jr, Deremee RA. Allergic granulomatosis and angiitis (Churg–Strauss syndrome). *Proc Mayo Clin* 1977; **52**: 477.
38. Cohen-Tervaert JW, Limburg PC, Elema JD et al. Detection of autoantibodies against myeloid lysosomal enzymes: a useful adjunct to classification of patients with biopsy-proven necrotizing arteritis. *Am J Med* 1991; **91**: 1991.

39. Hattori N, Ichimura M, Nagamatsu M et al. Clinico-pathological features of Churg–Strauss syndrome-associated neuropathy. *Brain* 1999; **122**: 427–39.

40. Wattiaux MJ, Kahn MF, Thevenet JP, Sauvezie B, Imbert JC. L'atteinte vasculaire de Ia polyarthrite rhumatoïde: étude retrospective de 37 polyarthrites rhumatoïdes avec atteinte vasculaire et revue de Ia littérature. *Ann Med lnt* 1987; **138**(8): 566–587.

41. Puechal X, Said G, Hilliquin P, et al. Peripheral neuropathy with necrotizing vasculitis in rheumatoid arthritis: a clincopathological and prognostic study of 32 patients. *Arthritis Rheum* 1995; **38**: 1618–1629.

42. Sergent JS, Lockshin MD, Christian CL, Gocke DJ. Vasculitis with hepatitis B antigenemia: long term observations in nine patients. *Medicine* 1976; **55**: 1–8.

43. Anonymous. Systemic vasculitis. *Lancet* 1985; **1**: 1252–1254.

44. Drueke T, Barbanel C, Jungers P et al. Hepatitis B antigen associated periarteritis nodosa in patients undergoing long-term hemodialysis. *Am J Med* 1980; **68**: 86–90.

45. Shusterman N, London WT. Hepatitis B and immune-complex disease. *N Engl J Med* 1984; **313**: 43–45

46. Diaz-Perez J, Winkelmann RK. Cutaneous periarteritis nodosa: a study of 33 cases. In: Vasculitis. Wolff K, Winkelmann RK, eds. London: Lloyd-Luke Ltd, 1980: 273–284.

47. Wees SJ, Sunwood LN, Oh SJ. Sural nerve biopsy in systemic necrotizing vasculitis. *Am J Med* 1981; **71**: 525–532.

48. Ropert A, Metral S. Conduction block in neuropathies with necrotizing arteritis. *Muscle Nerve* 1990; **13**: 102–105.

49. Mohamed A, Davies L, Pollard J. Conduction block in vasculitic neuropathy. *Muscle Nerve* 1998; **21**: 1084–1088.

50. Maxeiner SR, McDonald JR, Kirlklin JW. Muscle biopsy in the diagnosis of periarteritis nodosa: an evaluation. *Surg Clin North Am* 1952; **32**: 1225-1235.

51. Parry GJ, Brown MJ, Asbury AK. Diagnostic value of nerve biopsy in mononeuritis multiplex. *Neurology* 1981; **31**: 129–130.

52. Pages M, Pages AM. La biopsie nerveuse au cours de la périartérite noueuse. Son intêret diagnostique. *Semin Hop Paris* 1984; **60**: 3295–3299.

53. Fujimura H, Lacroix C, Said G. Vulnerability of nerve fibers to ischaemia. *Brain* 1991; **114**: 1929–1942.

54. Wolff SM, Fauci AS, Horn RG, Dale DC. Wegener's granulomatosis. *Ann Intern Med* 1974; **81**: 513–525.

55. Nishino H, Rubino FA, DeRemee RA, Swanson JW, Parisi JE. Neurological involvement in Wegener's granulomatosis: an analysis of 324 consecutive patients at the Mayo Clinic. *Ann Neurol* 1993; **33**: 4–9.

56. Paulley JW, Hughes JP. Giant cell arteritis or arthritis of the aged. *BMJ* 1960; **2**: 1562–1567.

57. Caselli RJ, Hunder GG, Whisnant JP. Neurologic disease in biopsy-proven giant cell (temporal) arteritis. *Neurology* 1988; **38**: 352–359.

58. Kelin RG, Hunder GG, Stanson AW, Sheps SG. Large artery involvement in giant cell (temporal) arteritis. *Ann Intern Med* 1975; **83**: 806–812.

59. Frayha RA, Abu-Haiclar F. Polyarteritis nodosa masquerading as temporal arteritis. *J Rheumatol* 1979; **6**: 76–9.

60. Sams WM Jr, Harville DD, Winkelmann RK. Necrotizing vasculitis associated with lethal reticuloendothelial diseases. *Br J Dermatol* 1968; **80**: 555–560.

61. Jaffe ES. Pathologic and clinical spectrum of post-thymic T cell malignancies. *Cancer Invest* 1984; **2**: 413–426.

62. Liebow AA, Carrington CRB, Friedman PJ. Lymphoma-toid granulomatosis. *Hum Pathol* 1972; **3**: 457.

63. Katzenstein AA, Carrington GB, Liebow AA. Lymphomatoid granulomatosis: a clinicopathologic study. *Cancer* 1979; **43**: 360–373.

64. Chung-Hong H, Winkelmann RK. Lymphomatoid granu-lomatosis of the skin. In: Vasculitis. Wolff K, Winkelmann RK, eds. London: Lloyd-Luke Ltd, 1980: 249–259.

65. Myers JL. Lymphomatoid granulomatosis: past, present . . . future? *Mayo Clin Proc* 1990; **565**: 274.

66. Jaffe ES. Pulmonary lymphocytic angiitis: a nosologic quandary. *Mayo Gun Proc* 1988; **63**: 411–413.

67. Calabrese LH, Estes M, Yen-Lieberman B et al. Systemic vasculitis in association with human immunodeficiency virus infection. *Arthritis Rheum* 1989; **32**: 569–576.

68. Said G. Inflammatory neuropathies associated with known infections (HIV, leprosy, Chagas' disease, Lyme disease). *Baillière's Clin Neurol* 1994; **3**: 149–171.

69. Said G, Lacroix C, Andrieu JM et al. Necrotizing arteri-tis in patients with inflammatory neuropathy and immunodeficiency virus infection (Abstract). *Neurology*, 1997; **37**(1): 176.

70. Said G, Goulon-Goeau C, Noulonguet A. Proximal diabetic neuropathy: Clinical aspects and morphological findings in biopsy specimens of the intermediate cutaneous nerve of the thigh. *Ann Neurol* 1994; **35**: 559–69.

71. Costigan DA, Krendel DA, Hopkins LC, Crittenden J. Inflammatory neuropathy in diabetes. *Ann Neurol* 1990; **28**: 272 (abst).

72. Duchen LW, Anjorin A, Watkins PJ, Mackay JD. Pathol-ogy of autonomic neuropathy in diabetes mellitus. *Ann Intern Med* 1980; **92**: 301–303.

73. Raff MC, Sangalang V, Asbury AK. Ischemic mono-neuropathy and mononeuropathy multiplex in diabetes mellitus. *Arch Neurol* 1968; **18**: 487–499.

74. Said G, Elgrably F, Lacroix C et al. Painful proximal diabetic neuropathy: Inflammatory nerve lesions and spontaneous favourable outcome. *Ann Neurol* 1997; **41**: 762–70.

75. Caplan L, Corbett J, Goodwin J et al. Neuro-ophthal-mologic signs in the angiitic form of neurosarcoidosis. *Neurology* 1983; **33**: 1130–1136.

76. Urich H. Neurosarcoidosis or granulomatous angiitis: a problem of definition. *Mt Sinai J Med* 1977; **44**: 718–725.

77. DeReeme RA. Sarcoidosis and Wegener's granulomato-sis: a comparative analysis. *Sarcoidosis* 1994; **11**: 7–18.

78. Jaynes DRW, Davies MJ, Fox CJV, Black CM, Lockwood CM. Treatment of systemic vasculitis with pooled intra-venous immunoglobulin. *Lancet* 1991; **337**: 1137–1139.

79. Mathieson PW, Cobbold SP, Hale G et al. Monoclonal antibody therapy in systemic vasculitis. *N Engl J Med* 1990; **323**: 250–254.

37

Acquired demyelinating neuropathies: molecular mechanisms and novel therapeutic approaches

Andreas J Steck, David Leppert, Peter Fuhr, Alexander J Radziwill, Susanne Renaud and Nicole Schaeren-Wiemers

OVERVIEW

Historically, chronic inflammatory demyelinating polyradiculoneuropathies (CIDPs) have constituted the major group of well-documented patients with symmetrical acquired demyelinating polyneuropathy. Diagnostic criteria for CIDP are both clinical, with a pattern of disease tending to affect distal and proximal limbs, and electrophysiological, with defined criteria specifying for a primary demyelinating polyneuropathy.[1] These patients respond well to corticosteroids or immunosuppressive agents, and it is understood that they should have no other concomitant disorder, though patients with serum paraproteins have also been included.[2]

Another well-documented group of patients with symmetrical acquired demyelinating polyneuropathy is characterized by predominantly distal involvement. Sensory symptoms are usually predominant, and when weakness is present, it is limited to distal muscle groups in a length-dependent fashion.[3] In contrast to classic CIDP, these patients often fail to respond to standard regimens of oral prednisone or intravenous immunoglobulin.[4] It has recently been proposed that this phenotype be called distal acquired demyelinating symmetric (DADS) neuropathy.[5] In this category of patients, which is distinguished primarily by clinical and electrodiagnostic features, there is a high proportion of patients with monoclonal protein.

NEURAL ANTIGENS IMPLICATED IN IMMUNE-MEDIATED NEUROPATHIES

Patients with polyneuropathy and serum M-protein often have antibodies directed against peripheral nerve constituents, and it has also been customary to categorize these patients on the basis of their antibody reactivity.[6] Antibodies with defined specificities have been implicated in particular subsets of these disorders.[7] Some of the major antigens and characteristics of the neuropathies with which they are associated are summarized in Table 37.1. Grouping patients with distinct clinical polyneuropathy syndromes primarily by antibodies is justified if there is evidence of a clear pathogenic mechanism. While this is true for some antibodies like the anti-MAG or anti-GQ1b antibodies, it is less clear for other antibodies such as anti-sulfatide antibodies.[8] Furthermore, antibodies such as GM1 antibodies are associated with heterogeneous clinical syndromes, including Guillain–Barré syndrome[9] and chronic motor neuropathies.[10]

There is widespread variation in relative reactivities, even within a specific target antigen. The development, evaluation and reporting of diagnostic tests is unstandardized.[11] Various test methodologies such as ELISA, Western blot or immunofluorescence may reveal considerable differences in reactivity or specificity patterns of antibodies. It is assumed that the way in which a given epitope is presented in an assay is an important factor affecting or modulating antibody reactivity. Furthermore, measurements in vitro are only an approximation of the in vivo situation. Factors affecting access of antibodies to the peripheral nervous system (PNS) include the presence of the blood–nerve barrier, the local accessibility, the target antigens, the membrane microenvironment and the temperature. The blood–nerve barrier is incomplete and absent at the most proximal and at the distal part of the nerve. Potentially pathogenic antibodies find easy access to peripheral

Table 37.1 Summary of neural antigens associated with immune-mediated peripheral neuropathies[7]

Antigen	Ig class	Neuropathy	Clinical features	Electrophysiology
MAG (and cross-reacting glycoconjugates including PO, PMP22 and SGPG)	IgM-M	DADS-M	Chronic Sensory > motor Symmetrical Distal > proximal	Predominantly demyelinating Reduced SNAP and CMAP Decreased velocities Prolonged distal latencies (TLI often reduced)
GM1 ganglioside	IgM polyclonal	MMN	Chronic Purely motor Distal > proximal Asymmetrical	Demyelinating or mixed Reduced CMAP CB and decreased velocities Limited to motor nerves
GM1 ganglioside	IgG polyclonal	AMAN	Acute Motor ≫ sensory Symmetrical Proximal > distal	Axonal Reduced CMAP Mildly decreased velocities
Ganglioside with polysialosyl moieties (GD1b, GD2, GD3, GT1b, GQ1b)	IgM-M	CANOMAD	Chronic Purely sensory Ataxia Ophthalmoplegia Symmetrical Proximal and distal	Axonal or demyelinating Absent or reduced SNAP Midly decreased velocities
GQ1b and other gangliosides with disialosyl moieties	IgG polyclonal	MFS	Acute Ataxia Ophthalmoplegia Areflexia	Predominantly demyelinating Limbs: reduced SNAP and decreased velocities Cranial nerves: reduced CMAP and decreased velocities
Sulfatide antigens: sulfatide or chondroitin sulfate	IgM or IgG polyclonal or monoclonal	SAN	Chronic Predominantly sensory Ataxia Symmetrical	Axonal or demyelinating Reduced SNAP Prolonged distal latencies Decreased velocities

DADS-M, distal acquired demyelinating symmetrical neuropathy with monoclonal protein; MMN, multifocal motor neuropathy; AMAN, acute motor axonal neuropathy; CANOMAD, chronic ataxic neuropathy with ophthalmoplegia, monoclonal protein, agglutination and disialosyl antibodies; MFS, Miller–Fischer syndrome; SAN, sensory ataxic neuropathy; SNAP, sensory nerve action potential; CMAP, compound muscle action potential; CB, conduction block; TLI, terminal latency index.

nerve fibers at these sites. The combination of absent blood–nerve barrier at the distal part of nerves together with lower temperature distally that may increase antibody binding could be responsible for the length-dependent demyelination observed in the anti-MAG neuropathy. However, much remains to be learned in terms of understanding the molecular pathogenesis of autoantibody-mediated neuropathies. In addition, proper evaluation of antibody tests will require the application of methodological standards.

MOLECULAR ORGANIZATION OF THE MYELIN MEMBRANE IN THE PERIPHERAL NERVOUS SYSTEM

Myelin is a multilamellar spiral of membrane that surrounds axons and promotes saltatory conduction.

Myelin formation is a complex, developmentally regulated process involving the coordinated expression of genes coding for myelin proteins and for enzymes associated with the synthesis of myelin-specific lipids. Seventy-five per cent of PNS myelin, formed by Schwann cells, consists of lipids. Cholesterol accounts for 20–30% of total lipids. Sphingomyelin (10–35%), galactosylceramide (~25%), sulfatide (~4%) and gangliosides (sphingolipids with an oligosaccharide head group including one or more sialic acid residues) are highly enriched and located in the outer leaflet, whereas unsaturated long-chain fatty acids (~35%) are mainly located in the inner leaflet of the myelin membrane.[12,13] The initial contact between the proliferating myelinating cell and the axon, spiral wrapping of the processes around the axon, and transport systems for ions and essential molecules between myelin lamellae, all require specific membrane and membrane-associated proteins.[14] The coordinated expression of genes and their proteins involved in these particular steps is a prerequisite for normal function of this special membrane. While the individual components (proteins and lipids) may normally function as part of a macromolecular structure of compact or non-compact myelin, their functional role has been mainly examined in isolation. The proteins that are thought to be involved in the process of wrapping and compaction are adhesion proteins such as myelin-associated glycoprotein (MAG)[15] and protein P0,[16] hydrophobic proteins such as peripheral myelin protein 22 (PMP-22),[17] and membrane-associated cytoplasmic proteins like myelin basic protein (MBP).[18] The most abundant myelin protein in the PNS is P0,[13,19] a 28-kDa integral membrane glycoprotein with an immunoglobulin-like extracellular domain, which forms tetramers in the plane of the compact myelin membrane.[20] PMP-22[21] is a 22-kDa protein that consists of four hydrophobic domains and carries as P0 a HNK-1 glycoconjugate.[22]

Identification of new myelin genes

By a differential screening approach for genes which are specifically expressed during myelin formation, several genes have been identified coding for proteins with different biochemical and functional properties.[23] Interestingly, four of the identified genes, apolipoprotein D (ApoD), UDP-galactose-ceramide galactosyltransferase (CGT), myelin and lymphocyte protein (MAL) and stearyl-CoA-desaturase 2 (SCD2), are involved in lipid metabolism. ApoD was originally isolated as a gene upregulated after peripheral nerve injury.[24] ApoD is a member of

the lipocalin superfamily, which share a conserved tertiary structure and are thought to be involved in the transport of small hydrophobic ligands. Its specific ligand(s) is not yet known but it is believed that ApoD binds and transports lipids (e.g. cholesterol), steroid hormones (e.g. progesterone and pregnenolone) and arachidonic acid.[25] CGT is the key enzyme for the glycosphingolipid pathway and preferentially uses hydroxyceramide as a substrate for glycosylation for the most prominent glycolipid galactosylceramide.[26] The functional role of glycosphingolipids in myelin was addressed in transgenic mice lacking CGT. Although myelin appears to be morphologically normal (with the exception of the paranodal loops), nerve conduction velocity from these animals was drastically reduced, and later during adulthood myelin becomes focally unstable. Furthermore, these mice suffer from hind limb paralysis and have a shorter lifespan.[27-30] Specific interactions between myelin lipids and proteins must play an important role in myelin formation and especially myelin maintenance. However, our knowledge of protein–lipid interactions in myelin is still very limited. One particular protein, MAL, is a small hydrophobic proteolipid of 17 kDa with four putative transmembrane-spanning regions of central and peripheral myelin.[31] Besides its localization in myelin membranes, MAL was additionally localized in apical membranes of epithelial cells of kidney and stomach.[32] Myelin and apical membranes are enriched in glycosphingolipids and cholesterol, which are co-purified with MAL in detergent-insoluble glycolipid-enriched microdomains.[33] According to the prevailing view of cellular membrane structure, lipids in the bilayer function mainly as a solvent for membrane proteins. In myelin membranes, different lipid species and membrane proteins are asymmetrically distributed over the exoplasmic and cytoplasmic leaflets. The lateral organization of these lipids and proteins is likely to be a result of preferential packing and sorting mechanisms, as suggested by Simons and Ikonen.[34]

Molecular and structural organization of the myelin sheath

The myelin sheath is composed of two distinct domains, compact and non-compact myelin, each of which is characterized by a unique set of proteins. Compact myelin contains P0, PMP22, MBP, protein P2, $2',3'$-cyclic nucleotide $3'$-phosphodiesterase (CNP) and MAL, whereas non-compact myelin contains MAG, connexin 32 (Cx32), $\alpha_6\beta_4$ integrin and E-cadherin.[13] Non-compact myelin is found at the paranodes and incisures, known as Schmidt–Lanterman incisures, funnel-shaped non-compacted plasma membranes that traverse the compact myelin sheath and contain bits of cytoplasm.[35] These components are so highly organized that myelin forms an almost crystalline structure, in which individual components form macromolecular complexes with themselves and each other. Such a structure requires a precise stochiometric relationship of individual components, so that alterations of the amount or structure of one component may result in myelin perturbation.

Mutations in myelin genes

Demyelination can be caused by acquired inflammatory insults or be due to inherited genetic alterations. Mutation, gene duplication or loss of one or both copies of PMP22, P0 and Cx32 genes have been shown to cause dominantly inherited demyelinating neuropathies, such as Charcot–Marie–Tooth (CMT) disease type 1, Dejerine–Sottas syndrome (DSS) and hereditary neuropathy with liability to pressure palsies (HNPP).[36] Since mutations in the same gene cause widely different syndromes, the classification of these diseases has a number of inconsistencies. The availability of animal models of inherited demyelinating neuropathies has helped to pinpoint the role of myelin proteins in demyelinating neuropathies.[37,38] Altered gene dosage resulting in changing protein expression has been shown to be a mechanism leading to demyelination, possibly because myelin stability is dependent on an exact stochiometry of the myelin constituents.[39–42] The study of myelin and inherited demyelinating disorders has converged to a common point, namely the biology of myelin-forming cells. All so far known mutations causing demyelination have turned out to affect genes expressed by myelinating cells, while mutations of neuronal genes have not yet been shown to cause any inherited demyelinating disease. The molecular mechanisms leading to the range of different morphological phenotypes encountered in the demyelinating neuropathies such as onion bulbs, hypomyelinated fibers and widening of myelin lamellae are not yet fully understood with respect to myelin composition. Identification of the genes responsible for several PNS demyelinating diseases gave hope that treatments could be developed. Although the genetic causes of these diseases are now known and their morphology well documented, the biology of the myelin disturbance is still not clear, and there are no therapeutic options possible.

NEUROPATHY ASSOCIATED WITH ANTI-MAG IgM REACTIVITY

Somewhat more than half of the patients with neuropathy with IgM gammopathy have a progressive sensory or sensory motor demyelinating neuropathy and a monoclonal IgM antibody that reacts with MAG.[43] The electrophysiological findings generally indicate a predominantly demyelinating neuropathy, and in 90% of patients the motor peroneal conduction velocity is less than 35 m/s.[44] A characteristic feature of this neuropathy is a marked distal accentuation of conduction slowing, which is consistent with a distally pronounced impairment of predominantly sensory or motor functions.[45]

The epitope, which is targeted by the human antibodies, is also recognized by several mouse monoclonal antibodies, including HNK-1 and L2.[46] The reactive epitope is a carbohydrate part of MAG and is shared with a number of other neural glyco-conjugates, including the major P0 glycoprotein of myelin and PMP22 as well as with SGPG and related glycolipids.[47] Compared to the HNK-1 monoclonal antibody, the human IgM paraproteins have a higher affinity for MAG than for the other myelin glyco-proteins such as P0 and PMP22. The MAG preference is probably due to the relatively low intrinsic affinity of the IgM antibodies for the monovalent oligosaccharide and to cooperative binding of the multimeric IgM with up to eight HNK-1 epitopes per MAG molecule.[48]

The role of the anti-MAG antibodies as a main pathogenic factor in the neuropathy has been confirmed by several studies. Gabriel et al demonstrated by confocal microscopy that IgM antibody deposits were associated with sites of MAG localization, mainly Schmidt–Lanterman incisures and paranodal loops.[49] Nerve biopsies from these patients usually show severe loss of myelinated fibers and sometimes axonal damage.[50] Deposits of monoclonal IgM on the myelin sheaths and ultrastructural alterations consisting of a widening of myelin lamellae in peripheral nerve are characteristic features of the neuropathy with anti-MAG monoclonal IgM antibody.[51] A widening of myelin lamellae is observed in more than 90% of patients with neuropathies associated with anti-MAG IgM antibodies.

Myelin widening is attributed to direct binding of IgM protein to the myelin membrane with resulting permeability effects or with changes in adhesion properties of MAG, leading eventually to abnormal myelin spacing. In a recent study,[52] we found a good correlation between the penetration and localization of IgM in myelinated fibers and the myelin widening, suggesting that deposition of IgM between the myelin membranes is associated with a typical modification of myelin observed at the ultrastructural level. In addition, the massive accumulation of IgM deposits at the node of Ranvier may represent a major mechanism leading to paranodal demyelination.

IgM deposition of anti-MAG antibodies has also been observed in the periphery of myelinated fibers associated with basal lamina.[53] The binding of anti-MAG IgM autoantibody to the basal lamina of myelin-forming Schwann cells suggests that they are interacting with HNK-1-like components of the basement membrane. These non-MAG HNK-1-containing epitopes may be expressed by fibronectin, L1, J1, tenascin,[54] some integrins[55] or sulfoglucuronyl[56] and chondroitin sulfate proteoglycans.[57] The identity of these antigenic epitopes

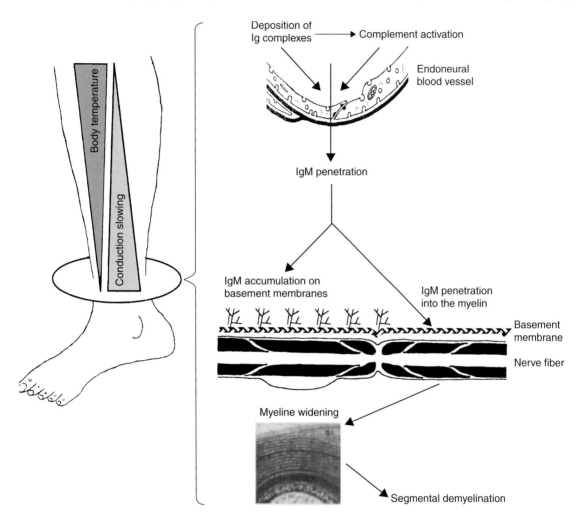

Figure 37.1 Pathogenesis of neuropathy associated with anti-MAG IgM reactivity. Electrophysiologically, there is a distal accentuation of conduction slowing in the anti-MAG polyneuropathy, suggesting a length-dependent neuropathic process that begins distally. This phenomenon may result from increased antibody binding at lower temperatures, since it is not unusual for anti-MAG IgM to also have cryoglobulinemic activity. The presence of terminal complement complex (TCC) in blood vessel walls suggests that TCC may initiate the penetration of IgM. Endothelial fenestrations have been observed in previous studies and may explain abnormal vascular permeability. IgM deposits are found on the basement membrane, and these sites may represent early targets for the uptake of antibody at the surface of myelinated fibers. Major areas of IgM deposits on the myelin sheaths are localized to regions of non-compact myelin, i.e. Schmidt–Lantermann incisures and paranodal loops. The IgM deposits in myelin are proportional to the myelin widening, suggesting that the IgM induces the separation of the myelin leaflets by blocking or interfering with the adhesion properties of MAG or other HNK-1-containing glycoconjugates.

associated with monoclonal anti-MAG IgM needs further investigation. These molecules, particularly on the basement membrane, recognized by anti-MAG monoclonal IgM may represent early targets (early antigens) for the uptake of antibody at the surface of myelinated fibers. Interestingly, the IgM penetration pattern into myelinated fibers was not correlated with the IgM anti-MAG titer[52], suggesting that other variables, such as affinity or other physicochemical properties of the antibody, are playing an important role.

Terminal complement complex (TCC) was not detectable in myelinated fibers in our study,[52] suggesting that it has already disappeared or that it may not be involved in the penetration of IgM through the basement membrane of myelinating Schwann cells. We do not rule out the possibility that other complement components (C3d or C5a) may contribute with IgM to the myelin damage. Indeed, other pathological studies have suggested a role for complement with deposits of C3d and TCC on myelin.[58,59] However, we found the presence of TCC only in blood vessel walls, suggesting that TCC may initiate the penetration of IgM from blood vessel into the endoneurial interstitium. Endothelial fenestrations have been observed in previous studies[60] and may explain abnormal vascular permeability and increased endoneural accumulation. The different pathogenetic steps and molecular features of the anti-MAG IgM neuropathy are schematically represented in Figure 37.1. Our findings indicate that the IgM deposits induce the myelin widening and that the widening is proportional to the penetration of IgM into the myelin sheaths. Interestingly, the basement membrane may be an early focus of the autoimmune attack. However, the components of the basement membrane involved in the binding of the anti-MAG IgM antibodies remain to be identified.

TREATMENT OF IgM PARAPROTEINEMIC NEUROPATHY

The rationale for treating IgM paraproteinemic neuropathy is based on the assumption that the paraprotein plays an etiological role in the neuropathy. This evidence is particularly compelling in the cases associated with antibodies directed against MAG. Current treatment strategies include conventional immunosuppressive or immunomodulating regimens such as steroids, intravenous immunoglobulin, plasma exchange, alkylating agents or other chemotherapeutic drugs such as cyclophosphamide or fludarabine. These treatments have produced inconsistent results. Most case series are small, and few randomized control trials have been published. Wilson et al[61] and Nobile-Orazio[4] et al have recently summarized treatment trials of IgM paraproteinemic neuropathy. Though IgM paraprotein concentration in response to therapy is not usually reported in most trials, antibody levels have been found to fall together with the clinical improvement.[62] Usually, a fall of at least 25% in the paraprotein concentration is associated with clinical improvement. Plasma exchange has been reported to lower serum IgM M-protein levels rapidly in these patients, but its effects are transient, because IgM levels rapidly rise to pretreatment levels after the exchanges are suspended.[63] These limitations explain the transient and inconsistent effects of this therapy on the neuropathy.

Combination of cyclophosphamide and plasma exchange has also been shown to be beneficial,[64] but repeated doses of cyclophosphamide may produce an increased risk of secondary malignancies. Because of the potentially severe side-effects, treatments cannot be maintained for prolonged periods of time and there are no data available on long-term effects. New treatments of paraproteinemic neuropathies with reduced side-effects would be desirable. Currently, two novel drugs are under evaluation. Both have shown promising results in small, uncontrolled trials.

Fludarabine, a fluorinated purine analog, has been shown to be efficacious in a wide variety of low-grade lymphoid malignancies.[65] Because of its activity in low-grade B-cell lymphoid malignancies and its favorable side-effect profile, fludarabine is a strong candidate for the treatment of IgM paraproteinemic neuropathy. Sherman et al[66] reported treating 10 patients with IgM paraproteinemic neuropathy with fludarabine. Seven of the eight MAG-positive patients improved clinically, six with a corresponding reduction in IgM titer of over 50%. Conversely, two patients with anti-GM1 antibodies did not improve. Recently, Wilson et al[61] treated four patients with IgM paraproteinemic neuropathy with intravenous pulses of fludarabine. Two of the four patients had antibodies to MAG. In all cases, subjective and objective clinical improvement occurred, associated with a significant fall in the IgM paraprotein concentration in three cases.

Rapid progress in recombinant biotechnology and protein engineering techniques has allowed the design of specific therapeutic strategies, replacing conventional immunosuppression. Rituximab, a new drug for the treatment of B-cell lymphoma, is a chimeric mouse–human monoclonal antibody directed against the CD20 protein.[67] The CD20 antigen is expressed on normal B-lymphocytes and on about 90% of B-lymphocytes derived from non-Hodgkin's lymphoma.[68] Rituximab produces antibody-dependent cell- and complement-mediated cytotoxicity in these cells. Rituximab was shown to reduce peripheral B-lymphocyte counts by about 90% within 3 days in patients with relapsed indolent lymphoma.[68] Counts remained depleted for 6 months and recovered by months 9–12 after four doses of rituximab 375 mg/m[2] once weekly. Rituximab seems to be well tolerated. The most common adverse event is a transient set of flu-like symptoms during the first infusion in approximately 50–80% of patients, generally resolving completely in less than 3 h.[69] In 10% of patients, the flu-like symptoms were accompanied by bronchospasms and/or hypotension.

In a preliminary study, Levine and Pestronk[70] treated five patients with neuropathy and immunoglobulin M antibodies to GM1 ganglioside or MAG by depleting B-cells with rituximab. Within 3–6 months after treatment, all five patients had improved function, significantly increased quantitative strength measurements, and reduced titers of serum autoantibodies. In an ongoing study, Renaud et al[71] have treated six patients with neuropathy and IgM antibodies to MAG with rituximab. Preliminary results show that B-lymphocyte counts were reduced by 90% in all patients and IgM levels were also reduced. Clinically, three patients showed some improvement. Because of its low toxicity profile and unique mechanism of action, rituximab may also be effective in combination with chemotherapy or other immunomodulatory agents in the treatment of B-cell neoplasm.

CHRONIC INFLAMMATORY DEMYELINATING POLYNEUROPATHY

CIDP is an immune-mediated disorder. Nerve biopsies or post-mortem studies have shown infiltration of inflammatory cells and macrophages associated with demyelination of spinal roots and peripheral nerves resembling the acute inflammatory form of Guillain–Barré syndrome. There is a clinical spectrum from acute through subacute to chronic inflammatory demyelinating polyneuropathy.[72] Support for the autoimmune hypothesis comes from the widespread evidence of aberrant immune responses to myelin antigens and the response of most patients to immunosuppressive treatment. Randomized, controlled trials have confirmed the value of oral prednisolone, intravenous immunoglobulin and plasma exchange, but as many as 30%

of patients do not improve with these treatments or may later become treatment resistant.[73]

MATRIX METALLOPROTEINASES IN CIDP

Matrix metalloproteinases (MMPs) are proteolytic enzymes that are involved in the remodeling of the extracellular matrix (ECM) in a variety of physiological and pathological processes.[74] The MMP family consists of at least 20 members. They are categorized into the collagenase, gelatinase, stromelysin and membrane-type subfamilies. Because MMPs can catalyze the degradation of all the protein constituents of the ECM, their activities are kept under tight control. MMPs are regulated in three ways: gene transcription, proenzyme activation and the action of tissue inhibitors of metalloproteinases (TIMPs).[75] Under physiological conditions, MMP activity is tightly controlled: however, excess MMP production and activation is thought to be a key feature of the pathology of many inflammatory diseases.[76]

MMPs are able to degrade subendothelial basement membranes and may therefore act as effector molecules of blood–nerve or blood–brain barrier disruption.[77] MMPs are upregulated in infiltrating immune cells in acute multiple sclerosis (MS) plaques and brain tissue in experimental autoimmune encephalitis.[78,79] Studies have shown that interferon beta (IFN-β) suppresses the production of MMPs in T-lymphocytes and thus downregulates transbasement membrane migration.[80] Consequently, inhibition of MMP activity seems to be one mechanism by which IFN-β down-modulates inflammatory activity. In experimental allergic neuritis (EAN), a model of acute inflammatory demyelinating polyneuropathy, an upregulation of MMPs has been described during the initial phase of the disease, with peak levels coincident with maximum clinical disease activity.[81] The potential consequences of elevated level of MMPs in EAN comprise blood–nerve barrier damage, leukocyte extravasation, enhancement of the release of the proinflammatory cytokine tumor necrosis factor alpha (TNF-α) and direct degradation of the myelin sheaths, though the latter effect is controversial. In a recent study, we quantitated MMPs in nerve biopsies from patients with CIDP and non-systemic vasculitic neuropathy (NSVN) by immunohistochemistry and correlated the expression levels with clinical and electrophysiological findings.[82] We have found that the expression of MMP-2 and MMP-9 is strongly enhanced in CIDP and NSVN. The results of dual-labeling experiments point to T-cells as a predominant source of MMP-2 and MMP-9 in CIDP, with weaker expression by macrophages. In NSVN, however, stromal nerve cells, presumably fibroblasts, showed strong expression of MMP-2. Thrombin is an activator of MMP-2 in stromal cells of blood vessels.[83] Thrombosis, during which thrombin can achieve high local concentrations, is a typical feature of vasculitic neuropathy and may therefore be a factor that leads to the pronounced upregulation of MMP2 observed in NSVN. These results suggest that MMP-2 and MMP-9 may be differentially regulated in CIDP and NSVN. An aspect of our findings raises doubts about the primary role of MMPs in demyelination in inflammatory neuropathies: although expression levels of MMPs were similar in CIDP and NSVN, demyelination is usually not observed in the latter condition.

Hydroxamic-type MMP inhibitors have been shown to attenuate disease symptoms and tissue damage in EAN.[84] Steroids and IFN-β are drugs that suppress the production of MMP-9, which is now considered one of the prominent factors contributing to their beneficial effect in acute and chronic MS respectively.[80] Accordingly, the same mechanism may be responsible for clinical improvement with corticosteroids and IFN-β in NSVN and CIDP. Furthermore, it is conceivable that the direct inhibition of MMP-9 activity by hydroxamic-acid type MMP inhibitors[84] would be more effective in chronic inflammatory neuropathies.

In summary, the aberrant expression of MMPs might be important in neuroinflammatory diseases of the PNS, and thus MMP inhibitors might enable advances to be made in the treatment of these diseases.

TYPE I INTERFERONS IN THE TREATMENT OF CIDP

IFN-β and IFN-α share components of the same receptor and are referred to as type I interferons.[85] In addition to antiviral activity, they have various immunomodulatory effects.[86] IFN-β downregulates MHC class II molecules. It upregulates interleukin-10 (IL-10) expression and inhibits the production of IL-12. Furthermore, IFN-β inhibits T-cell migration across basement membrane in vitro, presumably by decreasing the secretion of matrix-degrading enzymes.[80] All these effects should be beneficial in CIDP. IFN-β has been found, in controlled clinical trials, to have substantial activity in the prevention of relapses in MS.[87] Based on this rationale, a few studies have investigated the effect of interferon type I in CIDP. In an open label prospective study,

Gorson et al[88] treated 16 patients with CIDP with IFN-α for 6 weeks. All patients had failed to improve or had relapsed after treatment with conventional therapy. Assessment included clinical scores and electrodiagnostic studies. IFN-α_{2a} was given at a dosage of 3 million IU three times a week. Nine patients (56%) improved with IFN-α_{2a}, with gains in the mean motor and sensory scores, though mean grip strength and Rankin disability score did not change. In those patients who responded to IFN-α_{2a}, the clinical improvement generally began after several weeks. In a randomized, double-blind crossover study, Hadden et al[89] treated 10 CIDP patients inadequately controlled with current treatment with IFN-β_{1a} at a dosage of 6 million IU three times weekly for 10 weeks. The primary outcome measure was 'clinically important' improvement in three of eight clinical measures. There was no significant difference between IFN-β and placebo with regard to changes in any of the individual clinical measures between the beginning and the end of the treatment. The authors concluded that IFN-β is not efficacious in treatment-resistant CIDP. In a 6-month open label therapeutic trial in patients with CIDP who failed to achieve a prolonged response to conventional therapy, Kuntzer et al[90] administered IFN-β_{1a} at a dosage of 12 million IU three times a week. While there was no overall statistical benefit from therapy with IFN-β_{1a} alone, there was a statistically significant improvement in three of four patients in motor subscores. Combination therapy with IFN-β_{1a} and IVIG may induce a synergistic effect that could be of benefit for some patients.

In summary, based on the observations published so far, IFN-β but also IFN-α may provide an adjunctive therapy for patients who do not respond to first-line therapy. In the absence of further randomized, double-blind studies of IFN-α and IFN-β in patients with CIDP, only individual patients may be considered for this type of therapy.

REFERENCES

1. Barohn RJ, Kissel JT, Warmolts JR, Mendell JR. Chronic inflammatory demyelinating polyradiculoneuropathy. Clinical characteristics, course, and recommendations for diagnostic criteria. *Arch Neurol* 1989; **46**: 878–884.
2. Gorson KC, Allam G, Ropper AH. Chronic inflammatory demyelinating polyneuropathy: clinical features and response to treatment in 67 consecutive patients with and without a monoclonal gammopathy. *Neurology* 1997; **48**: 321–328.
3. Smith IS. The natural history of chronic demyelinating neuropathy associated with benign IgM paraproteinaemia. A clinical and neurophysiological study. *Brain* 1994; **117**: 949–957.

4. Nobile-Orazio E, Meucci N, Baldini L, Di Troia A, Scarlato G. Long-term prognosis of neuropathy associated with anti-MAG IgM M-proteins and its relationship to immune therapies. *Brain* 2000; **123**: 710–717.

5. Katz JS, Saperstein DS, Gronseth G, Amato AA, Barohn RJ. Distal acquired demyelinating symmetric neuropathy. *Neurology* 2000; **54**: 615–620.

6. Miescher GC, Steck AJ. Paraproteinaemic neuropathies. *Baillières Clin Neurol* 1996; **5**: 219–232.

7. Quarles RH, Weiss MD. Autoantibodies associated with peripheral neuropathy. *Muscle Nerve* 1999; **22**: 800–822.

8. Erb S, Ferracin F, Fuhr P et al. A comparison of polyneuropathy attributes between patients with anti-MAG and anti-sulfatide antibodies. *J Neurol* 2000; **247**: 767–772.

9. Yuki N, Ang CW, Koga M et al. Clinical features and response to treatment in Guillain–Barré syndrome associated with antibodies to GM1b ganglioside. *Ann Neurol* 2000; **47**: 314–321.

10. Kornberg AJ, Pestronk A. Chronic motor neuropathies and lower motor neurone syndromes. *Baillières Clin Neurol* 1995; **4**: 427–441.

11. Holloway RG, Feasby TE. To test or not to test? That is the question. *Neurology* 1999; **53**: 1905–1907.

12. Morell P. *Myelin*. New York: Plenum Publishing Corp, 1984.

13. Garbay B, Heape AM, Sargueil F, Cassagne C. Myelin synthesis in the peripheral nervous system. *Prog Neurobiol* 2000; **61**: 267–304.

14. Hudson L. Molecular biology of myelin proteins in the central and peripheral nervous system. *Neuroscientist* 1990; **2**: 483–496.

15. Salzer JL, Pedraza L, Brown M, Struyk A, Afar D, Bell J. Structure and function of the myelin-associated glycoproteins. *Ann NY Acad Sci* 1990; **605**: 302–312.

16. Filbin MT, Walsh FS, Trapp BD, Pizzey JA, Tennekoon GI. Role of myelin P0 protein as a homophilic adhesion molecule. *Nature* 1990; **344**: 871–872.

17. Suter U, Welcher AA, Snipes GJ. Progress in the molecular understanding of hereditary peripheral neuropathies reveals new insights into the biology of the peripheral nervous system. *Trends Neurosci* 1993; **16**: 50–56.

18. Moscarello M. Myelin basic protein, a dynamically changing structure. *Prog Clin Biol Res* 1990; **336**: 25–48.

19. Spiryda LB. Myelin protein zero and membrane adhesion. *J Neurosci Res* 1998; **54**: 137–146.

20. Shapiro L, Doyle JP, Hensley P, Colman DR, Hendrickson WA. Crystal structure of the extracellular domain from P0, the major structural protein of peripheral nerve myelin. *Neuron* 1996; **17**: 435–449.

21. Welcher AA, Suter U, De Leon M, Snipes GJ, Shooter EM. A myelin protein is encoded by the homologue of a growth arrest-specific gene. *Proc Natl Acad Sci USA* 1991; **88**: 7195–7199.

22. Snipes GJ, Suter U, Welcher AA, Shooter EM. Characterization of a novel peripheral nervous system myelin protein (PMP-22/SR13). *J Cell Biol* 1992; **117**: 225–238.

23. Schaeren-Wiemers N, Schaefer C, Valenzuela DM, Yancopoulos GD, Schwab ME. Identification of new oligodendrocyte- and myelin-specific genes by a differential screening approach. *J Neurochem* 1995; **65**: 10–22.

24. Spreyer P, Schaal H, Kuhn G et al. Regeneration-associated high level expression of apolipoprotein D mRNA in endoneurial fibroblasts of peripheral nerve. *EMBO J* 1990; **9**: 2479–2484.

25. Ong WY, He Y, Suresh S, Patel SC. Differential expression of apolipoprotein D and apolipoprotein E in the kainic acid-lesioned rat hippocampus. *Neuroscience* 1997; **79**: 359–367.

26. Schaeren-Wiemers N, van der Bijl P, Schwab ME. The UDP-galactose:ceramide galactosyltransferase: expression pattern in oligodendrocytes and Schwann cells during myelination and substrate preference for hydroxyceramide. *J Neurochem* 1995; **65**: 2267–2278.

27. Bosio A, Binczek E, Stoffel W. Functional breakdown of the lipid bilayer of the myelin membrane in central and peripheral nervous system by disrupted galactocerebroside synthesis. *Proc Natl Acad Sci USA* 1996; **93**: 13280–13285.

28. Coetzee T, Fujita N, Dupree J et al. Myelination in the absence of galactocerebroside and sulfatide: normal structure with abnormal function and regional instability. *Cell* 1996; **86**: 209–219.

29. Dupree JL, Coetzee T, Suzuki K, Popko B. Myelin abnormalities in mice deficient in galactocerebroside and sulfatide. *J Neurocytol* 1998; **27**: 649–659.

30. Dupree JL, Coetzee T, Blight A, Suzuki K, Popko B. Myelin galactolipids are essential for proper node of Ranvier formation in the CNS. *J Neurosci* 1998; **18**: 1642–1649.

31. Schaeren-Wiemers N, Valenzuela DM, Frank M, Schwab ME. Characterization of a rat gene, rMAL, encoding a protein with four hydrophobic domains in central and peripheral myelin. *J Neurosci* 1995; **15**: 5753–5764.

32. Frank M, van der Haar ME, Schaeren-Wiemers N, Schwab ME. rMAL is a glycosphingolipid-associated protein of myelin and apical membranes of epithelial cells in kidney and stomach. *J Neurosci* 1998; **18**: 4901–4913.

33. Frank M. MAL, a proteolipid in glycosphingolipid enriched domains: functional implications in myelin and beyond. *Prog Neurobiol* 2000; **60**: 531–544.

34. Simons K, Ikonen E. Functional rafts in cell membranes. *Nature* 1997; **387**: 569–572.

35. Scherer SS. Nodes, paranodes, and incisures: from form to function. *Ann NY Acad Sci* 1999; **883**: 131–142.

36. Suter U, Snipes GJ. Biology and genetics of hereditary motor and sensory neuropathies. *Annu Rev Neurosci* 1995; **18**: 45–75.

37. Griffiths IR. Myelin mutants: model systems for the study of normal and abnormal myelination. *Bioessays* 1996; **18**: 789–797.

38. Scherer SS. Molecular genetics of demyelination: new wrinkles on an old membrane. *Neuron* 1997; **18**: 13–16.

39. Gabriel JM, Erne B, Pareyson D, Sghirlanzoni A, Taroni F, Steck AJ. Gene dosage effects in hereditary peripheral neuropathy. Expression of peripheral myelin protein 22 in Charcot–Marie–Tooth disease type 1A and hereditary neuropathy with liability to pressure palsies nerve biopsies. *Neurology* 1997; **49**: 1635–1640.

40. Hodes ME, Dlouhy SR. The proteolipid protein gene: double, double, ... and trouble. *Am J Hum Genet* 1996; **59**: 12–15.

41. Magyar JP, Martini R, Ruelicke T et al. Impaired differentiation of Schwann cells in transgenic mice with increased PMP22 gene dosage. *J Neurosci* 1996; **16**: 5351–5360.

42. Sereda M, Griffiths I, Puhlhofer A et al. A transgenic rat model of Charcot-Marie-Tooth disease. *Neuron* 1996; **16**: 1049–1060.

43. Latov N, Hays AP, Sherman WH. Peripheral neuropathy and anti-MAG antibodies. *Crit Rev Neurobiol* 1988; **3**: 301–332.

44. Nobile-Orazio E, Manfredini E, Carpo M et al. Frequency and clinical correlates of anti-neural IgM antibodies in neuropathy associated with IgM monoclonal gammopathy. *Ann Neurol* 1994; **36**: 416–424.

45. Kaku DA, England JD, Sumner AJ. Distal accentuation of conduction slowing in polyneuropathy associated with antibodies to myelin-associated glycoprotein and sulphated glucuronyl paragloboside. *Brain* 1994; **117**: 941–947.

46. Hammer JA, O'Shannessy DJ, De Leon M et al. Immunoreactivity of PMP-22, P0, and other 19 to 28 kDa glycoproteins in peripheral nerve myelin of mammals and fish with HNK1 and related antibodies. *J Neurosci Res* 1993; **35**: 546–558.

47. Snipes GJ, Suter U, Shooter EM. Human peripheral myelin protein-22 carries the L2/HNK-1 carbohydrate adhesion epitope. *J Neurochem* 1993; **61**: 1961–1964.

48. Burger D, Pidoux L, Steck AJ. Identification of the glycosylated sequence of human myelin-associated glycoprotein. *Biochem Biophys Res Commun* 1993; **197**: 457–464.

49. Gabriel JM, Erne B, Miescher GC et al. Selective loss of myelin-associated glycoprotein from myelin correlates with anti-MAG antibody titre in demyelinating paraproteinaemic polyneuropathy. *Brain* 1996; **119**: 775–787.

50. Vital A, Vital C, Julien J et al. Polyneuropathy associated with IgM monoclonal gammopathy. Immunological and pathological study in 31 patients. *Acta Neuropathol* 1989; **79**: 160–7.

51. Ellie E, Vital A, Steck A, Boiron JM, Vital C, Julien J. Neuropathy associated with 'benign' anti-myelin-associated glycoprotein IgM gammopathy: clinical, immunological, neurophysiological, pathological findings and response to treatment in 33 cases. *J Neurol* 1996; **243**: 34–43.

52. Ritz MF, Erne B, Ferracin F, Vital A, Vital C, Steck AJ. Anti-MAG IgM penetration into myelinated fibers correlates with the extent of myelin widening. *Muscle Nerve* 1999; **22**: 1030–1037.

53. Gabriel JM, Erne B, Bernasconi L et al. Confocal microscopic localization of anti-MAG autoantibodies in a patient with peripheral neuropathy initially lacking a detectable IgM gammopathy. *Acta Neuropathol* 1998; **95**: 540–546.

54. Martini R. Expression and functional roles of neural cell surface molecules and extracellular matrix components during development and regeneration of peripheral nerves. *J Neurocytol* 1994; **23**: 1–28.

55. Pesheva P, Horwitz AF, Schachner M. Integrin, the cell surface receptor for fibronectin and laminin, expresses the L2/HNK-1 and L3 carbohydrate structures shared by adhesion molecules. *Neurosci Lett* 1987; **83**: 303–306.

56. Jungalwala FB. Expression and biological functions of sulfoglucuronyl glycolipids (SGGLs) in the nervous system. *Neurochem Res* 1994; **19**: 945–957.

57. Hoffman S, Edelman GM. A proteoglycan with HNK-1 antigenic determinants is a neuron-associated ligand for cytotactin. *Proc Natl Acad Sci USA* 1987; **84**: 2523–2527.

58. Hays AP, Lee SS, Latov N. Immune reactive C3d on the surface of myelin sheaths in neuropathy. *J Neuroimmunol* 1988; **18**: 231–244.

59. Monaco S, Bonetti B, Ferrari S et al. Complement-mediated demyelination in patients with IgM monoclonal gammopathy and polyneuropathy. *N Engl J Med* 1990; **322**: 649–652.

60. Mendell JR, Sahenk Z, Whitaker JN et al. Polyneuropathy and IgM monoclonal gammopathy: studies on the pathogenetic role of anti-myelin-associated glycoprotein antibody. *Ann Neurol* 1985; **17**: 243–254.

61. Wilson HC, Lunn MP, Schey S, Hughes RA. Successful treatment of IgM paraproteinaemic neuropathy with fludarabine. *J Neurol Neurosurg Psychiatry* 1999; **66**: 575–580.

62. Haas DC, Tatum AH. Plasmapheresis alleviates neuropathy accompanying IgM anti-myelin-associated glycoprotein paraproteinemia. *Ann Neurol* 1988; **23**: 394–396.

63. Ernerudh J, Brodtkorb E, Olsson T, Vedeler CA, Nyland H, Berlin G. Peripheral neuropathy and monoclonal IgM with antibody activity against peripheral nerve myelin; effect of plasma exchange. *J Neuroimmunol* 1986; **11**: 171–178.

64. Blume G, Pestronk A, Goodnough LT. Anti-MAG antibody-associated polyneuropathies: improvement following immunotherapy with monthly plasma exchange and IV cyclophosphamide. *Neurology* 1995; **45**: 1577–1580.

65. Keating MJ, O'Brien S, Plunkett W et al. Fludarabine phosphate: a new active agent in hematologic malignancies. *Semin Hematol* 1994; **31**: 28–39.

66. Sherman WH, Osserman EF, Latov N, Olarte MR, Rowland LP. Peripheral neuropathy, plasma cell dyscrasia, and hot blood. *Ann Neurol* 1982; **12**: 319.

67. Reff ME, Carner K, Chambers KS et al. Depletion of B cells in vivo by a chimeric mouse human monoclonal antibody to CD20. *Blood* 1994; **83**: 435–445.

68. Anderson KC, Bates MP, Slaughenhoupt BL, Pinkus GS, Schlossman SF, Nadler LM. Expression of human B cell-associated antigens on leukemias and lymphomas: a model of human B cell differentiation. *Blood* 1984; **63**: 1424–1433.

69. McLaughlin P, Grillo-Lopez AJ, Link BK et al. Rituximab chimeric anti-CD20 monoclonal antibody therapy for relapsed indolent lymphoma: half of patients respond to a four-dose treatment program. *J Clin Oncol* 1998; **16**: 2825–2833.

70. Levine TD, Pestronk A. IgM antibody-related polyneuropathies: B-cell depletion chemotherapy using Rituximab. *Neurology* 1999; **52**: 1701–1704.

71. Renaud S, Gregor M, Fuhr P, Steck AJ, Gratwohl A. Rituximab and anti-MAG-associated polyneuropathy—a pilot study. *J Neurol* 2000; **247**(suppl 3): 65.

72. Hadden RD, Hughes RA. Treatment of immune-mediated inflammatory neuropathies. *Curr Opin Neurol* 1999; **12**: 573–579.

73. Hahn AF, Bolton CF, Zochodne D, Feasby TE. Intravenous immunoglobulin treatment in chronic inflammatory demyelinating polyneuropathy. A double-blind, placebo-controlled, cross-over study. *Brain* 1996; **119**: 1067–1077.

74. Birkedal-Hansen H. Proteolytic remodeling of extracellular matrix. *Curr Opin Cell Biol* 1995; **7**: 728–735.

75. Ries C, Petrides PE. Cytokine regulation of matrix metalloproteinase activity and its regulatory dysfunction in disease. *Biol Chem Hoppe Seyler* 1995; **376**: 345–355.

76. Kieseier BC, Seifert T, Giovannoni G, Hartung HP. Matrix metalloproteinases in inflammatory demyelination: targets for treatment. *Neurology* 1999; **53**: 20–25.

77. Leppert D, Waubant E, Galardy R, Bunnett NW, Hauser SL. T-cell gelatinases mediate basement membrane transmigration in vitro. *J Immunol* 1995; **154**: 4379–4389.

78. Cossins JA, Clements JM, Ford J et al. Enhanced expression of MMP-7 and MMP-9 in demyelinating multiple sclerosis lesions. *Acta Neuropathol (Berl)* 1997; **94**: 590–598.

79. Kieseier BC, Clements JM, Pischel HB et al. Matrix metalloproteinases MMP-9 and MMP-7 are expressed in experimental autoimmune neuritis and the Guillain–Barré syndrome. *Ann Neurol* 1998; **43**: 427–434.

80. Leppert D, Waubant E, Burk MR, Oksenberg JR, Hauser SL. Interferon beta-1b inhibits gelatinase secretion and in vitro migration of human T-cells: a possible mechanism for treatment efficacy in multiple sclerosis. *Ann Neurol* 1996; **40**: 846–852.

81. Hughes PW, Clements G, Gearing J et al. Matrix metalloproteinase expression during experimental autoimmune neuritis. *Brain* 1998; **121**: 481–494.

82. Leppert D, Hughes P, Huber S et al. Matrix metalloproteinase upregulation in chronic inflammatory demyelinating polyneuropathy and nonsystemic vasculitic neuropathy. *Neurology* 1999; **53**: 62–70.

83. Galis ZS, Kranzhofer R, Fenton JW 2nd, Libby P. Thrombin promotes activation of matrix metalloproteinase-2 produced by cultured vascular smooth muscle cells. *Arterioscler Thromb Vasc Biol* 1997; **17**: 483–489.

84. Redford EJ, Smith KJ, Gregson NA et al. A combined inhibitor of matrix metalloproteinase activity and tumour necrosis factor-alpha processing attenuates experimental autoimmune neuritis. *Brain* 1997; **120**: 1895–1905.

85. Hohlfeld R. Biotechnological agents for the immunotherapy of multiple sclerosis. Principles, problems and perspectives. *Brain* 1997; **120**: 865–916.

86. Arnason BG. Interferon beta in multiple sclerosis. *Clin Immunol Immunopathol* 1996; **81**: 1–11.

87. PRISMS (Prevention of Relapses and Disability by Interferon beta-1a Subcutaneously in Multiple Sclerosis) Study Group. Randomised double-blind placebo-controlled study of interferon beta-1a in relapsing/remitting multiple sclerosis. *Lancet* 1998; **352**: 1498–1504.

88. Gorson KC, Ropper AH, Clark BD, Dew RB 3rd, Simovic D, Allam G. Treatment of chronic inflammatory demyelinating polyneuropathy with interferon-alpha 2a. *Neurology* 1998; **50**: 84–87.

89. Hadden RD, Sharrack B, Bensa S, Soudain SE, Hughes RA. Randomized trial of interferon beta-1a in chronic inflammatory demyelinating polyradiculoneuropathy. *Neurology* 1999; **53**: 57–61.

90. Kuntzer T, Radziwill AJ, Lettry-Trouillat R et al. Interferon-beta1a in chronic inflammatory demyelinating polyneuropathy. *Neurology* 1999; **53**: 1364–1365.

38

Radiation damage to peripheral nerves

Alexander Lossos and Ofer Merimsky

INTRODUCTION

Peripheral nerve damage is a rare but important complication of radiation therapy. In most instances, neurotoxicity is not an outcome of inappropriately planned treatment but rather a result of highly efficient modalities with narrow safety margins and imprecise tolerance doses inherent to a range of biological variables. Previous reviews extensively cover the topic and form the basis for this presentation.[1,2]

Ionizing radiation may directly affect the neural tissue or may indirectly compromise its function by damaging supporting cells, the microvasculature or adjacent structures. Since all but olfactory neurons are postmitotic, other elements associated with peripheral nerves, such as Schwann cells, fibroblasts and vascular endothelial and smooth muscle cells, are probably more radiosensitive.[2]

PATHOBIOLOGY AND KINETICS OF RADIATION INJURY IN PERIPHERAL NERVES

The radiation-induced lesion most detrimental to cell survival involves damage to the DNA, resulting in either cell death or, if the cell survives, in repair and recovery to a normal status, or misrepair, which may be subsequently associated with permanent mutations and induction of carcinogenesis. Absorption of the photon energy leads to molecular breaks or release of energetic electrons and secondary energy-attenuated photons, which may interact with other cellular molecules, leading to a chain reaction that produces a variety of short-lived ions and chemically unstable free radicals. Free radicals are extremely unstable and interact nearly instantaneously with neighboring molecules to produce chemically stable lesions. This process can be modified by free radical scavengers or by oxygen, which have opposing effects on the number of stable lesions and on the level of cellular radiosensitivity.[3]

Most normal tissue effects of radiation therapy can be attributed to cell killing, but there are some that cannot. The relevant example is the somnolence that can develop a few hours after cranial irradiation. Other symptoms include the nausea or vomiting that can occur within hours after irradiation of the upper abdomen, the acute edema or erythema that results from radiation-induced acute inflammation and associated vascular leakage, and the fatigability in patients receiving irradiation to a large volume, especially within the abdomen. These are most likely mediated by radiation-induced inflammatory cytokines.[4] Radiation-induced proliferative responses such as gliosis or certain forms of fibrosis could also cause late symptoms unrelated to cell depletion.

The type of the radiation beam is expected to be related to the acute and late side-effects. In other words, particle beams such as neutron, proton and electron beams are achieving their effect by bombardment of cellular molecules (DNA, RNA, proteins), whereas photons usually cause ionization of molecules and generate free radicals. The rate at which a charged particle such as an electron or proton deposits its energy along its track is described as its linear energy transfer (LET). The heavier the particle, the higher its LET. Electrons have a predominantly low LET, protons slightly higher, neutrons higher still, and heavy charged particles the highest LET of clinically used radiation. Neutrons deposit energy in a tissue through collisions with hydrogen nuclei rather than with electrons, as occurs with photon beams. Although neutrons are uncharged, they eject protons from the nucleus, and therefore the cellular injury they produce is through free radicals formed from ion pairs—the same basic mechanism as that for photons. The difference between neutrons and X-rays is that the column of ionization produced by the proton ejected from the nucleus by the neutron is much denser than that produced by an electron

Table 38.1   Peripheral nerve radiation injury grading scale[1]

	Grade I	Grade II	Grade III	Grade IV
Subjective				
Pain	Occasional	Intermittent	Persistent	Refractory to treatment
Paresthesia	Occasional	Intermittent	Persistent	Persistent
Weakness	Mild	Moderate	Severe	Complete paralysis
Function	Full	< 50% decrease	≥ 50% decrease	Complete loss
Objective				
Sensory deficit	Mild	Moderate	Severe	Complete
Motor deficit (MRC grade)	4–5/5	4/5	3/5	0–2/5
Muscle stretch reflexes	Decreased	Decreased/absent	Absent	Absent
Management				
Pain	Occasional non-narcotic	Regular non-narcotic	Narcotic	Invasive
Function		Physical therapy	Physical therapy	Surgical

ejected by a photon. Because of the density of resulting free radicals, neutron irradiation is more likely than X-irradiation to cause irreparable single-hit injury to a double strand of DNA.[5] The clinical significance of high-LET irradiation is increased acute and late toxicity along the particles' course within the tissue. For example, irradiation of the axilla by photons is expected to cause less late toxicity than irradiation of the same target by heavy particles. Hence the damage to peripheral nerves may be more severe with heavy particle beams.

The threshold for radiation-induced damage to peripheral nerves is 10–20 Gy in a single fraction. Other organ systems that respond to irradiation are the upper aerodigestive mucosa, kidney, heart, liver, spinal cord and brain, and skin is probably affected as well. These are deliberately listed as organs with effects related to both radiation damage to microcirculation and connective tissue interstitium, as well as parenchymal cells. When large single doses of irradiation are used, it is difficult to differentiate the impact of indirect vascular injury from the direct effects on parenchymal cells, which are often slow-cycling.[6]

After clinical doses of irradiation, cell death typically occurs only after one or more attempts at mitotic division. It follows that the time to development of most normal tissue injury will depend critically on the turnover time and differentiation kinetics of the involved tissue, reflected in the use of the terms 'acute,' 'subacute,' or 'late' to describe normal tissue effects of irradiation. Such imprecise

terms say little about the underlying pathogenesis of a response but do indicate times of functional inadequacy in an irradiated tissue. The terms are often loosely used to describe the tissues in which such effects are seen, as in 'acute effects tissue,' but this can be misleading because tissues and organs comprise more than one cell type, each with its own turnover rate. Any tissue can therefore express both acute and late symptoms of radiation damage, depending on the cell type that is limiting function at that time. Acute responses to radiation therapy are usually seen in tissues with rapid turnover. such as gastrointestinal mucosa, bone marrow, skin, and oropharyngeal and esophageal mucosa. Since the turnover of cells within the peripheral nervous system is very limited or very slow, acute effects due to radiation are not expected to occur at a high frequency. Certain tissues may display subacute effects several months after irradiation, reflecting failure of a critical cell population with a longer turnover time. Symptoms are generally reversible, although in some instances they may be associated with severe damage and even death. Examples of transient effects are Lhermitte's syndrome after spinal cord irradiation, or somnolence after brain irradiation. Subacute effects occur during the recovery phase in irradiated tissues and before the onset of late effects associated with slowly progressive damage. Late effects of radiation therapy can generally be considered as due to depletion of slowly proliferating 'target' cells with a slow rate of cell loss, e.g. in central oligodendroglia or peripheral

(Schwann cells) nervous tissue. Late demyelination after brain irradiation may be ascribed to loss of oligodendrocytes and subsequently neurons, but coincident with and preceding any neurologic changes, proliferation of astrocytes and microglial cells can be observed, as can vascular lesions with edema, hemorrhage, or inflammatory infiltrates. A cardinal feature of late effects is that they represent the end of an attempted healing process. Therefore, the extent of permanent damage depends on many factors, including the dose and the time since exposure. If severe injury develops early, recovery is often limited. Late effects of this type should be distinguished from 'consequential' late effects due to earlier damage, most often to an overlying acutely responding epithelial surface.[7] An example of consequential late effects due to earlier damage is entrapment of peripheral nerves in tissue fibrosis, e.g. entrapment of the sciatic nerve following irradiation of the thigh to more than 65 Gy or pelvis as adjuvant treatment for soft tissue sarcoma. This should be discriminated, however, from disease recurrence within the irradiated volume, which may be manifested by the same clinical picture. A second mechanism responsible for late damage to nerves is damage to the vascular supply of the nerve.

Blood capillaries and sinusoids, the narrowest and most ubiquitous elements of the vasculature, also appear to be the most radiosensitive parts of the vascular system. This is related to the sensitivity of endothelial cells, which constitute the most important part of their walls. Only some lesions of these vessels are appreciated by light microscopy. Dilatation is common and, when superficially located, can be detected clinically as telangiectasia of skin or mucous membranes, asymmetry with irregularity of the wall, focally prominent endothelial cells, and, rarely, thrombosis. These changes probably occur in many tissues, perhaps all, but have been documented in only a few.

Small arteries (up to 100 μm in external diameter) have a muscular wall, which gives some protection from rupture. These segments may develop necrosis in the delayed phase (e.g. fibrinoid necrosis of arterioles in the brain), but this is not observed often. More common are subendothelial or adventitial fibrosis, hyalinization of the media, and accumulation of lipid-laden macrophages in the intima. Thrombosis may occur with any of these changes.

Vasculitis may occur as a rare, delayed lesion. It is an exception to the general rule that cellular inflammatory exudate is absent or minimal in delayed radiation pathology. The infiltrate is generally lymphocytic, moderate to heavy, and localized in the media, adventitia, and, less frequently, the intima. In the intima, thrombosis may be present. In the acute cases, no generalized vasculitis has developed. Thus, it is believed that this radiation-associated vasculitis is probably focal and self-limited and heals without therapy.[8] The exact mechanism that is responsible for the damage to the vasa nervosum has not been determined, but it is conceivable that narrowing and thrombosis are the pathogenic processes.

CLINICAL SYNDROMES

Radiation-induced peripheral and cranial nerve injury has been conventionally classified according to the latent period from completion of radiotherapy and the clinical course.[2] Acute effects occur during the treatment and mainly consist of self-limited sensory symptoms in the distribution of nervous structures within the field of irradiation. Acute regional pain syndrome noted in up to 3.6% of patients after preoperative radiotherapy for rectal adenocarcinoma[9] and acute neuralgic amyotrophy occasionally reported in the setting of radiotherapy for Hodgkin's disease[10] may also be considered under this category. Early-delayed effects follow radiotherapy by a few weeks to months and are also at least partially reversible. Examples include brachial plexopathy reported in 1–1.4% of breast cancer patients after a latent period of 1.5–12 months (median 4.5)[11,12] and lumbar plexopathy documented in a patient with endocervical carcinoma 4 months after pelvic irradiation.[13] The former presents with hand and forearm paresthesias accompanied in some by mild shoulder pain and a variable degree of arm weakness and atrophy, while the latter case manifested symmetric proximal leg weakness and patellar areflexia with preserved sphincteric and sensory functions. The pathogenesis of acute and early-delayed reactions is not understood. Transient effects on the blood–nerve barrier with increased vascular permeability, electrochemical alterations with deranged saltatory conduction, and an autoimmune phenomenon have been suggested, but not confirmed.[1,2] Segmental slowing of nerve conduction velocity over the thoracic outlet as shown in cases with reversible brachial plexopathy[11] may suggest a possibility of a focal partial demyelination.

Late-delayed effects are the most serious complications of radiotherapy. They develop months to years after the treatment and typically follow a relentlessly progressive course leading to significant morbidity and functional disability. Any portion of the peripheral nervous system may be affected, depending on the field and dose of irradiation.

Brachial plexopathy (BP)

Radiation-induced BP (RBP) appears to be the most commonly reported syndrome of peripheral nerve injury caused by therapeutic irradiation. The disorder typically begins with hand and arm numbness and paresthesias followed by proximal weakness, and examination reveals sensory loss, reflex changes, weakness and atrophy in the distribution of the upper trunk, i.e. roots C5 and C6.[14] Ipsilateral limb lymphedema and cutaneous radiation changes may be present, but Horner's syndrome is rare and pain is not a dominant complaint. Onset is usually insidious but the course is unpredictable. Although preserved functional ability is seen in about 50% of the patients,[15,16] and there are occasional descriptions of spontaneous improvement, particularly of sensory symptoms,[17] many patients become severely disabled after a slowly progressive course over several years,[18] rarely with acute deterioration of motor functions.[19] Involvement of the upper as opposed to the lower trunk is considered by some to be particularly characteristic of RBP because of its longer course through the radiation port in the supraclavicular area and less absorptive protection provided by the clavicle and surrounding tissues with a presumed greater radiation exposure.[14,19,20] This feature, however, is not invariably documented, and others describe lower trunk plexopathy[21] or panplexopathy as a predominant finding.[15,16,18]

RBP may develop after radiotherapy for any tumor involving the neck, shoulder, upper thorax and axilla, but is mostly described in patients with breast or lung cancer and lymphoma, obviously related to their relative prevalence. Implicated radiation ports include supraclavicular, axillary and lower neck regions targeted to the site of original tumor, subclinical disease and lymphatic drainage. The latent period after treatment ranges from 3 months to 26 years,[14] with a median interval of 9 months, 4 years, 6 years and 9 years in four representative series,[14,17,21,22] and with 30–80% of the patients presenting within the first year.[14,17]

Earlier studies reported RBP in 15–70% of patients irradiated for breast cancer, largely depending on the total dose and fractionation schedule.[18,19] Thus, 24/33 patients (73%) treated with 63 Gy in 5.25 Gy fractions and 13/84 patients (15%) treated with 57.75 Gy in 5.25-Gy fractions developed RBP.[19] More recent estimations are based on less aggressive schedules and suggest a frequency of 1–35%.[12,15,16,23] Thus, 28/79 patients (35%) receiving 36.6–39.6 Gy in 3.05-Gy fractions and 19/128 patients (15%) receiving 50 Gy in 2-Gy fractions became neurologically

Table 38.2 Forms of brachial plexopathy in cancer patients
Neoplastic
Radiation-induced
Acute painful reversible form (Hodgkin's disease)[10]
Early-delayed reversible form (breast cancer)[11,12]
Late-delayed progressive form
Ischemic[35]
Peripheral nerve sheath tumors
Lymphedema (breast cancer)[81]
Paraneoplastic (Hodgkin's disease, lung cancer)[81,83]
Perioperative[84]
Chemotherapy
High-dose Ara-C[85]
Intra-arterial cisplatin[86]
Interleukin-2[87]
Unrelated causes

affected.[15,16] The actuarial incidence of RBP among 449 patients at 5.5 years was recently shown to be 1% for 1.8 Gy fractions and 5.9% for 3-Gy fractions using equivalent schedules.[23] As a general conclusion, radiation doses causing unacceptable risk of brachial plexus injury are usually greater than 60 Gy and fractions greater than 2 Gy.[1,16,23] A more accurate estimation can be made by calculating a cumulative radiation effect[24] and by using an isoeffect table of tolerance dosage limits;[25] individual host factors must also be taken into account.[2]

High radiation doses also seem to shorten the latent period[19] and to increase the severity of neurologic deficit,[16,19] but data interpretation is hampered by different treatment schedules, retrospective design, selection bias and often inadequate duration of follow-up. The effects of additional factors on the development of RBP were studied with no unanimously accepted conclusions.[23,26] Simultaneous or sequential administration of chemotherapy, younger age and greater extent of axillary surgery tend to increase the risk of RBP, whereas tumor size, number of infiltrated axillary lymph nodes and a prior early-delayed transient plexopathy do not.[12,15,16]

The pathogenesis of RBP is not well understood. Pathologic examinations, mainly performed for diagnostic purposes or at autopsy, document marked macroscopic fibrosis surrounding the brachial plexus and constricting the nerve bundles and, microscopically, thickened endoneurium, demyelination, axonal loss and hyalinization and obliteration of the blood vessels.[18,19] Which of these changes represents primary radiation-induced pathology and which is a secondary phenomenon remains uncertain, but both connective tissue fibrosis and decreased vascularity may in time destroy peripheral nerves and prevent regeneration of the proximal portions.[27]

The main differential diagnosis is from recurrent tumor involving the plexus. Selected case-comparison series analyzing the distinctive features of both disorders describe RBP in 22–56% of the studied cancer patients with BP.[14,17,18,21,22,28] These figures become higher if only previously irradiated patients are counted but probably do not represent true frequency because of a selection bias. Diagnostic criteria mostly rely on negative surgical exploration or biopsy and on an observation period of 2 years or more without evidence of metastatic disease. Patients irradiated for non-cancer causes or because of incorrect diagnosis are also sometimes included.[14,18] It is of note that the local plexus lesion may be the only site of tumor recurrence for a prolonged period, while radiation osteonecrosis may be interpreted as metastatic involvement.[14] Furthermore, patients with distant metastases may develop RBP, or metastasis may complicate established RBP[20] and may be associated with epidural spinal and radicular extension.[14]

The most important single clinical clue is pain.[2] Prominent early and persistent pain is an indicator of tumor infiltration, while late reappearance of pain in previously stable RBP suggests a recurrence.[20] Horner's syndrome and lower plexus deficit also suggest a metastasis, whereas relatively painless upper trunk plexopathy and panplexopathy are more consistent with RBP. Arm lymphedema, radiation skin changes, radiation pneumonitis and mediastinitis are probably of no diagnostic value and must be considered in accord with other findings.

The need for diagnostic certainty always requires auxiliary evaluation. In comparison to plain X-ray and bone scan, CT was the first useful diagnostic technique to define imaging findings in RBP with the aim of distinction from tumor infiltration. Ipsilateral diffuse loss of normal soft tissue planes in the region of the brachial plexus is seen in 44–80% of the patients with RBP, whereas associated bony erosion or soft tissue mass, either local, paravertebral or epidural, is typical for metastatic plexopathy.[28,29] MRI has several advantages over CT with respect to the brachial plexus imaging, but still yields incorrect diagnoses in 29% of patients with RBP.[23] A mass in or near the brachial plexus, displacement of adjacent structures, lymphadenopathy and bone lesions indicate tumor infiltration and their absence in the appropriate clinical setting suggests RBP. Contrast enhancement, T2 signal intensity changes and loss of soft tissue planes represent non-specific changes.[22,30,31] Newer MRI techniques[32] and [18]FDG-PET[33] will probably aid in difficult cases. Detailed electrophysiologic testing is helpful in delineating the site of nerve damage but cannot definitely distinguish RBP from tumor infiltration.[12,22,28,34] Common findings include reduced amplitude of CMAP and SNAP, prolonged or absent F-waves, conduction block across the brachial plexus and neurogenic pattern MUPs on needle EMG, i.e. large-amplitude, long-duration polyphasic MUPs, fibrillation and fasciculation potentials. However, only myokymic discharges, if found, are more characteristic of RBP.[28] In conclusion, the distinction from neoplastic BP may be difficult and must rely on the combination of clinical and laboratory findings. Diagnostic surgical exploration or biopsy may be considered when indicated by inconclusive results.[27] Otherwise, close follow-up with repeat evaluation is advocated.[22]

Less common causes of radiation-related brachial plexus dysfunction include post-irradiation peripheral nerve sheath tumors and a distinct form of acute painless BP due to radiation-induced large-vessel occlusion.[35]

Treatment of RBP remains disappointing. Splinting the arm to prevent shoulder joint subluxation, lymphedema-reducing measures, adequate pain control and intensive physical and occupational therapy are the mainstays of RBP management.[27,36] Therapeutic surgical exploration with neurolysis and pedicled omentoplasty, angiolysis and local muscle release is occasionally performed, with the aim of reducing the pain and halting the ongoing functional deterioration.[2,18,23] Results are uncertain and the procedure requires considerable surgical skill and intraoperative neurophysiologic monitoring to prevent possible complications.[37–39]

Lumbosacral plexopathy (LSP)

Radiation-induced LSP (RLSP) is less common than RBP. A recent frequency estimate in a large-scale study of gynecologic tumors was less than 1%.[40] Both prophylactic and therapeutic external-beam irradiation for various abdominal and pelvic neoplasms may cause RLSP when a portal includes the cauda equina or the lumbosacral plexus.[41] Addition of intracavitary implants, as for gynecologic malignancies, concomitant chemotherapy and a pre-existing neurologic deficit may be contributing factors.[9,42]

Table 38.3 Forms of lumbosacral plexopathy/radiculopathy in cancer patients

Neoplastic
Radiation-induced
Acute painful reversible form (adenocarcinoma of rectum)[9]
Early-delayed reversible form (carcinoma of cervix)[13]
Late-delayed progressive form
Peripheral nerve sheath tumors
Sacral osteoradionecrosis[56]
Perioperative[84]
Intra-arterial chemotherapy[44]
Unrelated causes

Implicated midplane doses range from 30 to 62 Gy,[41] and the total calculated dose to the plexus is about 57–70 Gy.[40,42]

Typically, the disorder starts insidiously with leg weakness, numbness and paresthesias several months to 31 years (median, 5 years) after the treatment,[41] although rare cases with acute, painful and early onset have been described,[42] especially with preoperative daily irradiation fractions of 5.0–5.1 Gy for rectal adenocarcinoma.[9] Slow progression and, finally, stabilization with a variable degree of functional disability characterize the following course. Pain is uncommon at the initial presentation but may develop later. Examination reveals asymmetric or symmetric lower motor neuron deficit in the L2–S1 or L5–S1 distribution associated with sensory loss but sparing sphincteric functions. Instances of urinary incontinence may be related to radiation-induced proctitis or bladder fibrosis,[41] and, on rare occasions, fecal incontinence has been ascribed to RLSP in patients with cervical cancer.[43] In contrast to RLSP, early and prominent pain, unilateral neurologic deficit, sphincter dysfunction and a rapid progression characterize tumor-related LSP.[41,44]

Diagnosis in a previously irradiated patient relies on the exclusion of local pelvic or retroperitoneal tumor mass, plexus infiltration, bone erosion, lymphadenopathy, spinal epidural extension or leptomeningeal involvement by the appropriate neuroimaging and cerebrospinal fluid (CSF) studies, and requires prolonged clinical follow-up. Myelography, CT and, more recently, MRI have been effective in the setting of cancer-related LSP,[44,45] but have not been systematically studied in RLSP. Electro-physiologic testing is helpful in delineating the site of nerve damage but yields no diagnosis-specific findings, except for myokymic discharges observed in up to 57% of RLSP cases.[41,46] Elevated CSF protein is present in some patients.[41] Surgical exploration or biopsy may be indicated by inconclusive results.[2,41]

As in RBP, the pathogenesis of RLSP is probably related to local fibrosis and vascular changes.[2,47,48] On the basis of target volume planning, and clinical, electrophysiologic and pathologic findings, involvement of the lumbosacral plexus and its nerves[40,48] as well as of the intraspinal and extraspinal portions of the motor and sensory caudal nerve roots,[41,49,50] has been suggested to underlie the neurologic deficit. In addition, injury to the anterior horn cells in the lower spinal cord was suspected after irradiation to the inguinal, iliac and para-aortic lymph nodes for testicular tumors exposing the spinal canal to the level of T11.[49,51] These cases with a predominantly lower motor neuron syndrome and only subtle sensory and sphincteric abnormalities have been variously termed 'post-irradiation lumbosacral myelopathy' or 'motor neuronopathy'.[49,51] More recent works favor 'radiculoplexopathy'[35] or 'radiculopathy'[44,46] to indicate the caudal nerve roots as the site of radiation damage leading to fibrosis, axonal loss and microvasculopathy. Both RLSP and post-irradiation lumbosacral radiculopathy probably represent a spectrum of radiation injury to the lumbosacral region in relation to several radiotherapy variables or to other as yet unknown factors.

No specific treatment is available for RLSP. Pain control and rehabilitation provide symptomatic relief and improve functional ability. Steroids have been ineffective in isolated cases,[49,53] and therapeutic surgical exploration with neurolysis has been only occasionally mentioned.[41,48] A recent beneficial trial of intravenous immunoglobulin in a 70-year-old patient with RLSP 5 years after 45-Gy external irradiation for endometrial carcinoma[54] raises the possibility of an immune-mediated mechanism or represents a diagnostic artifact. Modestly successful low-intensity anticoagulation with heparin and warfarin in two patients with RLSP after treatment for colon adenocarcinoma merits further evaluation considering the possible role for radiation-induced vasculopathy.[55] Hyperbaric oxygen therapy may be considered in osteoradionecrosis-related sacral plexopathy.[56]

Cranial nerve injury

Any cranial nerve within the irradiation field may be damaged by a sufficient dose of radiotherapy.

Anosmia, ageusia, xerophthalmia and xerostomia may develop during or early after the treatment, but do not constitute a neuropathy in a clinically strict sense and are related to the olfactory neuron taste bud and secretory cell dysfunction.[2] Serous otitis media due to eustachian tube dysfunction is the cause of early conductive hearing loss, whereas late-delayed sensorineural hearing loss results from damage to the organ of Corti with secondary acoustic nerve atrophy.[57] It may develop in up to 35% of patients 1–5 years after external radiotherapy for nasopharyngeal carcinoma.[58]

Visual loss related to the anterior visual pathway may be caused by radiation-induced optic neuropathy (RON), glaucoma, cataract or retinopathy.[2] Anterior RON complicates brachytherapy for uveal melanoma, whereas retrobulbar or posterior RON occurs after whole brain radiotherapy and after irradiation of the skull base, orbit, pituitary gland, cavernous sinuses, paranasal sinuses and nasopharynx.[59] The latent period ranges from 0.5 to 4 years and is inversely related to radiation dose. Being extensions of the central nervous system, anterior visual pathways are more sensitive to irradiation than the other cranial nerves, with an approximate tolerance of 55 Gy total dose and 2 Gy per fraction.[60] RON may also follow stereotactic radiosurgery in more than 20% of patients treated for skull base tumors after a single exposure to more than 8–10 Gy.[59] Detailed neurophthalmologic testing, visual evoked responses and MRI confirm the diagnosis; treatment with steroids might be helpful, and hyperbaric oxygen therapy seems promising.[59]

Ocular motor, trigeminal and facial nerves are rarely involved by conventional fractionated radiotherapy[61] and are more vulnerable to stereotactic radiosurgery. Trigeminal nerve exposure to more than 19 Gy after skull base meningioma radiosurgery[62] and facial nerve exposure to more than 18 Gy with acoustic schwannoma radiosurgery[63] significantly increase the risk of injury being manifested within a few months after the treatment. Important considerations include pre-existing nerve damage and the length of an exposed nerve segment. Ocular neuromyotonia is a rare disorder, with spontaneous ocular misalignment leading to episodic diplopia that occurs after radiotherapy to the sellar and parasellar regions.[64] It probably reflects impaired muscle relaxation due to inappropriate ocular motor nerve discharges and responds well to carbamazepine. A similar disorder involves facial and trigeminal nerves or lower cranial nerves, and is manifested by episodic involuntary contrac-

tions in the lower facial and masseter muscles,[65] or by a slowly progressive bulbar palsy.[65] EMG shows complex repetitive discharges, myokymia and neuromyotonia.

Intra- and extracranial portions of the lower cranial nerves may be affected by radiotherapy to the upper chest, neck, oral cavity and tonsillar region, with hypoglossal nerve injury being the commonest.[61,67] Doses greater than 60 Gy are usually used to treat head and neck tumors, but unilateral hypoglossal nerve palsy has been noted in only 1/400 irradiated patients.[68] The latent period ranges from 1 to 14 years and is inversely related to the radiation dose. MRI demonstrates denervated muscle changes in the distribution of the affected nerve.[69]

Intraoperative irradiation

Intraoperative radiotherapy (IORT) involves a large single-dose irradiation at the time of surgical exploration and is used in conjunction with chemotherapy and postoperative external radiotherapy to treat tumors with high risk for local recurrence.[70] Peripheral neuropathy is the dose-limiting toxicity of IORT. It develops in 30% of the patients 6–18 months after the treatment and involves nerves within the IORT field.[71] A single dose of 20 Gy is considered a maximum tolerable dose for peripheral nerve injury but additional factors may enhance its toxic effect.[71] Experimental animal studies of lumbosacral and sciatic nerve IORT-induced injury demonstrate loss of large myelinated fibers, endoneural fibrosis, and endo- and epineural vessel thickening[70] as well as small-vessel necrosis, hyalinization, thrombosis and hemorrhage.[70] Schwann cells and vasa nervosum have been implicated in the development of the observed changes.[73]

Radiation-induced tumors

Radiogenic tumors of the peripheral and cranial nerves are infrequent, but are an important consideration after therapeutic irradiation at conventional doses,[74] stereotactic radiotherapy,[75] or low-grade cranial irradiation (1.5 Gy) for tinea capitis in old age.[76] Increased risk of second primaries in cancer patients and genetic predisposition, such as in neurofibromatosis, are contributing factors.[74] Malignant peripheral nerve sheath tumors (MPNSTs) are the main histologic variant,[77] although atypical neurofibroma[74] and benign schwannoma[20,76,78] are also encountered. Non-neural sheath post-irradiation sarcoma may also involve neural structures.[22]

Radiogenic MPNSTs constitute about 5% of all post-irradiation sarcomas[77] and 10% of all MPNSTs.[79] Any previously irradiated site may be involved, but cervicobrachial and lumbosacral plexuses and retroperitoneal locations are the commonest. Painful mass lesion accompanied by progressive neurologic deficit is the characteristic initial manifestation.[74] Diagnosis requires demonstration of an in-field tumor that develops several years after the initial radiotherapy and that is of a different histological type from the original neoplasm.[2] Neuroimaging using MRI and possibly PET usually identifies the lesion,[22,77,80] but surgical excision is essential for tissue diagnosis and treatment.

REFERENCES

1. Gillette EL, Mahler PA, Powers BE, Gillette SM, Vujaskovic Z. Late radiation injury to muscle and peripheral nerves. *Int J Radiat Oncol Biol Phys* 1995; **31**: 1309–1318.

2. Posner JB. Side effects of radiation therapy. In: Posner JB, ed. *Neurologic Complications of Cancer*. Philadelphia: FA Davis Company, 1995: 311–337.

3. Ward JF. The yield of DNA double-strand breaks produced intracellularly by ionizing radiation: a review. *Int J Radiat Biol* 1990; **57**: 1141.

4. Hong J, Chiang C, Campbell IL et al. Induction of acute phase gene expression by brain irradiation. *Int J Radiat Oncol Biol Phys* 1996; **33**: 619.

5. Carlos A, Perez CA, Brady LW, Roti Roti JL. Overview. In: Perez CA, Brady LW, eds. *Principles and Practice of Radiation Oncology*, 3rd edn. Philadelphia: Lippincott-Raven, 1997: 1–78.

6. Philip Rubin P, Constine LS, Williams JP. Late effects of cancer treatment: radiation and drug toxicity. In: Perez CA, Brady LW, eds. *Principles and Practice of Radiation Oncology*, 3rd edn. Philadelphia: Lippincott-Raven, 1997: 155–211.

7. Withers HR, McBride WH. Biologic basis of radiation therapy. In: Perez CA, Brady LW, eds. *Principles and Practice of Radiation Oncology*, 3rd edn. Philadelphia: Lippincott-Raven, 1997: 79–118.

8. Luis Felipe Fajardo L-G. Morphology of radiation effects on normal tissues. In: Perez CA, Brady LW, eds. *Principles and Practice of Radiation Oncology*, 3rd edn. Philadelphia: Lippincott-Raven, 1997: 143–154.

9. Frykholm GJ, Sintorn K, Montelius A et al. Acute lumbosacral plexopathy during and after preoperative radiotherapy of rectal adenocarcinoma. *Radiother Oncol* 1996; **38**: 121–130.

10. Malow BA, Dawson DM. Neuralgic amyotrophy in association with radiation therapy for Hodgkin's disease. *Neurology* 1991; **41**: 440–441.

11. Salner AL, Botnick LE, Herzog AG et al. Reversible brachial plexopathy following primary radiation therapy for breast cancer. *Cancer Treat Rep* 1981; **65**: 797–802.

12. Pierce SM, Recht A, Lingos TI et al. Long-term complications following conservative surgery (CS) and radiation therapy (RT) in patients with early stage breast cancer. *Int J Radiat Oncol Biol Phys* 1992; **23**: 915–923.

13. Enevoldson TP, Scadding JW, Rustin GJS, Senanayake LFN. Spontaneous resolution of a postirradiation lumbosacral plexopathy. *Neurology* 1992; **42**: 2224–2225.

14. Kori SH, Foley KM, Posner JB. Brachial plexus lesions in patients with cancer: 100 cases. *Neurology* 1981; **31**: 45–50.

15. Olsen NK, Pfeiffer P, Mondrup K, Rose C. Radiation-induced brachial plexus neuropathy in breast cancer patients. *Acta Oncol* 1990; **29**: 885–890.

16. Olsen NK, Pfeiffer P, Johannsen L, Schroder H, Rose C. Radiation-induced brachial plexopathy: neurological follow-up in 161 recurrence-free breast cancer patients. *Int J Radiat Oncol Biol Phys* 1993; **26**: 43–49.

17. Bagley FH, Walsh JW, Cady B et al. Carcinomatous versus radiation-induced brachial plexus neuropathy in breast cancer. *Cancer* 1978; **41**: 2154–2157.

18. Thomas JE, Colby MY. Radiation-induced or metastatic brachial plexopathy? A diagnostic dilemma. *JAMA* 1972; **222**: 1392–1395.

19. Stoll BA, Andrews JT. Radiation-induced peripheral neuropathy. *BMJ* 1966; **1**: 834–837.

20. Brennan MJ. Breast cancer recurrence in a patient with a previous history of radiation injury of the brachial plexus: a case report. *Arch Phys Med Rehabil* 1995; **76**: 974–976.

21. Lederman RJ, Wilbourn AJ. Brachial plexopathy: recurrent cancer or radiation? *Neurology* 1984; **34**: 1331–1335.

22. Thyagarajan D, Cascino T, Harms G. Magnetic resonance imaging in brachial plexopathy of cancer. *Neurology* 1995; **45**: 421–427.

23. Powell S, Cooke J, Parsons C. Radiation-induced brachial plexus injury: follow-up of two different fractionation schedules. *Radiother Oncol* 1990; **18**: 213–220.

24. Svensson H, Westling P, Larsson L-G. Radiation-induced lesions of the brachial plexus correlated to the dose–time–fraction schedule. *Acta Radiol Ther Phys Biol* 1975; **14**: 228–238.

25. Cohen L, Svensson H. Cell population kinetics and dose–time relationships for post-irradiation injury of the brachial plexus in man. *Acta Radiol Oncol* 1978; **17**: 161–166.

26. Hardenbergh PH, Recht A, Gollamudi S et al. Treatment-related toxicity from a randomized trial of the sequencing of doxorubicin and radiation therapy in patients treated for early stage breast cancer. *Int J Radiat Oncol Biol Phys* 1999; **45**: 69–72.

27. Cherny NI, Foley KM. Brachial plexopathy in patients with breast cancer. In: Harris JR, Lippman ME, Morrow M, Hellman S, eds. *Diseases of the Breast*. Philadelphia: Lippincott-Raven, 1996: 797–808.

28. Harper CM, Thomas JE, Cascino TL, Litchy WJ. Distinction between neoplastic and radiation-induced brachial plexopathy, with emphasis on the role of EMG. *Neurology* 1989; **39**: 502–506.

29. Cascino TL, Kori S, Krol G, Foley KM. CT of the brachial plexus in patients with cancer. *Neurology* 1983; **33**: 1553–1557.

30. Wouter van Es H, Engelen AM, Witkamp TD, Ramos LMP, Feldberg MAM. Radiation-induced brachial plexopathy: MR imaging. *Skelet Radiol* 1997; **26**: 284–288.

31. Bowen BC, Verma A, Brandon AH, Fiedler JA. Radiation-induced brachial plexopathy: MR and clinical findings. *Am J Neuroradiol* 1996; **17**: 1932–1936.

32. Qayyum A, MacVicar AD, Padhani AR, Revell P, Husband JES. Symptomatic brachial plexopathy follow-

ing treatment for breast cancer: utility of MR imaging with surface-coil techniques. *Radiology* 2000; **214**: 837–842.

33. Ahmad A, Barrington S, Maisey M, Rubens RD. Use of positron emission tomography in evaluation of brachial plexopathy in breast cancer patients. *Br J Cancer* 1999; **79**: 478–482.

34. Mondrup K, Olsen NK, Pfeiffer P, Rose C. Clinical and electrodiagnostic findings in breast cancer patients with radiation-induced brachial plexus neuropathy. *Acta Neurol Scand* 1990; **81**: 153–158.

35. Gerard JM, Franck N, Moussa Z, Hildebrand J. Acute ischemic brachial plexus neuropathy following radiation therapy. *Neurology* 1989; **39**: 450–451.

36. Cooper J. Occupational therapy intervention with radiation-induced brachial plexopathy. *Eur J Cancer Care* 1998; **7**: 88–92.

37. Match RM. Radiation-induced brachial plexus paralysis. *Arch Surg* 1975; **110**: 384–386.

38. Killer HE, Hess K. Natural history of radiation-induced brachial plexopathy compared with surgically treated patients. *J Neurol* 1990; **237**: 247–250.

39. LeQuang C. Postirradiation lesions of the brachial plexus. Results of surgical treatment. *Hand Clin* 1989; **5**: 23–32.

40. Georgiou A, Grigsby PW, Perez CA. Radiation induced lumbosacral plexopathy in gynecologic tumors: clinical findings and dosimetric analysis. *Int J Radiat Oncol Biol Phys* 1993; **26**: 479–482.

41. Thomas JE, Cascino TL, Earle JD. Differential diagnosis between radiation and tumor plexopathy of the pelvis. *Neurology* 1985; **35**: 1–7.

42. Abu-Rustum NR, Rajbhandari D, Glusman S, Massad LS. Acute lower extremity paralysis following radiation therapy for cervical cancer. *Gynecol Oncol* 1999; **75**: 152–154.

43. Iglicki F, Coffin B, Ille O et al. Fecal incontinence after pelvic radiotherapy: evidence for a lumbosacral plexopathy. Report of a case. *Dis Colon Rectum* 1996; **39**: 465–467.

44. Pettigrew LC, Glass JP, Maor M, Zornoza J. Diagnosis and treatment of lumbosacral plexopathies in patients with cancer. *Arch Neurol* 1984; **41**: 1282–1285.

45. Taylor BV, Kimmel DW, Krecke KN, Cascino TL. Magnetic resonance imaging in cancer-related lumbosacral plexopathy. *Mayo Clin Proc* 1997; **72**: 823–829.

46. Aho K, Sainio K. Late irradiation-induced lesions of the lumbosacral plexus. *Neurology* 1983; **33**: 953–955.

47. Ashenhurst EM, Quartey GRC, Starreveld A. Lumbosacral radiculopathy induced by radiation. *Can J Neurol Sci* 1977; **4**: 259–263.

48. Mendes DG, Nawalkar RR, Eldar S. Post-irradiation femoral neuropathy. *J Bone Joint Surg* 1991; **73-A**: 137–140.

49. Berlit P, Schwechheimer K. Neuropathological findings in radiation myelopathy of the lumbosacral cord. *Eur Neurol* 1987; **27**: 29–34.

50. Feistner H, Weissenborn K, Munte TF, Heinze H-J, Malin JP. Post-irradiation lesions of the caudal roots. *Acta Neurol Scand* 1989; **80**: 277–281.

51. Maier JG, Perry RH, Saylor W, Sulak MH. Radiation myelitis of the dorsolumbar spinal cord. *Radiology* 1969; **93**: 153–160.

52. Bowen J, Gregory R, Squier M, Donaghy M. The post-irradiation lower motor neuron syndrome. Neuronopathy or radiculopathy? *Brain* 1996; **119**: 1429–1439.

53. Kristensen O, Melgard B, Schiodt A. Radiation myelopathy of the lumbo-sacral spinal cord. *Acta Neurol Scand* 1977; **56**: 217–222.

54. Morovati A, Engel WK. Postirradiation delayed progressive lumbosacral plexopathy responsive to intravenous immunoglobulin treatment: a dysimmune mechanism may sometimes be involved. *Ann Neurol* 1998; **44**: 478 (abstr).

55. Glantz MJ, Burger PC, Friedman AH et al. Treatment of radiation-induced nervous system injury with heparin and warfarin. *Neurology* 1994; **44**: 2020–2027.

56. Videtic GM, Venkatesan VM. Hyperbaric oxygen corrects sacral plexopathy due to osteoradionecrosis appearing 15 years after pelvic irradiation. *Clin Oncol* 1999; **11**: 198–199.

57. Grau C, Overgaard J. Postirradiation sensorineural hearing loss: a common but ignored late radiation complication. *Int J Radiat Oncol Biol Phys* 1996; **36**: 515–517.

58. Kwong DLW, Wei WI, Sham JST et al. Sensorineural hearing loss in patients treated for nasopharyngeal carcinoma: a prospective study of the effect of radiation and cisplatin treatment. *Int J Radiat Oncol Biol Phys* 1996; **36**: 281–289.

59. Leber KA, Bergloff J, Pendl G. Dose–response tolerance of the visual pathways and cranial nerves of the cavernous sinus to stereotactic radiosurgery. *J Neurosurg* 1998; **88**: 43–50.

60. Tachibana O, Yamaguchi N, Yamashima T, Yamashima J. Radiation necrosis of the optic chiasm, optic tract, hypothalamus, and upper pons after radiotherapy for pituitary adenoma, detected by gadolinium-enhanced, T1-weighted magnetic resonance imaging: case report. *Neurosurgery* 1990; **27**: 640–643.

61. Berger PS, Bataini JP. Radiation-induced cranial nerve palsy. *Cancer* 1977; **40**: 152–155.

62. Morita A, Coffey RJ, Foote RL, Schiff D, Gorman D. Risk of injury to cranial nerves after gamma knife radiosurgery for skull base meningiomas: experience in 88 patients. *J Neurosurg* 1999; **90**: 42–49.

63. Miller RC, Foote RL, Coffey RJ et al. Decrease in cranial nerve complications after radiosurgery for acoustic neuromas: a prospective study of dose and volume. *Int J Radiat Oncol Biol Phys* 1999; **43**: 305–311.

64. Frohman EM, Zee DS. Ocular neuromyotonia: clinical features, physiological mechanisms, and response to therapy. *Ann Neurol* 1995; **37**: 620–626.

65. Marti-Fabregas J, Montero J, Lopez-Villegas D, Quer M. Post-irradiation neuromyotonia in bilateral facial and trigeminal nerve distribution. *Neurology* 1997; **48**: 1107–1109.

66. Shapiro BE, Rordorf G, Schwamm L, Preston DC. Delayed radiation-induced bulbar palsy. *Neurology* 1996; **46**: 1604–1606.

67. Cheng VST, Schultz MD. Unilateral hypoglossal nerve atrophy as a late complication of radiation therapy of head and neck carcinoma: a report of four cases and a review of the literature on peripheral and cranial nerve damage after radiation therapy. *Cancer* 1975; **35**: 1537–1544.

68. Takimoto T, Saito Y, Suzuki M, Nishimura T. Radiation-induced cranial nerve palsy: hypoglossal nerve and vocal cord palsies. *J Laryngol Otolaryngol* 1991; **105**: 44–45.

69. King AD, Ahuja A, Leung SF et al. MR features of the denervated tongue in radiation induced neuropathy. *Br J Radiol* 1999; **72**: 349–353.

70. Kinsella TJ, Sindelar WF, DeLuca AM et al. Tolerance of peripheral nerve to intraoperative radiotherapy (IORT): clinical and experimental studies. *Int J Radiat Oncol Biol Phys* 1985; **11**: 1579–1585.

71. Vujaskovic Z, Powers BE, Paardekoper G et al. Effects of intraoperative irradiation (IORT) and intraoperative hyperthermia (IOHT) on canine sciatic nerve: histopathologic and morphometric studies. *Int J Radiat Oncol Biol Phys* 1999; **43**: 1103–1109.

72. LeCouter RA, Gillette EL, Powers BE et al. Peripheral neuropathies following experimental intraoperative radiation therapy (IORT). *Int J Radiat Oncol Biol Phys* 1989; **17**: 583–590.

73. Vujaskovic Z, Gillette SM, Powers BE et al. Intraoperative radiation (IORT) injury to sciatic nerve in a large animal model. *Radiother Oncol* 1994; **30**: 133–139.

74. Foley KM, Woodruff JM, Ellis FT, Posner JB. Radiation-induced malignant and atypical peripheral nerve sheath tumors. *Ann Neurol* 1980; **7**: 311–318.

75. Glass J, Silverman CL, Corn B, Hoenig E, Andrews DW. Possible early emergence of in-field second neoplasms following cranial irradiation, chemotherapy, and stereotactic irradiation: report of two cases. *J Radiosurg* 1998; **1**: 59–62.

76. Ron E, Modan B, Boice JD et al. Tumors of the brain and nervous tissue after radiotherapy in childhood. *N Engl J Med* 1988; **319**: 1033–1039.

77. Hussussian CJ, Mackinnon SE. Postirradiation neural sheath sarcoma of the brachial plexus: a case report. *Ann Plast Surg* 1999; **43**: 313–317.

78. Rubinstein AB, Reichenthal E, Borohov H. Radiation-induced schwannomas. *Neurosurgery* 1989; **24**: 929–932.

79. Woodruff JM, Kourea HP, Louis DN, Scheithauer BW. Malignant peripheral nerve sheath tumors (MPNST). In: Kleihues P, Cavenee WK, eds. *Pathology and Genetics. Tumors of the Nervous System.* Lyon: IARC Press, 2000: 172–174.

80. Maravilla KR, Bowen BC. Imaging of the peripheral nervous system: evaluation of peripheral neuropathy and plexopathy. *AJNR Am J Neuroradiol* 1998; **19**: 1011–1023.

81. Ganel A, Engel J, Sela M, Brooks M. Nerve entrapments associated with postmastectomy lymphedema. *Cancer* 1979; **44**: 2254–2259.

82. Lachance DH, O'Neill BP, Harper CM, Banks PM, Cascino TL. Paraneoplastic brachial plexopathy in a patient with Hodgkin's disease. *Mayo Clin Proc* 1991; **66**: 97–101.

83. Meador KJ, Richards B, Hunter S, Nichols FT, Watson RT. Bibrachial palsy due to paraneoplastic encephalomyelitis. *South Med J* 1989; **82**: 1053–1055.

84. Warner MA. Perioperative neuropathies. *Mayo Clin Proc* 1998; **73**: 567–574.

85. Scherokman B, Filling-Katz MR, Tell D. Brachial plexus neuropathy following high-dose cytarabine in acute monoblastic leukemia. *Cancer Treat Rep* 1985; **69**: 1005–1006.

86. Kahn CE, Messersmith RN, Samuels BL. Brachial plexopathy as a complication of intraarterial cisplatin chemotherapy. *Cardiovasc Intervent Radiol* 1989; **12**: 47–49.

87. Loh FL, Herskovitz S, Berger AR, Swerdlow ML. Brachial plexopathy associated with interleukin-2 therapy. *Neurology* 1992; **42**: 462–463.

39

Neuropathy due to malignant hematological diseases

Austin J Sumner

CHRONIC LYMPHOCYTIC LEUKEMIA

The chronic lymphocytic leukemias are hematological malignancies characterized by the proliferation of small, immunologically mature lymphoid cells. In more than 90% of the cases, these are B-cell in origin and are classified as B-cell chronic lymphatic leukemia (B-CLL). Other types include prolymphocytic leukemia, large granular lymphocytic leukemia, hairy cell leukemia, and the leukemic phase of lymphoma.

B-CLL in the USA has an average annual incidence of 2.7 cases per 100 000 population. The male to female ratio is approximately 2 : 1, and the usual age of onset is between 55 and 60 years. The diagnosis is usually made incidental to a routine blood screen, and confirmed by the laboratory finding of monoclonal B-cells in the setting of peripheral lymphocytosis. Prognosis is related to clinical staging at the time of diagnosis. Rai stage 0 correlates with a median survival of more than 10 years, Rai stage 2 or 3 a median survival of 7 years, and Rai stages 3 and 4 a median survival of less than 4 years.

The incidence of neurological complications associated with this disorder was recently reviewed by Mayo Clinic physicians.[1] The medical records of 962 patients met diagnostic criteria, and 109 (11.3%) had related neurological diagnoses. Idiopathic peripheral neuropathies and cerebral ischemic events were specifically excluded as specific complications because of the difficulties in proving a relationship. This study shows that the overall incidence of neurological complications in B-CLL is low, and non-zoster complications are rare within 6 years of the diagnosis (see Table 39.1).

A relationship between CLL and idiopathic polyneuropathy remains unclear, as a recent case report illustrates.[2] A 65-year-old man with CLL

Table 39.1   Incidence of neurologic complications in chronic lymphoid leukemia.

Herpes zoster infections (69 cases, 7.2%)	
Limited dermatomes	59
Cutaneous disseminated	6
Meningoencephalitis	2
Lumbosacral polyradiculopathy	2
Other opportunistic infections (17 cases, 1.8%)	
PML	5
Cryptococcal meningitis	4
Pneumococcal meningitis	3
Indeterminate CNS disease	3
Candida meningitis	1
Aspergillosis brain emboli	1
Treatment-related conditions (14 cases, 1.5%)	
Vincristine-induced neuropathy	10
Steroid myopathy	3
Steroid psychosis	1
Direct leukemic involvement of neural structures (8 cases, 0.8%)	
Intracranial hemorrhage (9 cases, 0.1%)	

CNS, central nervous system; PML, progressive multifocal leukoencephalopathy.

slowly developed progressive paresthesias and muscle weakness over the 2 years prior to his diagnosis with B-CLL. Examination confirmed the clinical findings of sensorimotor polyneuropathy: he was areflexic but had Babinski's sign bilaterally. Electrophysiological findings were absent sensory potentials, and slowed motor conduction velocities (MCVs) with low compound motor actions potential (CMAP) amplitudes (left median 33 m/s, 2.6 mV; right median 38 m/s, 1.8 mV; left posterior tibial 22 m/s, 0.4 mV, and right posterior tibial 35 m/s, 1.0 mV). In addition, there were temporal dispersion and prolonged terminal latencies, all consistent with a demyelinating polyneuropathy. A monoclonal paraprotein could not be detected, but serum IgM levels were elevated. ELISA assay confirmed that the serum had high titers of IgM antibody activity against GD1a, GT1b, and GQ1 band GD3, but not against other glycolipid antigens. Immunohistochemical studies showed IgM deposition in the sural nerve by direct immunofluorescence, and binding of the patient's serum IgM to normal nerve by indirect immunofluorescence. Another factor was the high serum and CSF antibody titers to HTLV-1. This case raises more questions than it answers. What was the relationship between the B-CLL and the monoclonal IgM? Is the IgM pathogenic with respect to the polyneuropathy and was this mediated via glycoprotein antigens? It seems likely that the patient also had HTLV-1-associated myelopathy (HAM). Did the HTLV-1 activate B-cell function? Finally, did the HTLV-1 play a more direct role in the pathogenesis of the polyneuropathy?

CHRONIC MYELOID LEUKEMIA

Perineurial and fascicular infiltrations of leukemia cells into the peripheral nerve is a rarely reported complication of CML.

LYMPHOMA

Direct infiltration of peripheral nerves can occur even when lymphoma is in hematological remission.[3] A 52-year-old patient with diffuse non-cleaved small cell, non-Hodgkin's lymphoma had been treated with extensive chemotherapy and was free of discernible disease when she developed diplopia and bilateral lower extremity weakness. She had a progressive mononeuritis multiplex which at autopsy was associated with lymphomatous infiltration of the femoral nerves and infiltrates in the right cerebral peduncle. There was no evidence of nerve root or meningeal infiltration, and nor was there evidence of lymphoma outside the nervous system.

Intraneural lymphoma infiltration tends to occur in three particular settings: (1) metastases to nerve in the setting of widespread systemic and neuraxis metastases; (2) focal nerve infiltration as the predominant or sole site of involvement with systemic spread; and, as in this case, (3) with isolated nerve lesions in a setting of system disease in hematological remission.

OSTEOSCLEROTIC MYELOMA

Osteosclerotic myeloma is a rare plasma cell dyscrasia accounting for less than 3% of myeloma cases. Fully one-half of these cases are associated with a demyelinating polyneuropathy. POEMS syndrome (polyneuropathy, organomegaly, endocrinopathy, monoclonal gammopathy and skin changes) is present in a proportion of these cases. Improvement in the polyneuropathy has been shown following surgery or irradiation of solitary bone lesions.[4–6] Responses in patients with multiple lesions have been less encouraging, but some patients have responded to systemic chemotherapy. Rotta and Bradley[7] reported a patient with severe polyneuropathy associated with multifocal osteosclerotic myeloma who improved remarkably following combined surgical, radiation and chemotherapy treatment. The 41-year-old man presented with 3 years of progressive weakness and numbness. Electrophysiological studies revealed a demyelinating polyneuropathy (e.g. median MCV 35.2 m/s) with secondary axonal degeneration. Cerebrospinal fluid (CSF) protein was 300 mg/dl. The patient was treated for chronic inflammatory demyelinating polyneuropathy (CIDP) with prednisone 60 mg daily and azathioprine 50 mg t.i.d., with modest response. Intravenous immunoglobin (IVIg) 0.8 g/kg per day for 5 days produced good but temporary improvement and, despite continued periodic treatments, the patient continued to deteriorate, until 2½ years later he was wheelchair-bound and unable to feed himself because of upper extremity weakness. After hospital admission for a pathological fracture, bone survey showed lytic lesions with sclerotic borders in the right humerus, and right coracoid and first lumbar vertebrae. Excisional biopsy showed neoplastic plasma cell proliferation. Serum electrophoresis and immunofixation showed a monoclonal IgG lambda paraprotein. Treatment at this time consisted of plasmapheresis, IVIg, focal irradiation of the bony lesions and chemotherapy with chlorambucil 3 mg per os q.d., danzol 200 mg per os t.i.d. and hydrocortisone 20 mg per os q.d. Thereafter, he made a steady improvement with only mild residual findings of polyneuropathy after two years. Aggressive local irradiation and systemic chemotherapy is indicated in patients with solitary plasmacytomas or multiple osteosclerotic lesions. Adjunctive immunosuppressive therapies like plasma exchange and IVIg may also be beneficial in these cases.

POLYCYTHEMIA VERA

Frank polyneuropathy is a rare complication of polycythemia vera. Paresthesias of the extremities are, however, a frequent symptom and have been reported as occurring in 10–20% of patients.

WALDENSTROM MACROGLOBULINEMIA

Uncontrolled proliferation of lymphocytes and plasma cells in this disorder results in IgM monoclonal protein production. A sensorimotor polyneuropathy commonly occurs which has similar characteristics to that associated with monoclonal gammopathy of unknown significance (MGUS). The systemic disease is characterized by weakness, fatigue, oronasal bleeding, anemia, hepatosplenomegaly and neurological symptoms of visual, auditory, cerebral and spinal origin. Serum protein electrophoresis is characterized by a prominent, tall, narrow peak within the gamma-globulin region. The paraprotein is IgM kappa light chain in 75% of cases and it is also found in the urine in most cases.

POLYNEUROPATHIES WITH MONOCLONAL GAMMOPATHIES

The polyneuropathies associated with monoclonal gammopathies exhibit heterogeneous clinical, electrophysiological and pathological features. Within this group, however, there is a chronic demyelinating polyneuropathy associated with IgM antibodies which appears to be a relatively specific entity. In these cases, monoclonal IgM antibodies react with a carbohydrate epitope shared by peripheral nerve glycoproteins, including myelin-associated glycoprotein (MAG), and two sulfated glycuronyl-containing glycosphingolipids, sulfated glucuronyl paragloboside (SGPG) and sulfated glucuronyl lactosaminyl paragloboside. This subgroup (anti-MAG/SGPG polyneuropathy) accounts for approximately one-half of IgM-associated polyneuropathies, which in turn, account for about 70% of polyneuropathies associated with monoclonal gammopathy. Clinical deficits in patients with anti-MAG/SGPG polyneuropathy evolve slowly in a distal, symmetrical fiber-length-dependent pattern. Initial symptoms are predominantly sensory, but distal weakness and atrophy are usually evident on examination. Tremor can be a prominent late feature. Uniform nerve conduction slowing with predictable distal accentuation has been described as a useful electrodiagnostic feature.[8] A quantitative relationship between proximal and distal conduction can be calculated by using a terminal latency index (TLI).[9] These electrophysiological features indicate a generalized fiber-length-dependent demyelination and axonal degeneration consistent with a disorder of axon–myelin interaction. Myelin-associated glycoprotein has been localized to specialized regions of the myelin sheath, the peripheral axonal membrane, inner and outer mesaxons, and Schmidt–Lantermann incisures. In areas of uncompacted myelin, MAG probably acts as a membrane spacer and as an adhesion molecule with axolemma in the periaxonal space, as suggested by its homology to the immunoglobulin supergene family.

REFERENCES

1. Bower JH, Hammack JE, McDonnell SK, Tefferi A. The neurologic complications of B-cell chronic lymphocytic leukemia. *Neurology* 1997; **48**: 407–412.
2. Mitsui Y, Kusunoki S, Hiruma S et al. Sensorimotor polyneuropathy associated with chronic lymphocytic leukemia, IgM antigangliosides antibody and human T-cell leukemia virus I infection. *Muscle Nerve* 1999; **22**(10): 1461–1465.
3. Walk D, Handelsman A, Beckmann E, Kozloff M, Shapiro C. Mononeuropathy multiplex due to infiltration of lymphoma in hematologic remission. *Muscle Nerve* 1998; **21**(6): 823–826.
4. Kelly JJ, Kyle RA, Miles JM, Dyck PJ. Osteosclerotic myeloma and peripheral neuropathy. *Neurology* 1983; **33**: 202–210.
5. Nakanishi T, Sobue I, Toyokura Y et al. The Crow–Fukase syndrome: a study of 102 cases in Japan. *Neurology* 1984; **34**: 712–720.
6. Soubrier MJ, Dubost JJ, Sauvezie BJM, the French Study Group on POEMS Syndrome. POEMS syndrome: a study of 25 cases and review of literature. *Am J Med* 1994; **97**: 543–553.
7. Rotta FT, Bradley WG. Marked improvement of severe polyneuropathy associated with multifocal osteosclerotic myeloma following surgery, radiation, and chemotherapy. *Muscle Nerve* 1997; **20**(8): 1035–1037.
8. Kaku DA, England JD, Sumner AJ. Distal accentuation of conduction showing in polyneuropathy associated with antibodies to myelin-associated glycoprotein and sulphated glucuronyl paraglobosicle. *Brain* 1994; **117**: 941–7.
9. Shahani BT, Young RR, Potts F, Maccabee P. Terminal latency index (TLI) and late response studies in motor neuron disease (MND), peripheral neuropathies and entrapment syndromes. *Acta Neurol* 1979; **73**: 118.

40

Hereditary inclusion body myopathies: clinical and genetic features

Zohar Argov

The term inclusion body myositis (IBM) was introduced three decades ago to describe an adult-onset, acquired (sporadic) inflammatory myopathy with two unique histological features:[1] cytoplasmic 'rimmed' vacuoles containing whorls of cytomembranes, and typical cytoplasmic and nuclear inclusions. Electron microscopy (EM) shows that these inclusions are composed of clusters of tubular filaments with a diameter of 14–18 nm. The vacuoles are not membrane bound, for the term rimmed refers to the extra basophilic stain around many of these vacuoles on hematoxylin and eosin staining. During the same period, a group of hereditary myopathies, each with its unique clinical features and ethnic cluster, was described. The histological and ultrastructural picture in these diverse myopathies is very reminiscent of sporadic IBM, with one clear exception: the absence of inflammation.[1] This heterogeneous group is now called hereditary inclusion body myopathy (HIBM).

The clinical–histological criteria shown in Table 40.1 are essential to diagnose an HIBM syndrome in a family.[2] Although features like facial weakness, joint contractures and ophthalmoplegia have been reported

in HIBM, the limb muscles are those that show the main involvement. The age of onset may vary, but in order to separate HIBM from the late adult-onset sporadic IBM, which might be familial,[3] I have set this age criterion. In some cases of sporadic IBM, inflammation is not detected by the first biopsy, and thus in a single family the diagnosis of HIBM requires more than one patient. However, a typical clinical syndrome in a single patient belonging to a known ethnic cluster suffices. Still, the most important criterion separating HIBM from familial, inflammatory IBM (which mimics Mendelian inheritance) is the lack of inflammation. The histological criteria have not been quantified, but think that at least three fibers in a medium-magnitude field should show vacuoles. The absence of other major structural changes is required because a few rimmed vacuoles may appear in many myopathies, associated with other pathological abnormalities. In some disorders, 'dystrophic' changes (necrosis, regeneration and fibrosis) may be seen in association with the rimmed vacuoles. The cytoplasmic or nuclear inclusions are sometimes hard to find. Whether lack of inclusions excludes this diagnosis is unclear. There are several hereditary myopathies with rimmed vacuoles without the typical inclusions and without other features. In some, EM was not done, and in others a thorough search for the inclusions was performed. Since the filaments are so typical, I suggest that HIBM should only be defined when they are present. The hereditary rimmed vacuole myopathies without filaments will be mentioned here too, as these may be 'possible' HIBM.

CLINICAL SYNDROMES OF HIBM

Currently, the classification of HIBM still relies on the clinical picture and clinical genetics. I will describe the various phenotypes associated with HIBM or 'possible' HIBM (Table 40.2).

Table 40.1   Diagnostic criteria for hereditary inclusion body myopathies

Primarily limb muscle weakness

Onset in teenage or early adulthood

At least two affected members in the same family

Numerous rimmed vacuoles, without other structural changes

No inflammation in affected muscle biopsy

Detection of 14–18-nm filamentous inclusions by electron microscopy

HIBM1 (dominant forms)

A. At least six families have been reported.[4,5] In all of them, patients have adult-onset (4th or 5th decade) proximal and distal muscle weakness, either in the upper or in the lower limbs. The quadriceps is affected. Serum creatine kinase (CK) is normal or mildly elevated. Brain magnetic resonance imaging (MRI) was not reported.

B. A single French-Canadian family, with a fascioscapulohumeral dystrophy-like HIBM starting distally in hand muscles at early childhood in the mother and proximally in the legs in her two adolescent boys, has been reported.[6] Facial weakness appeared early and was severe. Brain MRI was normal.

C. A single large Swedish family with proximal muscle weakness affecting primarily the pectoral and quadriceps muscles and with various degrees of external ophthalmoplegia has been reported.[7] Congenital joint contracture is the first sign, although this abnormality improves with time. In several patients, the onset of weakness could be traced to early childhood, but it seemed non-progressive. Further deterioration was noted at adulthood (after age 30).

D. Several disorders with adult-onset distal muscular weakness with rimmed vacuoles are prevalent in Scandinavia. The most common is Welander distal myopathy. Onset is in the hands during adulthood.[8] The Finnish tibial muscular dystrophy has distal onset, but in the legs.[9]

E. A large kindred with rimmed vacuole neuromyopathy was described from Italy. Onset was variable, from the teenage years to the early 6th decade of life with distal weakness in the legs. Progression was associated with spreading to the proximal musculature and bulbar muscles.[10]

F. A distal myopathy of late onset (around age 60) with early involvement in the posterior leg and thigh muscles was identified in a French family.[11]

Some of these dominantly inherited distal myopathies may be related to HIBM, sharing common pathophysiological processes. However, most represent what I call 'possible' HIBM.

HIBM2 (recessive)

A. Quadriceps-sparing myopathy (QSM) is a very unique neuromuscular disorder, starting in young adulthood and slowly progressing to affect all lower limb muscles but not the quadriceps. This muscle remains very strong even in old, wheelchair-bound patients.[12,13] This disorder was first described in Iranian Jews; currently I am aware of at least 120 patients belonging to 40 families of Iranian (Persian) Jewish descent with this disorder. This translates to an estimated prevalence of about 1 : 1500 in this community.[14] QSM type of HIBM exists not only in Iranian Jews. It was also diagnosed in five families of Afghani and two families of Iraqi Jewish origin.[15,16] At least eight non-Jewish families have been reported: two from India,[4,16] two Caucasian from the USA,[4,17] two from Mexico[18] and two from Denmark (Vissing, personal communication). Since this is the prototype of HIBM-1, I will describe the clinical and laboratory features in more detail.

Age at onset
This varies widely, even within the same family, being as early as 17 and as late as 48 years of age. The mean age at onset in our patients is around 30 years.

Mode of onset
Practically all my patients noted the first symptoms of weakness in their legs, most commonly in the foot extensors. In many patients, however, this was associated with hip flexor weakness, leading to difficulties in climbing stairs as well as frequent stumbling.

Weakness distribution
Although weakness at onset may be limited to the peroneal muscles and the hip flexors, the most common pattern in an established case is symmetrical, marked weakness of similar degree (usually 3/5 or less on the Medical Research Council (MRC) scale) of the hip flexors (iliopsoas), extensors (the glutei group) and knee flexors (hamstrings). The foot extensors are usually very weak or paralyzed at this stage, with the foot flexors (gastrocnemius–soleus) being either similarly involved or at times only partly affected. The hip extensors (quadriceps) are unaffected even at very advanced stages of the disease (age above 70 in two patients). In the upper limbs, involvement is usually initially limited to the scapular muscles. This pattern of scapular involvement with peroneal weakness led to the descriptive diagnosis of scapuloperoneal syndrome in some patients. Distal hand muscles also become involved, but in the later stages. Tendon reflexes may be absent in the Achilles, and subjective distal sensory impairment is sometimes reported.

Progression and prognosis
As patients were examined at various stages of their disease, it is hard to draw conclusions. QSM in Iranian Jews is a very slowly progressive neuromuscular disorder. Seven patients are in their 7th decade of life, and two are over 70 years of age. Most of the

patients still walk outdoors after 15–20 years of disease. Many of the patients in their fifties can still walk on flat, level terrain short distances, and only the very old patients with about 40 years of disease history are bedridden. Death related to complications of diffuse muscle weakness was reported in only three of our patients.

Other features

None of my patients had signs of central nervous system disease. Brain MRI in three patients did not show white matter disease. Even my two older patients had no evidence of dementia or other central nervous system (CNS) abnormal signs on clinical testing. ECG was normal.

Muscle CT

In 12 patients, this confirmed the lack of involvement of the quadriceps muscle. In very advanced stages, however, only the vastus lateralis is truly spared. Computer tomography (CT) of the calf muscles demonstrates that the soleus is much more affected than the gastrocnemius. Paraspinal and anterior abdominal muscles are clearly affected too.

Creatine kinase

In most patients, the serum levels of CK were only mildly elevated (about twice the upper limit of control values). In a few (<15%), they were normal. Only one patient had CK activity greater than 4 times the upper control value.

Electrophysiology

Nerve conduction studies (motor and sensory) are normal even in patients with sensory complaints and reduced tendon reflexes. Conventional concentric needle EMG shows spontaneous activity (abundant fibrillations and positive sharp waves and, at times, bizarre high-fequency discharges) in the tibialis anterior of most tested patients. Spontaneous activity is rare in other muscles. In most tested muscles, many units are small and polyphasic. However, reduced recruitment with prolonged, large or even polyphasic units is also recorded in a few affected muscles. Thus, the EMG picture can be interpreted as a mixture of 'neurogenic' and 'myopathic' patterns. Quantitative EMG studies showed a reduction in the size and duration of motor unit action potentials, more pronounced in the severely affected muscles. In the most affected tibialis anterior muscle, the turns/amplitude analysis also suggested an increase in polyphasia and small amplitude. Single-fiber EMG showed only a mild increase of fiber density. These electrophysiological observations led to the conclusion that this disorder is primary myopathic.

Histology

The most informative muscles are either the tibialis anterior in the leg or the biceps in the upper limb. The number of fibers with vacuoles varies from very few in lower-magnification fields to 20% of the total. In many fibers, a few, usually small, basophilic-rimmed vacuoles are seen, while in a few fibers a large single vacuole may occupy the center of the fiber. Many vacuoles contain concentric structures reminiscent of 'autophagic' vacuoles; however, the vacuoles are not membrane-bound, and the term 'autophagic' may be incorrect in HIBM. Only occasional fibers undergoing necrosis may be seen, and fibrosis is not an early feature. Amyloid deposits are rare in HIBM, unlike sporadic IBM. Muscle EM shows the typical inclusions composed of filamentous structures mainly in the cytoplasm. Nuclear filaments are harder to detect.

B. We followed several patients of three Egyptian Jewish families with QSM and typical HIBM pathology, where clear, mild–moderate facial weakness is seen.[19] Facial muscle involvement was not detected in any of my Middle Eastern Jewish patients with HIBM belonging to other ethnic communities.

C. Many patients of several Japanese families with adult-onset, rimmed-vacuole distal myopathy (DMRV), who have all of the typical histological features of HIBM, have been reported.[20] The main difference from QSM is the weakness distribution and its progression. Onset is in the middle of the third decade with preferential involvement of the anterior tibial (peroneal) muscles. Loss of ambulation occurs about 12 years later, probably because the quadriceps becomes involved within 5–10 years of onset in DMRV. There is no involvement of the brain or heart.

D. Several families in which patients with HIBM-like myopathy had white matter abnormalities on brain MRI (usually without clinical features of CNS disease) have been reported. Such families have been described among French-Canadians[21] and among Arabs from Tunisia,[22] only the latter showing a QSM pattern. The family from Canada had weakness onset in early childhood with delayed motor milestones. There is very slow progression over the years, with the patients still walking in their 4th decade. There are no detailed clinical reports of the Tunisian patients.

E. A small consanguineous Japanese family had two siblings with oculopharyngodistal myopathy and all the histological features of HIBM. The clinical picture is different from DMRV (and from oculo-pharyngeal muscular dystrophy).[23]

We have received sketchy reports of families with a scapuloperoneal syndrome and rimmed vacuoles that may be defined as HIBM. This is not surprising, as it was the mode of presentation in two families of Iranian Jewish decent.[12]

GENETIC LINKAGE STUDIES IN HIBM (Table 40.2)

The first report of genetic linkage of HIBM came in 1996, mapping the Iranian Jewish cluster to the 10-cM region on chromosome 9p1–1.[24] The disease interval has now been further narrowed to a 0.5-cM region. Some of the microsatellite markers (e.g. D9S1791) show a strong linkage disequilibrium with the disease site.[25] It has also been shown that the same genetic location is involved in the HIBM appearing in other Jewish communities, such as Afghani, Iraqi and Egyptian.[16] These findings are consistent with the migration currents and the strong historical ties between the Persian Jewish

community and Babylonian and Egyptian Jewry which go back at least 2000 years.[14]

QSM diagnosed in a non-Jewish family originating from East India has also been mapped to the same chromosomal locus.[16] Furthermore, the same chromosomal location has been reported for the distal myopathy (DMRV) diagnosed in Japanese patients (HIBM2C).[26] The Tunisian Arab disorder is probably also linked (Hentati, personal communication).[27] It seems that the recessive HIBM forms in the different communities are allelic variations. On the other hand, linkage studies have allowed the exclusion of the 9p1–q1 locus in the recessive disease described in the French-Canadian family with brain MRI abnormalities.[16] Thus, not all recessive forms of HIBM map to chromosome 9p1.

Some of the dominant disorders have been mapped. Both the Welander and the tibial muscular dystrophy are now linked to different sites on chromosome 2.[28,29] A family of the form described as HIBM1A (Denver family) was briefly reported to have linkage to a site on chromosome 8.[30] The HIBM1C reported from Sweden has been mapped to chromosome 17p13.1.[31] The Italian family (HIBM1E) is linked to chromosome 19p13.[10] In the disorder called limb girdle muscular dystrophy type 2G, which is linked to chromosome 17q11–12,[32] many fibers contain rimmed vacuoles, but dystrophic changes are also abundant (another 'possible' HIBM).

Table 40.2 Gene location by linkage analysis of various forms of HIBM	
Dominant	
HIBM1A	Chromosome 8
HIBM1B	Unknown
HIBM1C	Chromosome 17p13.1
HIBM1D	Chromosome 2p13 (Welander)
(possible HIBM)	Chromosome 2q (Finnish tibial muscular dystrophy)
HIBM1E	Chromosome 19p13
HIBM1F	Unknown
Recessive	
HIBM2A	Chromosome 9p1
HIBM2B	Chromosome 9p1–q1
HIBM2C	Chromosome 9p1–q1
HIBM2D	Chromosome 9p1–q1 (Tunisians)
	Unknown (French-Canadians)
HIBM2E	Unknown
HIBM2F	Unknown

The various designated names follow the classification of other disorders, like limb girdle muscular dystrophies, where 1 is dominant and 2 is recessive. The letters are arbitrary.

DISCUSSION

The eventual identification of the gene responsible for HIBM in Persian Jews may also have an impact on the other forms of HIBM as described above. Defects in different genes encoding proteins belonging to the same 'functional family' may lead to similar myopathological alterations (as in the case of membrane sarcoglycan complex), resulting in the unique form of cell death in various HIBM types. The ultimate characterization of the HIBM gene(s) may also give some insights into the pathogenesis of the similar structural abnormalities of the more common sporadic IBM. It should be noted that cellular abnormalities in IBM, both sporadic and hereditary, have many features common to degenerative brain diseases.[33] The similarity in structure of the IBM tubofilaments and the neurofibrillary tangles and the precipitation of amyloid and tau protein are the more obvious of these.[33] It may be speculated that the muscle cell degeneration in IBM goes through a similar cascade of events as the neurons in Alzheimer and other brain diseases. Should this hypothesis be confirmed, understanding HIBM may have much wider implications.

ACKNOWLEDGEMENT

Professor Argov's research in hereditary neuro-muscular diseases in Jews is supported by a special donation in memory of Nataly Hollo-Bencze.

REFERENCES

1. Criggs RC, Askanas V, DiMauro S et al. Inclusion body myositis and myopathies. *Ann Neurol* 1995; **38**: 705–715.
2. Argov Z, Sadeh M. Recessively-inherited inclusion body myopathies: clinical and laboratory features. *Acta Myol* 1998; **1**: 41–44.
3. Rider LG, Gurley RC, Pandey JP et al. Clinical, serologic, and immunogenetic features of familial idiopathic inflammatory myopathy. *Arthritis Rheum* 1998; **41**: 710–719.
4. Sivakumar K, Dalakas MC. The spectrum of familial inclusion body myopathies in 13 families and a description of a quadriceps-sparing phenotype in non-Iranian Jews. *Neurology* 1996; **47**: 977–984.
5. Neville HE, Baumbach LL, Ringel SP, Russo LS, Sujansky E, Garcia CA. Familial inclusion body myositis: evidence for autosomal dominant inheritance. *Neurology* 1992; **42**: 897–902.
6. McKee D, Karpati G, Johnson W, Carpenter S. Familial inclusion body myositis (IBM) mimics fascioscapulo-humeral dystrophy (FSHD). *Neurology* 1992; **42**(suppl): A302 (abst).
7. Oldfors A, Darin N, Wahlstrom J, Kylleman M. Early onset autosomal dominant myopathy with external ophthalmoplegia and rimmed vacuoles in muscle fibers. *Acta Myol* 1997; **1**: 35 (abst).
8. Borg K, Ahlberg G, Borg J, Edstrom L. Welander's distal myopathy: clinical, neurophysiological and muscle biopsy observations in young and middle-aged adults with early symptoms. *J Neurol Neurosurg Psychiatry* 1991; **54**: 494–498.
9. Udd B, Partanen J, Halonen P et al. Tibial muscular dystrophy. Late adult onset distal myopathy in 66 Finnish patients. *Arch Neurol* 1993; **50**: 604–608.
10. Servidei S, Capon F, Spinazzola A et al. A distinctive autosomal dominant vacuolar neuromyopathy linked to 19p13. *Neurology* 1999; 830–837.
11. Penisson-Besnier I, Dumez C, Chateau D, Dubas F, Fardeau M. Autosomal dominant late onset distal leg myopathy. *Neuromusc Dis* 1998; **8**: 459–466.
12. Sadeh M, Argov Z. Hereditary inclusion body myopathy in Jews of Persian origin: clinical and laboratory data. In: Askanas V, Engel WK, Serratrice G, eds. *Inclusion Body Myositis and Myopathies*. Cambridge: Cambridge University Press, 1997: 191–199.
13. Argov Z, Yarom R. 'Rimmed vacuole myopathy' sparing the quadriceps: a unique disorder in Iranian Jews. *J Neurol Sci* 1984; **64**: 33–43.
14. Argov Z, Mitrani-Rosenbaum S. Hereditary inclusion body myopathy (H-IBM) with quadriceps sparing: epidemiology and genetics. In: Askanas V, Engel WK, Serratrice G, eds. *Inclusion Body Myositis and Myopathies*. Cambridge: Cambridge University Press, 1997: 200–210.
15. Sadeh M, Gadoth M, Hadar H, Ben David E. Vacuolar myopathy sparing the quadriceps. *Brain* 1993; **16**: 217–232.
16. Argov Z, Tiram E, Eisenberg I et al. Various types of hereditary inclusion body myopathies map to chromosome 9p1–q1. *Ann Neurol* 1997; **41**: 548–551.
17. Bertorini TE, Homer LH, Halford H. Characteristics of magnetic resonance imaging in limb and axial weakness in myopathies. *Neurology* 1996; **46**(suppl): A345 (abst).
18. Askanas V, Engel WK. Recent progress and classification of the hereditary inclusion-body mopathies. *Acta Myol* 1998; **1**: 21–25.
19. Argov Z, Sadeh M, Eisenberg I, Karpati G, Mitrani-Rosenbaum S. Facial involvement in hereditary inclusion body myositis. *Neurology* 1998; **50**: 1925–1926.
20. Nonaka I, Sunohara N, Ishiura S, Satayoshi E. Familial distal myopathy with rimmed vacuoles and lamellar (myeloid) body formation. *J Neurol Sci* 1981; **51**: 141–145.
21. Cole AJ, Kuzniecky RR, Karpati G, Carpenter S, Andermann E, Andermann F. Familial myopathy with changes resembling inclusion body myositis and periventicular leucoencephalopathy. *Brain* 1988; **11**: 1025–1037.
22. Hentati F, Ben Hamida C, Tome F, Queslati F, Fardeau M, Ben Hamida M. Familial inclusion body myositis sparing the quadriceps with asymptomatic leuko-encephalopathy in a Tunisian kindred. *Neurology* 1991; **41**(suppl 1): 422 (abst).
23. Uyama E, Uchino M, Chateau D, Tome F. Autosomal recessive oculopharyngodistal myopathy in light of distal myopathy with rimmed vacuoles and oculopharyngeal dystrophy. *Neuromusc Discord* 1998; **8**: 119–125.
24. Mitrani-Rosenbaum S, Argov Z, Blumenfeld A, Seidman CE, Seidman JG. Hereditary inclusion myopathy maps to chromosome 9p1–q1. *Hum Mol Genet* 1996; **5**: 159–163.
25. Eisenberg I, Thiel C, Levi T et al. Fine-structure mapping of the hereditary inclusion body myopathy locus. *Genomics* 1999; **55**: 43–48.
26. Ikeuchi T, Asaka T, Saito M et al. Gene locus for autosomal recessive distal myopathy with rimmed vacuoles maps to chromosome 9. *Ann Neurol* 1997; **41**: 432–437.
27. Amouri R, Zouari M, Driss A et al. Heterogeneite genetique des myopathies a inclusions autosomales recessives en Tunisie. Abstract presented at Myology 2000 meeting in Nice, France.
28. Ahlberg G, von-Tell D, Borg K, Edstrom L, Anvret M. Genetic linkage of Welander distal myopathy to chromosome 2p13. *Ann Neurol* 1999; **6**: 399–404.
29. Haravuori H, Makela-Bengs P, Udd B et al. Assignment of the tibial muscular dystrophy locus to chromosome 2q31. *Am J Hum Genet* 1998; **62**: 620–626.
30. Clancy KP, Whaley LW, Baumbach LL et al. Autosomal dominant inclusion body myositis. *Muscle Nerve* 1998; 21 Suppl 7: S91 (abst).
31. Martinsson T, Darlin K, Kyllerman M, Oldfors A, Hallberg B, Washlstrom J. Dominant hereditary inclusion-body myopathy gene (IBM3) maps to chromosome region 17p13.1. *Am J Hum Genet* 1999; **64**: 1420–1426.
32. Moreira ES, Vainzof M, Marie SK, Sertie AL, Zatz M, Passos-Bueno MR. The seventh form of autosomal recessive limb-girdle muscular dystrophy is mapped to 17q11–12. *Am J Hum Genet* 1997; **61**: 151–159.
33. Askanas V, Engel WK. Newest approches to diagnosis of sporadic inclusion-body myositis and hereditary inclusion-body myopathies, including molecular-pathologic similarities to Alzheimer disease. In: Askanas V, Engel WK, Serratrice G, eds. *Inclusion Body Myositis and Myopathies*. Cambridge: Cambridge University Press, 1997: 3–78.

41

Exercise testing in muscle disease

John Vissing

INTRODUCTION

An invariable consequence of muscle disease is impaired motor function. In the majority of cases, this impairment is due to weakness caused by loss of muscle mass. In a number of cases, however, symptoms are caused by premature exertional fatigue related to disturbed muscle metabolism or neuromuscular transmission. In these conditions, which include mitochondrial and metabolic myopathies, myasthenia gravis and Lambert–Eaton's syndrome, symptoms are dynamic and exercise-related, whereas muscle mass is not necessarily affected. Likewise, patients with muscle diseases caused by ion-transport deficiencies across cellular membranes (the so-called channelopathies) also typically have normal muscle mass, but disturbed motor function related to either periodic weakness/paralysis or prolonged duration of muscle contraction (myotonia).

In order to recognize diagnosis, and to be able to monitor the course of a muscle disease or the effect of a treatment, exercise testing is crucial. After all, what could be more appropriate than to investigate the primary consequence of muscle disease, i.e. impaired muscle contraction and its effects on muscle strength and exercise capacity? In the following, different exercise tests used in the management of muscle disease will be reviewed. Special emphasis will be put on the diagnostic exercise tests used to evaluate patients with exertional myoglobinuria, premature exertional fatigue and exercise-induced muscle cramps and pain. First, other commonly used tests will briefly be reviewed.

A key element of a neurological examination is an assessment of muscle strength, based on manual static exercise testing. Muscle strength is usually scored using the MRC scale developed by the Medical Research Council of Great Britain.[1] This test enables the investigator to recognize the distribution and pattern of muscle weakness that can give important clues to diagnosis, and, in a clinical setting, can be helpful in the follow-up of treatment and clinical course of different muscle diseases. The disadvantage of the test is that the quantification of muscle strength is crude and subject to substantial interobserver variation. For scientific evaluation of the treatment and natural course of a disease, more sensitive measures of muscle strength testing have been developed, which are too complicated and time-consuming to use in normal clinical practice. These involve either isokinetic or static muscle testing, using dynamometers to assess muscle strength over multiple joints.[2-4] The dynamometer tests, however, still require optimal cooperation from the patient to be successful, and an investigator who is familiar with dynamometer testing.

In testing neuromuscular transmission defects, it is not so much the static muscle strength which is of interest as the endurance of the muscle contraction. This can either be done manually, where the time for which a patient can hold a contraction is monitored, or it can be tested neurophysiologically by repetitive stimulation of a motor nerve.[5]

In the muscle conditions associated with periodic weakness, registration of the compound muscle action potential (CMAP) over the hypothenar muscles before and after maximal handgrip exercise may be helpful in diagnosing disorders with potassium-sensitive periodic weakness.[6] In this test, CMAP elicited by stimulation of the ulnar nerve increases after exercise in most conditions with periodic paralysis compared to no change in healthy subjects.[6] However, the test cannot distinguish between the different types of periodic paralysis. Hyperkalemic periodic paralysis can be diagnosed by a cycle test where plasma potassium is measured after 30 min of exercise at a heart rate of around 140. Unlike healthy subjects, patients with hyperkalemic periodic paralysis have a second hyperkalemic episode 10–20 min after exercise, in which they can become symptomatic.

DIAGNOSTIC EXERCISE TESTING IN PATIENTS WITH EXERTIONAL MYOGLOBINURIA, PREMATURE EXERTIONAL FATIGUE AND EXERCISE-INDUCED MUSCLE CRAMPS AND PAIN

Exertional myoglobinuria, premature fatigue and exercise-induced muscle cramps and pain are typical features of patients with inborn errors of muscle metabolism. Exercise tests are usually the simplest, cheapest and least traumatic procedures that will give conclusive evidence about a possible diagnosis of disturbed muscle metabolism. Besides these considerations, there are several additional reasons to evaluate patients with exercise tests. First, the number of patients with these conditions is substantial. Mitochondrial myopathies are now recognized as one of the most common muscle diseases, with an estimated prevalence of 1 per 8000 in western Europe and the USA. Second, although individual defects of muscle glucose and fat metabolism are more rare than mitochondrial myopathies, they also affect a large group of patients, because the conditions cover more than 25 different metabolic defects. Also, this group of diseases is underdiagnosed, which may relate to the fact that patients often appear physically normal and can present with non-specific symptoms of exercise intolerance. Third, more than 1% of the population in developed countries suffer from muscle pain and exertional fatigue which are not caused by a neuromuscular condition, but rather a more non-specific muscle pain syndrome, like fibromyalgia. A simple exercise test is usually the best way to exclude or confirm a diagnosis of disturbed muscle metabolism.

Exercise tests are particularly useful in diagnosing disorders of muscle carbohydrate metabolism and defects of mitochondrial metabolism, whereas defects in fat metabolism typically are not easily diagnosed by these tests. Patients with partial enzymatic defects of fat metabolism may appear normal at rest and can have normal short-term exercise capacity and routine cycle ergometry findings. This is true of carnitine palmitoyltransferase II deficiency, which is the most common cause of exertional myoglobinuria. In this condition, only more sophisticated methods, i.e. substrate turnover measurements, are able to unmask a deficiency of fat mobilization during exercise.[7]

FOREARM EXERCISE TEST

Five decades ago, McArdle designed an exercise protocol aimed at studying muscle glycolysis, which led him to define the first metabolic myopathy.[8] He originally suggested that the defect was due to a defect in muscle glycogen breakdown,[8] and later it was found that the primary defect in this condition was a deficiency of myophosphorylase.[9,10] The disease, now called myophosphorylase deficiency or McArdle's disease, is the most common of the disorders of muscle carbohydrate metabolism, with an estimated prevalence of approximately 1 per 100 000. The general principles of the handgrip exercise test to diagnose defects of muscle glycolysis are:

(1) application of ischemia during exercise to maximally stimulate anaerobic glycolysis by applying a blood pressure cuff on the exercised arm, inflated to well above systolic pressure
(2) intermittent static handgrip exercise alternating between intended maximal handgrip for 1 s and rest for 1 s, for 1 min, after which exercise stops and the blood pressure cuff is released
(3) sampling of blood in the median cubital vein of the exercised arm to monitor changes in lactate and ammonia, and preferably also pyruvate, in the effluent venous blood.

Interpretation of results obtained with the ischemic forearm test

The metabolic basis for measuring lactate and pyruvate is straightforward, as glycolysis is blocked or impaired in these conditions. Lactate and pyruvate levels, therefore, are low during exercise in these conditions, except in lactate dehydrogenase deficiency, where pyruvate is elevated. It is just as important to measure ammonia in venous effluent blood as lactate. With ischemic exercise, ammonia is produced via deamination of AMP. In glycolytic defects, ammonia is produced in excess owing to increased accumulation of ADP during exercise, because ADP phosphorylation via glycolysis is impaired. In turn, high ADP levels lead to high levels of AMP, which is deaminated, resulting in high ammonia production in muscle glycolytic defects compared to that in healthy subjects.[11–16]

A sluggish increase of both lactate and ammonia with exercise does not indicate that the studied subject has a metabolic defect, but rather that either the work effort was too low or that a vein other than the median cubital vein was used to sample blood. Sampling from the basilic vein at the elbow level gives low lactate and ammonia responses, because the proportion of skin and inactive muscle drained by this vein is larger than from the median cubital vein. An abolished rise, or even a small drop in

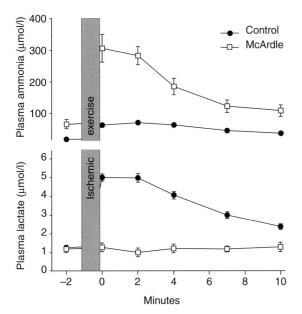

Figure 41.1 Plasma ammonia and lactate responses to an ischemic forearm exercise test in eight patients with McArdle's disease and nine healthy subjects (control). Values are means ± SEM.

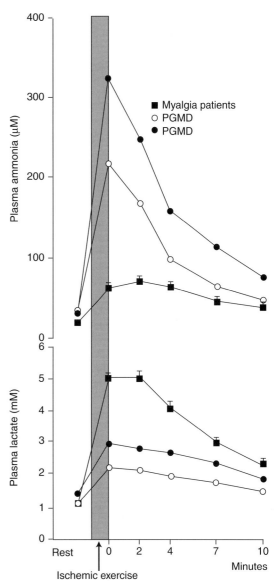

Figure 41.2 Changes in plasma ammonia and lactate concentrations after ischemic forearm exercise in two patients with phosphoglycerate mutase deficiency (PGMD) and in 16 patients with myalgia, but no evidence of neuromuscular disease.

plasma lactate, together with an exaggerated increase in plasma ammonia, is strong evidence for a complete block in muscle glycolysis (McArdle's disease and Tarui's disease (phosphofructokinase deficiency)) (Fig. 41.1).[8,11–17] An attenuated increase in lactate (1.5–3-fold resting values) together with a highly exaggerated increase in ammonia is indicative of a glycolytic defect with some residual enzyme activity left (phosphoglycerate mutase, phosphoglycerate kinase and lactate dehydrogenase deficiencies) (Fig. 41.2).[18] In summary, the test can conclusively distinguish between a complete block in muscle glycolysis and a partial deficiency, but cannot distinguish between the conditions within these groups.

Finally, approximately 1% of all people have a complete deficiency of myoadenylate deaminase, which results in an abolished rise in ammonia during the ischemic exercise test. By chance, some patients have combined defects of myoadenylate deaminase and glycolysis, and in a few cases it has been suggested that this could represent 'double trouble' for the patient.[19–21] However, although a pathogenic role has been suggested for myoadenylate deaminase deficiency,[22] no convincing data have been presented that support the clinical significance of this defect.[23,24]

Patients with glycolytic disorders of muscle metabolism almost invariably experience muscle cramps, pain and potential muscle injury during the ischemic forearm exercise test. It is, therefore, of interest that it has recently been shown that a forearm test identical to the one described above, but without ischemia, has the same diagnostic power as the ischemic test to identify patients with glycolytic muscle disorders.[17] The patients, at the same time, experience almost no discomfort from the test, suggesting that the ischemic test should be replaced by a non-ischemic test.[17]

Recently, it has been shown that a forearm exercise test can also be used to screen for mitochondrial myopathy.[25] Unlike the ischemic handgrip test used to stimulate muscle anaerobic metabolism to detect muscle glycolytic defects, this test is aimed at exploring the primary oxidative defect in these conditions. Therefore, the test is performed without arterial occlusion and with static handgrip exercise at 40% of maximal voluntary contraction force, alternating every second between contraction and relaxation. The parameter of interest with this test is not lactate and ammonia, as in the test for glycolytic disorders, but oxygen tension in the venous effluent blood. In patients with a clinically significant oxidative defect due to a mitochondrial disorder, oxygen tension does not drop, and may even paradoxically increase during exercise in venous effluent blood, compared to a consistent drop in oxygen tension in healthy subjects.[25] These findings are consistent with the lack of changes in deoxyhemoglobin concentration during forearm exercise in muscles of these patients as assessed by the more expensive and technically complicated near-infrared spectroscopy technique.[26–29]

CYCLE ERGOMETRY

Metabolism during cycle exercise is aerobic, except at maximal exertion. Cycle ergometry is, therefore, ideal to use in the diagnosis of muscle disease where muscle oxidative phosphorylation is severely impaired during exercise, as in patients with mitochondrial myopathies and patients with complete enzymatic blocks in muscle carbohydrate metabolism.[30] In the partial defects of glycolysis and in partial enzymatic defects of fat metabolism, aerobic capacity is almost normal, and routine measurements during cycling are usually unremarkable.[7,31] Therefore, cycle ergometry is primarily used for diagnosing McArdle's disease, phosphofructokinase deficiency and mitochondrial myopathies.

As a diagnostic test for muscle metabolic disorders, cycle ergometry has to be performed on a cycle ergometer that can be precisely adjusted in the 0–50-W range, since patients with mitochondrial myopathy and McArdle's and Tarui's diseases have very low work capacities.[32–34] To get a good sense of the

patient's exercise limitation, it is often advisable to start cycle testing with an incremental workload test, in which the workload is ramped upward with 5–10 W every other minute. In this way, the maximal oxidative capacity can be determined. An endless list of primarily metabolic parameters can be measured in these cycle tests, and although many of these are very interesting and may be diagnostic for the studied condition, it is prudent in a purely clinical setting to focus on measuring a few parameters. Measurements of gas exchanges (oxygen consumption (VO_2), carbon dioxide production (VCO_2) and the derived respiratory exchange ratio (VCO_2/VO_2)), heart rate, workload and plasma lactate obtained from a cubital vein are sufficient parameters to monitor in a clinical diagnostic setting.

Interpretation of cycle ergometry findings

In mitochondrial myopathy patients, the cycle testing may often suggest the diagnosis, due to exaggerated increases in plasma lactate at very low VO_2 (Fig. 41.3).[33,35–37] Likewise, the heart rate is exaggerated compared to healthy controls at a given VO_2.[33] If the initial incremetal cycle test to exhaustion

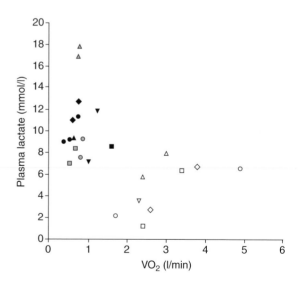

Figure 41.3 Plasma lactate concentration versus oxygen consumption during cycle exercise in eight patients with mitochondrial myopathy (closed symbols) and in five healthy subjects (open symbols). Two values are plotted for each subject representing plasma lactate and oxygen consumption values after 15 min of exercise at 65% of VO_{2max}, and at peak exercise capacity.

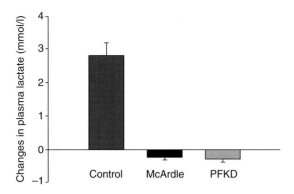

Figure 41.4 Changes in plasma lactate concentration after 15 min of cycle exercise at 65% of VO_{2max} in three patients with phosphofructokinase deficiency (PFKD), seven patients with McArdle's disease (McArdle) and 10 matched healthy control subjects (control).

was associated with no increase in lactate, then in all likelihood the patient has McArdle's or Tarui's disease (Fig. 41.4). To distinguish between these two conditions, a constant workload protocol at approximately 40% of VO_{2max} must be performed. In McArdle patients, this exercise is associated with an initial high heart rate and a high level of perceived exertion until the 8th–10th minute of exercise, when patients experience the so-called 'second wind' phenomenon. With the 'second wind', patients experience a dramatic drop in heart rate and perceived exertion at an unchanged workload (Fig. 41.5).[38–40] This effect relates to better extramuscular delivery of blood-borne fuels to muscle, which can partly substitute for the absent muscle glycogen breakdown.[34] This phenomenon is exclusively related to McArdle's disease, and is diagnostic for this condition. A double check of the McArdle diagnosis can be made by continuing the exercise test at a higher workload, so that the patient reaches the peak heart rate that was obtained before the 'second wind', and then give intravenous glucose (50 ml of a 50% solution). In McArdle patients, this will elicit a second 'second wind',[41] i.e. a drop in heart rate and perceived exertion at unchanged workload (Fig. 41.5). In Tarui's disease, no spontaneous 'second wind' occurs in exercise,[32] and in contrast to McArdle's disease, a glucose infusion worsens exercise tolerance.[42] Patients with partial glycolytic defects have no second wind and have no effect of a glucose infusion during exercise.

^{31}P-MAGNETIC RESONANCE SPECTROSCOPY

With ^{31}P-MRS, the content of skeletal muscle phosphorus-containing energy-rich molecules can be monitored at rest and during exercise. This is very helpful in diagnosing all the glycolytic disorders and mitochondrial myopathies. Obviously, this diagnostic

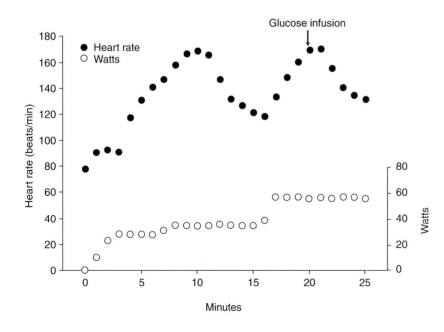

Figure 41.5 Heart rate (closed circles) and workload (open circles) in a 25-year-old man with McArdle's disease. During exercise, the patient experiences a spontaneous and then a glucose-induced second wind. See text for further explanation of the second wind phenomenon.

test requires more skills and expensive equipment than the forearm exercise and cycle ergometry tests, which limits this kind of investigation to specialized centers. The molecules of interest to test with ^{31}P-MRS are inorganic phosphate (P$_i$), phosphocreatine (PCr) and phosphomonoesters (PMEs). PMEs represent phosphorylated intermediates of glycolysis that can not be detected by ^{31}P-MRS in healthy muscle, except in low concentrations during very intense exercise. In glycolytic muscle disorders, however, PMEs accumulate behind the metabolic block and, therefore, constitute a prominent feature of phosphofructokinase deficiency and partial glycolytic defects.

Muscle pH can also be estimated from the distance between the P$_i$ and PCr peaks.[43] Different exercise protocols can be used, but commonly a protocol of rhythmic forearm, quadriceps, gastrocnemius or tibialis anterior muscle contraction to exhaustion is used.

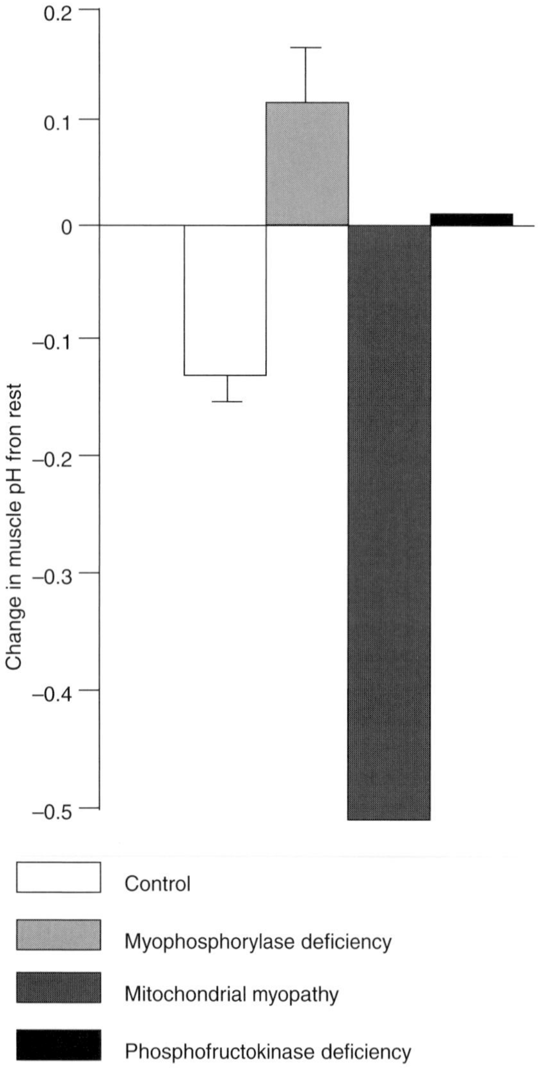

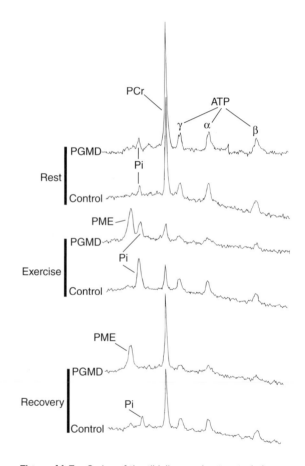

Figure 41.6 Changes from rest to exhaustion in ^{31}P-MRS-assessed forearm muscle pH in seven patients with McArdle's disease, in a patient with mitochondrial myopathy (MELAS), in a patient with phosphofructokinase deficiency and in five healthy subjects (control). The exercise paradigm was handgrip exercise at 30% of maximal voluntary contraction force. Reprinted with permission from Vissing et al.[46]

Figure 41.7 Series of the tibialis muscle at rest, during exhaustive exercise and during the 4th minute of recovery from exercise in a patient with phosphoglycerate mutase deficiency (PGMD) and a matched healthy subject (control). At rest, the ^{31}P-MRS spectrum is normal in the PGMD patient, but during exercise a phosphomonoester peak (PME) appears, representing accumulation of phosphorylated sugar behind the metabolic block. During recovery, the PME peak is maintained in the patient and inorganic phosphate (P$_i$) is trapped by the PME.

Interpretation of ^{31}P-MRS investigations

Mitochondrial myopathy

In mitochondrial myopathy, the normal resting PCr/P$_i$ ratio of about 10 is often decreased to about half.[44,45] In contrast to findings during cycle exercise, lactate accumulation and thus exaggerated acidification of working muscle in patients with mitochondrial myopathy is not a common feature,[44,45] although it may occur in patients with high resting plasma lactate levels.[46] The essentially normal pH response to exercise in muscle is probably related to an enhanced lactate extrusion capacity of muscle in these conditions.[45] Depletion of PCr in exercise, however, may be accelerated,[47] and, more importantly, when PCr has been depleted at the end of exercise, the recovery of PCr after exercise in mitochondrial myopathies is delayed, and is an indicator of impaired oxidative capacity.[44,45]

Glycolytic muscle disorders

^{31}P-MRS investigation of exercising muscle is able to group glycolytic disorders into McArdle's disease, Tarui's disease and partial glycolytic disorders. At rest, all these conditions show normal findings with ^{31}P-MRS. In McArdle's and Tauri's diseases, muscle does not acidify, because of absent lactate production, and accordingly pH does not drop during exercise (Fig 41.6).[44,48–52] In fact, pH increases a little during exercise in both conditions, because the absent acidification impairs PCr degradation. The two conditions can be distinguished from each other by ^{31}P-MRS, because in McArdle's disease, no phosphorylated sugar intermediates build up during exercise owing to the proximal block, whereas a high PME peak is characteristic of patients with Tarui's disease.[53,54] Partial glycolytic disorders all show the same pattern of a high PME peak at high exercise intensities (Fig 41.7),[55,56] and normal or slightly blunted muscle acidification during exercise. ^{31}P-MRS investigation of defects in muscle fat metabolism is usually unremarkable.

A flow-chart for exercise evaluation of patients with exertional myoglobinuria, premature exertional fatigue, muscle cramps or pain is provided in Fig 41.8.

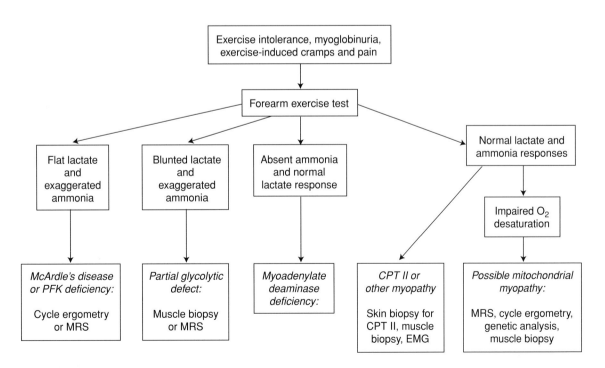

Figure 41.8 A flow chart for the evaluation of patients with exercise intolerance, myoglobinuria and exercise-induced muscle cramps and pain. PFK, phosphofructokinase; CPT II, carnitine palmitoyltransferase II deficiency.

REFERENCES

1. Medical Research Council. *Aids to the Investigation of Peripheral Nerve Injuries.* London: Her Majesty's Stationery Office, 1976.
2. Merlini L, Dell'Accio D, Holzl A, Granata C. Isokinetic muscle testing (IMT) in neuromuscular diseases. Preliminary report. *Neuromusc Disord* 1992; **2**: 201–207.
3. Mawdsley RH, Knapik JJ. Comparison of isokinetic measurements with test repetitions. *Phys Ther* 1982; **62**: 169–172.
4. Edwards RH, Hyde S. Methods of measuring muscle strength and fatigue. *Physiotherapy* 1977; **63**: 51–55.
5. Lambert EH. Neurophysiological techniques useful in the study of neuromuscular disorders. *Res Publ Assoc Res Nerv Ment Dis* 1960; **38**: 247.
6. McManis PG, Lambert EH, Daube JR. The exercise test in periodic paralysis. *Muscle Nerve* 1986; **9**: 704–710.
7. Haller RG, Vissing J, Sidossis LS, Wolfe RR. Impaired fat oxidation in adult carnitine palmitoyltransferase II deficiency is specific to exercise. *Neurology* 1999; **52**(6 suppl 2): A463–A464 (abstr)
8. McArdle B. Myopathy due to a defect in muscle glycogen breakdown. *Clin Sci Lond* 1951; **10**: 13–32.
9. Mommaerts W, Illingworth B, Pearson C, Guillory R, Seraydarian K. A functional disorder of muscle associated with the absence of phosphorylase. *Proc Natl Acad Sci USA* 1959; **45**: 791–797.
10. Schmid R, Mahler R. Chronic progressive myopathy with myoglobinuria: demonstration of a glycogenolytic defect in muscle. *J Clin Invest* 1959; **38**: 2044–2058.
11. Rumpf KW, Wagner H, Kaiser H, Meinck H-M, Goebel HH, Scheler F. Increased ammonia production during forearm ischemic work test in McArdle's disease. *Klin Wochenschr* 1981; **59**: 1319–1320.
12. Barcroft H, Greenwood B, McArdle B et al. The effect of exercise on forearm blood flow and on venous blood pH, PCO_2 and lactate in a subject with phosphorylase deficiency in skeletal muscle. *J Physiol* 1966; **189**: 44P–46P.
13. Haller RG, Bertocci LA. Exercise evaluation of metabolic myopathies. In: Engel AG, Franzini-Armstrong C, eds. *Myology*, 2nd edn. New York: McGraw-Hill, 1994: 807–821.
14. Sinkeler SP, Wevers RA, Joosten EM et al. Improvement of screening in exertional myalgia with a standardized ischemic forearm test. *Muscle Nerve* 1986; **9**: 731–737.
15. Coleman RA, Stajich JM, Pact VW, Periack-Vance MA. The ischaemic exercise test in normal adults and in patients with weakness and cramps. *Muscle Nerve* 1986; **9**: 216–221.
16. Mineo I, Kono N, Hara N et al. Myogenic hyperuricemia: a common pathophysiologic feature of glycogenosis types III, V and VII. *N Engl J Med* 1987; **317**: 75–80.
17. Kazemi-Esfarjani P, Skomorowska E, Jensen TD, Haller RG, Vissing J. No need for ischemia in the forearm exercise test for McArdle's disease. *Neurology* 2000; **54**(7 suppl 3): A332 (abstr).
18. Vissing J, Schmalbruch H, Haller RG, Clausen T. Muscle phosphoglycerate mutase deficiency with tubular aggregates: effect of dantrolene. *Ann Neurol* 1999; **46**: 274–277.
19. Bruno C, Minetti C, Shanske S et al. Combined defects of muscle phosphofructokinase and AMP deaminase in a child with myoglobinuria. *Neurology* 1998; **50**: 296–298.

20. Rubio JC, Martín MA, Bautista J, Campos Y, Segua D, Arenas J. Association of genetically proven deficiencies of myophosphorylase and AMP deaminase: a second case of 'double trouble'. *Neuromusc Disord* 1997; **7**: 387–389.
21. Tsujino S, Shanske S, Carroll JE, Sabina RL, DiMauro S. Double trouble: Combined myophosphorylase and AMP deaminase deficiency in a child homozygous for nonsense mutations at both loci. *Neuromusc Disord* 1995; **5**: 263–266.
22. Gross M. Clinical heterogeneity and molecular mechanisms in inborn muscle AMP deaminase deficiency. *J Inher Metab Dis* 1997; **20**: 186–192.
23. Verzijl HTFM, van Engelen BGM, Luyten JAFM et al. Genetic characteristics of myoadenylate deaminase deficiency. *Ann Neurol* 1998; **44**: 140–143.
24. Heller SL, Kaiser KK, Planer GJ, Hagberg JM, Brooke MH. McArdle's disease with myoadenylate deaminase deficiency: observations in a combined enzyme deficiency. *Neurology* 1987; **37**: 1039–1042.
25. Dysgaard Jensen T, Kazemi P, Skomorowska E, Vissing J. A diagnostic forearm test for mitochondrial myopathy. *Eur J Neurol* 2000; **7**(suppl 3): 50 (abstr).
26. Bank W, Chance B. An oxidative defect in metabolic myopathies: diagnosis by non-invasive tissue oxymetry. *Ann Neurol* 1994; **36**: 830–837.
27. Bank W, Chance B. Diagnosis of defects in oxidative muscle metabolism by non-invasive tissue oximetry. *Mol Cell Biochem* 1997; **174**: 7–10.
28. Abe K, Matsuo Y, Kadekawa J, Inoue S, Yanagihara T. Measurement of tissue oxygen consumption in patients with mitochondrial myopathy by non-invasive tissue oximetry. *Neurology* 1997; **49**: 837–841.
29. Van Beekvelt MC, Colier WN, Wevers RA, Van Engelen BG. Quantitative measurement of oxygen consumption and forearm blood flow in patients with mitochondrial myopathies. *Adv Exp Med Biol* 1999; **471**: 313–319.
30. Haller RG, Vissing J. Circulatory regulation in muscle disease. In: Saltin B, Boushel R, Secher N, Mitchell JH, eds. *Exercise and Circulation in Health and Disease.* Champaign, Illinois: Human Kinetics, 1999: 271–282.
31. Kissel JT, Beam W, Bresolin N, Gibbons G, DiMauro S, Mendell JR. Physiologic assessment of phosphoglycerate mutase deficiency: incremental exercise tests. *Neurology* 1985; **35**: 828–833.
32. Vissing J, Galbo H, Haller RG. Paradoxically enhanced glucose production during exercise in humans with blocked glycolysis due to muscle phosphofructokinase deficiency. *Neurology* 1996; **47**: 766–771.
33. Vissing J, Galbo H, Haller RG. Exercise fuel mobilization in mitochondrial myopathy: a metabolic dilemma. *Ann Neurol* 1996; **40**: 655–662.
34. Vissing J, Lewis SF, Galbo H, Haller RG. Effect of deficient muscular glycogenolysis on extra muscular fuel production in exercise. *J Appl Physiol* 1992; **72**(5): 1773–1779.
35. Finsterer J, Shorny S, Capek J et al. Lactate stress test in the diagnosis of mitochondrial myopathy. *J Neurol Sci* 1998; **159**(2): 176–180.
36. Siciliano G, Rossi B, Manca L et al. Residual muscle cytochrome c oxidase activity accounts for submaximal exercise lactate threshold in chronic progressive external ophthalmoplegia. *Muscle Nerve* 1996; **9**(3): 342–349.
37. Siciliano G, Renna M, Manca LM et al. The relationship of plasma catecholamine and lactate during anaerobic threshold exercise in mitochondrial myopathies. *Neuromusc Disord* 1999; **9**: 411–416.

38. Andersen KL, Lund-Johansen P, Clausen G. Metabolic and circulatory responses to muscular exercise in a subject with glycogen storage disease (McArdle's disease). *Scand J Clin Lab Invest* 1969; **24**: 105–113.

39. Braakhekke JP, deBruin MI, Stegeman DF, Wevers RA, Binkhorst RA, Joosten EMG. The second wind phenomenon in McArdle's disease. *Brain* 1986; **109**: 1087–1101.

40. Pernow BB, Havel RJ, Jennings DB. The second wind phenomenon in McArdle's syndrome. *Acta Med Scand Suppl* 1967; **472**: 294–307.

41. Haller RG, Vissing J. A glucose-induced second 'second wind' in McArdle's disease: implications for muscle oxidative metabolism. *Ann Neurol* 1997; **42**: 413 (abstr).

42. Haller RG, Lewis SF. Glucose-induced exertional fatigue in muscle phosphofructokinase deficiency. *N Engl J Med* 1991; **324**: 364–369.

43. Taylor DJ, Borc PJ, Styles P, Gadia DG, Radda GK. Bioenergetics of intact human muscle. A ^{31}P nuclear magnetic resonance study. *Mol Biol Med* 1983; **1**: 77–94.

44. Arnold DL, Matthews PM, Radda GK. Metabolic recovery after exercise and the assessment of mitochondrial function in vivo in human skeletal muscle by means of ^{31}P NMR. *Magn Reson Med* 1984; **1**: 307–315.

45. Arnold DL, Taylor DJ, Radda GK. Investigation of human mitochondrial myopathies by phosphorus magnetic resonance spectroscopy. *Ann Neurol* 1985; **18**: 189–196.

46. Vissing J, Vissing S, MacLean DA, Saltin B, Quistorff B, Haller RG. Sympathetic activation in exercise is not dependent on muscle acidosis: direct evidence from studies in metabolic myopathies. *J Clin Invest* 1998; **101**: 1654–1660.

47. Taylor DJ, Kemp GJ, Radda GK. Bioenergetics of skeletal muscle in mitochondrial myopathy. *J Neurol Sci* 1994; **127**: 198–206.

48. Duboc D, Jehenson P, Dinh S, Marsac C, Syrota A, Fardeau M. Phosphorus NMR spectroscopy study of muscular enzyme deficiencies involving glycogenolysis and glycolysis. *Neurology* 1987; **37**: 663–674.

49. Lewis SF, Haller RG, Cook JD, Nunnally RL. Muscle fatigue in McArdle's disease studied by ^{31}P NMR: effect of glucose infusion. *J Appl Physiol* 1985; **59**: 1991–1994.

50. Bendahan D, Confort-Gouny S, Kozak Ribbens G, Cozzone PJ. Investigation of metabolic myopathies by P-31 MRS using a standardized rest–exercise–recovery protocol: a survey of 800 explorations. *MAGMA* 1993; **1**: 91–104.

51. Ross BD, Radda GK, Gadian DG et al. Examination of a case of suspected McArdle's syndrome by ^{31}P nuclear magnetic resonance. *N Engl J Med* 1981; **304**: 1338–1342.

52. Argov Z, Bank WJ, Maris J, Chance B. Muscle energy metabolism in McArdle's syndrome by in vivo phosphorus magnetic resonance spectroscopy. *Neurology* 1987; **37**: 1720–1724.

53. Argov Z, Bank WJ, Leigh JSJ, Chance B. Muscle energy metabolism in human phosphofructokinase deficiency as recorded by ^{31}P NMR. *Ann Neurol* 1986; **22**: 46–51.

54. Bertocci L, Haller RG, Lewis SF, Fleckenstein JL, Nunnally RL. Abnormal high-energy phosphate metabolism in human muscle phosphofructokinase deficiency. *J Appl Physiol* 1991; **70**: 1201–1207.

55. Argov Z, Bank WJ, Boden B, Ro Y-I, Chance B. Phosphorus magnetic resonance spectroscopy of partially blocked muscle glycolysis. An in vivo study of phosphoglycerate mutase deficiency. *Arch Neurol* 1987; **44**: 614–617.

56. Vita G, Toscana A, Bresolin N et al. Muscle phosphoglycerate mutase (PGAM) deficiency in the first Caucasian patient: biochemistry, muscle culture and ^{31}P-MR spectroscopy. *J Neurol* 1994; **241**: 289–294.

Part 7

Specific neurological symptoms

42

Disorders of emotional behaviour

JP Newman

The Decade of the Brain (1990–2000) bore witness to exciting developments in the investigation of brain-based disorders of emotional behaviour. These developments centred on: adopting a consensual taxonomy of these disorders; investigating their neural bases; and developing treatment and rehabilitation strategies. A terse summary of these developments, however, easily falls prey to a good news–bad news format. The good news is that our taxonomy is quite adequate; our knowledge of the neural substrates is expanding rapidly. Sadly, our treatment and rehabilitation strategies lag far behind. In our examination of these developments, we will focus on brain-based, specifically neurological disorders of emotional behaviour. Psychiatric disorders with emotional components that have brain bases, such as schizophrenia, as well as emotional reactions to neurological illness, such as depressive reactions to exacerbation of multiple sclerosis, deserve separate treatment. So, too, do primarily neurological disorders that have in part emotional manifestations, such as Huntington's disease.

TAXONOMY AND LOCALIZATION

It is possible to divide brain-based disorders of emotional behaviour into two subcategories: disorders of overt emotional behaviour and disorders of emotional experience and communication.[1] In summarizing the taxonomy of disorders of emotional behaviour, attention will be paid to the existing literature regarding the localization of brain lesions heretofore reported for each disorder. It thereby becomes apparent that the aspirations of the early neurologists and clinical neuropsychologists to find single, specific lumps of brain tissue that, when damaged, cause particular symptoms have been laid to rest.[2] Even so, certain generalizations regarding localization of cortical cognitive functions in the normative dextral subject are possible. Several are

relevant to the present discussion: the frontal lobes are strongly implicated in the initiation and cessation of behaviours as well as cognitive flexibility, problem-solving and motor speech (Broca's area). The left parietal lobe is particularly essential to praxis; a portion of it, along with a portion of the temporal lobe (collectively referred to as Wernicke's area), comprehends language. The right parietal lobe performs visual–spatial functions such as orientation and navigation in space, and visual–spatial manipulations, and, when lesioned, can produce neglect phenomena. The temporal lobes recognize and comprehend auditory input and are critical in memory and learning. The occipital lobes recognize and process visual inputs. Certain functions, such as attention and concentration, depend upon widespread networks. In addition, subcortical structures such as the basal ganglia and thalamus are heavily implicated in language and memory functions.

DISORDERS OF OVERT EMOTIONAL BEHAVIOUR

Abulia

Abulia is characterized by loss of interest in and motivation to engage in purposeful behaviour. The abulic patient is passive, initiates little, lacks spontaneity, and finds no pleasure in former pursuits. However, affective and cognitive components of major depression, such as dysphoria, loss of optimism, guilt feelings and suicidal ideation, are lacking. Initial symptom onset follows brain disease or trauma.

Abulia is most commonly seen in left hemispheric lesions, particularly of the dorsolateral aspect of the frontal lobe.[3–6] However, it is also seen in lesions of the temporal lobes; parietal and occipital lobes together;[7] the internal capsule;[8–10] the dorsolateral caudate;[11–14] the thalamus;[5,15–17] the corpus callosum;[5]

the pons;[5] the midbrain;[5] and the periventricular white matter.[18]

Anosodiaphoria

Anosodiaphoria is characterized by indifference to medical illness or physical disability in spite of awareness of the illness or disability itself. This indifference has its onset after brain disease or trauma and represents a change in the patient's premorbid emotional assessment of his condition. A diagnosis of anosodiaphoria rules out unawareness or denial of the illness or stoicism as a coping style. It may be accompanied by unilateral or bilateral neglect.

Anosodiaphoria is most commonly seen in right-hemispheric lesions,[19,20] notably of the inferior frontal gyrus.[21] However, it is also seen in temporo-parietal lesions[20] as well as combined lesions of the putamen and internal capsule.[22]

Moria

Moria is the term applied to mood elevation (excitement or euphoria), often of a very caustic nature, occurring as a result of (and in spite of) brain disease or injury that results in significant disability or injury. It occurs in the absence of a premorbid history of hypomania or bipolar disorder. It must not result from pharmacological treatment or illicit drug use. Moria is commonly the result of right-hemispheric,[3] especially orbitofrontal parenchymal, lesions.[23] However, it has been reported after lesioning of the ventromedial caudate nucleus[14] as well as long-standing right frontoparietal hypoperfusion.[23] It is often accompanied by *Witzelsucht* (crass facetiousness and the repetitive telling of inappropriate, often sexual jokes).[23]

Pathological laughing and crying

Pathological laughing and crying[24–26] is the quite descriptive term for sudden, involuntary outbursts of laughter or crying in the absence of corresponding subjective feelings of happiness or sadness. They must occur as a result of brain disease or injury, and cannot have resulted from mood-altering prescription or illicit drug use, nor may they be the result of mental illness. They may be accompanied by exaggerated and involuntary facial expressions as well (though not by the weakness of facial muscles seen during reflexive or automatic movement in pseudobulbar palsy).

Pathological laughing and crying, reports of which date back at least to the 16th century,[27] typically result from bilateral lesions. Pathological crying more commonly results from left-hemispheric lesions, whereas pathological laughing is more common in right-hemispheric lesions.[28] (This parallels the depressive–catastrophic versus euphoric or indifferent responses that form part of clinical lore in hemispheric stroke.[29,30]) It most typically results from lesions of the corticobulbar tract, typically in the pons or ventral to it;[31–35] however, it also occurs in lesioning of the inferior frontal lobe with or without extension into the temporal or parietal lobe or basal ganglia,[36,37] the middle or inferior temporal gyri,[38,39] basilar artery occlusion,[40] and bilateral opercular lesions.[41]

DISORDERS OF EMOTIONAL EXPERIENCE AND COMMUNICATION

Alexithymia

Alexithymia is a cognitive–affective disturbance of the ability to recognize and describe one's own feelings and emotional states. It can occur after brain injury or disease, although it is also well described in the psychiatric literature.[42] Alexithymics have a poverty of inner fantasy life, constricted emotional activity, and few if any expressive facial movements, and sometimes have rigid posture as well.[43] It has been reported in cases of agenesis of the corpus callosum[44] as well as other defects of interhemispheric transfer;[45] it may also result from isolation of the anterior cingulate cortex (thereby disrupting transmission of interoceptive emotional information)[46] as well as diffuse right-hemispheric dysfunction.[47]

Auditory affective agnosia

Auditory affective agnosia, sometimes called sensory aprosody, is the impaired discrimination and identification of affective prosody. Its sufferers are unable to perceive the emotional tone of others' spoken speech, and sometimes facial expression as well. However, the patient's own expression of emotional tone via speech (and facial expression) is preserved. Auditory affective agnosia is the result of brain disease or injury, and is observed particularly in patients with temporoparietal lesions of the right hemisphere,[48,49] especially the posterior temporal and parietal opercula.[37,50] It also occurs as a result of combined lesions of the thalamus and posterior limb of the internal capsule[51] and combined lesions of the basal ganglia and posterior internal capsule.[52]

Motor aprosody

Motor aprosody is the term for impairment in the ability to incorporate affective modulation into motor speech, both on demand and in imitation of others. It may be accompanied by impairment in the ability to express emotion through facial expression as well. It follows brain disease or injury, represents a change in speech prosody production by the affected individual, and gives rise to monotonous speech devoid of the emotional intonation that is a crucial element in communication.[52,53] It must not be the result of depression or hypophonia.

Motor aprosody is typically seen in anterior right-hemispheric lesions corresponding to Broca's area in the left hemisphere[37] as well as combined frontal and anterior parietal opercular lesions.[37,48,52] It may also be seen in lesions of the internal capsule,[54] diverse basal ganglia loops and transcallosal projections.[52] Some reports also describe interhemispheric mixing of propositional and prosodic speech elements.[55] Finally, in addition to classic motor aprosody, there exists a well-known syndrome of dysprosody that manifests itself as a seeming foreign accent. However, this appears to be an apraxia of speech.[48,56]

Global aprosody

Global aprosody, as the term suggests, is impairment in all aspects of emotional communication: the patient neither uses nor perceives others' usage of emotional tone of voice or facial gestures, nor can the patient imitate modelled vocal emotional communication. It is typically the result of large right-hemisphere lesions encompassing the frontal, temporal and parietal perisylvian areas, essentially the same territories that result in global aphasia when lesioned in the left hemisphere.[6,48,50]

In the context of the aprosodies, we note that claims have been advanced for the existence of transcortical sensory, transcortical motor and mixed transcortical aprosodies as well as conduction aprosody and pure affective deafness, parallel to those of the aphasias.[37,52] However, few convincing cases have been reported, and the existence of these conditions has not as yet gained wide acceptance. It is possible that cases have not been widely recognized and reported because they have not been systematically sought by clinicians and are not readily apparent to patients.

THE NEURAL SUBSTRATES OF DISORDERS OF EMOTIONAL BEHAVIOUR

How have theorists attempted to integrate the wealth of clinical reports on brain lesions and disorders of emotional behaviour? Certainly, a comprehensive neuroanatomical and histological treatise on the brain bases of emotional behaviour is beyond the scope of this brief chapter. However, it is possible to paint a broad picture of current thinking as it has evolved over the course of the past decade and more.[57,58] This thinking can be summarized succinctly as follows: well-regulated, appropriate emotional behaviour is the final product of multiple complex modular neural networks encompassing the cerebral cortices, the basal ganglia, the limbic system, the reticular system and associated white matter tracts. Modulation of these networks is accomplished in ways that are only partly understood by the various neurotransmitter systems.

As put forth by leading theorists,[1,59,60] present-day models divide emotional experience into three component systems: arousal, valence and motor activation. The structures of the reticular formation and limbic system and their role in activation and arousal are reasonably well understood by neurologists; a standard textbook may be consulted for their description.[61] The cerebral cortices, the primary focus of recent theorization, are seen to regulate the functioning of the reticular system, the limbic system and the basal ganglia. The frontal cortices process and organize valence properties—the left mediating positive emotions, the right mediating negative emotions. The right hemisphere, especially the parietal lobe, plays a leading role in activating arousal systems. The left hemisphere modulates and inhibits these arousal systems. The right hemisphere is also critical in motor activation. The orbitofrontal projections of the frontal lobes mediate avoidance behaviours; the dorsomedial projections, as well as parietal lobe areas, mediate approach behaviours. The left cerebral hemisphere mediates the comprehension and expression of propositional language. The right cerebral hemisphere mediates the comprehension and expression of emotional gestures, including facial expression and emotional prosody. Just as the posterior left neocortex mediates the comprehension of propositional language and the anterior portions its production, so too does the posterior right neocortex mediate the comprehension of emotional expression (prosody and facial expression) and the anterior portion its production. Emotional experience and behaviour depend upon neural activation patterns within these modular systems. Derangement at any points in these modular systems can either inhibit or release various emotional behaviours. Lesions can result in focal dysfunction, contralateral cortical functional disinhibition, and/or ipsilateral subcortical disinhibition.

In their seminal 1995 paper, Tucker et al[62] presented a theoretical framework for understanding the integration and control of emotional behaviour networks. They emphasized the central role of the dual corticolimbic, primarily frontal pathways that diverge in terms of structural architecture, neurotransmitter systems, motivational biases and processing styles. They discuss social and emotional functions of the frontal lobes in terms of three anatomical dimensions: first, vertical integration of lower (brainstem and limbic) functions with higher (cognitive and motor planning) functions, which sustain the capacity for engaging and maintaining levels of activation and arousal in the service of goal-directed behaviour; second, functional differentiation of the dorsal and ventral anatomical pathways linking frontal cortex with limbic structures—lesions of the dorsomedial pathways lead to apathy and loss of initiative, whereas ventral (orbitofrontal) lesions lead to behavioural disinhibition; and third, lateral hemispheric specialization for emotion, as discussed above.

Underpinning these frontal structures lie brainstem neuromodulator systems that regulate activation and arousal in fundamentally different ways: a dopaminergic activation system that operates on the basis of a redundancy bias that routinizes actions and focuses attention; and a noradrenergic arousal system that is able to allocate attention to a broad array of novel events. The former operates in a tightly focused attentional mode, and the latter in a global, holistic perceptual mode. Overlying these systems are limbic networks that are essential to both emotional behaviour and working memory. Corticolimbic connections in the posterior brain are primarily from the sensory neocortex to limbic structures, whereas those of the anterior brain are primarily from limbic structures to the motor neocortex. The paralimbic networks are densely interconnected, further enabling more global, holistic perceptual modalities. However, interconnectivity for the widespread neocortical networks is comparatively sparse, further engendering focused, localized processing.

Tucker et al reviewed the evidence for different motivational biases of the ventral and dorsomedial pathways. They argued that the ventrolateral motor system, with its limbic cortical base in the orbital frontal lobe and its extensive connections with the amygdala, insula and temporal cortices, as well as the extensive visceroautonomic links of the insula, is particularly well suited for assessing the motivational significance of external stimuli in relation to internal states. By contrast, the dorsal pathway,

including the anterior cingulate and its afferent fibres from the amygdala, plays a dominant role in monitoring the emotional significance of stimuli, not just in terms of aversive initiation of action but also in assessing hedonic value. They argue that an understanding of these different motivational biases (assessment of the motivational significance of external stimuli versus their emotional significance) and processing styles (tightly focused and analytic versus global and holistic), based on differences in structural architecture and neurotransmitter systems, is essential to elucidating the roles of lateral and local hemispheric specialization in the regulation of emotional behaviour.[63]

TREATMENT STRATEGIES

There exist three primary treatment strategies for disorders of emotional behaviour: pharmacological treatment, neuropsychological rehabilitation and ecological manipulation. Alas, few disorders of emotional behaviour have proven amenable to drug treatment. Three major exceptions are abulia, moria and pathological laughing and crying. Abulia may be responsive to low doses of stimulants such as methylphenidate,[64] as well as dopamine agonists such as bromocriptine and lisuride.[10,65] Moria may respond to standard pharmacological treatments for bipolar disorder. Pathological laughing and crying are often responsive to antidepressants of the selective serotonin reuptake inhibitor class, especially paroxetine and citalopram.[66,67]

Neuropsychological rehabilitation is often by default a primary treatment strategy. Patients (and occasionally their primary-care physicians) readily attribute paresis, aphasia or hemispatial neglect to brain injury but often need to be educated to the fact that disorders of emotional behaviour, too, can be the direct result of brain injury rather than a purely psychological reaction to newly acquired deficits. This knowledge promotes acceptance, reduces guilt, and facilitates symptom-oriented problem-solving. It is difficult to overemphasize the utility of simple education. Detailed explanations of the type and location of brain injury, replete with pictures, diagrams and imaging studies, lend the message all-important scientific gravitas. Beyond that, intensive cognitive rehabilitation can often improve the patient's perception of affective cues; intensive re-education can improve output of or control over overt emotional expression. For example, biofeedback and modelling have been used to treat motor aprosodia.[68] Auditory affective agnosia can be treated using paired associate learning techniques: repeatedly pairing pictures of facial cues of specific emotional content (such as anger) with labels ('ANGER'); the labels can then be slowly withdrawn as the patient learns to associate the visual cue with the label. Abulic patients sometimes respond to external incentives as a replacement for internal motivation. Such a reward system must be tangible and accompanied by much encouragement or even cajoling, however. Even so, no clear-cut rules for rehabilitation can be conveyed in these few sentences. It is important to build a specific intervention strategy tailored to each individual patient's strengths and deficits.

Ecological manipulations typically centre on family members and care-takers, and are aimed at circumventing the patient's specific disability. For example, patients with an agnosia for auditory affective cues should be spoken to in clear, declarative language in order to communicate affect. Family members of patients with motor aprosody must learn to attend very carefully to the propositional components of speech, rather than assuming that 'the absence of emotional expression implies the absence of emotional experience'. In addition, simple education of family members can reduce their apprehension regarding the patient's behaviour. For example, it is very helpful to know that pathological laughing and crying are not, in fact, accompanied by subjective feelings of happiness or sadness and they need not be responded to as if the patient is excessively euphoric or depressed. In fact, such episodes are often best ignored, unless the patient is embarrassed and needs reassurance. Patients become more accepting of themselves when family members demonstrate acceptance. Finally, it is important to impart to patients and their family members a sense of hope that some degree of symptom improvement usually comes about in time and as a result of the collaborative efforts of all. Loss of hope is a powerful disincentive, and must be avoided whenever possible.

REFERENCES

1. Heilman KM, Gilmore RL. Cortical influences in emotion. *J Clin Neurophysiol* 1998; **15**: 409–423.
2. Goetz CG. Battle of the titans: Charcot and Brown-Sequard on cerebral localization. *Neurology* 2000; **54**: 1840–1847.
3. Belyi BI. Mental impairment in unilateral frontal tumours: role of the laterality of the lesion. *Int J Neurosci* 1987; **32**: 799–810.
4. Vilkki J. Amnestic syndromes after surgery of anterior communicating artery aneurysms. *Cortex* 1985; **21**: 431–444.
5. Fisher CM. Honored guest presentation: abulia minor versus agitated behavior. *Clin Neurosurg* 1983; **31**: 9–31.
6. Gautier JC, Awada A, Loron P. A cerebrovascular accident with unusual features. *Stroke* 1983; **14**: 808–810.
7. Lilly R, Cummings JL, Benson DF, Frankel M. The human Klüver–Bucy syndrome. *Neurology* 1983; **33**: 1141–1145.
8. Madureira S, Guerreiro M, Ferro M. A follow-up study of cognitive impairment due to inferior capsular genu infarction. *J Neurol* 1999; **246**: 764–769.
9. Tatemichi TK, Desmond DW, Prohovnik I et al. Confusion and memory loss from capsular genu infarction: a thalamocortical disconnection syndrome? *Neurology* 1992; **42**: 1966–1979.
10. Barrett K. Treating organic abulia with bromocriptine and lisuride: Four case studies. *J Neurol Neurosurg Psychiatry* 1991; **54**: 718–721.
11. Lim JK, Yap KB. Bilateral caudate infarct—a case report. *Ann Acad Med Singapore* 1999; **28**: 569–571.
12. Kumral E, Evyapan D, Balkir K. Acute caudate vascular lesions. *Stroke* 1999; **30**: 100–108.
13. Caplan LR, Schmahmann JD, Kase CS et al. Caudate infarcts. *Arch Neurol* 1990; **47**: 133–143.
14. Mendez MF, Adams NL, Lewandowski KS. Neurobehavioral changes associated with caudate lesions. *Neurology* 1989; **39**: 349–354.
15. Fox MW, Ahlskog JE, Kelly PJ. Stereotactic ventrolateralis thalamotomy for medically refractory tremor in post-levadopa era Parkinson's disease patients. *J Neurosurg* 1991; **75**: 723–730.
16. Haley EC Jr, Brashar HR, Barth JT, Cail WS, Kassel NF. Deep cerebral vein thrombosis. Clinical, neuroradiological and neuropsychological correlates. *Arch Neurol* 1989; **46**: 337–340.
17. Waxman SG, Ricaurte GA, Tucker SB. Thalamic hemorrhage with neglect and memory disorder. *J Neurol Sci* 1986; **75**: 105–112.
18. So NK, O'Neill BP, Frytak S. Delayed leukoencephalopathy in survivors with small cell lung cancer. *Neurology* 1987; **37**: 1198–1201.
19. Ishiai S. Neuropsychological disorders in minor hemisphere damage. *Rinsho Shinkeigaku* 1997; **37**: 1122–1124.
20. Stone SP, Halligan PW, Greenwood RJ. The incidence of neglect phenomena and related disorders in patients with an acute right or left hemisphere stroke. *Age Ageing* 1993; **22**: 46–52.
21. Mesulam MM, Waxman SG, Geschwind N, Sabin TD. Acute confusional states with right middle cerebral artery infarctions. *J Neurol Neurosurg Psychiatry* 1976; **39**: 84–89.
22. Ortiz N, Barraquer-Bordas L. Place disorientation as a clinical feature of a right capsulo-putamenal hematoma. *Neurologia* 1991; **6**: 103–107.
23. Vardi J, Finkelstein Y, Zlotogorski Z, Hod I. L'homme qui rit: inappropriate laughter and release phenomena of the frontal subdominant lobe. *Behav Med* 1994; **20**: 44–46.
24. Colover J. Pathological laughing and crying. *Lancet* 2000; **355**: 238.
25. McCullagh S, Moore M, Gawel M, Feinstein A. Pathological laughing and crying in amyotrophic lateral sclerosis: an association with prefrontal cognitive dysfunction. *J Neurol Sci* 1999; **169**: 43–48.
26. Arlazaroff A, Mester R, Spivak B, Klein C, Toren P. Pathological laughter: common versus unusual aetiology and presentation. *Int J Psychiatry Relat Sci* 1998; **35**: 184–189.

27. Altschuler EL, Wisdom S. An old case of pathological laughing and crying. *Lancet* 1999; **354**: 1736.

28. Sackeim HA, Greenber MS, Weiman AL et al. Hemispheric asymmetry in the expression of positive and negative emotions. Neurological evidence. *Arch Neurol* 1982; **39**: 210–218.

29. Babinski J. Contribution à l'étude des troubles mentaux dans l'hémiplégie organique cérébrale (anosognosie). *Rev Neurol* 1914; **27**: 845–848.

30. Goldstein K. *Language and Language Disturbances.* New York: Grune and Stratton, 1948.

31. Asfora WT, DeSalles AA, Abe M, Kjelberg RN. Is the syndrome of pathological laughing and crying a manifestation of pseudo-bulbar palsy? *J Neurol Neurosurg Psychiatry* 1989; **52**: 523–525.

32. van Hilten JJ, Buruma OJ, Kessing P, Vlasveld LT. Pathological crying as a prominent behavioral manifestation of central pontine myelinolysis. *Arch Neurol* 1988; **46**: 936.

33. Green RL, McAllister TW, Bernat JL. A study of crying in medically and surgically hospitalized patients. *Am J Psychiatry* 1987; **144**: 442–447.

34. Bouvier A, Chevalier JF, Brion S. Pathological laughing and posterior fossa tumours. *Encephale* 1981; **7**: 83–94.

35. Bauer G, Gerstenbrand F, Hengl W. Involuntary motor phenomena in the locked-in syndrome. *J Neurol* 1980; **223**: 191–198.

36. Ross ED, Stewart RS. Pathological display of affect in patients with depression and right frontal brain damage. *J Nerv Ment Dis* 1987; **175**: 165–172.

37. Ross ED. The aprosodias. Functional–anatomic organization of the affective components of language in the right hemisphere. *Arch Neurol* 1981; **38**: 561–569.

38. Sethi PK, Rao TS. Gelastic, quiritarian and cursive epilepsy. A clinicopathological appraisal. *J Neurol Neurosurg Psychiatry* 1976; **39**: 823–828.

39. Gascon GG, Lombroso CT. Epileptic (gelastic) laughter. *Epilepsia* 1971; **12**: 63–76.

40. Larner AJ. Basilar artery occlusion associated with pathological crying: 'folles larmes prodromiques'? *Neurology* 1998; **51**: 916–917.

41. Laurent-Vannier A, Fadda G, Laigle P, Dusser A, Leroy-Malherbe V. Syndrome de Foix-Chavany-Marie d'origine traumatique chez l'enfant. *Rev Neurol (Paris)* 1999; **155**: 387–390.

42. Taylor GJ. Recent developments in alexithymia theory and research. *Can J Psychiatry* 2000; **45**: 134–142.

43. Fricchione G, Howanitz E. Aprosodia and alexithymia—a case report. *Psychother Psychosom* 1985; **43**: 156–160.

44. Ernst H, Key JD, Koval MS. Alexithymia in an adolescent with agenesis of the corpus callosum and chronic pain. *J Am Acad Child Adolesc Psychiatry* 1999; **38**: 1212–1213.

45. Parker JD, Keighthley ML, Smith CT, Taylor GJ. Interhemispheric transfer deficit in alexithymia: an experimental study. *Psychosom Med* 1999; **61**: 464–468.

46. Lane RD, Ahern GL, Schwartz GE, Kaszniak AW. Is alexithymia the emotional equivalent of blindsight? *Biol Psychiatry* 1997; **42**: 834–844.

47. Jessimer M, Markham R. Alexithymia: a right hemisphere dysfunction specific to recognition of certain facial expressions? *Brain Cogn* 1997; **34**: 246–258.

48. Ackermann H, Hertrich I, Ziegler W. Prosodic disorders in neurologic diseases—a review of the literature. *Fortschr Neurol Psychiatry* 1993; **61**: 241–253.

49. Heilman KM, Scholes R, Watson RT. Auditory affective agnosia. Disturbed comprehension of affective speech. *J Neurol Neurosurg Psychiatry* 1975; **38**: 69–72.

50. Ross ED. Affective prosody and the aprosodias. In: Mesulam MM, (ed.) *Principles of Behavioral Neurology.* (2nd edn.) Oxford University Press, New York, 2000 (316–331).

51. Wolfe GI, Ross ED. Sensory aprosodia with left hemiparesis from subcortical infarction. Right hemisphere analogue of sensory-type aphasia with right hemiparesis? *Arch Neurol* 1987; **44**: 668–671.

52. Gorelick PB, Ross ED. The aprosodias: further functional–anatomic evidence for the organization of affective language in the right hemisphere. *J Neurol Neurosurg Psychiatry* 1987; **50**: 553–560.

53. Bell WL, Davis DL, Morgan-Fisher A, Ross ED. Acquired aprosodia in children. *J Child Neurol* 1990; **5**: 19–26.

54. Ross ED, Harney JH, deLacoste-Utamsing C, Purdy PD. How the brain integrates affective and propositional language into a unified behavioral function. Hypothesis based on clinicoanatomic evidence. *Arch Neurol* 1981; **38**: 745–748.

55. Speedie LJ, Coslett HB, Heilman KM. Repetition of affective prosody in mixed transcortical aphasia. *Arch Neurol* 1984; **41**: 268–270.

56. Ross ED. Nonverbal aspects of language. *Neurol Clin* 1993; **11**: 9–23.

57. Tucker DM. Lateral brain function, emotion and conceptualization. *Psychol Bull* 1981; **89**: 19–46.

58. Kolb B, Taylor L. Neocortical substrates of emotional behavior. In: Stein NL, Leventhal B, eds. *Psychological and Biological Approaches to Emotion.* Hillsdale, NJ: Lawrence Erlbaum Associates, 1990.

59. Fox NA. Dynamic cerebral processes underlying emotional regulation. *Monogr Soc Res Child Dev* 1994; **59**: 152–166, 250–283.

60. Heilman KM. The neurobiology of emotional experience. *J Neuropsychiatry Clin Neurosci* 1997; **9**: 439–448.

61. Adams RD, Victor M, Ropper AH (eds.) *Adams' & Victor's Principles of Neurology,* 6th edn. New York: McGraw Hill Text, 1997.

62. Tucker DM, Luu P, Pribram KH. Social and emotional self-regulation. *Ann NY Acad Sci* 1995; **769**: 213–239.

63. Newman JP. Effects of characterological anxiety and situational arousal on the solving of a color–word interference task: hemispheric processing implications. *Int J Neurosci* 1990; **52**: 1–9.

64. Mehta MA, Owen AM, Sahakian BJ, Mavaddat N, Pickard JD, Robbins TW. Methylphenidate enhances working memory by modulating discrete frontal and parietal lobe regions in the human brain. *J Neurosci* 2000; **20**: RC65.

65. Karli DC, Burke DT, Kim HJ et al. Effects of dopaminergic combination therapy for frontal lobe dysfunction in traumatic brain injury rehabilitation. *Brain Injury* 1999; **13**: 63–68.

66. McCullagh S, Feinstein A. Treatment of pathological affect: variability of response for laughter and crying. *J Neuropsychiatry Clin Neurosci* 2000; **12**: 100–102.

67. Muller U, Murai T, Bauer-Wittmund T, von Cramon DY. Paroxetine versus citalopram treatment of pathological crying after brain injury. *Brain Injury* 1999; **13**: 805–811.

68. Stringer AY. Treatment of motor aprosodia with pitch biofeedback and expression modeling. *Brain Injury* 1996; **10**: 583–590.

43

Cognitive and affective disturbances in multiple sclerosis

Jürg Kesselring and Ulrike Klement

The emotional and relationship problems associated with MS have not always been fully appreciated by the medical profession, which has tended to concentrate on the physical aspects of this disease. Yet the psychological problems of MS often cause more suffering than physical effects.[1]

Neuropsychological disturbances and psychiatric problems are common in multiple sclerosis (MS).[2-7] It is difficult to differentiate which of the disturbances are due to organic disease and which are psychological reactions to a disease which is always an enormous psychological burden, with its unpredictable course and potential to lead to severe disability and handicap.

PREMORBID PERSONALITY

Repeated attempts have been made, in retrospective investigations of patients already affected, to characterize a premorbid personality, and to determine characteristics of personality which dispose to the disease. Such investigations[8] claimed that the premorbid personality of MS patients should be characterized by hysterical aspects, as notes on 'hysteria' are frequently found in case reports of MS patients. In fact, MS may manifest itself in earlier phases of the disease by various symptoms which may be found in hysterical ('histrionics') personalities: sensory disturbances, emotional instability, and particularly fatigue. If, from such observations, the inference is made that hysterical characteristics of personality may dispose to the development of MS, it only discloses a lack of ability to diagnose early manifestations of MS. 'In its infancy multiple sclerosis used to be called hysteria' said the famous Queen Square physician Farquhard Buzzard more than 100 years ago. Usually the term 'hysteria' is used imprecisely and includes conversion phenomena, dissociations, or only characteristics of individual personalities. Generally, it discloses more about the way in which physicians think about their patients than depending on clinically relevant data.[9]

COGNITIVE FUNCTIONS

Reports of the frequency of disturbances of cognitive functions in MS patients are very variable, and depend on the methods used and on the types of patients examined. In about half of the patients in whom no mental disturbances are found on routine neurological examination, cognitive deficits may be detected during detailed neuropsychological examination.[4,6] Discrete or moderate impairment of cognitive functions may be found on neuropsychological testing in 60% of patients with a disease duration of less than 2 years,[10] without leading to disability in daily life. If such impairments are found, it is very likely that they will further decline over the next 3 years, whereas unimpaired cognitive functions indicate that they will remain stable over the next 3 years.[11]

The most frequently impaired cognitive function in patients with MS is memory. Patients with MS often show problems in tasks of working memory, but short-term memory—assessed by memory span tasks—often remains unimpaired. In long-term memory—a relatively unlimited and permanent memory store—impairment is commonly observed if spontaneous and free recall is required. Recognition memory is normal or less impaired than free recall. This special pattern in memory deficits in MS patients is put forward by some authors as evidence that in MS patients the encoding of information is unimpaired but they have problems in retrieving the stored information.[5] Beatty et al,[12] however, showed that only 53% of the MS patients examined exhibited a pattern of memory impairment in which the most marked feature was their inconsistent retrieval. Thornton and Raz[13] found in their quantitative review that MS patients show impairments across all memory domains and that long-term memory dysfunctions are not only based on retrieval deficits. Visuospatial processes, motor speed and reaction time, reading aloud and figure-copying are also affected in MS patients when compared to normal individuals and patients with other neurological diseases. MS appears to produce a general slowing of cognitive processes.[14] Patients with MS may also have problems in executive functions and planning skills. On specialized tests of abstract or conceptual reasoning, such as the Wisconsin Card Sorting Test (WCST) or the Tower of London, patients with MS show perseveration errors and more problems in profiting from feedback. MS patients perform as well as controls with regard to accuracy, but not speed, of tasks of divided or automatic attention, but they perform significantly worse on more effortful measures of attention. Patients with MS are more often distracted from tasks in which learning capabilities and memory are tested, although, in the absence of distraction, learning capabilities remain intact. Visuospatial processes, motor speed and reaction time, reading aloud and figure-copying, and memory appear to be more affected than verbal functions when compared to normal individuals and to patients with other neurological diseases. MS appears to produce a general slowing of cognitive processes,[14] but not a uniform pattern of cognitive deficits. In earlier phases of the disease, disturbances of memory are found in a great number of MS patients when tested adequately, but more discrete disturbances of memory, at least partly, may be due to depression and are frequently associated with changes of personality.[15] Attentional functions should be assessed in detail and treated selectively.[16] After a longer duration of the disease, disturbances of learning of verbal and non-verbal material are frequent.

More recent studies in MS have been devoted to the investigation of subgroups, e.g. primary versus secondary progressive MS,[17,18] or isolated clinical syndromes suggestive of MS.[19] A moderate correlation may be found with lesion burden on proton density-weighted MRI and with magnetization transfer-derived measures: overall macroscopic and microscopic brain damage is more important than the corresponding regional brain disease in determining deficits of selective cognitive domains.[20] In primary progressive MS, the disease process is more confined to the spinal cord and therefore leads to less cognitive impairment than the secondary, progressive form, in spite of comparable disability as determined on the Expanded Disability Status Scale[20a] (EDSS).

Usually there are no or only weak correlations between cognitive deficits and the degree of physical disability, the duration of illness or depression. Good et al,[15] however, suggested that even more discrete disturbances of memory, at least partly, may be due to depression and are frequently associated with changes of personality. Cognitive deficits are not usually correlated with anxiety symptoms but sometimes they are connected with the experience of apathy, indifference and euphoria. Some authors describe correlations between cognitive dysfunctions in MS and the amount and location of white matter disease as determined by MRI (indices: total cerebral lesion, cerebral metabolism, size of the lateral and third ventricles, size of the corpus callosum).[21,22]

Cognitive problems have a negative impact on the quality of life. MS patients with impaired cognitive functions are less likely to be working, are less engaged in social or vocational activities, and have more difficulties in performing household tasks. They are more often dependent on other persons in activities of daily living than MS patients without cognitive deficits. A recent study showed that MS patients with impaired autobiographical memory are more content with their quality of life than unimpaired patients.[23]

Being able to detect cognitive dysfunctions in MS patients by carrying out neuropsychological testing early will help to determine the work status of MS patients and to adapt the working settings to the remaining abilities of the patients. Thereby, more patients should be able to keep their jobs. It is also important to inform family members about the relationship between MS and cognitive dysfunctions. Not uncommonly, cognitive problems of patients are incorrectly attributed to obstinacy or depression. This causes additional stress, and which should be avoided.

AFFECTIVE DISORDERS

For decades, it was taken for granted that the mood of MS patients was typically euphoric, as described by many authors since Charcot. 'Euphoria' describes a type of mood which is characterized by inappropriate/inadequate serenity (in view of the physical disability). Comparative investigations in patients with muscle diseases and similar physical disabilities demonstrated that euphoria in MS patients occurs only after long disease duration, and with very marked neurological deficits, and is part of an 'organic psycho-syndrome' caused by extensive cerebral lesions. Even in very disabled MS patients, this type of mood does not occur in more than 10%. Anosognosia (a lack of insight into the disease) may be a blessing for severely disabled patients and their care-givers. It is, however, as rare as euphoria in early and middle phases of the disease.

So-called 'affect incontinence' (i.e. abruptly changing affective expressions which do not correspond to inner mood) may be very disabling for patients and those around them. They may occur as paroxysmal phenomena and are considered to be due to organic lesions.[9] Many patients describe a type of 'internal disconnection' which does not allow them to express verbally or non-verbally affects which they feel interiorly. Pathological laughing and crying may affect 1 in 10 patients with MS and occurs more often in severely physically disabled patients with long-standing disease. The presence of cognitive deficits in these cases relative to controls implies more extensive brain involvement.[24]

However, the most important affective disorder in MS patients is depression.[3,9,25] It is characterized by an 'inability to mourn', loss of hope, and pessimism, and is often associated with general loss of energy, sleep disturbances, weight loss, and lack of interest. Such episodes may precede neurological manifestations in MS. They may occur in most patients at some stage of their disease, and are occasionally considered a major symptom. In 20–25% of patients, depression may be so marked as to require treatment by a specialist.[25] The risk of suicide, particularly in the earlier stages of the disease, is markedly increased compared to that of the general population.[26] When comparing MS patients with similarly disabled patients with muscle diseases, depressive symptoms were equally frequent, and are therefore interpreted as being a reaction to the disease and its consequences. On the other hand, the observation that depressive episodes in MS patients are often associated with 'endogenous signs' such as vegetative disturbances and diurnal changes of mood is an argument for an organic basis. Depressive disturbances in MS are so frequent and of such importance that they have to be analysed and treated with particular care, sympathy, and persistence. When MS patients are interviewed regarding the subjective experiences of the psychosocial consequences of MS, three areas emerge: demoralization, deteriorated partnership, and benefit-finding. The latter includes deepening of relationships, enhanced appreciation of life, and an increase in spiritual interests, and is related to adaptive coping strategies such as positive reappraisal and seeking social support.[7]

REFERENCES

1. Burnfield A, Burnfield P. Common psychological problems in multiple sclerosis. *BMJ* 1978; **i**: 1193–1194.
2. Jambor KL. Cognitive functioning in multiple sclerosis. *Br J Psychiatry* 1969; **115**: 765–775.
3. Minden SL, Schiffer RB. Affective disorders in multiple sclerosis. Review and recommendations for clinical research. *Arch Neurol* 1990; **47**: 98–104.
4. Prosiegel M, Michael C. Neuropsychology and multiple sclerosis: diagnostic and rehabilitative approaches. *J Neurol Sci* 1993; **115**: S51–S54.
5. Rao SM. Neuropsychology of multiple sclerosis. *Curr Opin Neurol* 1995; **8**: 216–220.
6. Brassington JC, Marsh N. Neuropsychological aspects of multiple sclerosis. *Neuropsychol Rev* 1998; **8**: 43–77.
7. Mohr DC, Dick LP, Russo D et al. The psychosocial impact of multiple sclerosis: exploring the patient's perspective. *Health Psychol* 1999; **18**: 376–382.
8. Paulley JW. Psychological management of multiple sclerosis. *Psychother Psychosom* 1976/77; **27**: 26–40.
9. Kesselring J. *Multiple Sclerosis*. Cambridge University Press, Cambridge, UK 1997.
10. Lyon-Caën O, Jouvent R, Hauser S et al. Cognitive functions in recent-onset demyelinating diseases. *Arch Neurol* 1986; **43**: 1138–1141.
11. Kujala P, Portin R, Ruutiainen J. The progress of cognitive decline in multiple sclerosis. A controlled 3-year follow-up. *Brain* 1997; **120**: 289–297.
12. Beatty WW, Wilbanks SL, Blanco CR et al. Memory disturbance in multiple sclerosis: Reconsideration of performance on the Selective Reminding Test. *J Clin Exp Neuropsychol* 1996; **18**(1): 56–62.
13. Thornton AE, Raz N. Memory impairment in multiple sclerosis. A quantitative review. *Neuropsychology* 1997; **11**: 357–366.
14. Kail R. Speed of information processing in patients with multiple sclerosis. *J Clin Exp Neuropsychol* 1998; **20**: 98–106.
15. Good D, Clark CM, Oger JL, Paty D, Klonoff H. Cognitive impairment and depression in mild multiple sclerosis. *J Nerv Ment Dis* 1992; **180**: 730–732.
16. Plohmann AM, Kappos L, Ammann W et al. Computer assisted retraining of attentional impairments in patients with multiple sclerosis. *J Neurol Neurosurg Psychiatry* 1998; **64**: 455–462.
17. Comi G, Filippi M, Martinelli V et al. Brain MRI correlates of cognitive impairment in primary and secondary progressive multiple sclerosis. *J Neurol Sci* 1995; **132**: 222–227.
18. Camp SJ, Stevenson VL, Thompson AJ et al. Cognitive function in primary and transitional progressive multiple sclerosis: a controlled study with MRI correlates. *Brain* 1999; **122**: 1341–1348.
19. Feinstein A, Kartsounis LD, Miller DH, Youl BD, Ron MA. Clinically isolated lesions of the type seen in multiple sclerosis: a cognitive, psychiatric, and MRI follow-up study. *J Neurol Neurosurg Psychiatry* 1992; **55**: 869–876.
20. Rovaris M, Filippi M, Falautano M et al. Relation between MR abnormalities and patterns of cognitive impairment in multiple sclerosis. *Neurology* 1999; **50**: 1601–1608.

20a.Kutzke JF. *Neurology* 1983; **33**: 1444–52.

21. Blinkenber M, Rune K, Jensen CV et al. Cortical cerebral metabolism correlates with MRI lesion load and cognitive dysfunction in MS. *Neurology* 2000; **54**: 558–564.

22. Möller A, Wiedemann G, Rohde U, Backmund H, Sonntag A. Correlates of cognitive impairment and depressive mood disorder in multiple sclerosis. *Acta Psychiatr Scand* 1994; **89**: 117–121.

23. Kenealy PM, Beaumont JG, Lintern T, Murrell R. Autobiographical memory, depression and quality of life in multiple sclerosis. *J Clin Exp Neuropsychol* **22**: 125–131.

24. Feinstein A, Feinstein K, Gray T, O'Connor P. Prevalence and neurobehavioral correlates of pathological laughing and crying in multiple sclerosis. *Arch Neurol* 1997; **54**: 1116–1121.

25. Schubert DS, Foliart RH. Increased depression in multiple sclerosis patients. A meta-analysis. *Psychosomatics* 1993; **34**: 124–130.

26. Stenager EN, Stenager E, Koch Henricksen N et al. Suicide and multiple sclerosis: an epidemiological investigation. *J Neurol Neurosurg Psychiatry* 1992; **55**: 542–545.

44

From spinal shock to spasticity

Volker Dietz, Armin Curt and Lutz-Peter Hiersemenzel

INTRODUCTION

Recovery of locomotor function after spinal cord injury (SCI) is in an exciting phase of research development. This chapter highlights some of the recent developments emerging from animal and clinical studies on spinal lesions, as well as on novel approaches to enhance locomotor function in spinal cord-injured subjects.

The vertebrate central nervous system (CNS) has a limited capacity for regeneration. Much of the research effort aimed at improving functional recovery after SCI is directed towards enhancing the limited ability of CNS neurons to restore damaged connections between the spinal cord and brain. After many SCIs there is some preservation of anatomical continuity across the injury site, even in patients with minimal function below the lesion.[1] The problem then becomes one of maximizing the functional contribution of the preserved pathways and, if axonal regeneration also becomes possible, of newly regenerated projections.

After SCI, restoration of normal function, such as locomotion, will depend to a certain extent upon reorganization of existing spinal circuitry. This capacity for reorganization, generally referred to as plasticity, is a well-known property of the CNS, and is thought to underly many instances of functional recovery after injury, as well as learning and memory in the undamaged CNS. While plasticity has been well documented in many parts of the supraspinal CNS, the prevalent view of spinal cord function has been that it is relatively non-plastic and serves simply as a hardwired relay for supraspinal commands. This view has been changing with the accumulation of physiological and behavioural evidence that adaptive processes can also occur within spinal circuits. The potential ability of the spinal cord to 'learn' has obvious implications for altering and improving locomotor function after injury.

The neural mechanisms responsible for learning and adaptive processes are thought to involve changes in both the efficacy of synaptic function and the pattern of synaptic connections within neural circuits. In the uninjured CNS, these changes occur as a result of alteration in the amount of neural activity within circuits and are therefore termed activity-dependent. After CNS injury, there also appears to be reorganization of spared neural circuits. The mechanisms underlying this injury-induced plasticity are not understood fully, although it is possible that some of these changes are also guided in an activity-dependent manner (review: Muir and Steves[2]).

SCI can produce a number of significant changes in the anatomy and physiology of spinal cord neuronal circuitries. Sprouting of spared axons is perhaps the best-studied anatomical change after injury. In this instance, sprouting refers to the expansion of the terminal fields of undamaged axons when the terminals of injured axons degenerate. Although there has been some controversy over the extent of terminal sprouting and the conditions under which it takes place, results indicate that, caudal to a spinal hemisection in cats or monkeys, the central terminal projections of dorsal root afferents can increase the density and extent of their distribution.[3-5]

The clinical recovery from spinal shock is characterized by the reappearance of tendon tap reflexes and of muscle tone. These clinical signs are reflected by a change in the excitability of neuronal correlates.[6]

COURSE OF RECOVERY OF SPINAL NEURONAL ACTIVITY AFTER SCI

Possible neuronal correlates of tendon tap relexes are F-waves and H-reflexes. These parameters have been recorded over time after SCI.[6]

Fig. 44.1 shows the relationship between the excitability of tendon tap reflexes, F-waves and H-reflexes over time after SCI. The mean values of 18

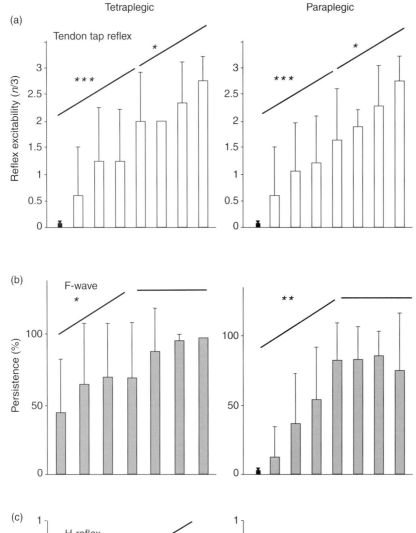

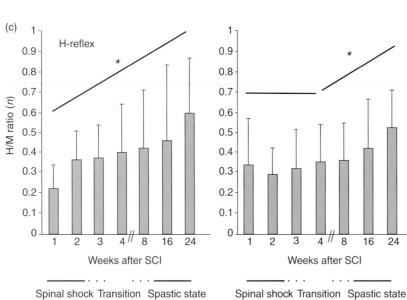

Figure 44.1 Mean values of excitability tendon tap reflexes (a); F-wave persistence (b) and H/M ratio (c) over time after SCI plotted from 18 patients. Levels of significance: *$P < 0.05$; **$P < 0.01$; ***$P < 0.01$.[6]

patients are plotted. The slope of increase in excitability of tendon reflexes over time was similar to that of F-wave persistence. In contrast, during spinal shock, all patients except one presented well-elicitable H-reflexes (range H/M ratio 0.1–0.7, mean 0.31). Also, in three patients whose first recordings were performed early after injury, a well-elicitable H-reflex could be obtained. H-reflex excitability remained approximately stable up to 8 weeks after SCI. During weeks 8–24, i.e. when spastic signs became established, the H/M ratio became significantly higher in paraplegic, but not in tetraplegic, patients (not shown). However, in this context one has to bear in mind that a decrease of M-wave amplitude occurred at this stage in paraplegic but not in tetraplegic patients. Therefore, changes in the excitability of tendon tap reflexes paralleled the recovery of F-waves, but not of the slope of H/M ratio.

The relationship between the clinically assessed muscle tone and spasm frequency by the Ashworth and Penn Scales,[7] and the electrophysiological recordings of flexor reflexes in TA (evoked at twice MT) over time after SCI, are shown in Fig. 44.2. The results of 18 patients are plotted. Muscle tone increased continuously over time. The frequency of muscle spasms increased after spinal shock and remained stable from the fourth week on after SCI. Flexor reflexes (amplitude and number of bursts) increased up to the fourth week ('transition'). However, after that RMS amplitude decreased significantly, while the number of bursts remained stable. Consequently, increase in muscle tone and spasms was associated with an increase in flexor reflex activity during the first weeks after SCI, but not at a later stage.

Examples of original recordings of a paraplegic patient (level of lesion Th6) and of a tetraplegic patient (level of lesion C4) during the three periods following an SCI are plotted in Figs 44.3b and 44.3c respectively. For comparison, a typical flexor reflex response obtained in a healthy subject is shown (Fig. 44.3a). During the first week after SCI, no flexor reflex could be elicited. During the second week after SCI, i.e. still during spinal shock, usually one flexor reflex burst could be elicited in most patients. During the development of spastic signs in most patients, two flexor reflex bursts were recorded. However, after the fourth week, the flexor reflex amplitude and number of bursts decreased continuously in the paraplegic patients. A contralateral reflex response was never found in para- and tetraplegic patients.

The relationship between the parameters plotted in Fig. 44.2 (Ashworth and Penn Scores and flexor

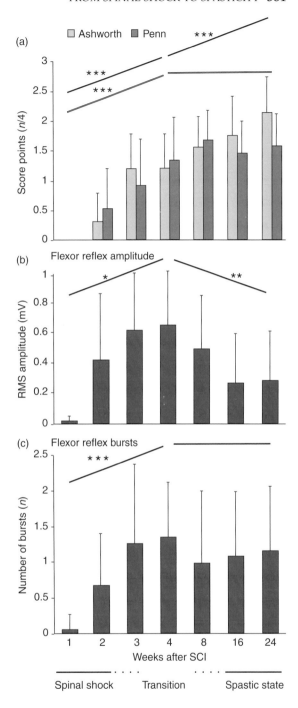

Figure 44.2 Mean values of muscle tone (Ashworth scale) and muscle spasm frequency (Penn scale) (a). Grand means of normalized RMS amplitude of tibialis anterior flexor reflex response (b) and number of flexor reflex bursts (c) over time after SCI from all patients. For significance levels see Fig. 44.1.[6]

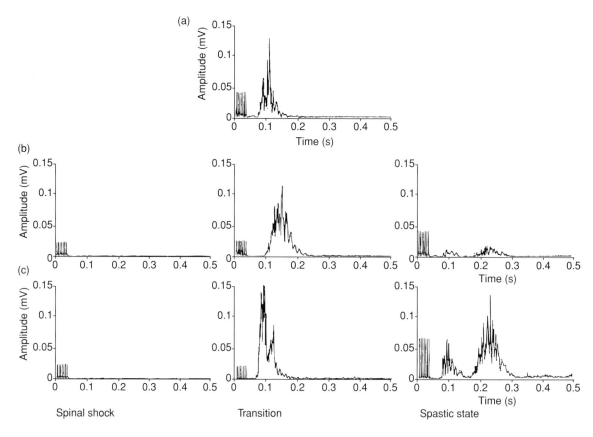

Figure 44.3 Typical examples of averaged (*n* = 5) flexor reflex responses in a healthy subject (a), a paraplegic (b) (level of lesion Th6, no. 15 in Table 1) and a tetraplegic (c) level of lesion C4) patient during the three periods after SCI.[6]

reflexes) are presented according to the level of lesion in Fig. 44.4. In this figure, the patients were attributed to one of the following groups: (1) tetraplegic patients, i.e. level of lesion above Th1 (*n* = 5); (2) high paraplegic patients, i.e. level of lesion Th1–Th4 (*n* = 6); and (3) low paraplegic patients, i.e. level of lesion at and below Th5 (*n* = 5). The mean values (with standard deviation) are shown. In all three groups, a similar increase of Ashworth and Penn scores took place over time up to 6 months. In contrast, in all groups, flexor reflex amplitude and number of bursts increased only up to about the fourth week after SCI. Afterwards, the number of bursts remained approximately constant in tetraplegic and high paraplegic patients and decreased significantly in low paraplegic patients. The flexor reflex amplitude decreased in all patients after the fourth week, but the decrease was only significant for the low paraplegic patients, with a tendency to significance in high paraplegic patients.

Higher stimulation intensity (3 × MT) resulted in a generally larger reflex amplitude. However, the decay in amplitude over time was about the same. These results indicate a divergent course of clinical signs and electrophysiological recordings from the fourth week after SCI on. This divergence obviously depends on the level of lesion and is most pronounced in low paraplegic patients.

Flexor reflexes were recorded once in three complete chronic tetraplegic patients (ASIA A). The reflex amplitudes were in the range of the responses obtained after 6 months in the tetraplegic patients.

NEURONAL ACTIVITY AFTER ACUTE SCI: SPINAL SHOCK

Clinical and neurophysiological background

More than 100 years ago, the term 'spinal shock' was introduced to describe the clinical state in patients

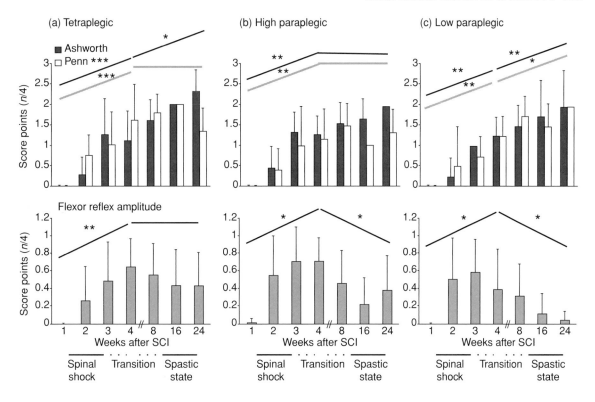

Figure 44.4 Mean values of Ashworth and Penn scale scores (a), grand averages of normalized RMS values of tibialis anterior flexor reflex response (b), and number of flexor reflex bursts (c), from tetraplegic ($n = 5$), high paraplegic (level over Th5, $n = 6$) and low paraplegic (level below Th4, $n = 5$) patients. For significance levels see Fig. 44.1.

with acute SCI presenting muscle paralysis with flaccid muscle tone and loss of tendon reflexes below the level of the lesion.[8] Although complete loss of sensorimotor function persists, spinal shock ends after some weeks, and during the following months a 'spastic syndrome' develops with exaggerated tendon reflexes, increased muscle tone and involuntary muscle spasms. The development of a spastic syndrome is a common finding in surgically or pathologically confirmed complete spinal cord transection;[9] that is, changes in the excitability of spinal cord neuronal circuits occur independently of supraspinal influences.

In order to explain these changes, several hypotheses have been put forward based on clinical observations, neurophysiological recordings, intracellular studies and theoretical considerations. A change from hypoexcitability of alpha-motoneurons (alpha-MN) during spinal shock to hyperexcitability during spasticity was presumed.[10] According to this concept, the alpha-MN hypoexcitability in spinal

shock is due to an acute loss of supraspinal excitatory input resulting in a hyperpolarized alpha-MN.[11] Such a hyperpolarization of spinal MN was observed in spinalized cats.[12]

In contrast to this, well-elicitable H-reflexes were described in humans early after SCI,[13,14] contradicting strong alpha-MN depression as a single cause for the loss of tendon tap reflexes during spinal shock. The latter observation led to the concept of concomitant gamma-motoneuron (gamma-MN) depression:[14] while a mechanical tap does not elicit a tendon tap reflex, electrical stimulation of group I afferent nerve fibres leads to an H-reflex response.

Furthermore, interneuron (IN) activity and excitability has an important influence on spinal neuronal activity. It is known that most of the supraspinal descending tracts impinge on spinal interneurons.[15] Interruption of these tracts will influence spinal IN function. However, little is currently known about the changes in IN activity that occur during spinal shock and the transition to spasticity.

Relationship between clinical and electrophysiological parameters

In a recent study,[6] clinical and electrophysiological parameters were systematically assessed in patients after an acute SCI.

The period of spinal shock was electrophysiologically associated with a reduced excitability of alpha-MN reflected by a low persistence of F-waves, which is in line with previous studies.[16,17] This observation may be related to the clinical signs found at this stage: the loss of tendon reflexes and muscle hypotonia. The neurophysiological basis of the reduced alpha-MN excitability may be the sudden loss of tonic input and/or trophic support from supraspinal to spinal neuronal centres. For instance, noradrenergic pathways were suggested to be responsible for the excitability level of alpha-motoneurons.[18] In view of other data on the effects of serotonin (5-hydroxytryptamine; 5-HT) on spinal motoneurons, both 5-HT and other descending pathways might be involved as well (review: Kiehn[19]).

The results of the electrophysiological measurements in humans fit well with the data obtained in animal cellular recordings, which show hyperpolarization of resting membrane potential.[12,20] In light of the close interaction between MN and muscle,[21] the initial reduction of M-wave amplitude[14] might be seen as a consequence of the changed MN behaviour.

In contrast to the neuronal depression reported above, H-reflexes could already be elicited at an early stage after SCI, which is in accordance with earlier reports.[10,14] The discrepancy between preserved H-reflex and the loss of tendon reflexes as a typical clinical sign might at least partially be due to a reduced activity of gamma-MN. However, one has to keep in mind that the level of fusimotor drive is not the only factor affecting muscle spindle responsiveness.[22]

Nevertheless, the early excitability of the H-reflex does not fit well with the assumption of an overall depression of neuronal activity including all motoneurons as a common final pathway of spinal neuronal activity. Several mechanisms could account for this discrepancy. First, the present observations are in line with the view described earlier for chronic paraplegic patients that presynaptic inhibition of group Ia afferents is, at least partially, removed after SCI.[23,24] Previous studies have shown a supraspinal influence on presynaptic inhibition of Ia afferents.[25] The decrease in presynaptic inhibition may compensate for the decreased excitability of alpha-MN. Consequently, early after SCI up to the spastic state a maximal H-reflex may be obtained which overrides the decreased excitability of alpha-MN assessed by F-waves. Second, one has to keep in mind that F-waves are caused by backfiring of only about 1% of motoneurons[26] and that H-reflex and F-wave were not investigated in the same muscle. Therefore, H-reflexes and F-waves may reflect the excitation of different populations of alpha-MN which only partially overlap, with the consequence that the excitability of the H-reflex does not parallel the persistence of the F-wave.

While H-reflex was present early and F-wave persistence was low (but usually F-waves could be recorded), there was a loss of flexor reflex activity in the TA early after SCI. The latter observation indicates a suppression of IN activity mediating this polysynaptic reflex (review: Lundberg[27]). However, we are aware that comparisons between the three types of responses have to be made with caution, as they were obtained (for physiological reasons) from different leg muscles.

TRANSITION PHASE

The recovery from spinal shock is reflected by an increase in the excitability of tendon tap reflexes and in muscle tone (assessed by the Ashworth scale) as well as more frequently occurring muscle spasms (assessed by the Penn spasm frequency scale).[7] These clinical changes were associated in the electrophysiological recordings by an increase of F-wave persistence and flexor reflex activity.[6] There was only a minor change in H-reflex excitability during this time period. It may be suggested that the increase in tendon tap reflex excitability is at least partially due to a recovery of alpha-MN and probably also of gamma-MN function mediating this reflex.

The increase in flexor reflex activity should be due not only to a recovery of alpha-MN excitability, but also to the function of spinal interneuronal circuits (see spinal shock). The fact that the flexor reflex is more difficult to elicit in healthy subjects than in paraplegic/tetraplegic patients[28] indicates an increased excitability of interneuronal circuits some weeks after SCI. The pathway underlying the flexor reflex is a polysynaptic spinal one and allows the integration of inputs from muscles, joints and cutaneous afferents on common interneurons (review: Kiehn[19]).

The changes in flexor reflex excitability may at least partly be reflected in the appearance of muscle spasms. The increase in muscle tone may be due to a more general recovery of spinal neuronal (alpha-MN and IN) activity. Nevertheless, for both clinical parameters reflecting recovery from spinal shock (Penn spasm frequency and Ashworth scale), it cannot be ruled out that other factors than the neuronal activity recorded here, as well as changes in muscle biomechanics, contribute to the development of spasticity.

SPASTIC STATE

Clinically, the development of the spastic syndrome is characterized by exaggerated muscle tendon tap reflexes, increased muscle tone and involuntary muscle contractions. The onset of spastic signs is difficult to determine because there is a smooth transition to a clearly established spasticity.

During this stage, both M-wave and flexor reflex amplitudes remained approximately stable in tetraplegic or decreased in amplitude in paraplegic patients, i.e. developed opposite to the clinical signs.[6] The latter observation was not due to a change in threshold, as the decrease in flexor reflex amplitude was the same with higher stimulation intensity (3 × instead of 2 × MT). The slight increase of H/M ratio, which is in line with an earlier study,[23] might contribute to exaggerated tendon tap reflexes. However, this increase, which was thought to be well correlated with the spastic state, must be considered cautiously: (1) the high H/M ratio can represent a decrease of M-wave (as found here) rather than an increase in reflex excitability; (2) short latency reflex hyperexcitability was shown to be little related to spastic muscle tone.[29]

The fact that the decrease of M-wave and flexor reflex amplitude was more pronounced in paraplegic than in tetraplegic patients indicates that several weeks after a SCI secondary degenerations of spinal tracts occur, including pre-motoneuronal circuits and alpha-MN. One may argue that some of the tetraplegic patients were sensory incomplete. However, there was no difference in flexor reflex amplitudes between sensory complete and incomplete, and chronic complete tetraplegic patients.

The decline of M-wave amplitude (i.e. loss of alpha-MN) was about equally distributed over all paraplegics, i.e. was little related to the decrease in flexor reflex excitability. Also, direct damage of alpha-MN as an underlying cause is rather unlikely, because M-wave amplitude increased up to the fourth week after SCI. Furthermore, entrapment of peripheral nerves could largely be excluded by electrophysiological examinations. Therefore, secondary degenerations are likely to depend on the level of the lesion, i.e. are less pronounced with a higher level of lesion.

On the basis of the observations made in the study of Hiersemenzel et al,[6] clinical signs of increasing spasticity, such as muscle tone and spasms, can hardly be related to the electrophysiological recordings. Secondary changes of motor units might contribute to the syndrome of spasticity, especially in respect of muscle tone and spasms.

Several studies claim that 'peripheral changes' (e.g. chronic transformation of muscle in spasticity) contribute to the increased muscle tone.[30,31] A decrease of M-wave in patients with a SCI[32] or those with a cerebral lesion[33] indicates an affection of spinal MN in the case of a disconnection from supraspinal input. Furthermore, signs of denervation are reported to occur during the first 2 months after SCI.[34] It has become obvious during recent years that, following a central motor lesion, changes in mechanical muscle fiber properties occur starting early after a lesion with the consequence of a significant contribution to muscle tone in the active (review: Dietz[35]) and passive muscles[36] (review: O'Dwyer and Ada[29]).

This study can only give a limited view of the neuronal adaptations occurring after a SCI. Spinal neuronal networks and reflex mechanisms may remain which were not assessed by our electrophysiological recordings. Therefore, the correlations made with the clinical signs have to remain to some extent speculative. Nevertheless, some of the results may be helpful for a better understanding of pathophysiological changes underlying spinal shock and the transition to the spastic syndrome with consequences for appropriate treatment.

CONCLUSIONS

Functional recovery from CNS injury may depend, in part, upon reorganization of undamaged neural pathways. Spinal cord circuits are capable of significant reorganization in the form of both activity-dependent and injury-induced plasticity. This plasticity is manifest behaviourally in the ability of spinal-injured animals to learn new locomotor tasks. Recent work with spinal-injured humans has demonstrated that training can improve functional locomotor abilities. New methodologies to enhance limb movement are designed to exploit further the plastic capabilities of the spinal cord by reinforcing appropriate connections in an activity-dependent manner.

Activity-dependent processes play a significant role in appropriate remodelling in CNS pathways such as in the visual system.[5,37] Thus, it is feasible that provision of appropriate patterns of activity within spinal cord circuits will assist in establishing functional connectivity between regenerating supraspinal axons and spinal neurons. Locomotor training, in combination wih appropriate physiological and pharmacological stimulation, can provide appropriate neural activity within spinal locomotor circuits and therefore has the potential to modify and refine the pattern of regenerating synaptic connections in an activity-dependent manner. Thus, the methods described for enhancing locomotor recovery after spinal injury in the absence of axonal regeneration might also play an important role in optimizing the functional contribution of regenerated spinal pathways.

Based on animal experiments, recent investigations have shown that the isolated human spinal cord contains neuronal centres which are able to generate complex movements. Nevertheless, the activation of these centres, with the aim of improving the mobility of paraplegic patients, is still limited.

After an acute SCI, basic changes in the spinal neuronal activity take place, which in part are associated with alterations of signs assessed by the clinical examination. The changes seen in the clinical signs from spinal shock to spasticity were shown to be only partially reflected by the neuronal correlates assessed by electrophysiological recordings, e.g. when increased muscle tone becomes established and muscle spasms appear. The divergent course of clinical signs of spasticity and the probable neuronal correlates indicates the occurrence of non-neuronal changes contributing to spasticity. However, one has to be aware that at present we are able to evaluate only a part of the spinal neuronal activity.

In complete paraplegic/tetraplegic patients, the level of lesion determines the locomotor activity in spinal-injured humans. The higher the level of spinal cord lesion, the more 'normal' is the locomotor pattern. This suggests that neuronal circuits underlying locomotor pattern generation extend from thoracolumbar to cervical levels. This observation may have important therapeutic implications in the future, when it might become possible to induce some regeneration of spinal tract fibres.

ACKNOWLEDGEMENT

This work was supported by the International Institute for Research on Paraplegia (P49/99) and the Swiss National Research Foundation (No. 31–53526.98).

REFERENCES

1. Dimitrijevic MR. Residual motor functions in spinal cord injury. *Adv Neurol* 1988; **47**: 138–155.
2. Muir GD, Steeves JD. Sensorimotor stimulation to improve locomotor recovery after spinal cord injury. *Trends Neurosci* 1997; **20**: 72–77.
3. Helgren ME, Goldberger ME. The recovery of postural reflexes and locomotion following low thoracic hemisection in adult cats involves compensation by undamaged primary afferent pathways. *Exp Neurol* 1993; **12**: 17–34.
4. Goldberger ME, Murray M. Patterns of sprouting and implications for recovery of function. *Adv Neurol* 1988; **47**: 361–385.
5. Goodman CS, Shatz CJ. Developmental mechanisms that generate precise patterns of neuronal connectivity. *Cell* 1993; **72**: 77–98.
6. Hiersemenzel LP, Curt A, Dietz V. From spinal shock to spasticity: neuronal adaptation to a spinal cord injury. *Neurology* 2000; **54**: 1574–1582.
7. Priebe MM, Sherwood AM, Thomby JL, Kharas NF, Markowski J. Clinical assessment of spasticity in spinal cord injury: a multidimensional problem. *Arch Phys Med Rehab* 1996; **77**: 713–716.
8. Bastian HC. On the symptomatology of total transverse lesions of the spinal cord, with special reference to the condition of the various reflexes. *Med Chir Trans (Lond)* 1890; **73**: 151–217.
9. Kuhn R. Functional capacity of isolated human spinal cord. *Brain* 1950; **73**: 1–51.
10. Diamantopoulos E. Excitability of motor neurones in spinal shock in man. *J Neurol Neurosurg Psychiatry* 1967; **30**: 427–431.
11. Ashby P, Verrier M, Lightfoot E. Segmental reflex pathways in spinal shock and spinal spasticity in man. *J Neurol Neurosurg Psychiatry* 1974; **37**: 1352–1360.
12. Schadt JC, Barnes CD. Motoneuron membrane changes associated with spinal shock and the Schiff–Sherrington phenomenon. *Brain Res* 1980; **201**: 373–383.
13. Leis AA, Zhou HH, Mehta M, Harkey HL, Paske WC. Behavior of the H-reflex in humans following mechanical perturbation or injury to rostral spinal cord. *Muscle Nerve* 1996; **19**: 1373–1382.
14. Weaver R, Landau W, Higgins J. Fusimotor function. Part 2: Evidence of fusimotor depression in human spinal shock. *Arch Neurol* 1963; **9**: 127–132.
15. Baldissera F, Hultborn H, Illert M. Integration in spinal neuronal system. In: *Handbook of Physiology. The Nervous System, Motor Control*, Section 1, Vol. 2, part 1. Washington, DC: American Physiological Society, 1981: 509–595.
16. Leis AA, Stetkarova I, Beric A, Stokic DS. The relative sensitivity of F wave and H reflex to changes in motoneuronal excitability. *Muscle Nerve* 1996; **19**: 1342–1344.
17. Curt A, Keck ME, Dietz V. Clinical value of F-wave recordings in traumatic cervical spinal cord injury. *Electroencephalogr Clin Neurophysiol* 1997; **105**: 189–193.
18. Grillner S. Interaction between sensory signals and the central networks controlling locomotion, in lamprey, dogfish and cat. In: Grillner S, Stein PSG, Stuart DG, Forssberg H, Herman RM, eds. *Neurobiology of Vertebrate Locomotion*. Wenner-Gren International Symposium Series, Vol. 45. London: Macmillan, 1986: 505–512.

19. Kiehn O. Plateau potentials and active integration in the 'final common pathway' for motor behaviour. *Trends Neurosci* 1991; **14**: 68–73.

20. Barnes C, Joynt R, Schottelius B. Motoneuron resting potential in spinal shock. *Am J Physiol* 1962; **203**: 1113–1116.

21. Buller AJ, Eccles JC, Eccles RM. Interactions between motoneurones and muscles in respect of the characteristic speeds of their responses. *J Physiol (Lond)* 1960; **150**: 417–439.

22. Burke D. Critical examination of the case for or against fusimotor involvement in disorders of muscle tone. *Adv Neurol* 1983; **39**: 133–150.

23. Faist M, Mazevet D, Dietz V, Pierrot-Deseilligny E. A quantitative assessment of presynaptic inhibition of Ia afferents in spastics. Differences in hemiplegics and paraplegics. *Brain* 1997; **117**: 1449–1455.

24. Yang JF, Stein RB. Phase-dependent reflex reversal in human leg muscles during walking. *J Neurophysiol* 1990; **63**: 1109–1117.

25. Meunier S, Pierrot-Deseilligny E. Cortical control of presynaptic inhibition of Ia afferents in humans. *Exp Brain Res* 1998; **119**: 415–426.

26. Dengler R, Kossev A, Wohlfahrt K, Schubert M, Elek J, Wolf W. F-waves and motor unit size. *Muscle Nerve* 1992; **15**: 1138–1142.

27. Lundberg A. Multisensory control of spinal reflex pathways. *Prog Brain Res* 1979; **50**: 12–28.

28. Shahani BT, Young RR. Human flexor reflexes. *J Neurol Neurosurg Psychiatry* 1971; **34**: 616–627.

29. O'Dwyer NJ, Ada L. Reflex hyperexcitability and muscle contracture in relation to spastic hypertonia. *Curr Opin Neurol* 1996; **9**: 451–455.

30. Dietz V, Quintern J, Berger W. Electrophysiological studies of gait in spasticity. Evidence that altered mechanical properties of muscle contribute to hypertonia. *Brain* 1981; **104**: 431–449.

31. Edström L. Selective changes in the sizes of red and white muscle fibres in upper motor lesions and Parkinsonism. *J Neurol Sci* 1970; **11**: 537–550.

32. Taylor S, Ashby P, Verrier M. Neurophysiological changes following traumatic spinal lesions in man. *J Neurol Neurosurg Psychiatry* 1984; **47**: 1102–1108.

33. Fisher MA. F/M ratios in polyneuropathy and spastic hyperreflexia. *Muscle Nerve* 1988; **11**: 217–222.

34. Aisen ML, Brown W, Rubin M. Electrophysiologic changes in lumbar spinal cord after cervical cord injury. *Neurology* 1992; **42**: 623–626.

35. Dietz V. Neurophysiology of gait disorders: present and future applications. *Electroencephalogr Clin. Neurophysiol* 1997; **103**: 333–355.

36. Ibrahim IK, Berger W, Trippel M, Dietz V. Stretch-induced electromyographic activity and torque in spastic elbow muscles. Differential modulation of reflex activity in passive and active motor tasks. *Brain* 1993; **116**: 971–989.

37. Constantine-Paton M, Cline HT, Debski E. Patterned activity, synaptic convergence, and the NMDA receptor in developing visual pathways. *Annu Rev Neurosci* 1990; **13**: 129–154.

45

Pathophysiology and treatment of fatigue in multiple sclerosis

Giancarlo Comi, Letizia Leocani, Bruno Colombo and Paolo Rossi

INTRODUCTION

Fatigue is a common symptom in medicine. It is a frequent complaint of patients with infectious disorders, tumors, systemic diseases, depression and dysfunctions of the motor system. The occurrence of fatigue in such different disorders is partially explained by the fact that the term fatigue has been utilized to describe various physical and psychological conditions. Fatigue is a highly subjective and non-specific symptom which can be easily confused with weakness on the one hand and with depressed mood on the other. The fact that in some disorders, such as multiple sclerosis (MS), fatigue may be associated with motor disturbances and/or mood disorders makes it very difficult, and sometimes impossible, to define whether fatigue is an aspect of these complications or a complication per se. This chapter reviews the main aspects of fatigue in MS, and its pathophysiology and management.

DEFINITION

Fatigue is an overwhelming sense of tiredness, lack of energy, or feeling of exhaustion. It can be independent of both depressed mood and weakness. Fatigue is frequently already present at rest. The patient has the feeling that the effort required to perform a given action is disproportionately high.[1] As a consequence, patients tend to reduce their physical activity, even if the beneficial effects of rest are usually modest. Fatigue is usually predominant in the second part of the day and is worsened by stress. This condition must be distinguished from fatigability. Fatigability is a generalized sensation of exhaustion, not present at rest, affecting the patient after a few minutes of physical activity, that disappears after a short rest. Both fatigue and fatigability affect MS patients, and sometimes they are associated in the same patient.

The pathophysiology of the two disturbances is probably different: fatigability affects predominantly the lower limbs and is invariably associated with clinical or subclinical involvement of the motor pathways.

Fatigue is a common symptom in MS patients, being present in about one-third of patients,[2–4] and for many of them fatigue is the more disabling symptom.[5]. However, this high prevalence is influenced by the frequent occurrence in MS patients of motor problems, painful syndromes and mood abnormalities.[6] Fatigue may occur at any stage of MS, even if it is more frequent and severe in primary and secondary progressive patients than in relapsing remitting patients.[7,8] Occasionally, fatigue may be the onset symptom of MS and may occur weeks or months before the first attack. Fatigue may be a transient phenomenon, frequently associated with or preceding clinical relapses,[9,10] or chronic, being present all the time. It is unclear whether transitory and chronic fatigue are different types of fatigue or if they share a common pathophysiology. There is no clear correlation between disability and fatigue in MS; nevertheless, fatigue has a tremendous impact on the activities of daily living, interfering with work, family life and social activities.

Many factors may influence fatigue in MS. Heat worsens fatigue, while cold relieves the condition. The effect of increased body temperature is explained by the instability of the nervous conduction in partially demyelinated fibers: the increase of body temperature causes a conduction block at the level of the Ranvier's nodes, with a reduced density of sodium channels, and a consequent deterioration of neurological functions. Depression affects about 20% of MS patients, and, if present, may negatively influence fatigue.[6] Pain affects about 40% of MS patients; it correlates with fatigue in a number of chronic disorders, so we can expect a similar negative impact in

Table 45.1 Principal fatigue scales[45]		
Name of scale	Dimensions	No. of items
	Multidimensional	
Modified Fatigue Impact Scale (MFIS)	Cognitive, psychosocial, physical	21
Multidimensional Assessment of Fatigue (MAF)	Severity, timing, distress, interference	16
Multidimensional Fatigue Inventory (MFI)	General activity, mental, physical, motivation	24
Fatigue Scale (FS)	Physical, mental	14
	Unidimensional	
Fatigue Severity Scale (FSS)	Severity on daily living	9
Functional Assessment of Multiple Sclerosis (FAMS)	Tiredness-thinking subscale	9
Rand Index of Vitality (RIV)	Vitality	4

MS. The relationship between sleep disorders and fatigue is controversial. Most MS patients with fatigue complain of sleep abnormalities, but polygraphic studies have shown that the median sleep latency is normal and fatigue is not associated with nocturnal hypoxia or breathing-associated sleep fragmentations.[11] There are some objective, physiological measures of fatigue, which will be described later. There are reasonable doubts about whether these instrumental tests really do measure the phenomenon described by patients. Fatigue is a subjective experience, which is why self-report instruments are probably more appropriate to quantify the phenomenon, even if they have obvious limitations. Multidimensional scales (Table 45.1) allow the evaluation of different characteristics of fatigue. The most frequently used are the Multidimensional Assessment of Fatigue (MAF), developed for patients with rheumatoid arthritis and recently used in MS patients,[12] the Fatigue Assessment Instrument (FAI), which identifies both severity and situation-specific factors,[13] and the Modified Fatigue Impact Scale (MFIS), with 21 items, including cognitive, psychosocial and physical dimensions.[5] The Fatigue Severity Scale is the most utilized unidimensional scale: it measures the impact of fatigue in daily living.[8] It is very easy to administer and has been used in clinical trials.[14,15] The longitudinal utilization of these scales is not fully validated; in particular, some intrinsic characteristics of these scales, like proportionality and responsiveness, have not been defined.

According to Bigland-Ritchie et al,[16] the physiological definition of fatigue is 'the inability of a muscle or group of muscles to sustain the required or expected force'. It may occur because of a loss of force-generating capacity within the muscle itself (peripheral fatigue), or because of an inability to sustain the central drive to spinal motoneurons (central fatigue). The phenomenon of fatigue can be studied with various tools. Neurophysiologically, fatigue can be quantified by the curve that expresses the change of force over time, both to a maximal voluntary contraction and to maximal repetitive electrical stimulation. During maximal voluntary contraction, as the amount of force declines, the frequency of motor unit potentials on electromyography (EMG) decreases,[17] and the changes can be objectified by the spectral EMG analysis. Finally, metabolic changes in the muscle during activation (voluntary or stimulated) can be studied using nuclear magnetic resonance spectroscopy (NMRS).

MS patients frequently complain of marked difficulties in mental performance: a recent psychometric study suggests that mental fatigue does really occur. Elkin et al[18] submitted a group of patients to a battery of cognitive tests and found a striking decline on measures of memory and conceptual thinking across the testing session, whereas the control group continued to improve with practice. It would be interesting to see if these changes are associated with a subjective complaint of fatigue.

PATHOGENESIS

The ability to produce and maintain a given level of exercise requires an increase in heart and respiratory rate and a 20-fold increase in bloodflow to the muscle; the muscles must have normal metabolic activity and normal elastic properties. There is some evidence that peripheral abnormalities may

Table 45.2 Median (range) values of central motor conduction time (CMCT) in fatigable (F) and non-fatigable (NF) patients[26]

CMCT	F	NF	P
Right upper limb	6.4 (5.3–19.4)	6.6 (5.5–7.9)	NS
Left upper limb	6.7 (5.3–12.3)	6.8 (5.5–7.7)	NS
Right lower limb	16 (12.1–31.7)	15 (11.2–16.3)	NS
Left lower limb	16.6 (11.1–26)	14.8 (13–21.4)	NS

NS, not significant.

contribute to produce fatigue in MS. MS patients complaining of fatigue show a significant decline of maximal voluntary force during exercise compared to normal controls and patients affected by chronic fatigue syndrome.[19,20] Miller et al.[20] found in MS patients complaining of fatigue a decline of muscle force during repetitive peripheral nerve stimulation. Lenman et al.[21] assessed fatigue of the tibialis anterior muscle by repetitive electrical stimulation and found a decrease in muscle tension and an increase in the half-relaxation time during repetitive activity in MS patients compared to controls. They explained the observed changes as being due to a transformation of fatigue-resistant fibers into fatigable ones. NMRS confirmed the existence of peripheral components of the fatigue in MS: intramuscular phosphocreatine resynthesis following exercise is slowed in MS patients, probably as a consequence of disuse and deconditioning.[22]

Even if peripheral mechanisms may have some role in the pathogenesis of fatigue in MS there are clear indications that the most important role is played by 'central abnormalities'.[23] A very simple explanation is that impaired conduction along central motor pathways due to demyelination and secondary axonal degeneration may lead to a reduced recruitment of spinal motor units or to inability to drive the motoneuron pool at sufficient rates to generate full tetanic force.[24] The observation that, in MS patients with fatigue, the decrease of force over time is significantly higher in the presence of pyramidal signs[19] supports the involvement of corticospinal tracts. However, objective fatigue is not associated with a central motor conduction slowing[23,25,26] (Table 45.2). Brasil-Neto et al.[27,28] reported transient decreases of motor evoked potential (MEP) amplitude after exercise and a post-exercise decrement from the first to the fourth MEP amplitude during repetitive transcranial magnetic stimulation (rTMS). Galardi et al.[29] performed rTMS in a group of patients complaining of fatigue and in a control group: the amplitude of the MEP was significantly lower in MS patients, but the decrement during exercise and post-exercise was the same in patients with and without fatigue. The results of this study again indicate that a progressive conduction failure of large-diameter, fast-conducting pyramidal fibers activated by rTMS does not occur and cannot explain the phenomenon of fatigue in MS. There is the possibility that central fatigue may have developed in cortical pathways rostral to the pyramidal tract. Sandroni et al.[25] found that reaction times accompanying the performance of auditory memory tasks significantly increased when MS patients were fatigued, compared to the rest condition. Interestingly, both P300 latency and central motor conduction time were not significantly increased by fatigue, suggesting that fatigue affects neural processes acting before activation of the primary motor cortex. An impairment of volitional drive to the descending motor pathways has also been suggested to explain 'normal' central fatigue[30] and the chronic fatigue syndromes.[31] Possible mechanisms for the withdrawal of volitional drive include the involvement of demyelinating lesions[30] in pathways directing the motor cortex or in the facilitatory afferent pathways. Feedback from both muscular and cutaneous afferents influences motor drive, either at the spinal or supraspinal level. Colombo et al.[26] found that the T2 lesion load in magnetic resonance imaging of the brain was significantly higher in MS patients complaining of fatigue compared to MS patients not complaining of fatigue, the two groups being matched for age, sex, duration of disease, disability and pyramidal functional system score (Table 45.3). Moreover, the T2 lesion load correlated significantly with the Fatigue Severity Scale score. Roecke et al[33] in a PET-FDG study, found a significant

Table 45.3 Brain MRI lesion loads in fatigable (F) and non fatigable (NF) MS patients[26]		
	F	NF
Frontal lobe	6 (0–21)	1 (0–30)
Parietal lobe	2 (0–24)*	0 (0–3)
Temporal lobe	0 (0–4)	0 (0–2)
Internal capsule	0 (0–7)*	0 (0–2)
Basal ganglia	0 (0–4)	0 (0–02)
Periventricular	20 (3–46)	14 (4–53)
Trigone	4 (0–10)*	1 (0–8)
Total	32 (5–82)	22 (6–60)

*$P < 0.05$ or better.

reduction of metabolic activity, bilaterally in the lateral and medial prefrontal cortex, in the premotor cortex and putamen, and in the right supplementary motor area. These very interesting results clearly indicate that frontal cortex and basal ganglia play a role in MS fatigue.

Immune factors could also contribute to fatigue. In both human and animal studies, some cytokines, like tumor necrosis factor alpha and interleukin-1, have been associated with fatigue.[34,35] Patients treated with β-interferons frequently complain of fatigue, particularly in the first weeks of therapy. However, in a recent short-term longitudinal study, Mainero et al[36] using triple-dose delayed scans, did not find any correlation between brain MRI activity and fatigue in a group of 11 relapsing–remitting MS patients.

TREATMENT

Management of fatigue is a complex and difficult task, because multiple factors, variably combined in MS patients, may contribute to produce the symptom. The first step is to inform the patient and the family that the symptom is genuine. The recognition of the physical nature of the phenomenon is important, particularly when fatigue is not associated with other major symptoms and signs. The self-esteem of the patient is enhanced when they are informed that the sense of exhaustion does not depend on a psychological reaction to the disease, but, on the contrary, is due to the nervous tissue damage produced by the disease. Management strategies include medications, exercise, and behav-

ioral therapy; in most cases, a combined approach is suitable.

Exercise

Exercise is important to contrast deconditioning. Exercise programs must be individualized, because overexertion may be detrimental. For the same reason, the workload during the day should be carefully distributed, with adequate rest periods. Excessive physical activity is not tolerated, because of the easy exhaustion and the negative effects of even a small increase in body temperature. Working or living in warm environments can be intolerable for some patients: in hot climates, air-conditioning is very important. The positive effects of graded exercises on fatigue are more relevant in patients with weakness and spasticity. In these MS patients, a 1-year multidisciplinary rehabilitation program was found to significantly reduce fatigue.[37] In another study, 54 patients were randomly assigned to 15 weeks of aerobic exercise or non-exercise. Patients who underwent aerobic exercise had a significant reduction of fatigue and an improvement of quality of life.[38]

Behavioral therapy

Behavioral therapy is useful in patients with fatigue and associated mood disorders, as demonstrated by the positive results obtained in patients with chronic fatigue syndrome.[39,40] We can expect that MS patients may also benefit from this therapy, but controlled studies are lacking.

Medication

A certain number of medications are utilized in the management of fatigue, sometimes with a poor rationale. Most of the clinical trials have been uncontrolled, involved a small number of patients and have been too short. In the clinical setting, the response to drugs is quite variable from patient to patient.

The most widely used drug is amantadine. It is a synthetic chemical originally introduced to treat infections and later found to be beneficial in Parkinson's disease, probably by promoting the release of dopamine. In a Canadian multicenter placebo-controlled trial,[41] amantadine, 100 mg twice daily, significantly improved fatigue. Amantadine is relatively safe in long-term use; confusion and urinary retention occur seldom and predominantly in the elderly.

Pemoline is a central nervous system stimulant, used in attentional deficit disorders in children. It has been used to treat fatigue in MS, without evidence of physical or psychological dependence. A placebo-controlled study[42] failed to demonstrate significant effects of pemoline, although a trend was observed; moreover, poorly tolerated side-effects occurred in 25% of the patients. In a placebo-controlled randomized study, pemoline was compared to amantadine and placebo;[14] again, only a positive trend was found for pemoline, while amantadine showed a benefit over placebo in some fatigue measures. As a consequence, pemoline has to be considered as second-line therapy. The range of the doses used varied between 18.75 mg and 56.25 mg. Nervousness, insomnia and anxiety may occur at the highest doses. Other stimulants, such as methylphenidate and dextroamphetamine, have been anecdotally reported to be effective.

A totally different therapeutic approach is based on the restoration of nerve conduction in partially demyelinated fibers undergoing conduction block. The potassium channel blocker 4-aminopyridine showed clear benefit for fatigue.[43] An open pilot study with 3,4–aminopyridine performed in eight MS patients complaining of fatigue showed a subjective improvement in six, but no changes were observed in nerve conduction.[44]

Especially in patients with associated fatigue and depression, treatment with antidepressants may be useful. Fluoxetine and other selective serotonin reuptake inhibitors are preferable to other antidepressant agents, because they produce less sedation and less anticholinergic effects.

Patients with fatigue and sleep disorders require specific interventions to correct sleep abnormalities. The use of benzodiazepines for insomnia may have advantages; however, high doses should be avoided because they can increase fatigue.

REFERENCES

1. Krupp LB, Pollina DA. Measurement and management of fatigue in progressive neurological disorders. *Curr Opin Neurol* 1996; **9**: 456–460.
2. Freal JE, Kraft GH, Coryell JK. Symptomatic fatigue in multiple sclerosis. *Arch Phys Med Rehabil* 1984; **65**: 135–138.
3. Krupp LB, Alvarez LA, La Rocca NG, Scheinberg LC. Fatigue in multiple sclerosis. *Arch Neurol* 1988; **45**: 435–437.
4. Vercoulen JH, Hommes OR, Swanink CM et al. The measurement of fatigue in patients with multiple sclerosis. A multidimensional comparison with patients with chronic fatigue syndrome and healthy subjects. *Arch Neurol* 1996; **53**(7): 642–649.
5. Fisk JD, Pontefract A, Ritvo PG et al. The impact of fatigue in patient with multiple sclerosis. *Can J Neurol Sci* 1994; **21**: 9–14.
6. Schwartz CE, Coulthard Morris L, Zeng Q. Psychosocial correlates of fatigue in multiple sclerosis. *Arch Phys Med Rehabil* 1996; **77**(2): 165–170.
7. Bergamaschi R, Romani V, Versino M et al. Clinical aspects of fatigue in multiple sclerosis. *Funct Neurol* 1997; **12**: 247–251.
8. Krupp LB, La Rocca NG, Muir-Nash J, Steinberg AD. The Fatigue Severity Scale. Application to patients with multiple sclerosis and systemic lupus erythematosus. *Arch Neurol* 1989; **46**: 1121–1123.
9. Geisser B. Multiple sclerosis: current concepts in management. *Drugs* 1985; **29**: 88–95.
10. Murray TJ. Amantadine therapy for fatigue in multiple sclerosis. *Can J Neurol Sci* 1985; **12**: 251–254.
11. Bohr KC, Haas J. Sleep related breathing disorders do not explain daytime fatigue in multiple sclerosis. *Multiple Sclerosis* 1988; **4**: 289a.
12. Elza BL, Henke CJ, Yelin EH et al. Correlates of fatigue in older women with rheumatoid arthritis. *Nurs Res* 1993; **42**: 93–99.
13. Vercoluen JHMM, Swanink CMA, Fennis JFM et al. Dimensional assessment of chronic fatigue syndrome. *J Psychosom Res* 1994; **38**: 383–392.
14. Krupp LB, Coyle PK, Doscher C et al. Fatigue therapy in multiple sclerosis: results of a double blind randomized parallel trial of amantadine, pemoline and placebo. *Neurology* 1995; **45**: 1956–1961.
15. Cookfair DL, Fischer J, Rudick R et al. Fatigue severity in low disability MS patients participating in a phase III trial of Avonex for relapsing remitting multiple sclerosis. *Neurology* 1997; **48**: 173a.
16. Bigland-Ritchie B, Jones DA, Hosking GP et al. Central and peripheral fatigue in sustained maximum voluntary contraction of human quadriceps muscle. *Clin Sci Mol Med* 1978; **54**: 609–614.
17. Edwards RHT. Human muscle function and fatigue. In: *Human Muscle Fatigue: Physiological Mechanisms. CIBA Foundation Symposium 82*. London: Pittman Medical, 1981: 1–18.
18. Elkin LE, Pollina DA, Scheffer SR, Krupp LB. *Neurology* 1998; **50**(suppl): 126a.
19. Djaidetti R, Ziv I, Achiron A, Melamed E. Fatigue in multiple sclerosis compared with chronic fatigue syndrome: a quantitative assessment. *Neurology* 1996; **46**: 632–635.
20. Miller RG, Green AT, Moussavi RS et al. Excessive muscular fatigue in patients with spastic paraparesis. *Neurology* 1990; **40**: 1271–1274.
21. Lenman A, Tulley FM, Vrbova G et al. Muscle fatigue in some neurological disorders. *Muscle Nerve* 1989; **12**: 938–942.
22. Kent-Braun JA, Sharma KR, Weiner MW, Miller RG. Effects of exercise on muscle activation and metabolism in multiple sclerosis. *Muscle Nerve* 1994; **17**: 1162–1169.
23. Sheean GL, Murray NMF, Rothwell JC, Miller DH, Thompson AJ. An electrophysiological study of the mechanism of fatigue in multiple sclerosis. *Brain* 1997; **120**: 299–315.
24. Rice CL, Vollmer TL, Bigland-Ritchie B. Nueromuscular responses of patients with multiple sclerosis. *Muscle Nerve* 1992; **15**: 1123–1132.

25. Sandroni P, Walker C, Starr A. Fatigue in patients with multiple sclerosis. Motor pathway conduction and event-related potentials. *Arch Neurol* 1992; **49**: 517–524.

26. Colombo B, Boneschi FM, Rossi P et al. MRI and motor evoked potentials findings in non-disabled multiple sclerosis patients with and without symptoms of fatigue. *J Neurol* 2000; **247**: 506–509.

27. Brasil-Neto JP, Pascual Leone A, Valls-Sole J et al. Postexercise depression of motor evoked potentials: a measure of central nervous system fatigue. *Exp Brain Res* 1993; **93**: 181–184.

28. Brasil-Neto JP, Cohen LG, Hallet M. Central fatigue as revealed by postexercise decrement of motor evoked potentials. *Muscle Nerve* 1994; **17**: 713–719.

29. Galardi L, Maderna S, Amadio S et al. Assessment of central fatigue by transcranial magnetic stimulation in multiple sclerosis patients. In: Hermes HJ, Merletti R, Freriks B, eds. *European Activities on Surface Electromyography*, Proceedings of the 1st SENIAM Workshop, Torino 1996: 127–129.

30. Gandevia SC, Allen GM, Butler GE, Taylor JL. Supraspinal factors in human muscle fatigue: evidence for suboptimal output from the motor cortex. *J Physiol* 1996; **490**: 529–536.

31. Lloyd AR, Gandevia SC, Hales JP. Muscle performance, voluntary activation, twitch properties and perceived effort in normal subjects and patients with the chronic fatigue syndrome. *Brain* 1991; **114**: 85–98.

32. Gandevia SC, Macefield G, Burke D, McKenzie DK. Voluntary activation of human motor axons in the absence of muscle afferent feedback. The control of deafferented hand. *Brain* 1990; **113**: 1563–1581.

33. Roecke U, Kappos L, Lechner-Scott J et al. Reduced glucose metabolism in the frontal cortex and basal ganglia of multiple sclerosis patients with fatigue. *Neurology* 1997; **48**: 1566–1571.

34. Bertolone K, Coyle PK, Krupp LB et al. Cytokine correlates of fatigue in multiple sclerosis. *Neurology* 1993; **43**: A356.

35. Chao CC, DeLa Hunt M, Hu S et al. Immunologically mediated fatigue: a murine model. *Clin Immunopathol* 1992; **64**: 161–165.

36. Mainero C, Faroni J, Gasperini C et al. Fatigue and magnetic resonance imaging activity in multiple sclerosis. *J Neurol* 1999; **246**(6): 454–458.

37. Heilman KM, Watson RT. Fatigue. *Neurol Net Comm* 1997; **1**: 283–287.

38. Di Fabio RP, Sodeberg I, Choi T et al. Extended outpatient rehabilitation: its influence on symptom frequency, fatigue and functional status for persons with progressive multiple sclerosis. *Arch Phys Med Rehabil* 1998; **79**: 141–146.

39. Deale AM, Chalder T, Marks I, Wessely S. Cognitive behaviour therapy for chronic fatigue syndrome: a randomized controlled trial. *Am J Psychiatry* 1997; **54**: 408–414.

40. Butler S, Chalder T, Ron M, Wessely S. Cognitive behaviour therapy in CFS. *J Neurol Neurosurg Psychiatry* 1991; **54**: 153–158.

41. Canadian MS Research Group. A randomized controlled trial of amantadine in fatigue associated with multiple sclerosis. *Can J Neurol Sci* 1987; **14**: 273–278.

42. Wheinshenker BG, Penman M, Bass B. A double-blind randomized crossover trial of pemoline in fatigue associated with multiple sclerosis. *Neurology* 1992; **42**: 1468–1471.

43. Van Diemen HAM, Polman CH, von Dangen JMMM et al. The effects of 4-amino pyridine on clinical signs in multiple sclerosis: a randomised, placebo-controlled, double-blind crossover study. *Ann Neurol* 1992; **32**: 123–130.

44. Sheean G, Murray N, Rotwell J et al. An open label clinical and electrophysiological study of 3,4-diaminopyridine in the treatment of fatigue in multiple sclerosis. *Brain* 1998; **121**: 967–975.

45. Krupp LB. Treatment of fatigue in multiple sclerosis. In: Rudick A, Goodkin E, eds. *Multiple Sclerosis Therapeutics*. Martin Dunitz, 1999: 467–474.

46

Management of vertigo and vestibular disorders

Thomas Brandt

Vestibular syndromes are commonly characterized by a combination of phenomena involving perceived vertigo, nystagmus, ataxia, and nausea.[1] These four manifestations correlate with different aspects of vestibular function and emanate from different sites within the central nervous system.

- The vertigo itself results from a disturbance of cortical spatial orientation.
- Nystagmus is secondary to a direction-specific imbalance in the vestibulo-ocular reflex, which activates brainstem ocular motor neuronal circuitry.
- Vestibular ataxia and postural imbalance are caused by inappropriate or abnormal activation of mono- and polysynaptic vestibulospinal pathways.
- The unpleasant autonomic responses with nausea, vomiting and anxiety travel along ascending (anxiety) and descending vestibulo-autonomic pathways to activate the medullary vomiting center.

Vertigo, dizziness and disequilibrium are common complaints of patients of all ages, particularly the elderly. As presenting symptoms, they occur in 5–10% of all patients seen by general practitioners and 10–20% of all patients seen by neurologists and otolaryngologists. The clinical spectrum of vertigo is broad, extending from vestibular rotatory vertigo with nausea and vomiting to presyncope light-headedness, from drug intoxication to hypoglycemic dizziness, from visual vertigo to phobias and panic attacks, and from motion sickness to height vertigo. Appropriate preventions and treatments differ for different types of dizziness and vertigo.

The prevailing good prognosis of vertigo should be emphasized, because:

(1) many forms of vertigo have a benign cause and are characterized by spontaneous recovery of vestibular function or central compensation of a peripheral vestibular tone imbalance

(2) most forms of vertigo can be effectively relieved by pharmacological treatment (Table 46.1), physical therapy (Table 46.2), surgery (Table 46.3), or psychotherapy.[1]

Table 46.1   Pharmacological therapies for vertigo

Therapy	Vertigo
Vestibular suppressants	Symptomatic relief of nausea (in acute peripheral and vestibular nuclei lesions), prevention of motion sickness
Antiepileptic drugs	Vestibular epilepsy, vestibular paroxysmia (disabling positional vertigo), paroxysmal dysarthria and ataxia in multiple sclerosis, other central vestibular paroxysms, superior oblique myokymia
β-Receptor blockers	Basilar migraine (vestibular migraine; benign recurrent vertigo)
Betahistine	Menière's disease
Antibiotics	Infections of the ear and temporal bone
Ototoxic antibiotics	Menière's disease (Menière's drop attacks)
Corticosteroids	Vestibular neuritis, autoimmune inner ear disease
Baclofen	Downbeat or upbeat nystagmus or vertigo
Acetazolamide	Familial periodic ataxia or vertigo

Table 46.2	Physical therapies for vertigo
Therapy	**Vertigo**
Deliberate maneuvers	Benign paroxysmal positioning vertigo
Vestibular exercises	Vestibular rehabilitation, central compensation of acute vestibular loss, habituation for prevention of motion sickness, improvement of balance skills (e.g. in the elderly)
Physical therapy (neck collar)	Cervical vertigo (fiction or reality?)

There is, however, no common treatment, and vestibular suppressants (Table 46.4) provide only symptomatic relief of vertigo and nausea. A specific therapeutic approach thus requires recognition of the various particular pathomechanisms involved.[1–3] Such therapy can include causative, symptomatic or preventive approaches.

ANTIVERTIGINOUS AND ANTIEMETIC DRUGS

A variety of drugs used for symptomatic relief of vertigo and nausea (Table 46.4) have the major side-effect of general sedation.[4] Vestibular suppressants, including anticholinergics, antihistamines, and benzodiazepines, provide symptomatic relief of distressing symptoms by downregulating vestibular excitability. Antiemetics preferably control nausea and vomiting by acting on the medullary vomiting center, the chemoreceptor trigger zone, or the gastrointestinal tract itself. Vestibular suppressants are often acetylcholine and histamine antagonists, which act as acetylcholine antagonists by competitive inhibition at muscarinic receptors in the vestibular nuclei, their most likely site of action. Vestibular suppression by benzodiazepines is best explained by their $GABA_A$ agonistic effect, because GABA is the major neuroinhibitory transmitter for vestibular neurons. Antiemetics are effective mainly because of their dopamine (D_2) antagonist properties, but some antiemetics also have muscarinergic or antihistaminic (H_1) properties that may assist in vestibular suppression as well. Primary vestibular suppressants such as scopolamine also effectively suppress vomiting by virtue of their muscarinergic action. Antiemetics are more selective in action. They are primarily used to control nausea and vomiting; for treatment of severe vertigo with nausea, they are often combined with antivertiginous drugs.[4]

There are only four clear indications for the use of antivertiginous (vestibular suppressants) and antiemetic drugs to control vertigo, nausea, and vomiting:

(1) to prevent nausea due to acute peripheral vestibulopathy (for the first 1–3 days or as long as nausea lasts)
(2) to prevent severe vertigo and nausea due to acute brainstem or archicerebellar lesions near the vestibular nuclei
(3) to prevent severe vertigo attacks recurring on a frequent basis
(4) to prevent motion sickness.

For the first two of these conditions, fast-acting compounds with vestibular and general sedation

Table 46.3	Surgical interventions for vertigo
Surgery	**Causes of vertigo**
Surgical decompression of eighth nerve	Tumor (acoustic neurinoma) or cyst
Neurovascular decompression	Vestibular paroxysmia (disabling positional vertigo)
Ampullary nerve section or canal plugging	Benign paroxysmal positioning vertigo
Endolymphatic shunt	Menière's disease
Vestibular nerve section or labyrinthectomy	Intractable Menière's disease
Surgical patching	Perilymph fistula
Surgical decompression of vertebral artery	Rotational vertebral artery occlusion

Table 46.4   Commonly used antivertiginous and antiemetic drugs

Drug	Dosage	Action
Anticholinergics		Muscarine antagonist
Scopolamine	0.6 mg p.o. every 4–6 h or	
(Transderm Scop)	transdermal patch: 1 every 3 days	
Antihistamines		
Dimenhydrinate	50 mg p.o. every 4–6 h or	Histamine (H$_1$) antagonist
(Dramamine)	i.m. every 4–6 h or	Muscarine antagonist
	100 mg suppository every 8–10 h	
Meclizine	25 mg p.o. every 4–6 h	Histamine (H$_1$) antagonist
(Antivert, Bonine)		Muscarine antagonist
Promethazine	15 or 50 mg p.o. every 4–6 h or	Histamine (H$_1$) antagonist
(Phenergan)	i.m. every 4–6 h or	Muscarine antagonist
	suppository every 4–6 h	Dopamine (D$_2$) antagonist
Phenothiazine		
Prochlorperazine	5 or 10 mg p.o. every 4–6 h or	Muscarine antagonist
(Compazine)	i.m. every 6 h or	Dopamine (D$_2$) antagonist
	25 mg suppository every 12 h	
Butyrophenone		
Droperidol	2.5 or 5 mg i.m. every 12 h	Muscarine antagonist
(Inapsine)		Dopamine (D$_2$) antagonist
Benzodiazepines		
Diazepam	5 or 10 mg p.o. b.i.d.–q.i.d.	GABA$_A$ agonist
(Valium)	i.m. every 4–6 h or i.v. every 4–6 h	
Clonazepam	0.5 mg p.o. t.i.d.	GABA$_A$ agonist
(Klonopin)		

should preferably be administered, e.g. diazepam or promethazine combined with dimenhydrinate if nausea and vomiting are exceptionally severe. These drugs should not be given after nausea has disappeared, because they prolong the time course of central compensation of an acute vestibular tone imbalance.

Mobility and vestibular excitability are major requirements for recovery and vestibular rehabilitation. Readjustment of the vestibular reflexes, which act on eye and body muscles, requires sensory feedback from the sensory mismatch elicited by voluntary movements. Therefore, on the basis of our current knowledge of vestibular physiology, continued management should consist of vestibular exercises that promote central compensation. Antivertiginous and antiemetic drugs are not indicated for patients suffering from chronic dizziness. A prophylactic treatment with vestibular suppressants, e.g. scopolamine or dimenhydrinate,

is justified only in exceptional situations of rare patients who have frequent and severe vertigo attacks. In severe cases of benign paroxysmal positioning vertigo, it may become necessary to control nausea and vomiting when performing physical liberatory maneuvers. It is our own experience that severe central positioning vomiting is best controlled by benzodiazepines rather than antiemetics or typical vestibular suppressants.[5] Scopolamine administered transdermally as Transderm Scop provides a continuous blood level over a 3–day period and effectively prevents motion sickness. The selection of vestibular suppressants and antiemetic drugs should take into account the fact that those that reach a peak effect 7–9 h after ingestion[6] are ineffective for treating short vertigo attacks.

Other effective drugs can be expected to be developed from compounds that interfere with the presynaptic histamine receptor H$_3$ or GABA$_A$ receptors.

SPECIFIC DRUG TREATMENT FOR VESTIBULAR DISORDERS

Corticosteroids and virostatics are currently being tested in prospective studies to determine their value as treatment for vestibular neuritis, which is most likely caused by viral inflammation of the vestibular ganglion. Paroxysmal vestibular syndromes resulting from pathological excitation rather than loss of function due to a lesion can effectively be treated by antiepileptics such as carbamazepine or phenytoin. These conditions include vestibular epilepsy, vestibular paroxysmia due to neurovascular cross-compression or paroxysmal ataxia in multiple sclerosis. Familial episodic ataxia I and II are highly responsive to acetazolamide. Episodic vertigo occurring in the form of an aura with basilar or 'vestibular' migraine can be prevented by administering β-receptor blockers.

Some reliable pharmacological therapies are available for abnormal vestibular and non-vestibular eye movements, which override fixation and thus cause oscillopsia and impair vision.[7,8] The $GABA_B$ agonist baclofen suppresses periodic alternating nystagmus in patients[9] and animals with experimental lesions of the nodulus and uvula. The GABAergic anticonvulsant gabapentine[10] and the glutamate antagonist memantine[11] also effectively suppress acquired pendular nystagmus. Baclofen provides an effective treatment of some patients with downbeat or upbeat nystagmus;[12] occasional patients will also respond to gabapentine.[10]

SURGICAL TREATMENT

Surgical procedures for the treatment of dizzy patients primarily involve otolaryngologists but also to a minor extent neurosurgeons. There is no doubt that surgery is an appropriate therapy, e.g. for acoustic neurinomas, for an infratentorial cavernoma, or for patching a perilymph fistula, such as a dehiscence of the superior semicircular canal.[13] The same holds for the rotational vertebral artery syndrome, because of the danger of vertebral artery occlusion or embolism. In these cases, vertigo may be part of the clinical syndrome, but the indication for surgery is based mainly on the impending risk of brain and cranial nerve damage. Indications for surgical interventions based only on the goal of controlling recurrent or chronic vertigo are rare and should always be considered second choice after conservative management has failed. The multiple procedures can be classified as:

- non-destructive—decompression of the eighth nerve (acoustic neurinoma, cerebellopontine angle cyst); neurovascular decompression of the eighth nerve (vestibular paroxysmia); endolymphatic shunt in Menière's disease; surgical patching of perilymph fistulas
- selectively destructive—retrolabyrinthine or middle fossa vestibular nerve section in intractable Menière's disease; semicircular canal plugging or ampullary nerve section in intractable benign paroxysmal positioning vertigo
- destructive—oval window or transmastoid labyrinthectomy; translabyrinthine vestibular nerve section; laser labyrinthectomy.

Surgery is still most often considered for treatment of Menière's disease. Thomsen et al[14] have criticized endolymphatic sac surgery, since they found no statistical difference between endolymphatic sac surgery and placebo surgery. Many otolaryngologists continue to believe in the beneficial effect of this relatively safe, non-destructive procedure.[15] Vestibular nerve section is still performed in rare patients with disabling vertigo and preserved hearing in whom medical treatment and endolymphatic sac shunts have failed. Vestibular neurectomy poses risks of facial paresis, meningitis, cerebral fluid leakage, or epidural hematoma.[16] Labyrinthectomy of the affected ear can be performed only in cases with associated intractable hearing loss. Both procedures, vestibular neurectomy and labyrinthectomy, were found to be equally effective in relieving vertigo,[16] although deafferentation of the vestibular end-organ is sometimes incomplete, as shown for bilateral vestibular neurectomy.[17] Laser labyrinthectomy has also been performed in animals and patients,[18] with the aim of selectively destroying individual otolithic or semicircular canal structures. Despite vestibular compensation, vestibular neurectomy results in permanent dynamic vestibulo-ocular reflex deficits.[19,20] A considerable percentage of patients will never sufficiently compensate and will continue to suffer from chronic dizziness and disequilibrium.[21]

According to most available reports, the less effective results of destructive surgery for non-Menière's vertigo[22] are difficult to evaluate, since convincing analysis of the specific diagnoses is lacking.[23] These operations were based on such diagnoses as 'chronic vestibular neuronitis'[22] or 'uncompensated vestibular neuritis'.[23] Clinical experience has taught us that many of these so-called chronic conditions actually represent the transition of a peripheral vestibular dysfunction to a psychosomatic disease, e.g. phobic postural vertigo.

Transtympanic aminoglycoside treatment of Menière's disease[24] also offers control of vertigo at the risk of profound hearing loss. Aminoglycoside treatment is increasingly being preferred to surgery. Surgical procedures for benign paroxysmal positioning vertigo[25] include either transmeatal singular neurectomy or semicircular canal plugging. If physical liberatory maneuvers are performed correctly and continuously over a sufficiently long time, it is our experience that these procedures are required for only exceptional patients.

THERAPEUTIC AMINOGLYCOSIDE OTOTOXICITY

'Functional labyrinthectomy' with ototoxic aminoglycosides (gentamicin or streptomycin), proposed by Schuknecht in 1957,[26] was first tried in Europe with 8–24 mg gentamicin sulfate (Refobacin) instilled daily through a plastic tube inserted behind the anulus via the transmeatal approach.[27,28] At that time it was thought that it is possible to selectively damage the dark cells of the secretory epithelium (and thereby improve endolymphatic hydrops) before significantly affecting vestibular and cochlear function. Instillations were stopped when daily audiograms or a check of spontaneous nystagmus by using Frenzel's glasses indicated a beginning end-organ deafferentation. Since then, indications and recommendations for intratympanic gentamicin therapy[29–31] have changed, especially when Magnusson and Padoan[32] observed that the onset of ototoxic effects was delayed by a few days to a week after gentamicin instillation.

It is most likely that the route of transport of gentamicin from the middle to the inner ear is through the round window membrane to the perilymphatic space and from there to the hair cells in the endolymphatic space.[24] Ototoxicity was traditionally explained by reversible transduction channel blocking[33] and by damage to mitochondria due to excessive mitochondrial superoxide production that leads to cell death.[34] These multistage mechanisms of gentamicin ototoxicity are consistent with findings that the functional deficit was reversible at an early stage and became irreversible at a late stage.[30] There is, however, increasing evidence that aminoglycosides cause excitotoxicity in hair cells as a result of their agonist action at the polyamine site on the N-methyl-D-aspartate (NDMA) receptor.[35] This means that hair cells are excited to death. In animal experiments, regeneration of cochlear and vestibular hair cells[36] and protection from destruction when using neurotrophins[37,38] have been described. From these findings, new pharmacological strategies for preventing aminoglycoside ototoxicity

are emerging.[39] Reduction of aminoglycoside vestibulotoxicity was seen in rats when using the NMDA receptor/channel antagonist dizocilpine maleate.[40] As memantine overcomes the adverse side-effects of this drug, it may become an effective and better-tolerated alternative NMDA receptor antagonist.[41]

Thus, application of excessive gentamicin can cause unnecessary, inadvertent damage to the inner ear receptors, including the cochlear hair cells. Low-dose treatment—which does not even diminish or abolish caloric responses of the treated ear—has also been demonstrated to be effective[42–44] and is therefore recommended as the standard procedure.

Rare indications for intratympanic gentamicin therapy are the same as those for surgical labyrinthectomy:[24,29,43]

- conservatively or pharmacologically intractable course, with frequent vertigo attacks or drop attacks over more than 6 months, and hearing loss to a non-serviceable level (hearing loss > 60 dB) on the affected side
- continuing attacks despite selective vestibular nerve section (a rare failure of vestibular destructive procedures due to anatomical variants[45]).

Since severe hearing loss does not always occur when gentamicin is carefully instilled,[43,46,47] some otolaryngologists give ototoxic treatment even in patients with moderate hearing loss, if hearing in the opposite ear is unaffected. Bilateral manifestation of Menière's disease is a relative contraindication for ototoxic treatment.

There is no general agreement on the optimal concentration, temporal sequence and total dosage of intratympanic gentamicin instillations. Concentrations of 30 mg/ml gentamicin or less have usually been administered.[32,43,44,46] Two to three injections on consecutive days were effective and had fewer side-effects, such as chronic hearing loss[47] or vestibular insufficiency,[43] than four or more injections.

All the reported experience with this kind of treatment indicates that one injection per week (1–2 ml with concentrations less than 30 mg/ml) on an outpatient basis could be recommended in order to better monitor the delayed ototoxic effects.

BENIGN PAROXYSMAL POSITIONING VERTIGO (BPPV): POSITIONAL EXERCISES AND LIBERATORY MANEUVERS

The positional exercises proposed in 1980[48] were the first effective physical therapy for canalolithiasis in BPPV. The exercises comprised a sequence of rapid lateral head/trunk tilts, repeated serially to promote dispersion of the debris towards the utricular cavity. We instructed the patients to sit, to then move rapidly into the challenging position to induce the correct plane-specific stimulation of the posterior semicircular canal, to remain in the position until the evoked vertigo subsided, or for at least 30 s, and then to sit up for 30 s before assuming the opposite head-down position for an additional 30 s. Troost and Patton[49] reviewed and diagrammed this exercise protocol. The Semont[50] and Epley[51] liberatory maneuvers require only a single sequence, making them preferable to the multiple repetitions over many days required by the Brandt–Daroff exercises. With canalolithiasis as the established mechanism of BPPV, we can now explain the efficacy of the therapies according to anatomical and physical principles.

Fig. 46.1 illustrates the Semont maneuver in a patient with typical (posterior canal) left-sided BPPV. The clot causes no deflection of the cupula in the upright position. When the patient is quickly tilted towards the affected left ear with a 45° head rotation to the right (moving the left posterior canal to a plane corresponding to the plane of the head tilt), the clot gravitates towards the lower part of the canal, causing the cupula to deflect downwards (ampullofugal), and triggering a typical BPPV attack. These events explain the latency of a few seconds (the time needed for the clot-induced endolymph flow to develop by gravitational force), the ineffectiveness of a very slow positioning movement (the clot would then slowly gravitate along the undermost wall of the canal without plugging the canal and deflecting the cupula), and the short duration of the positional vertigo/nystagmus (the cupula deflection ends when the clot reaches its lowest position in the canal).[53] If the patient is swung towards the opposite right side with the nose down, the clot will gravitate downwards, causing stimulation of the posterior canal of the affected left ear (now uppermost). If no vertigo and nystagmus are elicited, we gently shake the patient's head in this position; this sometimes seems to facilitate loosening and gravitation of the clot. The patient is then slowly moved to the upright position; the clot will gravitate downwards through the common crus of the posterior and anterior canals and enter the utricular cavity, where it becomes harmless. We share the experience of others[54] that complete recovery after a single maneuver is achieved in about 50–70% of cases. Semont et al[50] recommended having the patient maintain the upright position for 48 h following the liberation, but we have not found this to be necessary.

In patients with rare horizontal canal BPPV, we first try 'barbecue rotation' and propose that

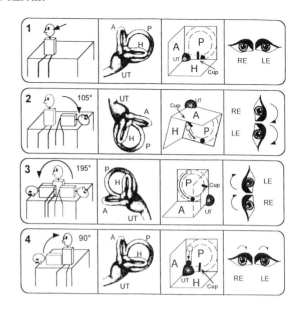

Figure 46.1 Schematic drawing of the Semont liberatory maneuver in a patient with typical BPPV of the left ear. Boxes from left to right: position of body and head, position of labyrinth in space, position and movement of the clot in the posterior canal and resulting cupula deflection, and direction of the rotatory nystagmus. The clot is depicted as an open circle within the canal; a black circle represents the final resting position of the clot. (1) In the sitting position, the head is turned horizontally 45° to the unaffected ear. The clot, which is heavier than endolymph, settles at the base of the left posterior semicircular canal. (2) The patient is tilted approximately 105° towards the left (affected) ear. The head position change, relative to gravity, causes the clot to gravitate to the lowermost part of the canal and the cupula to deflect downwards, inducing BPPV with rotatory nystagmus beating towards the undermost ear. The patient maintains this position for 3 min. (3) The patient is turned approximately 195° with the nose down, causing the clot to move towards the exit of the canal. The endolymphatic flow again deflects the cupula such that the nystagmus beats towards the left ear, now uppermost. The patient remains in this position for 3 min. (4) The patient is slowly moved to the sitting position; this causes the clot to enter the utricular cavity. A, anterior semicircular canal; P, posterior semicircular canal; H, horizontal semicircular canal; Cup, cupula, UT, utricular cavity; RE, right eye; LE, left eye.[52]

prolonged bedrest with the head turned towards the unaffected ear[55] be maintained for up to 12 h. If this is still unsuccessful after 2 days, we advise the patients to perform the Brandt–Daroff exercises. Both physical therapies can be performed at home and do not require the presence of a physical therapist.

VESTIBULAR COMPENSATION AND SUBSTITUTION: VESTIBULAR EXERCISES AND PHYSICAL THERAPY FOR VESTIBULAR REHABILITATION

Vestibular exercises are performed either to promote central habituation so as to prevent motion sickness or to readjust vestibulo-ocular and vestibulospinal reflexes as a form of retraining for exceptional patient populations (vestibular compensation).

Animal experiments have shown that exercise may facilitate vestibular compensation.[56–59] The special role of visual input has been convincingly demonstrated by Courjon and Jeannerod[60] and Lacour and Xerri.[61] Furthermore, animal experiments suggest that there is a critical period for functional recovery which is crucial for achieving either optimal or minimal repair.[28,62] The few available clinical control studies provide evidence that physical therapy is superior to general conditioning exercises.[63] Such physical therapy helps patients with chronic dizziness[64] and those after resection of an acoustic neuroma recover balance earlier than if not treated;[65] similarly, patients after acute unilateral vestibular neuritis exhibit normalization of postural sway within a significantly shorter time than the control group (Fig. 46.2).[66]

Vestibular compensation is no 'simple or single' process. It consists of multiple processes for perceptual, vestibulo-ocular and vestibulospinal readjustment, which have different time courses at different sites in the brain and the spinal cord.[67–69] Therefore, vestibular rehabilitation should incorporate different exercises that involve eye, head and body movements and the monitoring of patients' progress separately for the different perceptual, ocular motor and postural vestibular functions. A study on the efficacy of vestibular exercises for compensation and substitution after an acute unilateral partial vestibular loss (cases of vestibular neuritis without recovery of peripheral function during the training phase) found that only postural balance was significantly facilitated, not the time course of recovery of ocular torsion or tilts of perceived vertical as measured in degrees.[66] Recovery from bilateral labyrinthine loss was also demonstrated in animal experiments[70] and in patients with chronic bilateral vestibular deficits.[71] In such cases, recovery takes place more slowly and incompletely, leaving permanent instability during intensified balance tasks and in darkness as well as rapid head movements while walking. Up to now, no controlled studies have focused on the effects of physical exercise on the rehabilitation of patients

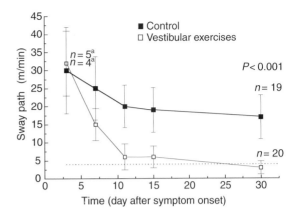

Figure 46.2 Efficacy of specific vestibular exercises for postural sway in patients with acute vestibular neuritis. Time course of the changes in total sway path (SP) values of the controls ($n = 20$) and physiotherapy ($n = 19$) groups: vestibular exercises improved central vestibulospinal compensation. For postural control, SP values (m/min, mean ± SD) were measured in patients with eyes closed and standing on a compliant foam-padded posturography platform. The total SP is the length of the path described by the center of force during a given time (20 s), which is generated by the inherent instability of a subject standing on a recording platform. SP is approximated by the sum of the distances between two consecutive sampling points in the anteroposterior (sagittal = x) plane, i.e. sagittal sway (calculated as $\sum|\Delta x|$), mediolateral (frontal = y) plane, i.e. frontal sway (calculated as $\sum|\Delta y|$), or for two dimensions as the total SP (calculated as $\sum\sqrt{(|\Delta x^2| + \sum|\Delta y^2|)}$). There was a significant difference (ANOVA, $P < 0.001$) between the two groups at the statistical endpoint (day 30 after symptom onset). The dotted line indicates the normal range.[66]

with central vestibular disorders. However, the patients' rapid recovery, e.g. from lateropulsion in Wallenberg's syndrome, when they become mobilized and are able to perform intensive physical therapy seems to support the efficacy of exercises, but provides no proof.

Vestibular compensation is less perfect than generally believed. For instance, after acute unilateral vestibular deafferentation, which occurs in vestibular neuritis, the process of normalization is impressive for *static* conditions in the absence of head motion: the initial rotatory vertigo, spontaneous nystagmus and postural imbalance subside. Compensation is, however, less impressive for *dynamic* conditions, especially when the vestibular system is exposed to high-frequency head accelerations.[68,72] The dynamic disequilibrium, i.e. VOR asymmetry, causes oscillopsia, the illusory movement of the environment due to excessive slip of images upon the retina during fast head movements or walking, because after uni- and bilateral peripheral vestibular lesions the VOR cannot generate fast compensatory eye rotations during high-frequency head rotations. The dynamic vestibular tone imbalance can be detected clinically by provoking a directional head-shaking nystagmus[73] or by bedside testing of the VOR with rapid head rotation.[74]

Thus, the so-called simple and complete vestibular compensation for peripheral deficits is only a legend. Nevertheless, the vestibular system provides an excellent and attractive model for investigations of neural and behavioral plasticity in humans and animals. Certain of its distinct features have several advantages:[67]

(1) the peripheral vestibular lesion can be precisely located, is restricted, and easy to reproduce without disturbing central parts of the vestibular system, which are important for plasticity.

(2) the recovery of function—as well as its time course—can be measured quantitatively at different levels (vestibulospinal reflex, vestibulo-ocular reflex, and perception).

(3) the anatomy, physiology and functions of the VOR network have been intensively studied.

Pharmacological and metabolic studies suggest that the process of compensation can be retarded by alcohol, phenobarbitol, chlorpromazine, diazepam, and adrenocorticotrophic hormone (ACTH) antagonists, whereas caffeine, amphetamines and steroids may accelerate it. Drug-induced modification of vestibular compensation continues to attract research interest, although without convincing proof.[75] Gingko biloba extract, for example, has been reported to accelerate compensation, but according to a recent study in guinea pigs it seems that the vehicle carrying the extract was the responsible agent.[76] Vestibular compensation is usually considered a central 'repair mechanism' for a vestibular tone imbalance secondary to a peripheral vestibular loss. However, central compensation is also possible for central vestibular tone imbalance. It is still poorly understood which central vestibular syndromes can be compensated and which cannot. Upbeat and downbeat nystagmus may serve as an example. Acquired upbeat nystagmus is rarely permanent, whereas acquired downbeat nystagmus may be permanent. All in all, however, we now know a lot about vestibular compensation and substitution.

REFERENCES

1. Brandt T. *Vertigo: its multisensory syndromes*, 2nd edn. London: Springer-Verlag, 1999.
2. Baloh RM, Halmagyi GM, eds. *Disorders of the Vestibular System*. New York: Oxford University Press, 1996.
3. Bronstein AM, Brandt T, Woollacott M. *Clinical Disorders of Balance, Posture and Gait*. London: Arnold, 1996.
4. Foster C, Baloh RW. Drug therapy for vertigo. In: Baloh RW, Halmagyi GM, eds. *Disorders of the Vestibular System*. New York: Oxford University Press, 1996, 541–550.
5. Arbusow V, Strupp M, Brandt T. Amiodarone-induced severe prolonged head-positional vertigo and vomiting. *Neurology* 1998; **51**: 917.
6. Manning C, Scandale L, Manning EJ, Gengo FM. Central nervous system effects of meclizine and dimenhydrinate: evidence of acute tolerance to antihistamines. *J Clin Pharmacol* 1992; **32**: 996–1002.
7. Leigh RJ, Averbuch-Heller L, Tomsak RL, Remler BF, Yaniglos SS, Dell'Osso LF. Treatment of abnormal eye movements that impair vision: strategies based on current concepts of physiology and pharmacology. *Ann Neurol* 1994; **36**: 129–141.
8. Leigh RJ, Ramat S. Neuropharmacologic aspects of the ocular motor system and the treatment of abnormal eye movements. *Curr Opin Neurol* 1999; **12**: 21–27.
9. Halmagyi GM, Rudge P, Gresty MA. Treatment of periodic alternating nystagmus. *Ann Neurol* 1980; **8**: 609–611.
10. Averbuch-Heller L, Tusa RJ, Fuhry L et al. A double-blind controlled study of gabapentin and baclofen as treatment for acquired nystagmus. *Ann Neurol* 1997; **41**: 818–825.
11. Starck M, Albrecht H, Pöllman W, Straube A, Dieterich M. Drug therapy for acquired pendular nystagmus in multiple sclerosis. *J Neurol* 1997; **244**: 9–16.
12. Dieterich M, Straube A, Brandt T, Paulus W, Büttner U. The effects of baclofen and anticholinergic drugs on upbeat and downbeat nystagmus. *J Neurol Neurosurg Psychiatry* 1991; **54**: 627–632.
13. Minor LB, Solomon D, Zinnreich JS, Zee DS. Sound-and/or pressure-induced vertigo due to dehiscence of the superior semicircular canal. *Arch Otolaryngol Head Neck Surg* 1998; **124**: 249–258.
14. Thomsen J, Bretlau P, Tos M, Johnsen NJ. Placebo effect in surgery for Meniere's disease. *Arch Otolaryngol* 1981; **107**: 271–277.
15. Brackmann DE. Surgical procedures: endolymphatic shunt, vestibular nerve section and labyrinthectomy. In: Baloh RW, Halmagyi GM, eds. *Disorders of the Vestibular System*. New York: Oxford University Press, 1996: 551–562.
16. Gacek RR, Gacek MR. Comparison of labyrinthectomy and vestibular neurectomy in the control of vertigo. *Laryngoscope* 1996; **106**: 225–230.
17. Böhmer A, Fisch U. Bilateral vestibular neurectomy for treatment of vertigo. *Otolaryngol Head Neck Surg* 1993; **109**: 101–107.
18. Nomura Y, Okuno T, Mizuno M. Treatment of vertigo using laser labyrinthectomy. *Acta Otolaryngol (Stockh)* 1993; **113**: 261–262.
19. Halmagyi GM, Curthoys IS, Todd MJ et al. Unilateral vestibular neurectomy in man causes a severe permanent horizontal vestibulo-ocular reflex deficit in response to high-acceleration ampullofugal stimulation. *Acta Otolaryngol (Stockh) Suppl* 1991; **481**: 411–414.

20. Kanayama R, Bronstein AM, Gresty MA, Brookes GB, Faldon ME, Nakamura T. Perceptual studies in patients with vestibular neurectomy. *Acta Otolaryngol (Stockh) Suppl* 1995; **520**: 408–411.

21. Halmagyi GM. Vestibular insufficiency following unilateral vestibular deafferentation. *Aust J Otolaryngol* 1994; **1**: 510–512.

22. Benecke JE. Surgery for non-Meniere's vertigo. *Acta Otolaryngol (Stockh) Suppl* 1994; **513**: 37–39.

23. Kemink JL, Telian SA, El-Kashlan H, Langman AW. Retrolabyrinthine vestibular nerve section: efficacy in disorders other than Meniere's disease. *Laryngoscope* 1991; **101**: 523–528.

24. Bergenius J, Ödkist LM. Transtympanic aminoglycoside treatment of Meniere's disease. In: Baloh RM, Halmagyi GM, eds. *Disorders of the Vestibular System*. New York: Oxford University Press, 1996: 575–582.

25. Pohl DV. Surgical procedures for benign positional vertigo. In: Baloh RW, Halmagyi GM, eds. *Disorders of the Vestibular System*. New York: Oxford University Press, 1996: 563–582.

26. Schuknecht HF. Ablation therapy in the management of Menière's disease. *Acta Otolaryngol (Stockh) Suppl* 1957; **132**: 1.

27. Beck C, Schmidt CL. Ten years of experience with intratympanally applied streptomycin (gentamicin) in the therapy of morbus Ménière. *Arch Otorhinolaryngol* 1978; **221**: 149–152.

28. Lacour M, Réapprentissage et période postopératoire sensible dans la restauration des fonctions nerveuses. Exemple de la compensation vestibulaire et implications cliniques. *Ann Oto-Laryngol (Paris)* 1984; **101**: 177–187.

29. Graham MD, Goldsmith MM. Labyrinthectomy. Indications and surgical technique. *Otolaryngol Clin North Am* 1994; **27**: 325–335.

30. Halmagyi GM, Fattore CM, Curthoys IS, Wade S. Gentamicin vestibulotoxicity. *Otolaryngol Head Neck Surg* 1994; **111**: 571–574.

31. Hellström S, Ödkvist L. Pharmacologic labyrinthectomy. *Otolaryngol Clin North Am* 1994; **27**: 307–315.

32. Magnusson M, Padoan S. Delayed onset of ototoxic effects of gentamicin in treatment of Ménière's disease. *Acta Otolaryngol (Stockh)* 1991; **111**: 671–676.

33. Kroese ABA, Das A, Hudspeth AJ. Blockage of transduction channels of hair cells in bullfrog's sacculus by aminoglycoside antibiotics. *Hear Res* 1989; **37**: 203–218.

34. Hutchin T, Cortopassi G. Proposed molecular and cellular mechanism for aminoglycoside ototoxicity. *Antimicrob Agents Chemother* 1994; **38**: 2517–2520.

35. Smith PF. Are vestibular hair cells excited to death by aminoglycoside antibiotics? *J Vestib Res* 2000; **10**: 1–5.

36. Forge A, Li L, Nevill G. Hair cell recovery in the vestibular sensory epithelia of mature guinea pigs. *J Comp Neurol* 1998; **397**: 69–88.

37. Kimura N, Nishizaki K, Orita Y, Masuda Y. 4-Methylcatechol, a potent inducer of nerve growth factor synthesis, protects spiral ganglion neurons from aminoglycoside ototoxicity—preliminary report. *Acta Otolaryngol (Stockh) Suppl* 1999; **540**: 12–15.

38. Staecker H, Kopke R, Malgrange B, Lefebre P, Van De Water TR. NT-3 and/or BDNF therapy prevents loss of auditory neurons following loss of hair cells. *Neuro Report* 1996; **7**: 889–894.

39. Smith PF. Pharmacology of the vestibular system. *Curr Opin Neurol* 2000; **13**: 31–37.

40. Basile AS, Brichta AM, Harris BD, Morse D, Coling D, Skolnick P. Dizocilpine attenuates streptomycin-induced vestibulotoxicity in rats. *Neurosci Lett* 1999; **265**: 71–74.

41. Parsons CG, Danysz W, Quack G. Memantine is a clinically well tolerated N-methyl-D-aspartate (NMDA) receptor antagonist—a review of preclinical data. *Neuropharmacology* 1999; **38**: 735–767.

42. Driscoll CLW, Kasperbauer JL, Facer GW, Harner SG, Beatty CW. Low-dose intratympanic gentamicin and the treatment of Meniere's disease: preliminary results. *Laryngoscope* 1997; **107**: 83–89.

43. Murofushi T, Halmagyi GM, Yavor RA. Intratympanic gentamicin in Ménière's disease: results of therapy. *Am J Otol* 1997; **18**: 52–57.

44. Yamazaki T, Hayashi M, Komatsuzaki A. Intratympanic gentamicin therapy for Meniere's disease placed by a tubal catheter with systemic isosorbide. *Acta Otolaryngol (Stockh) Suppl* 1991; **481**: 613–616.

45. Monsell EM, Brackmann DE, Linthicum FH Jr. Why do vestibular destructive procedures sometimes fail? *Otolaryngol Head Neck Surg* 1988; **99**: 472–479.

46. Nedzelski JM, Chiong CM, Fradet G, Schessel DA, Bryce GE, Pfeiderer AG. Intratympanic gentamicin instillation as treatment of unilateral Ménière's disease: update of an ongoing study. *Am J Otol* 1993; **14**: 278–282.

47. Ödkvist LM. Middle ear ototoxic treatment for inner ear disease. *Acta Otolaryngol (Stockh) Suppl* 1988; **457**: 83–86.

48. Brandt Th, Daroff RB. Physical therapy for benign paroxysmal positional vertigo. *Arch Otolaryngol* 1980; **106**: 484–485.

49. Troost BT, Patton JM. Exercise therapy for positional vertigo. *Neurology* 1992; **42**: 1441–1444.

50. Semont A, Freyss G, Vitte E. Curing the BPPV with a liberatory maneuver. *Adv Otorhinolaryngol* 1988; **42**: 290–293.

51. Epley JM. The canalith repositioning procedure: for treatment of benign paroxysmal positional vertigo. *Otolaryngol Head Neck Surg* 1992; **107**: 399–404.

52. Brandt Th, Steddin S, Daroff RB. Therapy for benign paroxysmal positioning vertigo, revisited. *Neurology* 1994; **44**: 796–800.

53. Brandt Th, Steddin S. Current view of the mechanism of benign paroxysmal positioning vertigo: cupulolithiasis or canalolithiasis? *J Vestib Res* 1993; **3**: 373–382.

54. Serafini G, Palmierei AMR, Simoncelli C. Benign paroxysmal positional vertigo of posterior semicircular canal: results in 160 cases treated with Semont's maneuver. *Ann Otol Rhinol Laryngol* 1996; **105**: 770–775.

55. Vannucchi P, Giaonnoni B, Pagnini P. Treatment of horizontal semicircular canal benign paroxysmal positional vertigo. *J Vestib Res* 1997; **7**: 1–6.

56. Courjon JH, Jeannerod M, Ossuzio I, Schmid R. The role of vision in compensation of vestibulo-ocular reflex after hemilabyrinthectomy in the cat. *Exp Brain Res* 1977; **28**: 235–248.

57. Fetter M, Zee DS. Recovery from unilateral labyrinthectomy in rhesus monkeys. *J Neurophysiol* 1988; **59**: 370–393.

58. Igarashi M. Compensation for peripheral vestibular disturbances—animal studies. In: Bles W, Brandt Th, eds. *Disorders of Posture and Gait*. Amsterdam: Elsevier, 1986: 337–351.

59. Lacour M, Roll JR, Apaix M. Modifications and development of spinal reflexes in the alert baboon (*Papio papio*) following unilateral vestibular neurectomy. *Brain Rev* 1976; **113**: 255–269.

60. Courjon JH, Jeannerod M. Visual substitution of labyrinthine defect. In: Granit R, Pompejiano O, eds. *Progress in Brain Research*, Vol. 50, *Reflex Control of Posture and Locomotion*. Amsterdam: Elsevier, 1979: 783–792.

61. Lacour M, Xerri C. Vestibular compensation: new perspectives. In: Flohr H, Precht W, eds. *Lesion-induced Neuronal Plasticity in Sensorimotor Systems*. Berlin: Springer, 1981: 240–253.

62. Xerri C, Lacour M. Compensation des déficits posturaux et cinétiques après neurectomie vestibulaire unilatérale chez le chat. *Acta Otolaryngol (Stockh)* 1980; **90**: 414–424.

63. Herdman SJ, Blatt PJ, Schubert MC. Vestibular rehabilitation of patients with vestibular hypofunction or with benign paroxysmal positional vertigo. *Curr Opin Neurol* 2000; **13**: 39–43.

64. Horak FB, Jones-Rycewicz C, Black O, Shumway-Cook A. Effects of vestibular rehabilitation on dizziness and imbalance. *Otolaryngol Head Neck Surg* 1992; **106**: 175–180.

65. Herdman SJ, Clendaniel RA, Mattox DE, Holiday M, Niparko JK. Vestibular adaptation exercises and recovery: acute stage following acoustic neuroma resection. *Otolaryngol Head Neck Surg* 1995; **113**: 71–77.

66. Strupp M, Arbusow V, Maag KP, Gall C, Brandt T. Vestibular exercises improve central vestibulo-spinal compensation after an acute unilateral peripheral vestibular lesion: a prospective clinical study. *Neurology* 1998; **51**: 838–844.

67. Brandt T, Strupp M, Arbusow V, Dieringer N. Plasticity of the vestibular system: central compensation and sensory substitution for vestibular deficits. *Ann Neurol* 1997; **73**: 297–309.

68. Curthoys IS, Halmagyi GM. Vestibular compensation: a review of the oculomotor, neural, and clinical consequences of unilateral vestibular loss. *J Vestib Res* 1994; **5**: 67–107.

69. Dieringer N. 'Vestibular compensation': neural plasticity and its relations to functional recovery after labyrinthine lesions in frogs and other vertebrates. *Prog Neurobiol* 1995; **46**: 97–129.

70. Igarashi M, Ishikawa K, Ishii M, Yamane H. Physical exercise and balance compensation after total ablation of vestibular organs. *Prog Brain Res* 1988; **76**: 395–401.

71. Krebs DE, Gill-Body KM, Riley PO, Parker SW. Double-blind placebo controlled trial of rehabilitation for bilateral vestibular hypofunction: preliminary report. *Otolaryngol Head Neck Surg* 1993; **109**: 735–741.

72. Halmagyi GM, Curthoys IS, Cremer PD et al. The human horizontal vestibulo-ocular reflex in response to high-acceleration stimulation before and after unilateral vestibular neurectomy. *Exp Brain Res* 1990; **81**: 479–490.

73. Hain TC, Fetter M, Zee DS. Head-shaking nystagmus in patients with unilateral peripheral vestibular lesions. *Am J Otolaryngol* 1987; **8**: 36–47.

74. Halmagyi GM, Curthoys IS. A clinical sign of canal paresis. *Arch Neurol* 1988; **45**: 737–739.

75. Curthoys IS. Vestibular compensation and substitution. *Curr Opin Neurol* 2000; **13**: 27–30.

76. Schlatter M, Kerr DR, Smith PF, Darlington CL. Evidence that the ginkgo biloba extract, Egb 761, neither accelerates nor enhances the rapid compensation of the static symptoms of unilateral vestibular deafferentation in guinea pig. *J Vestib Res* 1999; **9**: 111–118.

47

Eye movements: supranuclear mechanisms and their disorders

Lea Averbuch-Heller†

The ocular motor system is the best-understood motor system. Because three-dimensional eye rotations can be measured with precision and analyzed using mathematical models, eye movement research is an invaluable tool for investigating common mechanisms of motor systems. Over the last decade, a wealth of new data from animal studies has expanded and modified traditional schemes of premotor organization of the ocular motor system. In this chapter, I review functional mechanisms concerned with programming eye movements at the brainstem level and present current knowledge of their neural substrate, along with some clinical disorders of supranuclear gaze control.

MECHANISMS OF SUPRANUCLEAR CONTROL

Functional classes of eye movements

It is important to remember that eye movements are subordinate to vision; their purpose is to get an object of interest onto the fovea and to hold it there steadily. Whereas the ultimate command for moving the eye issues from the nuclei of cranial nerves III, IV and VI, multiple premotor signals converge on the nuclei. These signals derive from various functional classes of eye movements, aimed at optimizing vision during different activities (Table 47.1).[1]

Gaze-holding mechanisms act to prevent slip of images on the retina. Vestibulo-ocular reflexes are at work constantly when we are walking, producing compensatory eye movements to counteract high-frequency head perturbations that occur with each step. Their loss (e.g. due to aminoglycoside toxicity) causes blurred vision and severe oscillopsia during locomotion. Optokinetic eye movements can stabilize gaze during slow, sustained head rotations. Smooth pursuit contributes to holding the image steadily on the fovea while tracking a small moving target or during linear self-motion. The fixation system controls excessive slip of images on the retina and programs corrective responses; it also suppresses unwanted saccades. Neural integration is

Table 47.1 Functional classes of eye movements	
Class	**Principal function**
Fixation	Holds the image of a stationary object steadily on the fovea
Vestibulo-ocular reflex	Holds images steadily on the retina during brief head rotations
Optokinetic system	Holds images steadily on the retina during sustained head rotations
Smooth pursuit	Holds the image of a small moving target close to the fovea
Neural integrator	Holds the eyes steadily in an eccentric orbital position against elastic forces of orbital tissues
Saccades	Place images of eccentrically located objects on the fovea by moving the eyes in the same direction
Vergence	Places images of a single object on both foveae during gaze shifts in depth by moving the eyes in opposite directions

important for sustaining steady gaze in eccentric orbital positions. To neutralize the mechanical pull of the suspensory ligaments and fascia that tend to return the globe towards mid-position, there is a need for an appropriate neural command, achieved by 'integrating' velocity to position signal. When this mechanism is impaired, gaze-evoked nystagmus occurs.

Gaze-shifting mechanisms act to orient the line of sight to the next object of interest. Saccades are fast, conjugate movements which can be made voluntarily or in response to external (visual or other sensory) stimuli. Vergence, on the other hand, is slow; this is an inherently disconjugate system, which operates during gaze shifts in depth, between near and far targets. In contrast to all the aforementioned (version) eye movements, it shifts the eyes in opposite directions so that foveae of both eyes simultaneously acquire the images of an object.

In spite of this elaborate functional division, in real-life situations various classes of eye movements almost never work in isolation.[2] For example, we only rarely employ pure version or pure vergence: gaze shifts in depth calling for vergence are usually accompanied by saccades. This 'saccade–vergence interaction' requires common control of version and vergence mechanisms in which the properties of both systems undergo modification.[3,4]

Binocular coordination

Precise coordination between the movements of both eyes is needed in order to ensure depth perception and prevent diplopia. The mechanism of binocular coordination is unresolved. The prevailing theory today, Hering's law, claims that the brain treats the two eyes as a single 'cyclopean' eye, providing common innervation to both eyes. Such yoking may be embedded in the anatomical arrangement of projections of the excitatory burst neurons onto ocular motoneurons of both eyes.[5] An opposing opinion voiced by Helmholtz in the late 19th century maintains that each eye is governed independently.[6,7] Modern research appears to partly support this view. Thus, it was demonstrated that eye movements in monkeys during sleep are disconjugate or even monocular.[6] Moreover, premotor neurons in the paramedian pontine reticular formation were found to encode monocular saccadic commands.[7] Further evidence in support of monocular control comes from psychophysical experiments in humans. Study of prism-induced adaptation in normal human subjects established that both monocular and binocular mechanisms (i.e.

saccade–vergence interaction) take place in the disconjugate adaptation of eye movements.[8] Their relative contributions are yet to be determined.

BRAINSTEM ORGANIZATION OF SUPRANUCLEAR OCULAR MOTOR CONTROL

The planning and execution of ocular motor behavior involves the entire brain. Descending, centrally programmed saccadic, pursuit, and vergence commands, ascending vestibular commands, and cerebellar modulatory signals, all come together on ocular motoneurons. In considering the presumed profile of the system, we will start with immediate premotor structures responsible for carrying out all eye movement commands, then move on to cerebellar influences, and conclude with descending cortical pathways.

Immediate premotor control

Brainstem control of horizontal and vertical gaze is anatomically separated. Structures important for horizontal gaze are located in the lower pons and upper medulla, whereas those involved in vertical gaze occupy the rostral midbrain; vergence control is divided between the midbrain and pons.

Horizontal gaze
The abducens nucleus represents the ultimate horizontal 'gaze center'. It receives neural commands for all functional classes of eye movements (Fig. 47.1). In contrast to other motor nuclei, it controls not only the ipsilateral muscle to which it projects (lateral rectus) but also the contralateral agonist, yoke muscle (medial rectus). Two neuronal populations reside in the abducens nucleus: abducens motoneurons, the axons of which project to the ipsilateral VI nerve, and internuclear neurons. The latter send their axons across the midline, to join the contralateral medial longitudinal fasciculus (MLF) on their way to the contralateral medial rectus subnucleus (Fig. 47.1).[9,10] In the opposite direction, oculomotor internuclear neurons of the medial rectus subnucleus descend to the contralateral abducens nucleus.[11] Together, these two groups of internuclear neurons provide the anatomical basis for yoking of horizontal movements in both eyes—i.e. Hering's law.

Saccade signals reach the abducens nucleus from the pontine paramedian reticular formation (PPRF).[12–14] There are three types of neuron in the PPRF that are involved in saccade generation (Fig.

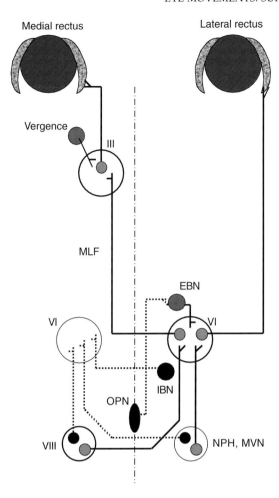

Figure 47.1 Anatomical scheme for brainstem control of horizontal gaze. The abducens nucleus (VI) is a horizontal gaze 'center'. It contains two neuronal populations: abducens motoneurons that project to the ipsilateral lateral rectus, and internuclear neurons that cross and project to the contralateral medial rectus subnucleus of the oculomotor nucleus (III) via contralateral medial longitudinal fasciculus (MLF). Saccadic, pursuit, vestibular and integrator commands all join on VI (for details see text); vergence signal accesses III directly. Note that pursuit signals reach VI via VIII. Black symbols and dotted lines represent inhibitory inputs. VIII, vestibular nucleus; NPH, nucleus prepositus hypoglossi; MVN, medial vestibular nucleus; EBN, excitatory burst neurons; IBN, inhibitory burst neurons; OPN, omnipause neurons. The dashed line indicates midline, in this and the following figures.

47.1). (1) Excitatory burst neurons receive their input mainly from the contralateral superior colliculus (SC); they project directly to the ipsilateral abducens nucleus and stimulate it for an ipsilateral saccade. (2)

Inhibitory burst neurons project to the contralateral abducens nucleus; they inhibit the antagonist, contralateral lateral rectus during ipsilateral abduction. (3) Omnipause neurons (OPNs) carry out suppression of saccades during visual fixation. OPNs reside in a paramedian nucleus raphe interpositus; they receive input from the rostral 'fixation' zone of the SC and project to both horizontal and vertical excitatory burst neurons.[15] OPN activity has to be suppressed in order for saccades to be made; lesions of OPNs may result in saccadic intrusions up to opsoclonus or slow saccades.

The eccentric gaze-holding commands arrive at the abducens nucleus from the nucleus prepositus hypoglossi (NPH) and the medial vestibular nucleus (MVN)—structures that function as a 'neural integrator' for horizontal gaze.[16] The NPH and MVN provide tonic eye-position signals for a sustained contraction of the extraocular muscles that is required for steady gaze-holding in an eccentric orbital position (Fig. 47.1). Smooth pursuit projections reach the abducens nucleus from the ipsilateral dorsolateral pontine nuclei via the contralateral vestibular and cerebellar nuclei. Excitatory vestibular and optokinetic signals derive from the contralateral vestibular nuclei.[17]

Vertical gaze

The analog of PPRF for vertical eye movements occupies the rostral interstitial nucleus of MLF (riMLF) at the mesodiencephalic junction (Fig. 47.2). The riMLF accommodates excitatory burst neurons for vertical and torsional saccades. In each riMLF, neurons discharge for both upward and downward eye movements but only for ipsilateral torsional saccades.[18–20] Motoneurons of eye elevator muscles receive bilateral projections from the riMLF, whereas those of depressor muscles receive only ipsilateral input. Yoke muscle pairs in the two eyes (e.g. right superior rectus–left inferior oblique, right inferior rectus–left superior oblique) get collaterals from the same burst neuron in the riMLF; this arrangement is the basis for fulfillment of Hering's law in the vertical plane.[5] In non-human primates, unilateral riMLF inactivations slow downward saccades and produce torsional nystagmus with contralesionally beating quick phase, while bilateral lesions abolish all vertical saccades.[21]

Neural integration (eccentric gaze-holding) in the vertical plane is accomplished by an interstitial nucleus of Cajal (INC).[22,23] The INC projects via the posterior commissure to motoneurons of the contralateral nuclei of cranial nerves III and IV and the contralateral INC (Fig. 47.2).[24] The INC also

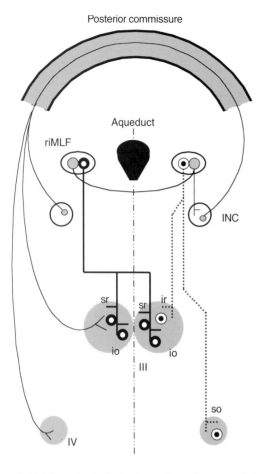

Figure 47.2 Anatomical scheme for brainstem control of vertical gaze. The rostral interstitial nucleus of the MLF (riMLF) on each side contains excitatory burst neurons for upward (black circles, white dots) and downward (white circles, black dots) saccades, and ipsitorsional saccades. Projections from the riMLF onto motoneurons of the depressor muscles subnuclei, inferior rectus (ir) and superior oblique (so), are ipsilateral (dotted lines); note that this arrangement assures simultaneous and equal innervation to a pair of agonists: ipsilateral ir and contralateral so muscle (since outputs of the trochlear nucleus decussate). Projections onto the elevator muscles subnuclei are bilateral (solid lines). Inputs of the interstitial nucleus of Cajal (INC) cross in the posterior commissure, while those of riMLF cross ventrally to the aqueduct. For simplicity of representation, vestibular and pursuit inputs are omitted. III, the oculomotor nucleus; IV, the trochlear nucleus; sr, superior rectus; io, inferior oblique.

receives ascending vertical vestibular and smooth pursuit inputs from the medulla and pons that run partly in the MLF and partly through alternative pathways.[25] INC dysfunction causes poor vertical

gaze-holding, hypometric vertical saccades, hypoactive vertical vestibulo-ocular reflexes, and torsional nystagmus.[26]

The posterior commissure (PC) receives axons from the nucleus of the posterior commissure (NPC), in addition to conveying the crossing fibers from the INC. The NPC contributes to upgaze generation and coordination between lid and eye movements.[27] PC lesions result in limited upgaze and lid retraction.[28] Pharmacological inactivation of neurons in the rostral part of the mesencephalic reticular formation causes slow and hypometric vertical saccades, along with downward displacement of the initial eye position—findings reminiscent of dorsal midbrain syndrome (see below).[29]

Vergence

Vergence motor commands are put forth by motoneurons of the medial rectus subnucleus in the oculomotor nuclear complex. A specific group of the medial rectus motoneurons (dorsomedial, rostral subgroup C) may be selectively involved in vergence responses.[30] Premotor commands for vergence arise in the rostral midbrain, the so-called 'midbrain near-response neurons' in the supraoculomotor area.[31] For tonically sustaining a particular vergence angle (the 'vergence integration'), the nucleus reticularis tegmenti pontis (NRTP) is important.[32] NRTP houses two types of neurons: those which fire for near targets, and those which fire for far targets. Stimulating NRTP produces changes in vergence angle and accommodation.

Cerebellar influence

The cerebellum is important for short-term and long-term regulation of all eye movements, including vestibulo-ocular responses, saccades, pursuit, and vergence. Two separate parts of the cerebellum contribute to ocular motor control: (1) the dorsal vermis of the posterior lobe and the fastigial nuclei; and (2) the vestibulocerebellum (flocculus, paraflocculus, nodulus, and ventral uvula). The dorsal vermis and the fastigial nuclei modulate voluntary gaze-shifting—saccades, pursuit and vergence—whereas the vestibulocerebellum contributes to stabilization of sight during motion.

The dorsal vermis controls contralateral saccades and pursuit.[33–35] A major input to cerebellum from cortical eye fields goes via pontine nuclei, particularly the NRTP (Fig. 47.3). Other inputs arrive from the ipsilateral structures responsible for saccades, pursuit and vestibulo-ocular reflexes; all those further project to the fastigial nucleus. Neurons in

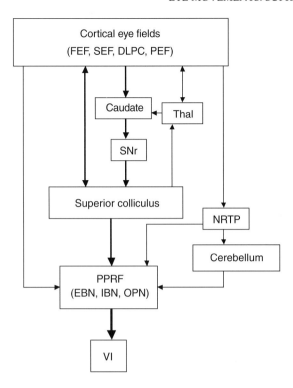

Figure 47.3 A block diagram of descending pathways involved in fixation and horizontal saccades generation. FEF, frontal eye fields; DLPC, dorsolateral prefrontal cortex; SEF, supplementary eye fields; PEF, parietal eye fields; Thal, thalamus; SNr, substantia nigra pars reticulata; NRTP, nucleus reticularis tegmenti pontis; PPRF, pontine paramedian reticular formation; EBN, excitatory burst neurons; IBN, inhibitory burst neurons; OPN, omnipause neurons; VI, the abducens nucleus. For details, see text.

the fastigial nucleus provide acceleration for contralateral saccades and pursuit. The fastigial nucleus projects via the uncinate fasciculus to the contralateral brainstem generators of horizontal and vertical saccades. Therefore, lesions of the medulla affecting inputs to the fastigial nucleus produce hypermetric ipsilateral saccades (i.e. 'lateropulsion'), whereas midbrain lesions affecting its outputs result in hypermetric contralateral saccades. Neurons in the fastigial nucleus and nucleus interpositus project to the midbrain vergence ('near-response') cells. A recent study using single-unit recording demonstrated a 'far-response' region within a posterior nucleus interpositus. Neurons there are active during divergence and accommodation, the response being elicited by both blur and disparity cues.[36] Their dysfunction may underlie the esotropia that occurs occasionally with cerebellar lesions.

The flocculus takes part in the adaptive control of the vestibulo-ocular reflex.[37] It receives inputs from structures important for 'neural integration' and projects to the vestibular nuclei. The nodulus and uvula are responsible for the 'velocity-storage' mechanism, by which secondary vestibular neurons prolong their responses beyond those of the primary vestibular neurons.[38] 'Velocity storage' is implicated in the pathogenesis of periodic alternating nystagmus.

Descending pathways

In general, reflexive eye movements of various types originate in posterior parts of the brain, whereas voluntary, self-initiated movements (saccades, pursuit and fixation) derive from frontal areas that include but are not limited to the frontal eye fields (FEFs).[1] Although cortical control of saccades is contralateral, the exact location of the notorious 'ocular motor decussation' is unknown, being somewhere between the level of nerve nuclei IV and VI. In contrast, pursuit control is mainly ipsilateral. The descending ocular motor projections defy the usual 'upper motor neuron—lower motor neuron' sequence; their cortical neurons do *not* directly project to ocular motoneurons in the brainstem. Moreover, very few of them end up directly on the PPRF. For both saccades and pursuit, the descending pathways are polysynaptic, with numerous intermediate stations on the way to their final destination. Similarly to skeletal motor control, internal feedback loops for saccades include the basal ganglia and thalamus (Fig. 47.3).

The SC mediates much of the frontal ocular motor influence.[39] The signals conveyed from the FEF to the SC are manifold, reflecting the diverse neuronal population within the FEF. The SC consists of several functionally and anatomically distinct zones. Its rostral pole is important for fixation; it receives direct input from fixation FEF neurons with foveal visual responses.[39–41] The caudal region contains neurons responsible for activation of saccades. The 'saccade-related' cells in the SC are under tonic inhibition of the substantia nigra pars reticulata (SNr); this inhibition is phasically removed by another inhibition from the caudate nucleus to the SNr, resulting in a disinhibition of the SC. The efferents of 'saccade-related' SC neurons reach the contralateral PPRF. While lesions restricted to the SC have relatively minor effects on eye movements,[42] combined damage to the frontal cortex and the SC causes severe ocular motor dysfunction by affecting all the descending projections.

Smooth pursuit pathways travel to the ipsilateral brainstem from the temporo–parieto–occipital junction and FEFs. A pretectal structure important for pursuit is the rostral part of the nucleus of optic tract (NOT).[43] Lesions there affect ipsilateral pursuit along with ipsilateral OKN, suggesting that processing of these two functions is closely related. The pursuit pathways further descend to the ipsilateral dorsolateral pontine nuclei whose efferents decussate to reach contralateral cerebellar flocculus, and from there to the vestibular nuclei. Vestibular projections cross again to finally end up on the abducens nucleus, ipsilateral to the cortex where the signal originated, which makes the pursuit pathway essentially ipsilateral.

DISORDERS OF SUPRANUCLEAR CONTROL OF EYE MOVEMENTS

We will consider here major disorders of conjugate horizontal and vertical gaze and some vergence disorders. Owing to space limitations, we are forced to leave out fixation disorders, such as most forms of nystagmus and saccadic intrusions; for them, the reader is referred to standard texts.[1,44]

Horizontal gaze disorders

Gaze palsy

Damage to the abducens nucleus results in a rare but fairly characteristic pattern of a 'nuclear VI': inability to activate the ipsilateral lateral rectus and contralateral medial rectus for all types of conjugate eye movements, including vestibulo-ocular reflexes ('doll's eyes' maneuvers).[45] Vergence movements, however, may be spared. 'Nuclear VI' is usually accompanied by ipsilateral peripheral facial weakness (because of the adjacent genu of the VII nerve) and esotropia (because of the possible concurrent involvement of the VI nerve fascicle on the side of the lesion). As opposed to the loss of all conjugate eye movements seen with the nuclear VI palsy, selective impairment of ipsilateral horizontal saccades (in both eyes) results from discrete lesions of the PPRF.[46,47] Bilateral damage to the PPRF results in slow vertical saccades, in addition to inability to produce horizontal saccades in both directions. Selective defects of horizontal saccades occur in degenerative conditions, such as various types of spinocerebellar degenerations or Gaucher's disease. Isolated deficits of ipsilateral smooth pursuit occur with pontine lesions affecting the dorsolateral pontine nuclei; cerebellar lesions can impair contralateral pursuit.[48,49]

Internuclear ophthalmoplegia (INO)

Lesions of the MLF result in impaired adduction during conjugate contralesional gaze and 'abducting nystagmus'. The MLF lesion is on the side of poor adduction. The dissociate nystagmus of the abducting eye (contralateral to the lesion) reflects central adaptation in response to the adduction weakness;[50] similar dissociated nystagmus may be observed in a healthy agonist muscle with extraocular muscle weakness of any etiology. Extensive damage to the MLF may be accompanied by skew deviation (see below) and dissociate vertical nystagmus. Subtle INO may manifest in slowing of adducting saccades, without range limitation. This discrepancy of the velocities between abducting and adducting can be readily demonstrated using an optokinetic tape. Although the medial rectus on the affected side appears weak, it can often be activated during convergence effort, since premotor vergence commands reach motoneurons of the medial rectus subnucleus from the rostral midbrain, and not via the MLF. However, in some INO patients convergence is not preserved (Cogan's 'anterior INO').

Unfortunately, this classification of INO into anterior and posterior types according to preservation of convergence does not help to localize the responsible lesion to either pons or midbrain. Patients with unilateral INO do not complain of diplopia on looking straight ahead, since they are orthotropic (or exophoric) unless accompanied by skew deviation. In contrast, patients with bilateral INO have exotropia—a syndrome termed WEBINO: 'wall-eyed bilateral INO'. The most frequent cause of bilateral INO, especially in young adults, is multiple sclerosis. Other causes include brainstem strokes, neoplastic processes and trauma.

'One-and-a-half' syndrome

Lesion involving the MLF and the abducens nucleus on the same side causes palsy of all conjugate horizontal movements except for abduction in the contralateral eye.[51] In its partial form restricted for saccadic impairment, the syndrome can arise from combined damage to the ipsilateral PPRF and MLF. Acutely, the patient may be exotropic ('paralytic pontine exotropia').[52] This syndrome has been described with various processes affecting the pons, such as stroke, multiple sclerosis, and tumors.

Impaired eccentric gaze-holding

Lesions affecting the medial vestibular nucleus (MVN) and adjacent nucleus prepositus hypoglossi (NPH) abolish the gaze-holding mechanism (neural integrator).[16,53] As a result, during attempted horizontal gaze, the eyes drift slowly towards the orbital mid-position; consequent corrective quick phases (saccades) produce the appearance of gaze-evoked nystagmus. The NPH and MVN are susceptible to toxic effects of numerous substances, among them antiepileptic medications and lithium; they also suffer early in the course of thiamin deficiency. Thus, gaze-evoked nystagmus may be a sensitive sign of Wernicke's encephalopathy or drug intoxication.

Saccadic lateropulsion

In lateral medullary infarction (Wallenberg's syndrome), there is a characteristic change in saccades: ipsilateral horizontal saccades become hypermetric and deviate towards the side of the lesion ('ipsipulsion').[54] A similar phenomenon affects vertical saccades, with unwanted horizontal, ipsilesional curving of the trajectories. An explanation for lateropulsion lies in impaired cerebellar modulation of saccadic metrics, secondary to dysfunction of the dorsal vermis and the fastigial nucleus. An infarcted inferior cerebellar peduncle in Wallenberg's syndrome results in inhibition of the ipsilateral fastigial nucleus, thus producing ipsipulsion of saccades.[33] In the same vein, lesions affecting crossed outputs of the fastigial nucleus via the superior cerebellar peduncle result in contrapulsion, such as seen with midbrain disease.

Gaze deviations

As a rule, with brainstem (pontine) lesions, gaze deviation is contralesional. However, medullary lesions producing Wallenberg's syndrome can cause the eyes to deviate ipsilesionally. In pontine gaze deviations, the eyes cannot be driven into the paretic field by vestibulo-ocular reflexes ('doll's eyes'); this can help to distinguish between hemispheric and pontine gaze deviations.

Vertical gaze disorders

Since generation of pure vertical gaze shifts requires bilateral activation of the corresponding cortical and brainstem areas, unilateral lesions along the pathway are expected to result in relatively mild changes in vertical eye movements. In order to produce noticeable deficits of vertical gaze, damage has to be either bilateral or midline, hence affecting the crossing fibers from both right and left counterparts. Indeed, unilateral lesions of the riMLF cause only a slowing of downward saccades; upward saccades remain unchanged (perhaps reflecting the bilateral projections of the riMLF to elevator muscles

but ipsilateral projections to depressor muscles). Nevertheless, ipsitorsional saccades become markedly impaired (e.g. damage to the right riMLF will cause inability to produce quick extorsion of the right eye and intorsion of the left eye), with tonic, contralesional torsional deviation.[47]

Bilateral experimental lesions of the riMLF in monkeys essentially abolish vertical saccades; other eye movements are spared, including vertical gaze-holding, vestibular eye movements and pursuit, as well as horizontal saccades.[21] Similarly, patients with discrete, bilateral lesions (e.g. infarctions in the territory of the posterior thalamo-subthalamic artery) of the riMLF have markedly abnormal vertical saccades in both upward and downward directions.[55] Certain degenerative, metabolic or even infectious disorders selectively affect the riMLF bilaterally, thus producing slow or even absent vertical saccades (e.g. progressive supranuclear palsy, Niemann–Pick type C, Whipple's disease).

Eccentric vertical gaze-holding can be impaired by unilateral experimental lesions of the INC. In addition, lesions there are associated with skew deviation (see below) and impaired vertical vestibulo-ocular reflex, as well as hypometric vertical saccades; these deficits are more pronounced with bilateral INC lesions.[26] In both patients and animal studies, lesions of the riMLF and INC are accompanied by torsional nystagmus. The direction of the nystagmus can help in localizing the lesion: with riMLF lesions, the nystagmus is contralesional, whereas with INC lesions, it is ipsilesional (in both cases, tonic torsional deviation is contralesional).[56]

The posterior commissure lesions result in loss of upward gaze,[57] with profound deficit of vertical gaze-holding (integrator failure)[27] due to dysfunction of the nucleus of the posterior commissure and the crossing fibers from the INC and the adjacent mesencephalic reticular formation. In its full form, dorsal midbrain syndrome (Parinaud syndrome) is characterized by limitation of upward eye movements, with downward bias of the resting eye position—'setting sun' sign; upper eyelid retraction on looking straight ahead (Collier's sign); convergence–retraction nystagmus at attempted upward gaze; pseudoabducens palsy; and mid-dilated pupils with light-near dissociation. 'Convergence-retraction nystagmus' can be provoked by making the patient watch a downwards moving optokinetic tape: refixation effort will stimulate a series of repetitive upward saccades, each being substituted by a convergence movement. Co-contraction of the horizontal recti produces globe retraction, which is best seen by observing the patient's eye in profile.

Increased vergence tone underlies bilateral limitation of abduction ('pseudoabducens palsy').[58] The most common causes of dorsal midbrain syndrome are pineal area tumors, midbrain infarction, and hydrocephalus (especially in children).

Skew deviation is a vertical ocular misalignment of supranuclear origin. Although classically comitant, the hypertropia may vary or even alternate as a function of orbital eye position. Non-comitant skew can be distinguished from IV nerve palsy by a usually negative head tilt and the direction of cyclorotation: with skew deviation, the hypertropic eye is incyclotorted, whereas with trochlear palsy, it is excyclotorted (Fig. 47.4). Skew deviation is a part of a more general ocular tilt reaction (OTR) that consists of head tilt, ocular torsion and vertical skew (all in the same direction), with the torsional deviation being the most sensitive and consistent sign (Fig. 47.4).[59] In addition, OTR patients have deviation of the subjective visual vertical. OTR reflects imbalance of otolithic inputs; it can occur with lesions anywhere along this pathway, from the otolithic organs in the inner ear, through the ipsilateral vestibular nuclei, and up to the contralateral INC. The common occurrence of skew deviation with peripheral VIII nerve lesions[60–62] such as vestibular nerve surgery or vestibular neuritis seemingly contradicts its definition as a supranuclear disorder. Yet, in this context, 'supranuclear' refers to the ocular motor nuclei, which may be affected by changes in otolithic inputs on any level, including peripheral. Since central otolithic projections cross at the lower pontine level and run in the MLF to reach the contralateral INC,[63] peripheral and lower brainstem lesions cause ipsilateral OTR, whereas high pontine and midbrain lesions produce contralateral OTR.[64] Thus, lesions of the vestibular nerve result in ipsilesional head tilt, hypotropia and excyclotorsion; lesions of the MLF and INC cause contralateral head tilt, hypotropia and excyclotorsion. In some patients with midbrain lesions, skew deviation may slowly alternate.[65]

Vergence disorders

Comitant esotropia occurs with structural and degenerative cerebellar disease, implying an increased vergence tone—perhaps as a result of impaired cerebellar control of divergence (see above).[66] Convergence spasm (spasm of the near reflex) is usually psychogenic, manifesting in unilateral or bilateral limitation of abduction that mimics VI nerve palsy. Once the diagnosis is suspected, pupils should be carefully examined: on attempted

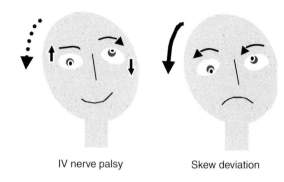

IV nerve palsy   Skew deviation

Figure 47.4 Skew deviation versus IV nerve palsy. The right panel illustrates right ocular tilt reaction (OTR), and the left panel illustrates left trochlear palsy. In both, left hypertropia (usually non-comitant) is accompanied by right head tilt. Torsional deviation of the hypertropic eye helps to distinguish between the two conditions: with IV nerve palsy, the hypertropic eye is excyclotorted and the hypotropic eye has no torsional deviation; with OTR, the hypertropic eye is incyclotorted and the hypotropic eye is excyclotorted (curved 'eyebrow' arrows). In OTR, spontaneous head tilt in the direction of torsional deviation (solid curved arrow) does not eliminate vertical diplopia, since it is not compensatory to ocular misalignment. In contrast, in IV nerve palsy, contralateral head tilt is compensatory (dotted curved arrow): it results in depression of the hypertropic eye and elevation of the hypotropic eye (vertical arrows), thus alleviating diplopia.

lateral gaze, miosis is observed, implying that the patient is using vergence instead of a version movement (the pupil constricts as a part of the near triad). Rarely, tonic spasm of the near reflex may occur with organic midbrain disease.[58,67]

Divergence insufficiency is a rare clinical entity, characterized by comitant esotropia at far distances; the patients complain of diplopia while viewing distant objects. A prerequisite of the diagnosis is exclusion of VI nerve dysfunction, i.e. normal velocities of abducting saccades. Divergence insufficiency has been reported in seizures, progressive supranuclear palsy, following viral infections, and in the course of recovery from the abducens palsy.[68] It is possible that lesions encroaching on an outer cap of the abducens nucleus may selectively affect neurons encoding for tonic eye position and thus result in pure static ocular misalignment, without slowing abducting saccades. Most patients benefit from base-out prisms incorporated in distant spectacle correction.

Convergence insufficiency is a common cause of diplopia in young adults, who complain of 'eye strain' and diplopia at near distances. Examination shows a full range of movements but poor convergence amplitudes and exotropia at near distances. Accommodation and pupillary constriction components of the 'near triad' are preserved and attest to patients' effort during near viewing. Precise eye movement recordings have confirmed that orthoptic 'vergence' exercises can improve vergence performance.[69] Selective loss of vergence has been reported with bilateral paramedian thalamic infarctions that presumably disrupt supranuclear projections onto midbrain vergence neurons.[70]

ACKNOWLEDGEMENT

Partially supported by German–Israeli Fund grant I-574.

REFERENCES

1. Leigh RJ, Zee DS. *The Neurology of Eye Movements*, 3rd edn. Oxford University Press, 1999.
2. Krauzlis RJ, Basso MA, Wurtz R. Shared motor error for multiple eye movements. *Science* 1997; **276**: 1693–1695.
3. Zee DS, FitzGibbon EJ, Optican LM. Saccade–vergence interactions in humans. *J Neurophysiol* 1992; **68**: 1624–1641.
4. Ramat S, Das VE, Somers JT, Leigh RJ. Tests of two hypotheses to account for different-sized saccades during disjunctive gaze shifts. *Exp Brain Res* 1999; **129**: 500–510.
5. Moschovakis AK, Scudder CA, Highstein SM. A structural basis for Hering's law: projections to extraocular motoneurons. *Science* 1990; **248**: 1118–1119.
6. Zhou W, King WM. Binocular eye movements not coordinated during REM sleep. *Exp Brain Res* 1997; **117**: 153–160.
7. Zhou W, King WM. Premotor commands encode monocular eye movements. *Nature* 1998; **393**: 692–695.
8. Averbuch-Heller L, Lewis RF, Zee DS. Disconjugate adaptation of saccades: contribution of binocular and monocular mechanisms. *Vision Res* 1999; **39**: 341–352.
9. King WM, Lisberger SG, Fuchs AF. Responses of fibers in medial longitudinal fasciculus of alert monkeys during horizontal and vertical conjugate eye movements evoked by vestibular or visual stimuli. *J Neurophysiol* 1976; **39**: 1135–1149.
10. Nguyen LT, Baker R, Spencer RF. Abducens internuclear and ascending tract of Deiters inputs to medial rectus motoneurons in the cat oculomotor nucleus: synaptic organization. *J Comp Neurol* 1999; **405**: 141–159.
11. Clendaniel RA, Mays LE. Characteristics of antidromically identified oculomotor internuclear neurons during vergence and versional eye movements. *J Neurophysiol* 1994; **71**: 1111–1127.
12. Strassman A, Highstein SM, McCrea RA. Anatomy and physiology of saccadic burst neurons in the alert squirrel monkey. I. Excitatory burst neurons. *J Comp Neurol* 1986; **249**: 337–357.

13. Strassman A, Highstein SM, McCrea RA. Anatomy and physiology of saccadic burst neurons in the alert squirrel monkey. II. Inhibitory burst neurons. *J Comp Neurol* 1986; **249**: 358–380.
14. Izawa Y, Sugiuchi Y, Shinoda Y. Neural organization from the superior colliculus to motoneurons in the horizontal oculomotor system of the cat. *J Neurophysiol* 1999; **81**: 2597–2611.
15. Büttner-Ennever JA, Horn AK, Henn V, Cohen B. Projections from the superior colliculus motor map to omnipause neurons in monkey. *J Comp Neurol* 1999; **413**: 55–67.
16. Straube A, Kurzan R, Büttner U. Differential effects of bicuculline and muscimol microinjections into the vestibular nuclei on simian eye movements. *Exp Brain Res* 1991; **86**: 347–358.
17. Langer T, Kaneko CRS, Scudder CA, Fuchs AF. Afferents to the abducens nucleus in the monkey and cat. *J Comp Neurol* 1986; **245**: 379–400.
18. Moschovakis AK, Scudder CA, Highstein SM. Structure of the primate oculomotor burst generator. I. Medium-lead burst neurons with upward on-directions. *J Neurophysiol* 1991; **65**: 203–217.
19. Moschovakis AK, Scudder CA, Highstein SM. Structure of the primate oculomotor burst generator. II. Medium-lead burst neurons with downward on-directions. *J Neurophysiol* 1991; **65**: 218–229.
20. Vilis T, Hepp K, Schwartz U, Henn V. On the generation of vertical and torsional rapid eye movements in the monkey. *Exp Brain Res* 1989; **77**: 1–11.
21. Suzuki Y, Büttner-Ennever J, Straumann D, Hepp K, Hess BMJ, Henn V. Deficits in torsional and vertical rapid eye movements and shift of the Listing's plane after uni- and bilateral lesions of the rostral interstitial nucleus of the medial longitudinal fasciculus. *Exp Brain Res* 1995; **106**: 215–232.
22. Dalezios Y, Scudder CA, Highstein SM, Moschovakis AK. Anatomy and physiology of the primate interstitial nucleus of Cajal. II. Discharge pattern of single efferent fibers. *J Neurophysiol* 1998; **80**: 3100–3111.
23. Kokkoroyannis T, Scudder CA, Balaban CD, Highstein SM, Moschovakis AK. Anatomy and physiology of the primate interstitial nucleus of Cajal. I: Efferent projections. *J Neurophysiol* 1996; **75**: 725–739.
24. Chimoto S, Iwamoto Y, Yoshida K. Projections and firing properties of down eye-movement neurons in the interstitial nucleus of Cajal in the cat. *J Neurophysiol* 1999; **81**: 1199–1211.
25. Cremer PD, Migliaccio AA, Halmagyi GM, Curthoys IS. Vestibulo-ocular reflex pathways in internuclear ophthalmoplegia. *Ann Neurol* 1999; **45**: 529–533.
26. Helmchen C, Rambold H, Fuhry L, Büttner U. Deficits in vertical and torsional eye movements after uni- and bilateral muscimol inactivation of the interstitial nucleus of Cajal of the alert monkey. *Exp Brain Res* 1998; **119**: 436–452.
27. Partsalis AM, Highstein SM, Moschovakis AK. Lesions of the posterior commissure disable the vertical neural integrator of the primate oculomotor system. *J Neurophysiol* 1994; **71**: 2582–2585.
28. Schmidtke K, Büttner-Ennever JA. Nervous control of eyelid function. A review of clinical, experimental and pathological data. *Brain* 1992; **115**: 227–247.
29. Waitzman DM, Silakov VL, DePalma-Bowles S, Ayers AS. Effects of reversible inactivation of the primate

mesencephalic reticular formation. II. Hypometric vertical saccades. *J Neurophysiol* 2000; **83**: 2285–2299.

30. Büttner-Ennever JA, Cohen B, Horn AK, Reisine H. Pretectal projections to the oculomotor complex of the monkey and their role in eye movements. *J Comp Neurol* 1996; **366**: 348–359.

31. Mays LE, Gamlin PD. Neuronal circuitry controlling the near response. *Curr Opin Neurobiol* 1995; **5**: 763–768.

32. Gamlin PD, Clarke RJ. Single-unit activity in the primate nucleus reticularis tegmenti pontis related to vergence and ocular accommodation. *J Neurophysiol* 1995; **73**: 2115–2119.

33. Fuchs AF, Robinson FR, Straube A. Role of caudal fastigial nucleus in saccade generation. I. Neuronal discharge patterns. *J Neurophysiol* 1993; **70**: 1723–1740.

34. Fuchs AF, Robinson FR, Straube A. Participation of the caudal fastigial nucleus in smooth-pursuit eye movements. I. Neuronal activity. *J Neurophysiol* 1994; **72**: 2714–2728.

35. Noda H, Fujikado T. Topography of the oculomotor area of the cerebellar vermis in macaques as determined by microstimulation. *J Neurophysiol* 1987; **58**: 359–378.

36. Zhang H, Gamlin PD. Neurons in the posterior interposed nucleus of the cerebellum related to vergence and accommodation. I. Steady-state characteristics. *J Neurophysiol* 1998; **79**: 1255–1269.

37. Lisberger SG, Miles FA, Zee DS. Signals used to compute errors in monkey vestibuloocular reflex: possible role of flocculus. *J Neurophysiol* 1984; **52**: 1140–1153.

38. Cohen B, Henn V, Raphan T, Dennett D. Velocity storage, nystagmus, and visual–vestibular interactions in humans. *Ann NY Acad Sci* 1981; **374**: 421–443.

39. Sommer MA, Wurtz RH. Composition and topographic organization of signals sent from the frontal eye field to the superior colliculus. *J Neurophysiol* 2000; **83**: 1979–2001.

40. Munoz DP, Wurtz RH. Saccade-related activity in monkey superior colliculus. I. Characteristics of burst and buildup cells. *J Neurophysiol* 1995; **73**: 2313–2333.

41. Munoz DP, Wurtz RH. Saccade-related activity in monkey superior colliculus. II. Spread of activity during saccades. *J Neurophysiol* 1995; **73**: 2334–2348.

42. Pierrot-Deseilligny C, Rosa A, Masmoudi K, Rivaud S, Gaymard B. Saccade deficits after a unilateral lesion affecting the superior colliculus. *J Neurol Neurosurg Psychiatry* 1991; **54**: 1106–1109.

43. Yakushin SB, Gizzi M, Reisine H, Raphan T, Büttner-Ennever J, Cohen B. Functions of the nucleus of the optic tract (NOT). II. Control of ocular pursuit. *Exp Brain Res* 2000; **131**: 433–447.

44. Leigh RJ, Averbuch-Heller L. Nystagmus and related disorders. In: Miller NR, Newman NJ, eds. *Walsh and Hoyt's Clinical Neuro-ophthalmology*, Vol. 1, 5th edn. Baltimore: Williams and Wilkins, 1998: 1461–1505.

45. Bronstein AM, Morris J, Du Boulay G, Gresty MA, Rudge P. Abnormalities of horizontal gaze. Clinical, oculographic and magnetic resonance imaging findings. I. Abducens palsy. *J Neurol Neurosurg Psychiatry* 1990; **53**: 194–199.

46. Henn V, Lang W, Hepp K, Reisine H. Experimental gaze palsies in monkeys and their relation to human pathology. *Brain* 1984; **107**: 619–636.

47. Henn V, Hepp K, Vilis T. Rapid eye movement generation in the primate. Physiology, pathophysiology, and clinical implications. *Rev Neurol (Paris)* 1989; **145**: 540–545.

48. Johnston JL, Sharpe JA, Morrow MJ. Paresis of contralateral smooth pursuit and normal vestibular smooth eye movements after unilateral brainstem lesions. *Ann Neurol* 1992; **31**: 495–502.

49. Thier P, Bachor A, Faiss J, Dichgans J, Koenig E. Selective impairment of smooth-pursuit eye movements due to an ischemic lesion of the basal pons. *Ann Neurol* 1991; **29**: 443–448.

50. Zee DS, Hain TC, Carl JR. Abduction nystagmus in internuclear ophthalmoplegia. *Ann Neurol* 1987; **21**: 383–388.

51. Pierrot-Deseilligny C, Chain F, Serdaru M, Gray F, Lhermitte F. The 'one-and-a-half' syndrome. Electro-oculographic analyses of five cases with deductions about the physiological mechanisms of lateral gaze. *Brain* 1981; **104**: 665–699.

52. Sharpe JA, Rosenberg MA, Hoyt WF, Daroff RB. Paralytic pontine exotropia. A sign of acute unilateral pontine gaze palsy and internuclear ophthalmoplegia. *Neurology* 1974; **24**: 1076–1081.

53. Cannon SC, Robinson DA. Loss of the neural integrator of the oculomotor system from brain stem lesions in monkey. *J Neurophysiol* 1987; **57**: 1383–1409.

54. Dieterich M, Brandt T. Wallenberg's syndrome: lateropulsion, cyclorotation and subjective visual vertical in 36 patients. *Ann Neurol* 1992; **31**: 399–408.

55. Büttner-Ennever JA, Büttner U, Cohen B, Baumgartner G. Vertical gaze paralysis and the rostral interstitial nucleus of the medial longitudinal fasciculus. *Brain* 1982; **105**: 125–149.

56. Helmchen C, Glasauer S, Bartl K, Büttner U. Contralesionally beating torsional nystagmus in a unilateral rostral midbrain lesion. *Neurology* 1996; **47**: 482–486.

57. Pasik P, Pasik T, Bender MB. The pretectal syndrome in monkeys. I. Disturbances of gaze and body posture. *Brain* 1969; **92**: 521–534.

58. Pullicino P, Lincoff N, Truax BT. Abnormal vergence with upper brainstem infarcts: pseudoabducens palsy. *Neurology* 2000; **55**: 352–358.

59. Brandt T, Dieterich M. Vestibular syndromes in the roll plane: topographic diagnosis from brainstem to cortex. *Ann Neurol* 1994; **36**: 337–347.

60. Wolfe GI, Taylor CL, Flamm ES, Gray LG, Raps EC, Galetta SL. Ocular tilt reaction resulting from vestibuloacoustic nerve surgery. *Neurosurgery* 1993; **32**: 417–420.

61. Safran AB, Vibert D, Issoua D, Hausler R. Skew deviation after vestibular neuritis. *Am J Ophthalmol* 1994; **118**: 238–245.

62. Riordan-Eva P, Harcourt JP, Faldon M, Brookes GB, Gresty MA. Skew deviation following vestibular nerve surgery. *Ann Neurol* 1997; **41**: 94–99.

63. Büttner-Ennever JA. A review of otolith pathways to brainstem and cerebellum. *Ann NY Acad Sci* 1999; **871**: 51–64.

64. Brandt T, Dieterich M. Pathological eye–head coordination in roll: tonic ocular tilt reaction in mesencephalic and medullary lesions. *Brain* 1987; **110**: 649–666.

65. Corbett JJ, Schatz NJ, Shults WT, Behrens M, Berry RG. Slowly alternating skew deviation: description of a pretectal syndrome in three patients. *Ann Neurol* 1981; **10**: 540–546.

66. Versino M, Hurko O, Zee DS. Disorders of binocular control of eye movements in patients with cerebellar dysfunction. *Brain* 1996; **119**: 1933–1950.

67. Dagli LR, Chrousos GA, Cogan DG. Spasm of the near reflex associated with organic disease. *Am J Ophthalmol* 1987; **103**: 582–585.

68. Stern RM, Tomsak RL. Magnetic resonance images in a case of 'divergence paralysis'. *Surv Ophthalmol* 1986; **30**: 397–401.

69. Van Leeuwen AF, Westen MJ, van der Steen J, de Faber JT, Collewijn H. Gaze-shift dynamics in subjects with and without symptoms of convergence insufficiency: influence of monocular preference and the effect of training. *Vision Res* 1999; **39**: 3095–3107.

70. Wiest G, Mallek R, Baumgartner C. Selective loss of vergence control secondary to bilateral paramedian thalamic infarction. *Neurology* 2000; **54**: 1997–1999.

Part 8

Imaging and clinical neurophysiology

48

The role of radionucleide brain scan and multimodality

Isabelle Berry, Pierre Duthil, Frédéric Courbon, Slimane Zerdoud, Monique Bessou, Michel Clanet and Claude Manelfe

Radionucleide brain scan has undergone recent advances mainly related to improved imaging technology and radiopharmaceutical developments. The introduction of technetium-labeled compounds, such as HMPAO (hexamethylpropyl amine oxime) and ECD (ethyl cysteinate dimer) as perfusion tracers has provided gains in the availability, safety and sensitivity of the method. Indeed, the radioactive compound is readily marked on site. With its short radioactive half-life (6 h), the dosimetry of technetium is quite favorable. The energy of the radioactive emission (140 keV) is well adapted to the detectors of the gamma-cameras. The implementation of the tomographic principle, by making the gamma-camera rotating, enables the acquisition of volumetric data sets in which any reconstruction plane can be obtained with a spatial resolution of 1–1.5 cm. The lipophilic perfusion tracers cross the intact blood–brain barrier and are subsequently retained in the brain because of local hydrophilic transformation. The remanence of the tracers eases the data acquisition which may be delayed from an acute episode, the picture of which is representative of the perfusion at the time of the injection.

Multimodality is the association of imaging modalities of different sources such as computed tomography (CT), magnetic resonance imaging (MRI), magnetic resonance spectroscopic imaging (MRSI), angiography, positron emission tomography (PET), and single photon emission computed tomography (SPECT). Each modality provides for a different physical interaction with the region imaged and reflects complementary information. For example, CT is based on the X-ray interaction with the electronic cloud of the atoms, reflects density and assesses at best the details of the bone. MRI is based on the radiofrequency interaction with the nucleus of the atoms and, moreover, on their release of

energy, reflecting the relaxation times. It assesses at best the soft tissues, but not the bone, because of its extremely short transverse relaxation time. The association of the information from CT and MRI, as well as from any pair of imaging modalities, may be done according to various procedures, ranging from combined inspection of the single-modality images to fusion of the information displayed in new mutiparametric images (Figs 48.1 and 48.2). The choice depends upon the needs of the application, the discrepancy between the spatial resolution of the two modalities to be associated, and the advancements in the available software and hardware.[1] The minimum requirement is that the images be correctly aligned for a reliable display of the same region. This can be achieved in many ways:

(1) match of the positioning of one data set acquisition to the other
(2) realignment of one data set to the other during image reconstruction
(3) realignment of one data set to the other or the two data sets together during post-processing.

Realignment methods share the requirement of common landmarks. Upon acquisition, external landmarks such as the nasion and the internal auditory canals are used. Data set rearrangements performed during reconstruction or post-processing require the recognition of points or contours on the two modalities. This is the limiting step of the procedure, particularly if functional images are involved.

The level of interaction between the information on the two images can be:

(1) Side-by-side inspection.
(2) Cursor pointing at matching pixels on the images or block of images of each modality. This aspect is most important in the stereotactic

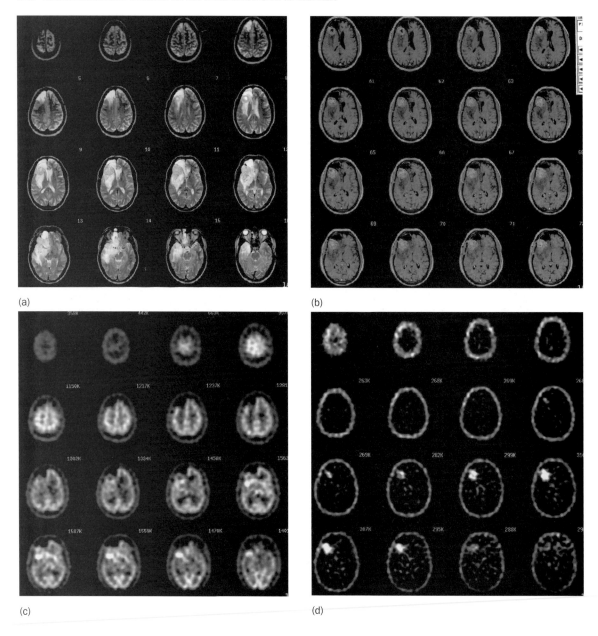

Figure 48.1   Source images of a recurrent oligodendroglioma. (a) Two-dimensional data set of T2-weighted MRI with inhomogeneous right frontal lesion, producing right frontal horn compression, invading the insula and infiltrating the right basal ganglia. (b) Three-dimensional data set of T1-weighted MRI after intravenous injection of gadolinium chelate. The inhomogeneous lesion is better analyzed and separated in a gadolinium-enhancing rounded and partly rim frontal lesion. Anteriorly is located a cavity from previous surgery. Posterior infiltration does not enhance after gadolinium and could correspond either to tumor or to edema. (c) Three-dimensional data set of perfusion SPECT after intravenous injection of Tc-ECD. A high focus of tracer uptake is identified in the right insula. (d) Three-dimensional data set of thallium SPECT, to identify viable tumor uptake of this atom, which is analogous to potassium.

applications, in which the simultaneous display of brain images from different imaging devices is obtained in different orientations. Dynamic multi-image environments allow for all modality images to be simultaneously displayed in multiple windows and adjusted for common

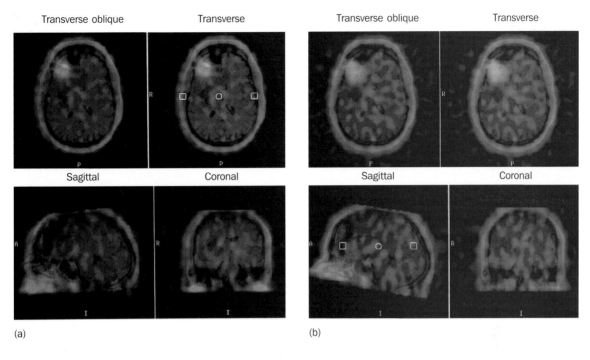

Transverse oblique   Transverse
Sagittal   Coronal
(a)

Transverse oblique   Transverse
Sagittal   Coronal
(b)

Transverse oblique   Transverse
Sagittal   Coronal
(c)

Figure 48.2 Multimodality images. (a) Volumetric realignment of thallium-SPECT three-dimensional data set to T1-weighted MRI three-dimensional data set. Adjustment has been achieved in the transverse and coronal planes and is in process in the sagittal plane. Note in this plane the mismatch of the SPECT, which requires upward tilt to match the MRI. (b) Completed realignment of thallium-SPECT three-dimensional data set onto T1-weighted MRI three-dimensional data set. The focus of thallium uptake corresponds to the location of the gadolinium enhancement on MRI. This pattern is likely to correspond to viable high-grade tumor. (c) Completed realignment of Tc-ECD-perfusion-SPECT three-dimensional data set onto T1-weighted MRI three-dimensional data set. The focus of ECD uptake is immediately posterior to the location of gadolinium enhancement. Although this region does not uptake thallium because of blood–brain barrier integrity, it is also likely to be viable tumor. On the other hand, the most posterior part of the lesion, hyperintense on T2-weighted sequence, hypointense on T1-weighted sequence, lacking thallium uptake and presenting with slightly decreased perfusion is likely to correspond to edema.

coordinates with reference to stereotactic frame fiducial markers.[2]

(3) Definition of regions of interest on one image automatically reported on the other modality by linkages between images allowing for information interchanges. This capability is of help in studying the focal inhomogeneities in lesions. For example, the comparison of gadolinium contrast enhancement on T1-weighted MRI and the thallium uptake of brain on SPECT benefits patients with acquired immunodeficiency syndrome who have intracranial mass lesions. It

can help to distinguish between lymphoma and infectious lesions such as *Toxoplasma* encephalitis. Both lesions enhance with gadolinium, but lymphoma only takes up thallium with a high sensitivity.[3] The uptake of thallium is best assessed with an index of fixation of the lesion related to that of the scalp.[4] The reliability of the SPECT index is improved when the definition of the regions of interest is done on the anatomical images, the scalp being better delineated.

(4) Definition of volumes of interest on one block automatically reported on the other modality.

(5) Fusion of information under various displays— plain superimposition, superimposition with different color scales, superimposition with variable proportion of each modality, altering display of the modalities (whole images, stripes, checkerboards, etc.).

(6) Fusion of statistically processed information from one of the modalities with information from the other. Brain activation imaging is an example in which statistically significant pixels of PET reflecting relevant increases of local cerebral bloodflow related to a task performance are fused on a morphological data set usually coming from volumetric MRI. One of the most widespread software packages used to achieve both the realignment of the data sets, the statistical extraction of the relevant pixels and the fusion of data is SPM (statistical parametric mapping).[5] Another example of this type of analysis is the fusion on MRI of epileptogenic foci identified in subtracting resting from critical perfusion SPECT. This data processing is known as SISCO.[6]

(7) Inclusion of multimodality parametric imaging in application software such as neuronavigation for surgical treatment planning, or systems for radiation treatment planning. For example, functional information is aimed at being registered in those systems for sparing eloquent areas during both surgery[7] and radiation therapy. In these, the planning system provides dose–volume histograms for volumes of interest and helps to produce treatment plans that spare functional brain while providing identical target coverage.[8]

Multimodality offers new applications for functional imaging techniques. It enhances their potential by improving their capability of localization. This is especially true in the case of SPECT, in which spatial resolution is very coarse. The capabilities, though, were limited when only CT and two-dimensional

SPECT were available. The only realignment achievable was to match the positions for the acquisitions, because the two-dimensional data sets containing only slices could not easily be rearranged during post-processing. Also, the software allowed at most the definition of regions of interest.[9] Now MRI is usually preferred as the morphological modality and can be acquired volumetrically in the three-dimensional mode as well as SPECT. This allows for powerful realignments of data sets with rigid or elastic transformations similar to the adjustment of 'a hat to the head'. Usually, the SPECT data set containing less digital data because of its coarser spatial resolution is realigned to the MRI data set by brain surface matching. Reported accuracy shows mismatches ranging from 2.1 to 4.3 mm.[10] Fully automated algorithms to register the images are being worked on.[11] Partitioning is added to co-registration and allows for tissue segmentation.[12]

SELECTED APPLICATION OF THE USE OF RADIONUCLEIDE BRAIN SCAN AND MULTIMODALITY: ALZHEIMER'S DISEASE

Alzheimer's disease (AD) is one application where multimodality explorations will be further emphasized because of recent developments. MRI volumetric sampling of SPECT perfusion has proven its success in preclinical prediction of AD. It was recently established that cingulate regions show significant perfusion abnormalities in the prodromal phase of AD and that the combination of structural and functional imaging methods may be particularly useful in identifying individuals in the earliest pathophysiological stages of AD.[13]

Of the many potential causes of dementia, AD is the most common and accounts for approximately two-thirds of cases in older populations. Typical clinical features help differentiate various other conditions. Neuropsychological measures are of high sensitivity, but their coupling with neuroimaging visualization improves specificity.[14] The typical SPECT pattern shows hypoperfusion in the posterior cerebral association cortices on both or one side. Atypical patterns are frequently encountered due to the wide spectrum of AD presentation.[15] Early brain atrophy has been recognized in AD and imaged on CT performed in the temporal lobe axis orientation to study the medial temporal lobe. In patients with histopathologically confirmed AD, the size of the medial temporal lobe is almost half that in age-matched controls, and the rate of atrophy shown by yearly scans (15% per year) is 10-fold greater. The degree of medial temporal lobe atrophy is related to the density of neurofibrillary tangles in the hippocampus. This was recognized as a useful guide to diagnosis and it was expected to have potential as a screening tool in populations. It was even proposed that measurement of the rate of atrophy in asymptomatic individuals may be a predictor of AD and could be used to monitor the effectiveness of therapies designed to retard the rate of neurodegeneration.[16] In fact, the measurements on CT suffer from lack of reproducibility and needed the improvements in volumetry brought about by the segmentation of tissue allowed by MRI. Automated hemispheric surface displays better assessed the cortical atrophy and permitted the quantification of the mean hemispheric-to-intracranial volume ratio: 58.4% in AD, significantly smaller than the ratio in the control subjects (66.0%).[17] Segmentation of brain compartments showed a decrease in gray matter (–6 84 ± 1.58%) and white matter fractions (–9.79 ± 2.47%) and an increase in cerebrospinal fluid fraction (+58.80 ± 10.37%).[18]

The combination of information from functional and structural imaging increases the specificity of the diagnosis and allows for a better quantitative data analysis.[19] One of the most important limiting factors in quantitative data analysis is partial volume averaging. This effect is increased in the case of atrophy and it influences measurement of the metabolic reduction as well as the perfusion reflecting it. In this case, interpretation can be biased, because cortical activity will be underestimated due to the atrophy. Although hypometabolic areas usually correspond to atrophic regions, they also occur without such changes. Thus, it is of importance to differentiate authentic hypometabolism and hypoperfusion from that due to partial volume effect from atrophy (cell loss). Consequently, methods for correction of SPECT data with three-dimensional MRI are of interest. They are based on a segmentation on the MRI of the cerebral structures, into gray matter, white matter and cerebrospinal fluid, and a superimposition of the SPECT images onto the MRI to obtain anatomofunctional correlations through a correction map. This method is derived from a PET method of correction for the cerebral metabolic rate of glucose, showing after correction that global cortical metabolism increases on average by 24–29%, whereas increases were 65–75% for the AD patients.[20]

The diagnostic value for AD of SPECT and MRI evaluated separately and in combination leads to the conclusion that adding SPECT to MRI seems useful only if a diagnosis of AD is suspected clinically and confirmation is needed.[21] Indeed, the sensitivity and specificity of MRI for AD are 70% and 76%. Those of SPECT are 30% and 71%. When both tests are positive, the combined sensitivity is low (20%), but the false-positive rate is also very low (5%). A negative result on MRI or SPECT yields a high specificity (93–98%) but also a high false-negative rate (60–80%).[21]

Preclinical prediction of the development of AD is the most important challenge for imaging. SPECT was reported by Johnson after clinical follow-up of four groups ($n = 136$), differing in cognitive status: group 1—normal controls at both baseline and follow-up; group 2—subjects with 'questionable' AD at both baseline and follow-up; group 3—subjects with questionable AD at baseline who converted to AD on follow-up (converters); and group 4—subjects with AD at baseline. All SPECT data in the analyses were gathered at baseline. The four groups could be distinguished on the basis of their baseline SPECT data ($P <$ or $= 0.00005$; hit rate = 83%). Regional decreases in perfusion were most prominent among converters in the hippocampal–amygdaloid complex, the posterior cingulate, the anterior thalamus, and the anterior cingulate. Inclusion of apolipoprotein E status did not significantly improve the discrimination.[22] SPECT data analyzed with the aid of MRI to determine volumetric measurements of perfusion improved the prediction value hit.

REFERENCES

1. Pietryzk U, Herholz K, Schuster A, von Stockhausen HM, Lucht H, Heiss WD. Clinical applications of registration and fusion of multimodality brain images from PET, SPECT, CT, and MRI. *Eur J Radiol* 1996; **21**: 174–182.
2. Zhang J, Levesque ME, Wilson CL et al. Multimodality imaging of brain structures for stereotactic surgery. *Radiology* 1990; **175**: 435–441.
3. Ruiz A, Ganz WI, Post MJ et al. Use of thallium-201 brain SPECT to differentiate cerebral lymphoma from toxoplasma encephalitis in AIDS patients. *Am J Neuroradiol* 1994; **15**: 1885–1894.
4. Holman BL, Zimmerman RE, Johnson KA et al. Computer-assisted superimposition of magnetic resonance and high-resolution technetium-99m-HMPAO and thallium-201 SPECT images of the brain. *J Nucl Med* 1991; **32**: 1478–1484.
5. Friston KJ, Holmes AP, Worsley KJ, Poline JB, Frith CD, Fracowiak RSJ. Statistical parametric maps in functional imaging: a general approach. *Hum Brain Mapp* 1995; **2**: 189–210.
6. Weder B, Oettli R, Maguire RP, Vonesch T. Partial epileptic seizure with versive movements examined by [99m Tc] HM-PAO brain single photon emission computed tomography: an early post study analyzed by computerized brain atlas methods. *Epilepsia* 1996; **37**: 68–75.

7. Schulder M, Maldjian JA, Liu WC et al. Functional image-guided surgery of intracranial tumors located in or near the sensorimotor cortex. *J Neurosurg* 1998; **89**: 412–418.

8. Hamilton RJ, Sweeney PJ, Pelizzari CA et al. Functional imaging in treatment planning of brain lesions. *Int J Radiat Oncol Biol Phys* 1997; **37**: 181–188.

9. Tzourio N, Joliot M, Mazoyer BM, Charlot V, Sutton D, Salamon G. Cortical region of interest definition on SPECT brain images using X-ray CT registration. *Neuroradiology* 1992; **34**: 510–516.

10. Hogan RE, Cook MJ, Kilpatrick CJ, Binns DW, Desmond PM, Morris K. Accuracy of coregistration of single-photon emission CT with MR via a brain surface matching technique. *Am J Neuroradiol* 1996; **17**: 793–797.

11. Nikou C, Heitz F, Armspach JP, Namer IJ, Grucker D. Registration of MR/MR and MR/SPECT brain images by fast stochastic optimization of robust voxel similarity measures. *Neuroimage* 1998; **8**: 30–43.

12. Ashburner J, Friston K. Multimodal image coregistration and partitioning—a unified framework. *Neuroimage* 1997; **6**: 209–217.

13. Johnson KA, Killiany R, Jones KJ et al. MRI volumetric sampling of SPECT perfusion in prodromal Alzheimer's disease. *Neurology* 2000; **54**: A78.

14. Small GW. Differential diagnosis and early detection of dementia. *Am J Geriatr Psychiatry* 1998; **6**: S26–S33.

15. Galton CJ, Patterson K, Xuereb JH, Hodges JR. Atypical and typical presentations of Alzheimer's disease: a clinical, neuropsychological, neuroimaging and pathological study of 13 cases. *Brain* 2000; **123**: 484–498.

16. Smith AD, Jobst KA. Use of structural imaging to study the progression of Alzheimer's disease. *Br Med Bull* 1996; **52**: 575–586.

17. Kitagaki H, Mori E, Yamaji S et al. Frontotemporal dementia and Alzheimer disease: evaluation of cortical atrophy with automated hemispheric surface display generated with MR images. *Radiology* 1998; **208**: 431–439.

18. Brunetti A, Postiglione A, Tedeschi E et al. Measurement of global brain atrophy in Alzheimer's disease with unsupervised segmentation of spin-echo MRI studies. *J Magn Reson Imag* 2000; **11**: 260–266.

19. Julin P, Lindqvist J, Svensson L, Slomka P, Wahlund LO. MRI-guided SPECT measurements of medial temporal lobe blood flow in Alzheimer's disease. *J Nucl Med* 1997; **38**: 914–919.

20. Labbe C, Froment JC, Kennedy A, Ashburner J, Cinotti L. Positron emission tomography metabolic data corrected for cortical atrophy using magnetic resonance imaging. *Alzheimer Dis Assoc Disord* 1996; **10**: 141–170.

21. Scheltens P, Launer LJ, Barkhof F, Weinstein HC, Jonker C. The diagnostic value of magnetic resonance imaging and technetium 99m-HMPAO single-photon-emission computed tomography for the diagnosis of Alzheimer disease in a community-dwelling elderly population. *Alzheimer Dis Assoc Disord* 1997; **11**: 63–70.

22. Johnson KA, Jones K, Holman BL et al. Preclinical prediction of Alzheimer's disease using SPECT. *Neurology* 1998; **50**: 1563–1571.

49

Imaging brain inflammation

Marco Rovaris and Massimo Filippi

INTRODUCTION

Brain inflammation is associated with a local increase of the blood–brain barrier (BBB) permeability.[1] The leakage of gadolinium (Gd) (a paramagnetic contrast material which does not cross the normal BBB) through the damaged BBB modifies the T1 relaxation time of the areas where it is concentrated and, as a consequence, makes it possible to image brain inflammation in vivo using magnetic resonance imaging (MRI).[2] In the last two decades, Gd-enhanced MRI has dramatically improved our understanding of the inflammatory processes taking place in the brain and of the pathophysiology of many neurological conditions.[3] It has also provided sensitive and reliable outcome measures to assess the efficacy of several drugs thought to interfere with brain inflammation and associated phenomena.[4]

Nevertheless, imaging brain inflammation with Gd-enhanced MRI is not without limitations. First, a large amount of brain inflammation goes undetected when using this technique.[5,6] This 'undetected' inflammation might be important in determining the clinical manifestations of different pathological processes, and its role in the pathophysiology of many neurological conditions warrants further investigation. Second, Gd enhancement lacks pathological specificity to the various tissue changes, such as demyelination and axonal loss, which can occur at the site of inflammation and which may influence the clinical outcome of the process.[7]

The development and application of cell-specific imaging[8] as well as the acquisition of Gd-enhanced MRI in association with other MR techniques,[4] thought to be more pathologically specific, are likely to go some way towards overcoming such limitations. These new techniques have the potential to increase our understanding of the cellular mechanisms of brain inflammation and to clarify the nature and quantify the amount of the tissue damage associated with inflammation.

This chapter outlines the major results achieved using MR technology in the understanding of brain inflammation in patients with multiple sclerosis (MS). MS can indeed serve as a useful model of how MRI of brain inflammation might be applied to other neurological conditions, since brain inflammation is one of the major pathological hallmarks of MS[9] and the application of MR techniques to the study of MS has dramatically changed our understanding of how MS evolves.[10]

IMAGING BRAIN INFLAMMATION IN MULTIPLE SCLEROSIS

Gadolinium-enhanced MRI

Gd is a rare element of the lanthanide series, with strong paramagnetic properties. When chelated with diethylenetriamine pentaacetic acid (DTPA), it is widely used as a contrast agent in MRI. Gd markedly decreases the T1 relaxation time of adjacent mobile water protons, thus producing focal high signal intensity on T1-weighted images in areas where it is concentrated.[2] The intensity and size of enhancement depend on the local concentration of Gd, which in turn depends on its intravascular concentration, the degree of BBB permeability and the size of the leakage space.[2] The pathophysiological mechanisms of Gd leakage are still not completely understood, though there is evidence supporting an active, energy-dependent, vescicular or microvescicular transport rather than an opening of the tight junctions between adjacent endothelial cells.[1,11,12]

Studies in animals[12] and in humans with MS[13,14] have demonstrated that Gd enhancement is consistent with histopathological findings of BBB breakdown. A study of chronic relapsing experimental allergic encephalomyelitis (EAE),[12] a model of immune-mediated demyelination, demonstrated that areas of Gd enhancement correspond to areas of

BBB breakdown labelled histochemically with horse-radish peroxidase. The pattern of BBB breakdown in acute and chronic inflammatory demyelination evolves from a diffuse short-lived disturbance in acute EAE to a more focal and prolonged breakdown in animals with the chronic relapsing form of the disease.[15] This indicates that prolonged BBB break-down and inflammation may result in chronic demyelinating lesions.[16] On the other hand, peri-vascular inflammation appears to be a necessary precondition for the development of enhancement, since non-inflammatory demyelination is unaccom-panied by changes in BBB permeability.[9,17] Recent studies in animals with EAE have shown that Gd enhancement correlates with the number of inflam-matory cells within the lesions[18,19] and mainly repre-sents macrophage activation.[20] Because chronic relapsing EAE and MS present similar morphologi-cal and functional changes, it is likely that enhance-ment in MS lesions may reflect active inflammation and that immunologically mediated inflammation is the cause of the initial vascular changes of acute lesions. This is confirmed by the post-mortem results obtained by Katz et al,[13] who found that Gd-enhanc-ing lesions correspond to areas with intense inflam-matory activity and mononuclear cell infiltration, and also by the evidence that intravenous steroids strongly suppress enhancement (possibly by reduc-ing the activity of the 92–kDa metalloproteinase involved in the trafficking of activated T-cells across the BBB,[21] whereas they have no effect on the devel-opment of MS lesions on T2-weighted images.[22,23]

Serial MRI studies confirm that enhancement often occurs in brain lesions from patients with relapsing–remitting (RR) or secondary progressive (SP) MS.[24] Studies with weekly MRI scans have shown that virtually all new lesions enhance during the earliest phases of their lives.[25] Enhancement may, however, also reappear in chronic lesions, with or without a concomitant increase in their sizes,[24] thus suggesting either partial repair of the BBB or possi-ble reactivation of the BBB abnormalities. The duration of enhancement, as measured by the administration of a standard dose (SD) of Gd, is, on average, between 4 and 8 weeks for most MS lesions,[24,26,27] even though a shorter enhancing period (less than 1 month) was described in 44% of lesions seen in longitudinal studies with weekly scanning.[25,28] The heterogeneity of MS inflammation is also reflected by the different morphological patterns of enhancement, i.e. nodular, patchy or ring-like. Nodular enhancing lesions may represent small areas of perivascular inflammation either at the edges of established lesions or in areas of formerly normal-appearing white matter (NAWM), whereas ring-enhancing areas are probably areas of acute inflammation at the edge of chronic lesions.[29,30] Lesions may, however, change their enhancing pattern from ring (2–5 min after Gd injection) to homogeneous (15–20 min later), thus suggesting that the BBB permeability is lower at the centre than at the periphery of these lesions.[29] Kermode et al.[29] also reported a gradual increase of the area of enhance-ment over several hours after Gd injection, which might be explained by the extension of the oedema beyond the region of active BBB breakdown and the subsequent diffusion of Gd into the extracellular space. Recently, Bruck et al.[31] and van Waesberghe et al.[32] found that ring enhancement is not restricted to reacti-vation of older MS lesions, but may be the first manifes-tation of new activity or the evolution of other enhancement patterns, especially in very large plaques.

Pathological reports[33] have described the presence of vascular damage and perivascular inflammation in the NAWM of MS patients. A recent study from Silver et al.[5] found that, after Gd injection, a persis-tent increase of signal intensity occurs both in unenhanced lesions and in the NAWM of MS patients. These changes are more evident and prolonged in patients with the progressive forms of the disease and are most likely the result of Gd leakage from the intravascular to the extracellular space via a dysfunctional BBB. This suggests that brain inflammation can occur in MS independently from focal enhancing lesions.

Although enhanced MRI with a SD of Gd is sensi-tive for detecting active MS lesions, there is evidence that a relevant amount of brain inflammation goes undetected when using this technique. Using a triple dose (TD) of Gd, 70–80% more enhancing lesions can be seen than when using a SD.[6,34,35] This may be due to the time course of the BBB leakage of these lesions, implying that these lesions might be detectable only with TD for a part of their inflammatory episode, or to the fact that BBB permeability is too modest for enhancement to be seen on SD scans. Reparative mechanisms are active soon after the appearance of a new MS lesion.[36] Thus, it is likely that lesions at the beginning or at the end of the inflammatory episode have a less permeable BBB, and that this subtle abnormality can be seen only by increasing the intravascular concentration of Gd or by allowing more time for the Gd molecules to diffuse.[2] However, in a recent longitudinal MRI study,[37] it has been demonstrated that lesions enhancing only after the injection of a TD of Gd have a shorter duration of enhancement, and that lesions enhancing after different Gd doses change their pattern of enhancement on follow-up scans only in a minority of cases. In addition, TD lesions have higher magnetization transfer ratio (MTR) values than SD lesions when they start to enhance, and the degree of MTR recovery observed during a 3-month follow-up period is higher for the former lesions.[34] This suggests that the extent of BBB opening is correlated with the degree of associated tissue damage. These findings indicate that enhancing MS lesions form a heterogeneous population and those enhancing only after a TD of Gd are characterized by a milder and shorter opening of the BBB, which is most probably associated with less severe inflammatory changes.

The correlation between the occurrence of brain inflammation and the development of permanent tissue damage in MS is still not completely elucidated. Longitudinal studies with monthly[24,38,39] or weekly[25,28] MRI scans indicate that only a minority of MS lesions appear without prior Gd enhancement. That the development of MS tissue damage may, however, occur in the absence of BBB breakdown is suggested by a study of Lee et al,[40] who found that the spatial distribution of Gd-enhancing lesions in the brain of MS patients significantly differs from that of T2-weighted abnormalities. While persistent and new T2-weighted lesions tend to occur more in the central than in the peripheral white matter, Gd-enhancing lesions are equally distributed between the two regions, thus suggesting that some periventricular MS lesions can develop without concomitant local inflammation. Molyneux et al[41] noted a correlation between the number of enhancing lesions and changes of T2 hyperintense lesion load in both RR MS and SP MS patients. Other longitudinal studies[42,43] have reported that the frequency and extent of enhancement only partially predict the accumulation of T1 hypointense lesions (i.e. the lesions with more severe demyelination and axonal loss) and is only poorly correlated with the rate of development of brain atrophy,[43] which can proceed despite the ability of some treatments to suppress the inflammatory activity.[44] Filippi et al,[45] in a 1-year follow-up study with monthly MRI scans, found a significant correlation between the number of enhancing lesions and the changes of T2-weighted and magnetization transfer imaging (MTI) lesion load in SP MS but not in RR MS patients. Patients with RR MS and SP MS have higher MRI activity than those with primary progressive (PP) or benign courses.[26,46,47] The low MRI activity of PP MS patients reflects a less intense degree of inflammation in lesions of these patients, as confirmed by a pathological study.[48] Recent studies have also suggested that the frequency and extent of enhancement is

lower in SP MS than in RR MS patients.[45,49] All these findings indicate that brain inflammation significantly, but not exclusively, contributes to the development of tissue damage in MS.

Several studies have found that the number of enhancing lesions increases shortly before and during clinical relapses[38,50,51] and correlates with the MRI activity in the subsequent few weeks.[41,50] In patients with clinically isolated syndromes suggestive of MS at the onset, the presence of one or more Gd-enhancing lesions is highly predictive of the subsequent conversion to clinically definite MS.[52] Koudriavtseva et al[50] reported that the presence of enhancing lesions in RR MS patients predicts the number of relapses in the subsequent 6 months. Stone et al[53] found a moderate correlation between the degree of clinical disability and the mean frequency of enhancing lesions over 3 months in a group of RR MS patients. Losseff et al[54] showed that in patients with SP MS, the number of enhancing lesions detected with monthly MRI scans over a 6-month period correlates with clinical progression 5 years later.

The sensitivity of MRI in revealing disease activity makes it a valuable tool with which to monitor the efficacy of treatments with the potential to modify the clinical course of MS.[4] Several studies,[38,39,46,55,56] have reported that enhanced brain MRI is 5–10 times more sensitive than clinical evaluation in detecting disease activity in patients with RR MS and SP MS, thus allowing clinical trials to be performed with reduced sample sizes and follow-up durations. The beneficial effect of steroids on BBB disruption and inflammation leads to a reduction in the duration and severity of MS relapses and has been confirmed by several MRI studies,[22,57,58] which found a positive, although transient, effect of high-dose intravenous methylprednisolone in reducing the number of enhancing lesions. At present, virtually all the large-scale, multicentre clinical trials in MS are using enhanced MRI as a primary (phase II) or secondary (phase III) outcome measure.[4,27]

Several strategies have been developed to increase the sensitivity of enhanced MRI for detecting active lesions in MS, with the ultimate goal of further reducing the numbers of patients and the durations of the follow-up needed to detect a treatment effect.[59] A first strategy tries to maximize the information that can be obtained by conventional scanning by using more frequent MRI scanning (i.e. weekly instead of monthly)[28] or an increased delay between Gd injection and image acquisition (20–30 minutes instead of the conventional 5–7 minutes).[60,61] These strategies only modestly improve (10–20%) the sensitivity of enhanced MRI, while increasing examination costs, patient discomfort and analysis time. A second strategy uses a high dose of Gd (0.3 mmol/kg (TD) instead of 0.1 mmol/kg (SD)).[6,35,60,62–64] While conflicting results have been reported in PP MS,[60,62] several cross-sectional studies have found that TD detects significantly more enhancing lesions and 'active' scans than SD in patients with benign, SP MS and RR MS.[6,63] In a recent, longitudinal study,[35] monthly SD and TD scans were obtained from patients with RR MS or SP MS for a 3-month period. This study showed that the serial use of TD enhanced MRI is safe and confirmed its increased sensitivity in detecting subclinical MS activity. As a consequence, the number of scans needed to show various treatment effects can be reduced by 30% or more.[35,65] The third strategy increases the likelihood of detecting enhancing lesions by reducing the signal of the background tissue with the application of an MT pulse to the conventional enhanced T-weighted scans.[60,64,66–68] Two cross-sectional[60,64] studies and one longitudinal[66] study recently compared the sensitivity of MRI obtained after a TD of Gd to that of MT T1-weighted scans obtained after SD injection, and found TD to be much more sensitive. The combination of TD, delayed scanning and MT pulse increased the detection of enhancing lesions by about 130%.[60]

Activity undetected by conventional Gd-enhanced MRI may contribute to disease evolution and explain some discrepancies previously found between MRI and other clinical and immunological markers of disease activity.[69–72] In addition, the increased sensitivity of new enhanced MRI techniques could improve our ability to understand how a treatment works. Using weekly MRI scanning, it is possible to show that interferon (IFN) beta-1b determines an immediate reduction of MS activity.[73] Using monthly SD and TD MRI, Filippi et al[74a] found that the effect of rh-IFN-β_{1a} on enhancing MS lesions varies according to the lesions' intrinsic nature and size (being more significant on small lesions and on those enhancing only after TD of Gd), thus suggesting that the effect of the drug is proportional to the degree of lesion inflammation.

Cell-specific imaging

Gd-enhanced MRI depicts active MS lesions, but it is not able to identify the presence of inflammatory cells. New methods for cell-specific imaging use markers for tracking various cell components of the immune system.[8] A superparamagnetic iron oxide contrast agent, also known as monocrystalline iron oxide nanoparticles (MION), can be used to label lymphocytes in vitro and in vivo for trafficking studies.[74b] This technique has been applied to the study of RR EAE in Lewis rats.[75–77] The histopathological analysis of EAE lesions showed the presence of macrophages at the sites were MION-enhanced abnormalities were seen on the MRI scans.[77] Another study[78] has demonstrated that human mononuclear cells labelled with MION can be detected by MRI in vitro, thus suggesting the possibility that the technique could provide new in vivo information on lymphocyte and monocyte trafficking in MS lesions.

Other potential techniques for cell-specific imaging may include antibody-linked paramagnetic molecules that could bind to specific cellular components or cytokines produced in the lesions. Magnetic resonance spectroscopy (MRS) also has the potential to be developed for specific imaging of spectral shifts designed to track lymphocytes, macrophages or compounds thought to be important in the development of MS lesions.[79]

Subtraction MT imaging

By applying image co-registration and subtraction post-processing techniques to serial MTI scans, it is possible to show as regions of 'pseudo-enhancement' the new active lesions which rapidly change their MTR values.[80] These areas of pseudo-enhancement correspond to MS lesions enhancing after a SD or a TD of Gd,[80] and no 'false-positive' lesions are visible in patients and healthy controls. This MTI-based method might, therefore, be used as a non-invasive and cost-effective technique to image brain inflammation.

IMAGING TISSUE DAMAGE ASSOCIATED WITH BRAIN INFLAMMATION

Magnetization transfer imaging

MTI has been used to evaluate the pathological characteristics and the evolution of enhancing MS lesions. Lower MT ratio (MTR) values, which indicate a more pronounced tissue disorganization,[10] were found in: (1) ring-enhancing compared to nodular-enhancing lesions;[67,68,81] (2) lesions enhancing only after the injection of a SD of Gd compared to those enhancing after a TD;[34] (3) lesions enhancing on at least two consecutive monthly scans compared to those enhancing on a single scan;[82] and (4) T1-weighted hypointense lesions at the time of their initial enhancement compared to isointense lesions.[34] In addition, two possible evolutions of the MTR of new enhancing lesions have been described.[83] In some lesions, a moderate decrease of MTR, with subsequent complete recovery within a few weeks, may reflect early oedema, demyelination and subsequent remyelination.[83,84] In other lesions, a marked reduction of MTR with only a partial recovery at follow-up may indicate the formation of lesions with severe pathological destruction and subsequent failure of the reparative mechanisms.[32,83,84] A recent, longitudinal study,[32] correlating MT and non-contrast T1-weighted images, described two additional patterns of MTR evolution in enhancing lesions, following an initial marked decrease. The first was a rapid restoration of MTR suggesting remyelination, and the second a complete failure of restoration of MTR values, suggesting concomitant destruction of oligodendrocytes and axons.

Variable changes of MTR may also be detected in the NAWM, which is subsequently involved by enhancement.[85–87] MTR reduction may reflect different but not mutually exclusive pathological substrates. These include: (1) increased amounts of NAWM degradation products;[33] (2) increased water content in the hyperplastic astrocytes participating in the demyelinating process,[33,88] and (3) demyelination and remyelination, which are both known to occur after the early phases of lesion formation.[34,89–91] Filippi et al[34] observed that the greatest reduction of MTR occurs about 1 month before enhancement. This interval is similar to the time between immune activation and clinical manifestations of the lesions in EAE,[92] and it may be the time necessary for immune activation and BBB transmigration of T-cells in the early phase of the pathological evolution of MS lesions.

Magnetic resonance spectroscopy

MRS allows in vivo identification of changes in the chemical composition of brain tissues.[93] Reduced *N*-acetyl aspartate (NAA) levels are associated with axonal dysfunction,[93] while changes in inositol, choline and lactate concentrations are correlated with inflammation and demyelination.

MRS studies of enhancing MS lesions[94] have shown that, in some lesions during the first 6–10 weeks following the onset of enhancement, elevated lactate levels can be found which might be due to the concomitant presence of inflammation, local ischaemia and neuronal mitochondrial dysfunction. In a recent study[95] correlating MRS and pathological findings, high lactate levels were found in MS lesions with marked inflammation and mononuclear cell infiltration. MR spectra from enhancing lesions

may also show an elevated choline peak returning to normal over a 4–6-month period, and lipid peaks suggesting increased membrane turnover due to demyelination.[94]

Data from several MRS studies support the hypothesis that, in MS, perivenous inflammation and demyelination may represent two partially separated pathological processes.[93,94,96,97] In enhancing lesions, lipid signal may persist for up to 4–8 months, whereas enhancement usually ceases within 2 months. Moreover, Coles et al[44] demonstrated that progressive brain atrophy can be seen in SP MS patients without evidence of ongoing inflammation and that this is associated with decreased NAA levels, thus suggesting axonal degeneration. This process can be conditioned by a previous high inflammatory load, but proceeds even when inflammation has been suppressed.

Recent studies[98,99] have demonstrated that MRS can detect transient NAA reductions which occur in the NAWM during a severe MS relapse[98] or when a large, solitary lesion develops in the contralateral hemisphere.[99] These findings indicate that a generalized and reversible axonal dysfunction may accompany MS relapses, even in the absence of MRI-visible inflammatory changes, and that the effects of damage to axons traversing inflammatory lesions can be transmitted over long distances. A longitudinal study[97] using MRS imaging reported that increased lipid peaks can be found both in unenhanced T2 lesions and in the NAWM of RR MS patients. Interestingly, NAWM regions where lipid levels increased subsequently developed macroscopic T2 abnormalities.

Diffusion-weighted imaging

Diffusion-weighted imaging (DWI) is sensitive to the presence of pathological processes which, by modifying the integrity of biological tissues, result in a loss of 'restricting' barriers and lead to an increase of water molecular motion and loss of tissue anisotropy.[100]

In EAE, DWI signal intensity increased before any detectable change on T2-weighted scans,[101] and an increased apparent diffusion coefficient (ADC) was seen in lesions,[101] with relatively preserved diffusion anisotropy in chronic compared to acute lesions.[102] The first report of water diffusion in MS showed that lesions had increased ADC values compared to NAWM.[103] Conflicting results have been achieved when comparing enhancing versus non-enhancing MS lesions: two studies[104,105] found a significantly increased mean diffusivity ($\bar{D}$) in non-enhancing compared to enhancing lesions, while another,[106] which assessed more patients, did not find any significant difference between the two lesion groups. Fractional anisotropy (FA) was found to be lower in enhancing versus non-enhancing lesions.[105]

All these data again suggest that, although the intrinsic nature of macroscopic MS lesions is heterogeneous, loss and disorganization of structural barriers to water motion can be detected during the early inflammatory phase of lesions. Since inflammatory cells are likely to restrict water molecular motion, demyelination or, less likely, axonal loss might contribute to the increased $\bar{D}$ and decreased FA in enhancing MS lesions.

CONCLUSIONS

Gd-enhanced MRI has provided relevant information about the inflammatory events related to MS lesion formation. The development and application of cell-specific imaging as well as the conduction of multiparametric MR studies should increase our understanding of the pathological steps between inflammation and irreversible tissue loss, and, as a consequence, our understanding of the mechanisms leading to neurological disability in MS. A similar MR approach is now warranted to define better the nature of brain inflammation in other neurological conditions, and, hopefully, to evaluate the efficacy of experimental treatments in preventing the formation of 'disabling' lesions.

REFERENCES

1. Bradbury M. *The Concept of Blood Brain Barrier*. Chichester: John Wiley, 1979: 351–382.
2. Tofts PS, Kermode AG. Measurement of the blood–brain barrier permeability and leakage space using dynamic MR imaging. I. Fundamental concepts. *Magn Reson Med* 1991; **17**: 357–367.
3. Carter EC, Cornick DMH. Contrast media in MRI. *Clin MRI* 1991; **1**: 34–35.
4. Rovaris M, Filippi M. Magnetic resonance techniques to monitor disease evolution and treatment trial outcomes in multiple sclerosis. *Curr Opin Neurol* 1999; **12**: 337–344.
5. Silver NC, Tofts PS, Symms MR, Barker GJ, Thompson AJ, Miller DH. Evidence of widespread subtle blood–brain barrier dysfunction associated with progressive MS. *Proc Int Soc Magn Reson Med* 1999; **7**: 628 (abstr).
6. Filippi M, Yousry T, Campi A et al. Comparison of triple dose versus standard dose gadolinium-DTPA for detection of MRI enhancing lesions in patients with MS. *Neurology* 1996; **46**: 379–384.
7. McDonald WI, Miller DH, Barnes D. The pathological evolution of multiple sclerosis. *Neuropathol Appl Neurobiol* 1992; **18**: 319–334.
8. Schoepf U, Marecos EM, Melder EJ et al. Intracellular magnetic labeling of lymphocytes for in vivo trafficking studies. *Biotechniques* 1998; **24**: 642–651.
9. Lusmden CE. The neuropathology of multiple sclerosis. In: Vinken PJ, Bruyn GW, eds. *Handbook of Clinical Neurology*. Amsterdam: North-Holland Publishing Company, 1970: 217–309.
10. Rovaris M, Filippi M. The value of new magnetic resonance techniques in multiple sclerosis. *Curr Opin Neurol* 2000; **13**: 249–254.
11. Brown WJ. The capillaries in acute and subacute multiple sclerosis plaques: a morphometric analysis. *Neurology* 1978; **28**: 89–92.
12. Hawkins CP, Munro PMG, Mackenzie F et al. Duration and selectivity of blood brain barrier breakdown in chronic relapsing experimental allergic encephalomyelitis studied by gadolinium-DTPA and protein markers. *Brain* 1990; **113**: 365–378.
13. Katz D, Taubenberger JK, Cannella B, McFarlin DE, Raine CS, McFarland HF. Correlation between magnetic resonance imaging findings and lesion development in chronic, active multiple sclerosis. *Ann Neurol* 1993; **34**: 661–669.
14. Nesbit GM, Forbes GS, Scheithauer BW et al. Multiple sclerosis: histopathological and MR and/or CT correlation in 37 cases at biopsy and 3 cases at autopsy. *Radiology* 1991; **180**: 467–474.
15. Hawkins CP, Mackenzie F, Tofts P et al. Patterns of blood brain barrier breakdown in inflammatory demyelination. *Brain* 1991; **114**: 801–810.
16. Lassman H. *Comparative Neuropathology of Chronic Experimental Allergic Encephalomyelitis and Multiple Sclerosis*. Berlin, Heidelberg, New York: Springer, 1983.
17. Dousset V, Brochet B, Vital A et al. Lysolecithin-induced demyelination in primates: preliminary in vivo study with MR and magnetization transfer. *AJNR Am J Neuroradiol* 1995; **16**: 225–231.
18. Seeldrayers PA, Syha J, Morrissey SP et al. Magnetic resonance imaging investigation of blood–brain barrier damage in adoptive transfer experimental autoimmune encephalomyelitis. *J Neuroimmunol* 1993; **46**: 199–206.
19. Namer IJ, Steibel J, Piddlesen SJ et al. Magnetic resonance imaging of antibody-mediated demyelinating experimental allergic encephalomyelitis. *J Neuroimmunol* 1994; **54**: 41–50.
20. Morrissey SP, Stodal H, Zettl U et al. In vivo MRI and its histological correlates in acute adoptive transfer experimental allergic encephalomyelitis. Quantification of inflammation and oedema. *Brain* 1996; **119**: 239–248.
21. Rosemberg GA, Dencoff JE, Correa N et al. Effects of steroids on CSF matrix metalloproteinase in multiple sclerosis: relation to blood–brain barrier injury. *Neurology* 1996; **46**: 1626–1632.
22. Barkhof F, Hommes OR, Scheltens P, Valk J. Quantitative MRI changes in gadolinium-DTPA enhancement after high-dose intravenous methylprednisolone in multiple sclerosis. *Neurology* 1991; **41**: 1219–1222.
23. Burnham JA, Wright RR, Dreisbach J et al. The effect of high-dose steroids on MRI gadolinium enhancement in acute demyelinating lesions. *Neurology* 1991; **41**: 1349–1354.
24. Miller DH, Rudge P, Johnson J et al. Serial gadolinium-enhanced magnetic resonance imaging in multiple sclerosis. *Brain* 1988; **111**: 927–939.

25. Tortorella C, Rocca MA, Codella M et al. Disease activity in multiple sclerosis studied with weekly triple dose magnetic resonance imaging. *J Neurol* 1999; **246**: 689–692.

26. Thompson AJ, Kermode AG, MacManus DG et al. Patterns of disease activity in multiple sclerosis: clinical and magnetic resonance imaging study. *BMJ* 1990; **300**: 631–634.

27. Harris JO, Frank JA, Patronas N, McFarlin DE, McFarland HF. Serial gadolinium-enhanced magnetic resonance imaging scans in patients with early, relapsing-remitting multiple sclerosis: implications for clinical trials and natural history. *Ann Neurol* 1991; **29**: 548–555.

28. Lai M, Hodgson T, Gawne-Cain M et al. A preliminary study into the sensitivity of disease activity detection by serial weekly magnetic resonance imaging in multiple sclerosis. *J Neurol Neurosurg Psychiatry* 1996; **60**: 339–341.

29. Kermode AG, Tofts P, Thompson AJ et al. Heterogeneity of blood–barrier changes in multiple sclerosis: an MRI study with gadolinium-DTPA enhancement. *Neurology* 1990; **40**: 229–235.

30. Prineas JW, Connel F. The fine structure of chronically active multiple sclerosis plaques. *Neurology* 1978; **28**(suppl): 68–75.

31. Bruck W, Bitsch A, Kolenda H, Bruck Y, Stiefel M, Lassmann H. Inflammatory central nervous system demyelination: correlation of magnetic resonance imaging findings with lesion pathology. *Ann Neurol* 1997; **42**: 783–793.

32. van Waesberghe JHTM, van Walderveen MAA, Castelijns JA et al. Patterns of lesion development in multiple sclerosis: longitudinal observations with T1-weighted spin-echo and magnetization transfer MR. *AJNR Am J Neuroradiol* 1998; **19**: 675–683.

33. Allen IV, McKeown SR. A histological, histochemical and biochemical study of the macroscopically normal white matter in multiple sclerosis. *J Neurol Sci* 1979; **41**: 81–91.

34. Filippi M, Rocca MA, Rizzo G et al. Magnetization transfer ratios in multiple sclerosis lesions enhancing after different dose of gadolinium. *Neurology* 1998; **50**: 1289–1293.

35. Filippi M, Rovaris M, Capra R et al. A multi-centre longitudinal study comparing the sensitivity of monthly MRI after standard and triple dose gadolinium-DTPA for monitoring disease activity in multiple sclerosis: implications for clinical trials. *Brain* 1998; **121**: 2011–2020.

36. Prineas JW, Barnard RO, Kwon EE et al. Multiple sclerosis: remyelination of nascent lesions. *Ann Neurol* 1993; **33**: 137–151.

37. Rovaris M, Mastronardo G, Gasperini C et al. MRI evolution of new MS lesions enhancing after different doses of gadolinium. *Acta Neurol Scand* 1998; **98**: 90–93.

38. McFarland HF, Frank JA, Albert PS et al. Using gadolinium-enhanced magnetic resonance imaging to monitor disease activity in multiple sclerosis. *Ann Neurol* 1992; **32**: 758–766.

39. Miller DH, Barkhof F, Nauta JJP. Gadolinium enhancement increased the sensitivity of MRI in detecting disease activity in MS. *Brain* 1993; **116**: 1077–1094.

40. Lee MA, Smith S, Palace J et al. Spatial mapping of T2 and gadolinium-enhancing T1 lesion volumes in multiple sclerosis: evidence for distinct mechanisms of lesion genesis? *Brain* 1999; **122**: 1261–1270.

41. Molyneux PD, Filippi M, Barkhof F et al. Correlations between monthly enhanced MRI lesion rate and changes in T2 lesion volume in multiple sclerosis. *Ann Neurol* 1998; **43**: 332–339.

42. van Walderveen MAA, Truyen L, van Oosten BW et al. Development of hypointense lesions on T1-weighted spin-echo magnetic resonance images in multiple sclerosis. Relation to inflammatory activity. *Arch Neurol* 1999; **56**: 345–351.

43. Ge Y, Grossman RI, Udupa JK et al. Brain atrophy in relapsing-remitting multiple sclerosis and secondary progressive multiple sclerosis: longitudinal quantitative analysis. *Radiology* 2000; **214**: 665–670.

44. Coles AJ, Wing MG, Molyneux P et al. Monoclonal antibody treatment exposes three mechanisms underlying the clinical course of multiple sclerosis. *Ann Neurol* 1999; **46**: 296–304.

45. Filippi M, Rocca MA, Horsfield MA, Comi G. A one year study of new lesions in multiple sclerosis using monthly gadolinium enhanced MRI: correlations with changes of T2 and magnetization transfer lesion loads. *J Neurol Sci* 1998; **158**: 203–208.

46. Thompson AJ, Miller DH, Youl BD et al. Serial gadolinium-enhanced MRI in relapsing/remitting multiple sclerosis of varying disease duration. *Neurology* 1992; **42**: 60–63.

47. Thompson AJ, Kermode AG, Wicks D et al. Major differences in the dynamics of primary and secondary progressive multiple sclerosis. *Ann Neurol* 1991; **29**: 53–62.

48. Revesz T, Kidd D, Thompson AJ, Barnard RO, McDonald WI. A comparison of the pathology of primary and secondary progressive multiple sclerosis. *Brain* 1994; **117**: 759–765.

49. Filippi M, Rossi P, Colombo B et al. Serial contrast-enhanced MR in patients with multiple sclerosis and varying levels of disability. *AJNR Am J Neuroradiol* 1997; **18**: 1549–1556.

50. Koudriavtseva T, Thompson AJ, Fiorelli M et al. Gadolinium enhanced MRI disease activity in relapsing-remitting multiple sclerosis. *J Neurol Neurosurg Psychiatry* 1997; **62**: 285–287

51. Smith ME, Stone LA, Albert PS et al. Clinical worsening in multiple sclerosis is associated with increased frequency and area of gadopentetate dimeglumine-enhancing magnetic resonance imaging lesions. *Ann Neurol* 1993; **33**: 480–489.

52. Brex PA, O'Riordan JI, Miszkiel KA et al. Multi-sequence MRI in clinically isolated syndromes and the early development of MS. *Neurology* 1999; **53**: 1184–1190.

53. Stone LA, Smith E, Albert PS et al. Blood–brain barrier disruption on contrast-enhanced MRI in patients with mild relapsing-remitting multiple sclerosis: relationship to course, gender and age. *Neurology* 1995; **45**: 1122–1126.

54. Losseff N, Kingsley D, McDonald WI et al. Clinical and magnetic resonance imaging predictors in primary and secondary progressive MS. *Multiple Sclerosis* 1996; **1**: 218–222.

55. Thorpe JW, Kidd D, Moseley IF et al. Serial gadolinium-enhanced MRI of the brain and spinal cord in early relapsing-remitting multiple sclerosis. *Neurology* 1996; **46**: 373–378.

56. Barkhof F, Scheltens P, Frequin STMF et al. Relapsing-remitting multiple sclerosis: sequential enhanced MR imaging vs clinical findings in determining disease activity. *Am J Roentgenol* 1992; **159**: 1041–1047.

57. Gasperini C, Pozzilli C, Bastianello S et al. The influence of clinical relapses and steroid therapy on the development of Gd-enhancing lesions: a longitudinal MRI study in relapsing-remitting patients. *Acta Neurol Scand* 1997; **95**: 201–207.

58. Miller DH, Thompson AJ, Morrissey SP et al. High dose steroids in acute relapses of multiple sclerosis: MRI evidence for a possible mechanism of therapeutic effect. *J Neurol Neurosurg Psychiatry* 1992; **55**: 450–453.

59. Barkhof F, Filippi M, Miller DH et al. Strategies for optimizing MRI techniques aimed at monitoring disease activity in multiple sclerosis. *J Neurol* 1997; **244**: 76–84.

60. Silver NC, Good CD, Barker GJ et al. Sensitivity of contrast enhanced MRI in multiple sclerosis: effects of gadolinium dose, magnetization transfer contrast and delayed imaging. *Brain* 1997; **120**: 1149–1161.

61. Filippi M, Yousry T, Rocca MA et al. Sensitivity of delayed gadolinium-enhanced MRI in multiple sclerosis. *Acta Neurol Scand* 1997; **95**: 331–334.

62. Filippi M, Campi A, Martinelli V et al. Comparison of triple dose versus standard dose gadolinium-DTPA for detection of MRI enhancing lesions in patients with primary progressive multiple sclerosis. *J Neurol Neurosurg Psychiatry* 1995; **59**: 540–544.

63. Filippi M, Capra R, Campi A et al. Triple dose of gadolinium-DTPA and delayed MRI in patients with benign multiple sclerosis. *J Neurol Neurosurg Psychiatry* 1996; **60**: 526–530.

64. van Waesberghe JHTM, Castelijns JA, Roser W et al. Single dose gadolinium with magnetization transfer contrast versus triple dose gadolinium in detecting enhancing multiple sclerosis lesions. *AJNR Am J Neuroradiol* 1997; **18**: 1279–1285.

65. Sormani MP, Molyneux PD, Gasperini C et al. Statistical power of MRI monitored trials in multiple sclerosis: new data and comparison with previous results. *J Neurol Neurosurg Psychiatry* 1999; **66**: 465–469.

66. Bastianello S, Gasperini C, Paolillo A et al. Sensitivity of enhanced MR in multiple sclerosis: effects of contrast doses and magnetization transfer contrast. *AJNR Am J Neuroradiology* 1998; **19**: 1863–1867.

67. Petrella JR, Grossman RI, McGowan JC, Campbell G, Cohen JA. Multiple sclerosis lesions: relationship between MR enhancement pattern and magnetization transfer effect. *AJNR Am J Neuroradiol* 1996; **17**: 1041–1049.

68. Hiehle JF, Grossman RI, Ramer NK et al. Magnetization transfer effect in MR-detected multiple sclerosis lesions: comparison with gadolinium-enhanced spin-echo images and non-enhanced T1-weighted images. *AJNR Am J Neuroradiol* 1995; **16**: 69–77.

69. Hartung HP, Reiners K, Archelos JJ et al. Circulating adhesion molecules and tumor necrosis factor receptor in multiple sclerosis: correlation with magnetic resonance imaging. *Ann Neurol* 1995; **38**: 186–193.

70. Martino G, Filippi M, Martinelli V et al. Clinical and radiological correlates of a novel T lymphocyte gamma-interferon-activated Ca^{2+} influx in patients with relapsing-remitting multiple sclerosis. *Neurology* 1996; **46**: 1416–1421.

71. Rieckmann P, Albrecht M, Kitze B et al. Tumor necrosis factor-alpha messenger RNA expression in patients with relapsing-remitting multiple sclerosis is associated with disease activity. *Ann Neurol* 1995; **37**: 82–88.

72. Rieckmann P, Altenhofen B, Riegel A et al. Soluble adhesion molecules (sVCAM-1 and sICAM-1) in cerebrospinal fluid and serum correlate with MRI activity in multiple sclerosis. *Ann Neurol* 1997; **41**: 326–333.

73. Calabresi P, Stone LA, Bash CN et al. Interferon beta results in immediate reduction of contrast-enhanced MRI lesions in multiple sclerosis patients followed by weekly MRI. *Neurology* 1997; **48**: 1446–1448.

74a. Filippi M, Rovaris M, Capra R et al. Interferon β treatment for multiple sclerosis has a graduated effect on MRI enhancing lesions according to their size and pathology. *J Neurol Neurosurg Psychiatry* 1999; **67**: 386–389.

74b. Yeh TC, Zhang W, Ildstad ST, Ho C. In vivo dynamic MRI tracking of rat T-cells labelled with superparamagnetic iron-oxide particles. *Magn Reson Med* 1995; **33**: 200–208.

75. Xu S, Jordan EK, Brocke ES et al. Study of relapsing remitting experimental allergic encephalomyelitis SJL mouse model using MION-46L enhanced in vivo MRI: early histopathological correlation. *J Neurosci Res* 1998; **52**: 549–558.

76. Dousset V, Delalande C, Ballarino L et al. In vivo macrophage activity imaging in the central nervous system detected by magnetic resonance. *Magn Reson Med* 1999; **41**: 329–333.

77. Dousset V, Ballarino L, Delalande C et al. Comparison of ultrasmall particles of iron oxide (USPIO)-enhanced T2-weighted, conventional T2-weighted and gadolinium-enhanced T1-weighted MR images in rats with experimental autoimmune encephalomyelitis. *AJNR Am J Neuroradiol* 1999; **20**: 223–227.

78. Sipe JC, Filippi M, Martino G et al. Method for intracellular magnetic labeling of human mononuclear cells using approved iron contrast agents. *Magn Reson Imaging* 1999; **17**: 1521–1523.

79. Dingley AJ, Veale MF, King NJ, King GF. Two-dimensional 1H NMR studies of membrane changes during the activation of primary T lymphocytes. *Immunomethods* 1994; **4**: 127–138.

80. Horsfield MA, Rocca MA, Cercignani M, Filippi M. Activity revealed in MRI of multiple sclerosis without contrast agent. A preliminary report. *Magn Reson Imaging* 2000; **18**: 139–142.

81. Campi A, Filippi M, Comi G et al. Magnetization transfer ratios of enhancing and non-enhancing lesions in multiple sclerosis. *Neuroradiology* 1996; **38**: 115–119.

82. Filippi M, Rocca MA, Comi G. Magnetization transfer ratios of multiple sclerosis lesions with variable durations of enhancement. *J Neurol Sci* 1998; **159**: 162–165.

83. Dousset V, Gayou A, Brochet B, Caille JM. Early structural changes in acute MS lesions assessed by serial magnetization transfer studies. *Neurology* 1998; **51**: 1150–1155.

84. Alonso J, Rovira A, Cucurella MG et al. Serial magnetization transfer imaging in multiple sclerosis lesions. *Proc Int Soc Magn Reson Med* 1997; **5**: 639 (abstr).

85. Filippi M, Rocca MA, Martino G et al. Magnetization transfer changes in the NAWM precede the appear-

ance of enhancing lesions in patient with multiple sclerosis. *Ann Neurol* 1998; **43**: 809–814.

86. Goodkin DE, Rooney WD, Sloan R et al. A serial study of new MS lesions and the white matter from which they arise. *Neurology* 1998; **51**: 1689–1697.

87. Pike GB, De Stefano N, Narayana S et al. A longitudinal study of magnetization transfer in multiple sclerosis. *Proc Int Soc Magn Reson Med* 1997; **5**: 122 (abstr).

88. McKeown SR, Allen IV. The cellular origin of lysosomal enzymes in the plaque in multiple sclerosis: a combined histological and biochemical study. *Neuropathol Appl Neurobiol* 1978; **4**: 471–482.

89. Lexa FJ, Grossman RI, Rosenquist AC. MR of wallerian degeneration in the feline visual system: characterization by magnetization transfer rate with histopathological correlation. *AJNR Am J Neuroradiol* 1994; **15**: 201–212.

90. Dousset V, Brochet B, Vital A et al. MR imaging including diffusion and magnetization transfer in chronic relapsing experimental encephalomyelitis: correlation with immunological and pathological data. *Proc Soc Magn Reson* 1994; **2**: 483 (abstr).

91. Thorpe JW, Barker GJ, Jones SJ et al. Quantitative MRI in optic neuritis: correlation with clinical findings and electrophysiology. *J Neurol Neurosurg Psychiatry* 1995; **59**: 487–492.

92. Cambi F, Lees MB, Williams RM et al. Chronic experimental encephalomyelitis produced by bovine proteolipid apoprotein: immunological studies in rabbits. *Ann Neurol* 1983; **13**: 303–308.

93. Grossman RI, Lenkinski RE, Ramer KN, Gonzales-Scarano F, Cohen JA. MR proton spectroscopy in multiple sclerosis. *AJNR Am J Neuroradiol* 1992; **13**: 1535–1543.

94. Davie CA, Hawkins CP, Barker GJ et al. Serial proton magnetic spectroscopy in acute multiple sclerosis lesions. *Brain* 1994; **117**: 49–54.

95. Bitsch A, Bruhn H, Vougioukas V et al. Inflammatory CNS demyelination; histopathologic correlation with in vivo quantitative proton MR spectroscopy. *AJNR Am J Neuroradiol* 1999; **20**: 1619–1627.

96. Narayana PA, Wolinsky JS, Jackson EF, McCarthy M. Proton MR spectroscopy of gadolinium-enhanced multiple sclerosis plaques. *J Magn Reson Imaging* 1992; **2**: 263–270.

97. Narayana PA, Doyle TJ, Lai D, Wolinsky JS. Serial proton magnetic resonance spectroscopic imaging, contrast-enhanced magnetic resonance imaging and quantitative lesion volumetry in multiple sclerosis. *Ann Neurol* 1998; **43**: 56–71.

98. De Stefano N, Matthews PM, Narayanan S, Francis GS, Antel JP, Arnold DL. Axonal dysfunction and disability in a relapse of multiple sclerosis: longitudinal study of a patient. *Neurology* 1997; **49**: 1138–1141.

99. De Stefano N, Narayanan S, Matthews PM, Francis GS, Antel JP, Arnold DL. *In vivo* evidence for axonal dysfunction remote from focal cerebral demyelination of the type seen in multiple sclerosis. *Brain* 1999; **122**: 1933–1939.

100. Le Bihan D. Separation of diffusion and perfusion in intravoxel incoherent motion (IVIM) MR imaging. *Radiology* 1988; **168**: 497–505.

101. Heide AC, Richards TL, Alvord EC et al. Diffusion imaging of experimental allergic encephalomyelitis. *Magn Reson Med* 1993; **4**: 478–484.

102. Verhoye MR, Gravenmade EJ, Raman ER et al. In vivo noninvasive determination of abnormal water diffusion in the rat brain studied in an animal model for multiple sclerosis by diffusion-weighted NMR imaging. *Magn Reson Imaging* 1996; **14**: 521–532.

103. Larsson HBW, Thomsen C, Frederiksen J et al. In vivo magnetic resonance diffusion measurement in the brain of patients with multiple sclerosis. *Magn Reson Imaging* 1992; **10**: 7–12.

104. Droogan AG, Clark CA, Werring DJ et al. Comparison of multiple sclerosis clinical subgroups using navigated spin echo diffusion-weighted imaging. *Magn Reson Imaging* 1999; **17**: 653–661.

105. Werring DJ, Clark CA, Barker GJ, Thompson AJ, Miller DH. Diffusion tensor imaging of lesions and normal-appearing white matter in multiple sclerosis. *Neurology* 1999; **52**: 1626–1632.

106. Filippi M, Iannucci G, Cercignani M, Rocca MA, Pratesi A, Comi G. A quantitative study of water diffusion in MS lesions and NAWM using echo-planar imaging. *Arch Neurol* 2000; **57**: 1017–1021.

50

Advances in neurosonology

Michael Hennerici and Stephen Meairs

INTRODUCTION

Ultrasound has been used for the evaluation of cerebrovascular diseases for over a decade and has made considerable progress since the introduction of simultaneous vessel wall and bloodflow imaging by means of duplex systems.[1] Not only is the initial diagnosis of early stages of atherosclerosis as the major source of arterial obstructive lesions now possible, but also its follow-up may be analyzed prospectively, whether it is spontaneous or during treatment in clinical trials and clinical practice. Ultrasound has become a standardized technology for screening patients who are at risk for atherosclerosis and for evaluation of advanced asymptomatic vascular disease. In addition, it has assumed a firm role in the investigation of patients in the acute phase of developing neurological symptoms, during acute treatment in stroke units and intensive care units, during surgery or percutaneous transluminal angioplasty, and in the follow-up of such events or procedures. The introduction of color and power Doppler flow imaging in transcranial applications has led to greater confidence in vessel identification and has added new dimensions to the assessment of small vessels of the brain and to insonation of the cerebral venous system.

Because of improvements in transducer technology and in digital image processing, the spatial resolution of ultrasound now approaches that of other non-invasive techniques, such as spiral computed tomography and magnetic resonance angiography (MRA), and three-dimensional and four-dimensional techniques are continuously improving.[2–5] Ultrasound remains superior in terms of temporal resolution. This allows the detection of high-intensity transient signals (HITS) as important indicators of ongoing cerebral microembolism, which are suspected to indicate an increased risk for cerebral ischemia in the individual patient. Monitoring of patients in stroke units, intensive care units or during carotid endarterectomy and percutaneous

transluminal angioplasty is another important topic, which is supposed to support secondary prevention in stroke patients.

Standardization of procedures and interpretation is a major issue and has been the focus of several recent consensus statements. Two important European consensus conferences[6,7] have established the basis for non-invasive diagnosis of extracranial carotid disease, which in experts' hands and in centers with close cooperation between neurologists and vascular surgeons forms the basis for a complete non-invasive work-up in the majority of patients who are to undergo carotid endarterectomy.

The major disadvantage of clinical stroke trials for the assessment of treatment regimens is the inability to identify patients who are particularly at risk. Rather than defining groups who benefit most from treatment versus those who have nothing to gain, we urgently need adequate criteria to identify the individual subject's prognosis. At present, approximately 80% of symptomatic and more than 95% of asymptomatic patients with severe carotid disease are operated on unnecessarily,[8–10] only 10 in 1000 benefit from early platelet-aggregating agent,[11,12] but 60%, who are likely to suffer cardio-embolic stroke from non-valvular atrial fibrillation, are not yet treated with anticoagulants.[13–16] It is therefore of the utmost importance to identify patients at highest risk who gain most and risk least from treatment, particularly if the treatment is invasive and potentially harmful. Ultrasound can be extremely useful for this purpose, and some recent studies indicate that ultrasound is on the way towards meeting this challenge.

CONSENSUS CONFERENCES

Quantification of carotid stenosis

The results of an international consensus conference on 'Quantification of atheromatous stenosis in the extracranial internal carotid artery' were published in 1995.[6] A review of the literature and expert analysis of validity and reproducibility led to the conclusion that, before carotid endarterectomy, X-ray angiography can be avoided if ultrasound and MRA concur in identifying severe stenosis. Ultrasound Doppler duplex methods can identify the degree of extracranial carotid artery stenosis, in terms of both diameter reduction according to the criteria established by recent surgical studies[9,10] and residual area in four sections. Technical requirements (e.g. carrier frequency, Doppler angle, sample volume) are a frequent source of incomparable data among different laboratories and should, therefore, be standardized. Peak Doppler frequency shift/flow velocities measured at the tightest point of the stenosis and the degree of poststenotic flow disturbances should be considered, as well as indirect indicators of the hemodynamic significance of obstruction. A value of 4 kHz (120 cm/s) identifies most stenoses more than 50% in local diameter reduction, and an end-diastolic value of 4.5 kHz (135 cm/s) identifies stenoses of more than 80%, whereas a carotid ratio (i.e. systolic velocity at the site of the stenosis versus that in the proximal common carotid artery) greater than 1.5 determines stenosis of more than 50% (threshold value of 4.4 for stenosis >70%). The area ratio between the total arterial lumen cross-section and the minimal residual lumen should be determined by echotomography with additional color Doppler flow imaging (CDFI). Indirect criteria, such as asymmetry of pulsatility of the common carotid artery, reduced vasomotor response of the middle cerebral artery signals and inverted flow of the ophthalmic artery or cross-flow in the anterior circle of Willis distinguish moderate from high-degree stenosis (>80% diameter reduction). MRA and spiral computed tomography can improve the preoperative diagnostic work-up in cases where continuous insonation of the carotid system is impossible (lack of exclusion of significant intracranial obstructive lesions, cases of calcified stenosis where ultrasound images are poor and application of echocontrast media failing to improve image quality).

In the light of consensus recommendations, newer studies have questioned the validity of MRA as a definitive imaging modality for carotid stenosis. Analysis has shown that CDFI offers superior accuracy to MRA, thus supporting non-invasive preoperative carotid imaging alone for detecting a threshold of greater than 60% stenosis.[17] Despite overwhelming consensus on the superiority of ultrasound for identification of carotid stenosis, the literature is still burdened by curious reports claiming

ultrasound as a mere screening technique with recommendations of routine angiography in all patients considered for carotid surgery.[18,19]

Recently, emphasis has been placed on laboratory-specific criteria for identification of patients with internal carotid artery stenoses.[20] Despite the use of similar equipment, ultrasound grading of carotid stenosis is operator-dependent and relies on different and individually validated criteria. Greater sensitivity of ultrasound screening can be achieved by applying diagnostic criteria specific to each laboratory, and multicenter studies should use laboratory-specific criteria with a local validation process.[21]

Characterization of carotid plaques

In a second international consensus meeting,[7] criteria were determined for the characterization of carotid plaques. Ultrasound B-mode is a useful technique for qualitative description of the composition, surface (from smooth to cavitated), echogenicity (from anechoic to hyperechoic) and texture (from homogeneous to heterogeneous) of plaques, whereas the thickness and length can reliably be measured down to a spatial resolution of <100 μm. Echogenicity has to be standardized, and luminal surfaces should be classified as regular, irregular (depth 0.4–2 mm) or ulcerated (depth >2 mm), the latter remaining a challenge for all imaging procedures. In addition, frequency-modulated and amplitude-modulated CDFI should be used to support plaque contour delineation and to identify secondary local flow irregularities and vortices. Magnetic resonance imaging (MRI), with or without angiography, does not yet play an important role, but may in the future become more valid in identifying intraplaque hemorrhage and lipid accumulation, both being important individual indicators of a high risk of plaque rupture and secondary embolism.

Microembolism detection

A recent consensus conference of microembolus detection by Transcranial Doppler (TCD)[22] noted that HITS may indicate solid microembolic material. Artifacts from gaseous particles, however, can occur quite often within intracranial cerebral arteries, in particular in patients with artificial heart valves, and should not be misinterpreted. Transient cellular formation, laminar condensation or bloodflow irregularities are further sources of error, and have contributed to discrediting this new technique when they are prematurely interpreted as cerebral microembolism. The members of the consensus group determined guidelines for proper use in clinical practice and scientific investigations. Their suggestion was that the standard be reported and validated in neurovascular laboratories to establish the required sensitivity and specificity for technical instruments (i.e. ultrasound device, transducer size and type, fast Fourier transform (FFT) size, FFT length, FFT overlap, high-pass filter settings), methodology (e.g. identification of arteries insonated, insonation depth, detection threshold, scale settings, axial extension of sample volume, recording time) and methods for analysis and interpretation (i.e. algorithms for signal intensity measurement, standardization of inter- and intraobserver variability and comparison of semi-automatic embolus detection algorithms).

ADVANCES IN TRANSCRANIAL APPLICATIONS

TCD monitoring in carotid surgery

A major focus of many studies is the accuracy of TCD in predicting cerebral protection during carotid surgery. Whereas results of intraoperative TCD as a monitoring modality to detect cross-clamp-dependent ischemia or ongoing embolism ipsilateral to the surgical procedure revealed inconsistent and highly variable sensitivities (60–85%) and somewhat more reliable specificities (70–95%), even the occurrence of microemboli during carotid surgery did not result in clinical sequelae in the majority of patients. Results from recent studies, however, showed that showers of HITS seemed to predict postoperative new ischemic lesions and identified the perioperative phase at the carotid endarterectomy as a potential source of cerebral complications. Lennard et al[23] and Levi et al[24] established that neurological events occurred in patients with major cerebral microembolization and showed a reasonable association between the acute development of a neurological deficit and a high number of HITS monitored in the middle cerebral artery immediately after endarterectomy. This was also confirmed by Cantelmo et al[25] by means of postoperative MRI ischemic changes. These studies have furthermore demonstrated that, in patients who have sustained embolization after carotid endarterectomy, intervention with hemodilution may significantly reduce perioperative morbidity and mortality rates, thus underscoring the important role of postoperative rather than intraoperative HITS monitoring in surgical patients.

Monitoring of vasospasm

TCD monitoring in patients after subarachnoid hemorrhage has been suggested to be useful since the infancy of TCD. It has been suggested that studies might enable identification of patients at particular risk of developing secondary vasospasm associated with ischemic events, which could be avoided by adequate early preventive medical treatment. Because this concept has been questioned by increasing evidence of potential pitfalls in the interpretation of bloodflow velocity alterations in these patients, and discrepancies between angiographically demonstrated vasospasm in the absence of elevated bloodflow velocities recorded by TCD monitoring and vice versa, the use of the test has been abandoned in many institutions.

A recent prospective study that included 186 patients admitted and examined with TCD by Wardlaw et al[26] showed that the diagnosis of the late ischemic event was predicted in 72% of patients with this complication, and this led to beneficial altered management in 43%. Although the number of individuals studied was small and hence the results are not final, these authors recommended regular TCD studies in the management of patients prone to post-subarachnoid hemorrhage vasospasm and cerebral ischemia, and speculated about potential improvement of recording the altered medical management. A randomized control trial may thus be necessary to assess these ideas finally.

The value of TCD monitoring does not seem to be limited to patients with subarachnoid hemorrhage. Hadani et al[27] have shown that after severe head injury, transiently increased basilar artery flow velocities are potential indicators of vasospasm, and hence may be monitored and patients treated to prevent unfavorable outcomes. Furthermore, patients with bacterial meningitis[28] have also been shown to benefit from repeat prospective TCD studies, if prophylactic treatment succeeds in preventing secondary stroke from associated early vasospasm.

Assessment of intracranial pressure

A more recent application of TCD deals with the assessment of intracranial pressure (ICP), which normally requires invasive methods. Increased ICP leads to changes of bloodflow velocity wave forms in intracranial arteries. It has therefore been suggested that, at least under certain conditions, a quantitative estimation of the ICP could be performed on the basis of consistent relationships between flow velocity parameters recorded from intracranial arteries and continuous but non-invasive arterial blood pressure measurement. Schmidt et al[29] supported this concept and showed that a mathematical model could predict ICP modulations from the shapes of arterial bloodflow and pulse non-invasively. These are preliminary but promising findings.

Functional transcranial Doppler investigations

The introduction of bilateral continuous TCD monitoring has resulted in the development of a variety of new sophisticated applications as supplementary tools to positron emission tomography and functional MRI studies. These include evaluation of functional recovery after stroke, investigation of perfusion asymmetries during complex spatial tasks or melody recognition, assessment of hemispheric dominance in candidates for epilepsy surgery and elucidation of temporal patterns of regional neuronal activity.

Recent studies have suggested that changes in cerebral perfusion during motor activity in stroke patients with early recovery of motor function may be monitored by TCD.[30] Increased flow velocities in both the contralateral and ipsilateral middle cerebral arteries during motor tasks have been demonstrated, suggesting that areas of the healthy hemisphere can be activated soon after a focal ischemic injury and contribute to the positive evolution of a functional deficit. This phenomenon of ipsilateral activation is not transient, because it is evident months after stroke onset. In patients with Broca aphasia following ischemic stroke, a similar increase in middle cerebral artery flow velocities has been detected after successful speech therapy, providing additional support for contralateral involvement in functional recovery after stroke.[31]

Evidence is increasing that supports the ability of non-invasive functional TCD to assess hemispheric dominance. One study, which compared intracarotid amobarbital anesthesia (Wada test) in patients evaluated for epilepsy surgery and continuous bilateral measurements of bloodflow velocities in the middle cerebral arteries during cued word-generation tasks known to activate lateralized language areas,[32] showed perfect concordance in determination of language dominance. Using another paradigm, Klingelhöfer et al[33] also provided evidence for non-invasive assessment of hemispheric dominance of language using functional TCD by detection of perfusion asymmetries caused by hemisphere-specific activation during complex spatial tasks.

Further clinical trials will be necessary to validate the impressive results of these recent studies.

Other new applications of functional TCD pertain to elucidation of complex brain functions. For example, it has been shown that, although melody perception requires bilateral activation of hemispheres, melody recognition involves activation primarily of the right hemisphere.[34] Reading induces task-specific temporal patterns of regional neuronal activity, which show habituation with longer duration of activation.[35]

UPDATE ON PATENT FORAMEN OVALE

Paradoxical embolism through a patent foramen ovale (PFO) is a known cause of embolic strokes and transient ischemic attacks in patients with stroke of uncertain etiology. Of considerable interest are recent reports on the variability of the detection of PFO when using different examination techniques. For example, the sensitivity of diagnosing PFO with both TCD and TEE is considerably higher when contrast media is injected into the femoral vein rather than into the antecubital vein, the current route for contrast media application.[36] This may be related to different inflow patterns to the right atrium, because inferior vena cava flow is directed to the right atrial septum and superior vena cava flow to the tricuspid valve. The timing of the Valsalva maneuver, the dose of the contrast medium and the patient's posture during the examination are further factors influencing detection of PFO.[37]

Evidence is mounting that migraine with aura is associated with patency of the foramen ovale, thus providing a possible explanation for the increased risk of stroke in this patient population.[38] Recently, multiple brain lesions imaged with MRI in sports divers without decompressive symptoms have been found to be associated with the presence of a large PFO as detected by echo-contrast transcranial Doppler ultrasonography.[39] A possible pathological mechanism for this association may be paradoxical gas embolism. Further large prospective studies will be necessary to validate these findings and to establish the importance of PFO as a possible risk factor for stroke.

PEDIATRIC APPLICATIONS IN NEUROSONOLOGY

Owing to its increased sensitivity for low flow perfusion, transcranial power Doppler imaging can improve demonstration of luxury perfusion after neonatal ischemic brain injury.[40] This technique is also useful for diagnosis of intracranial hemorrhage in the second trimester.[41] A major contribution to prevention of first stroke in children with sickle-cell anemia is the work by Adams et al,[42] which showed substantial benefit of transfusions in patients with abnormal TCD examinations (time-averaged mean bloodflow velocity in the internal carotid or middle cerebral arteries of 200 cm/s or higher).

ECHO-CONTRAST STUDIES IN CEREBROVASCULAR DISEASE

The ability of intravenous contrast media to increase the echogenicity of flowing blood has been known for some time.[43] Only recently, however, has there been an increasing demand for the use of echo-enhancing agents in assessment of cerebrovascular disease (e.g. transcranial ultrasound studies in patients with severe hyperostosis of the skull, quantification of internal carotid stenosis in the presence of calcification, differentiation between internal carotid occlusion and pseudo-occlusion, assessment of intracranial aneurysms and arterio-venous malformations, and investigation of the basilar and intracranial vertebral arteries).

Carotid artery stenosis

Clinical studies with Levovist have shown it to be safe and effective in improving diagnostic confi-dence for patients with carotid artery stenosis. Contrast enhancement helps to reduce operator variability, improves ultrasound images, and can aid in distinguishing between pseudo-occlusions and true occlusions, thus helping to identify patients who will benefit from surgery.[44] First reports on the use of ultrasonic contrast media to investigate carotid arteries demonstrated a significant improve-ment in characterization and quantification of severe internal carotid stenosis.[45] In further studies, Levovist considerably improved image quality in patients with high-grade carotid stenosis and allowed better visualization of the entire length of the intrastenotic residual flow lumen, suggesting that echo-contrast media might play an important role in the diagnosis of internal carotid occlusion.[46] Recent data suggest that power Doppler imaging (PDI) without contrast agents may approach the diagnostic yield achieved with the combined approach for assessment of carotid artery pseudo-occlusion.[47] Although contrast agents will continue to play an important role in ultrasonographic evalu-ation of high-grade carotid stenosis, further studies will be necessary to define the clinical setting in which their use is mandatory.

Transcranial Doppler examinations

In transcranial Doppler sonography, insonation through the transtemporal bone window is often impaired by an insufficient signal-to-noise ratio, especially in elderly patients. Echo-contrast agents have been shown to provide conclusive transcranial examinations in most patients with insufficient ultrasound penetration. Most studies have been performed with the galactose-based microbubble agent Levovist. Depending on the concentration of Levovist, the average maximal transcranial signal enhancement is approximately 12.0 ± 5.4 dB for 300 mg/ml.[48] Albunex has likewise been shown to improve the quality of transcranial Doppler exami-nations through better visualization of the internal carotid artery, the middle cerebral artery, and the circle of Willis,[49] although the relatively short duration of the contrast enhancement is a limiting factor.

Contrast agents have also been shown to enhance diagnoses when using transcranial CDFI in patients with poor tissue penetration, where imaging of vessels would otherwise be inadequate.[50] Other studies have confirmed these initial findings in patients whose basal arteries could not be assessed adequately with transcranial CDFI. After adminis-tration of Levovist, over 85% of examinations of the middle cerebral artery, the anterior cerebral artery, the P1 and P2 segments of the posterior cerebral artery, and the supraclinoid portion of the internal carotid artery siphon, were satisfactory.[51] Moreover, use of intravenous contrast material often enables the entire circle of Willis to be evaluated from a single temporal bone acoustic window when using both PDI and CDFI.[52] Recently, contrast agents have been used to enable intracranial insonation through lateral and paramedian frontal bone windows, thus offering a new approach to study the circle of Willis, the venous midline vasculature, and the frontal parenchyma.[53] The technical success rate of three-dimensional transcranial PDI investigations has also been improved with contrast agents.[54]

There is good evidence that echo-contrast agents may be valuable in transcranial Doppler examina-tions of patients with acute cerebrovascular disease. In an investigation of patients presenting with ischemic strokes and transient ischemic attacks who had insufficient temporal bone windows, 66% of contrast-enhanced transcranial CDFI studies were conclusive.[55] These findings have been confirmed by a similar study of acute stroke patients, in which native transcranial investigations were inadequate.[56]

The quality of transtemporal precontrast scans is strongly predictive of the potential diagnostic benefit that is to be expected from application of an intravenous contrast agent. In patients whose intracranial structures are not visible in B-mode imaging and whose vessel segments are not depicted with CDFI, there is little chance that the use of a contrast agent will provide diagnostic confidence.[57] This has also been shown in patients with acute cerebral ischemia. Precontrast identification of any cerebral artery provided an overall accuracy of 97% in predicting a conclusive investigation with contrast agent, while in those without precontrast vessel identification there were no conclusive studies.[55]

Basilar and intacranial vertebral arteries

Echo-contrast agents have been shown to be useful for examining the intracranial vertebral arteries and the basilar artery. Insonation through the foramen magnum when using color-coded duplex sonography and an echo-contrast agent has been reported to increase the depth at which vessels can be identified and improve the number of pathological findings not seen in native scans by about 20%.[58] Moreover, echo-contrast enhancement of the vertebral and basilar arteries may significantly increase diagnostic confidence. As in the examination of the carotid arteries, however, the relative merits of using contrast-enhanced CDFI (CE-CDFI) or PDI for assessing the intracranial vertebrobasilar system remain unclear. One study comparing these two modalities has concluded that contrast-enhanced transcranial CDFI and power Doppler sonography are equally effective in visualizing the vertebrobasilar system.[59] Conclusive studies on the role of contrast agents in investigation of the basilar artery are still lacking.

Intracranial aneurysms and arteriovenous malformations

In the last several years there has been growing interest in using transcranial CDFI and PDI as supplementary non-invasive techniques to arteriography in the detection and assessment of intracranial aneurysms. Recently, contrast-enhanced CDFI and contrast-enhanced power Doppler imaging (CE-PDI) employing Levovist have been used to detect and measure the size of intracranial aneurysms.[60] Although CE-PDI missed 4 of 36 angiographically verified aneurysms, measurements of aneurysm size correlated well with angiographic findings. Other ultrasound studies have suggested that aneurysm dimensions may vary with ICP, being larger and less pulsatile at low ICP and smaller but more pulsatile

at high ICP.[61] Intraoperative transcranial CDFI allows characterization and localization of aneurysms[62] as well as identification of vessels potentially threatened by clipping,[63] whereas intraoperative microvascular Doppler sonography has been shown to be an effective alternative to intraoperative angiography for assessment of vessel patency in aneurysm surgery.[64] An important question remains of whether in cases of acute subarachnoid hemorrhage, transcranial ultrasound is capable of detecting not only the bleeding aneurysm, but also additional asymptomatic aneurysms which may also require neurosurgical intervention.

Transcranial CE-PDI with Levovist has also been used to evaluate arteriovenous malformations (AVMs).[65] In this study, CE-PDI identified all angiographically confirmed AVMs in patients with adequate temporal bone windows. Although this technique slightly underestimated AVM size, it consistently showed feeding arteries. Coincidental blood supply from another intracranial or extracranial vessel, however, was missed by CE-PDI in all cases. These results are encouraging and demonstrate the potential of CE-PDI for evaluation and follow-up of AVM.

Sinus venous thrombosis

Recently, there has been increased interest in evaluation of the cerebral venous system with ultrasound.[66] Although transtemporal power-based and frequency-based color-coded duplex sonography enable imaging and velocity measurements in deep cerebral veins,[67] assessment of straight and transverse sinuses has been poor. Contrast-enhanced CDFI, however, can resolve these difficulties and may be of practical value in the initial work-up of patients with clinically suspected transverse sinus venous thrombosis.[68] This examination technique may also be useful for follow-up studies, in particular for monitoring of recanalization.

EMERGING APPLICATIONS IN B-MODE IMAGING OF THE BRAIN

Advances in transducer technology and image processing have enabled new applications of B-mode imaging of the brain. In patients with hereditary hemochromatosis without clinical signs of basal ganglia disorders, for example, hyperechogenic lesions of the lentiform nucleus have correlated well with both dense signals seen in cranial computed tomography and with corresponding findings in MRI.[69] Moreover, changes in the basal ganglia as visualized with transcranial ultrasonography have provoked new discussions regarding the pathophysiology of idiopathic dystonia.[70] In a recent study of 330 healthy volunteers, it was found that unilateral or bilateral hyperechogenic signals in the substantia nigra correlated to a marked decrease in the accumulation of [^{15}F]dopa in the caudate nucleus and putamen.[71] These results suggest that hyperechogenicity of the substantia nigra may indicate functional impairment of the nigrostriatal system. Further studies will be necessary to confirm these interesting findings.

CAROTID PLAQUE MOTION

One feature of carotid plaques which has received little attention is plaque motion, i.e. translational plaque movements coincident with those of arterial walls, plaque rotations and local, plaque-specific deformations. Experimental work has suggested that analysis of plaque motion may provide new insights into plaque modeling as well as into mechanisms of plaque rupture with subsequent embolism. Observations on the relative positions of fiduciary markers placed along plaque specimens during pressure loading, for example, have demonstrated that, prior to plaque fissuring, the markers display asymmetrical movement. It is thought that such plaque surface movement may be attributable to deformations resulting from crack propagation of multiple local internal tears in the plaque. Identification of local variations in surface deformability may therefore provide information on relative vulnerability to plaque fissuring or rupture.

An approach for studying plaque surface deformations has been recently reported.[72] This technique uses four-dimensional (4D) ultrasonography to acquire temporal three-dimensional ultrasound data on carotid artery plaques. The ultrasound data are then analyzed with motion detection algorithms to determine apparent velocity fields, also known as optical flow, of the plaque surface. Using this method, differences in plaque motion patterns between patients with symptomatic and asymptomatic carotid artery disease have been characterized.[72] Asymptomatic plaques showed a homogeneous orientation and magnitude of computed velocity vectors, corresponding to a global pattern of arterial motion without evidence of inherent plaque movement. Analysis of symptomatic plaques, however, demonstrated consistent evidence for plaque deformation, irrespective of arterial wall movements (Fig. 50.1). Whether analysis of plaque motion in patients with carotid artery stenosis may

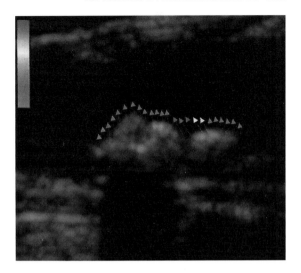

Figure 50.1 Results of plaque surface motion estimation between two digitized frame volumes of a symptomatic carotid artery plaque in systole at 80 ms and 120 ms following the ECG R-wave. Grey-scale coding of motion vectors on the plaque surface represents the magnitude of computed velocities. The vectors have been magnified (3×) for better visualization. The plaque shows a characteristic discrepant motion pattern (fast arrows at the center of the plaque) with a maximal discrepant surface velocity of 7.1 mm/s.

allow detection of motion patterns specific to patients with an increased risk for plaque complications must be addressed in new prospective studies.

ULTRASOUND THROMBOLYSIS

The experimental use of low-frequency ultrasound for direct intravascular clot lysis was first reported in 1974.[73] There was renewed interest in this novel approach when it was shown that low-frequency ultrasound could significantly accelerate the effect of thrombolytic drugs such as urokinase, streptokinase and rt-PA.[74–77] This effect is probably due to an enhancement of enzyme transport, thus enabling increased uptake of rt-PA with deeper penetration into the clot.[78] A recent study showing that low-frequency ultrasound increases rt-PA-mediated thrombolysis through the skull indicates that this technique may be applicable for treatment of acute ischemic stroke.[79] By reducing the time to recanalization of cerebral artery occlusions, adjunctive treatment with ultrasound could improve patient outcome by allowing increased salvage of viable brain tissue.

There is also evidence suggesting that low-frequency ultrasound in combination with ultrasound contrast agents can accelerate clot lysis,[80,81] even in the absence of thrombolytic drugs. Microbubble stability appears to play an important role in the enhancing effect of rt-PA-mediated thrombolysis, as shown recently in a comparison between dodecafluoropentane emulsion and sonicated albumin.[82]

SONOGRAPHIC IMAGING OF BRAIN PERFUSION

Harmonic imaging

Nonlinear oscillation of contrast agent microbubbles can produce ultrasound signals with harmonic frequency components, the relative amplitudes of which are dependent upon the amplitude of the incident pressure, the type of contrast agent, and the size of the microbubbles.[83] Because these harmonic components from microbubbles are several times larger than the harmonic signals scattered from biological tissues, they can be exploited to improve the contrast between microbubbles and tissue. Contrast harmonic imaging (CHI) is a recent ultrasound technology which uses transducers with broad bandwidths to transmit ultrasound at one frequency and receive signals at twice that frequency, thus enabling the detection of these microbubble harmonics.

The suitability of harmonic imaging for demonstration of myocardial tissue perfusion has been demonstrated in several studies. Non-invasive assessment of the intramyocardial coronary vasculature and measurement of coronary bloodflow reserve have been successfully performed using second harmonic contrast echocardiography.[84] Intermittent imaging has resulted in further improvement of harmonic imaging capabilities. By interrupting diagnostic ultrasound pulses instead of conventional 25–30-Hz frame rate imaging, very low doses of intravenous contrast medium can produce transient but significantly better myocardial contrast. This has been demonstrated in humans and can be produced safely with minute quantities of intravenous perfluorocarbon.[85]

The potential clinical value of harmonic imaging for evaluation of patients with cerebral perfusion abnormalities (i.e. those with acute cerebral ischemia) is significant, because this method would offer a unique opportunity to perform bedside monitoring of cerebral perfusion. Such a monitoring technique would be extremely helpful in the assessment of individual stroke therapy.

Two recent studies have used gray-scale second harmonic imaging with contrast agents to visualize intracranial blood perfusion.[86,87] Both have provided good evidence for the capability of ultrasound to assess regional differences in brain echo-contrast. Comparison of washout curves has shown a significant decrease in signal intensity in investigations of similar brain structures at different insonation depths. Because of this depth dependence of contrast enhancement, a quantitative analysis of brain perfusion through analysis of washout curves will require a sophisticated method to correct for this effect.[86,87]

Pulse inversion contrast harmonic imaging

Although CHI has been shown to be capable of imaging brain tissue perfusion, there remain important limitations. Significant energy loss, signal reverberations and aberrations occur when insonating through the transtemporal bone window. Moreover, in dual-frequency harmonic imaging, the bandwidths have to be narrow to avoid overlap between the fundamental and second harmonic frequencies. This leads to an inherent trade-off in image resolution, thus accentuating the problem of the transtemporal bone window.

Pulse inversion contrast harmonic imaging (PICHI) is a new ultrasound technique which significantly minimizes the shortcomings of CHI. It uses a two-pulse sequence with a 180° phase difference to cancel the effect of transmitted second harmonics on the received signal.[88] By preserving axial resolution and avoiding harmonic frequency overlaps, PICHI may open new possibilities for qualitative, as well as for quantitative, evaluation of the cerebral circulation.

First results with PICHI have demonstrated excellent ultrasonographic visualization of adult brain tissue.[89] Exceptional depth penetration has allowed simultaneous measurement of harmonic microbubble (Levovist) contrast enhancement in both ipsilateral and contralateral temporal lobes, thus providing a basis for qualitative comparison of perfusion characteristics with a single bolus injection of contrast agent (Figs 50.2 and 50.3). Although preliminary, the results provide evidence that PICHI may be very sensitive in characterization of brain perfusion. Should further studies confirm these initial findings, then a multitude of cerebrovascular applications aimed at characterization of abnormal cerebral perfusion states await this fascinating new, non-invasive ultrasound technology.

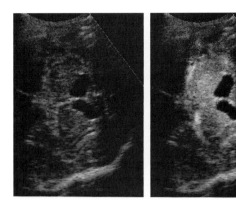

Figure 50.2 Pulse inversion contrast harmonic imaging of the brain. The left image shows a transverse section through the brain at the level of the frontal horns of the lateral ventricles, insonated with a 2–5 MHz dynamic range curved array transducer on a HDI 5000 platform (Advanced Technology Laboratories, Bothell, WA, USA). The right image demonstrates tissue contrast enhancement after an intravenous bolus injection of Levovist.

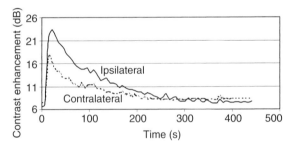

Figure 50.3 Time–intensity curves of intravenous bolus injection of Levovist from two 10-mm² regions of interest, placed symmetrically in the ipsilateral and contralateral temporal lobes of Fig. 50.2. Decreased amplitude in the contralateral lobe is due to beam attenuation. The time-to-peak intensity and the washout phase are identical in this normal subject.

CONCLUSION

Rapid progress in non-invasive ultrasound techniques has resulted in a wide variety of clinical applications for assessment of both extracranial and intracranial arterial diseases. Recent highlights in cerebrovascular ultrasound research include the use of echo-contrast agents for improved evaluation of acute stroke patients, three-dimensional imaging of the extra- and intracranial vessels, characterization of carotid artery plaque motion, and harmonic imaging techniques for depiction of brain perfusion. The important role of transcranial Doppler microembolism detection in carotid disease has been defined, new approaches to non-invasive Doppler measurement of intracranial pressure are progressing, and the clinical indications for transcranial Doppler monitoring of intracranial vasospasm to prevent secondary stroke have expanded. New functional transcranial Doppler applications, which are complementary to positron emission tomography and functional MRI studies, are evolving for evaluation of functional recovery after stroke, investigation of perfusion asymmetries during complex spatial tasks, assessment of hemispheric dominance in surgical candidates for epilepsy surgery, and elucidation of temporal patterns of regional neuronal activity. Rapid progress is likewise being made in the field of neurosonologic imaging of brain tissue. Emerging applications include assessment of the lenticular nucleus in dystonia and characterization of nigrostriatal alterations. With increasing sophistication of ultrasound methodology, it is essential that standards for data acquisition and interpretation be established. Three consensus meetings have provided detailed recommendations on quantification of carotid artery stenosis, on characterization of carotid artery plaques and on microembolism detection by transcranial Doppler.

REFERENCES

1. Hennerici M, Neuerburg-Heusler D. *Vascular Diagnosis with Ultrasound*. New York: Stuttgart, Thieme, 1998.
2. Delcker A, Tegeler C. Influence of ECG-triggered data acquisition on reliability for carotid plaque volume measurements with a magnetic sensor three-dimensional ultrasound system. *Ultrasound Med Biol* 1998; **24**(4): 601–605.
3. Griewing B, Schminke U, Morgenstern C, Walker ML, Kessler C. Three-dimensional ultrasound angiography (power mode) for the quantification of carotid artery atherosclerosis. *J Neuroimaging* 1997; **7**(1): 40–45.
4. Hayashi T, Ichiyama T, Nishikawa M, Kaneko J, Nakashima K, Furukawa S. Three-dimensional reconstruction of the power flow Doppler imaging of intracranial vascular structures in the neonate. *J Neuroimaging* 1998; **8**(2): 94–96.
5. Lyden PD, Nelson TR. Visualization of the cerebral circulation using three-dimensional transcranial power Doppler ultrasound imaging. *J Neuroimaging* 1997; **7**(1): 35–39.
6. De Bray JM, Glatt B. Quantification of atheromatous stenosis in the extracranial internal carotid artery. *Cerebrovasc Dis* 1995; **5**: 414–426.
7. De Bray JM, Baud JM, Dauzat M. Consensus concerning the morphology and the risk of carotid plaques. *Cerebrovasc Dis* 1997; **7**: 289–296.
8. Executive Committee for the Asymptomatic Carotid Atherosclerosis Study. Endarterectomy for asymptomatic carotid artery stenosis. *JAMA* 1995; **273**: 1421–1428.

9. North American Symptomatic Carotid Endarterectomy Trial Collaborators. Beneficial effect of carotid endarterectomy in symptomatic patients with high-grade stenosis. *N Engl J Med* 1991; **325**: 445–453.

10. European Carotid Surgery Trialists' Collaborative Group. MRC European Surgery Trial: interim results for symptomatic patients with severe (70–99%) or mild (0–29%) carotid stenosis. *Lancet* 1991; **19**: 45–57.

11. International Stroke Trial Collaborative Group. The International Stroke Trial (IST): a randomised trial of aspirin, subcutaneous heparin, both, or neither among 19 435 patients with acute ischaemic stroke. *Lancet* 1997; **349**(9065): 1569–1581.

12. CAST (Chinese Acute Stroke Trial) Collaborative Group. CAST: randomised placebo-controlled trial of early aspirin use in 20,000 patients with acute ischaemic stroke. *Lancet* 1997; **349**(9066): 1641–1649.

13. Connolly SJ, Laupacis A, Gent M, Roberts RS, Cairns JA, Joyner C. Canadian Atrial Fibrillation Anticoagulation (CAFA) Study. *J Am Coll Cardiol* 1991; **18**(2): 349–355.

14. Stroke Prevention in Atrial Fibrillation Study Investigators. The Stroke Prevention in Atrial Fibrillation Study: final results. *Circulation* 1991; **84**: 527–539.

15. Veterans Affairs Stroke Prevention in Nonrheumatic Atrial Fibrillation Investigators. Warfarin in the prevention of stroke associated with nonrheumatic atrial fibrillation. *N Engl J Med* 1992; **327**: 1406–1412.

16. Boston Area Anticoagulation Trial for Atrial Fibrillation Investigators. The effect of low-dose warfarin on the risk of stroke in nonrheumatic atrial fibrillation. *N Engl J Med* 1998; **323**: 1505–1511.

17. Jackson MR, Chang AS, Robles HA et al. Determination of 60% or greater carotid stenosis: a prospective comparison of magnetic resonance angiography and duplex ultrasound with conventional angiography. *Ann Vasc Surg* 1998; **12**(3): 236–243.

18. Chen JC, Salvian AJ, Taylor DC, Teal PA, Marotta TR, Hsiang YN. Can duplex ultrasonography select appropriate patients for carotid endarterectomy? *Eur J Vasc Endovasc Surg* 1997; **14**(6): 451–456.

19. Worthy SA, Henderson J, Griffiths PD, Oates CP, Gholkar A. The role of duplex sonography and angiography in the investigation of carotid artery disease. *Neuroradiology* 1997; **39**(2): 122–126.

20. Kuntz KM, Polak JF, Whittemore AD, Skillman JJ, Kent KC. Duplex ultrasound criteria for the identification of carotid stenosis should be laboratory specific. *Stroke* 1997; **28**(3): 597–602.

21. Alexandrov AV, Vital D, Brodie DS, Hamilton P, Grotta JC. Grading carotid stenosis with ultrasound. An interlaboratory comparison. *Stroke* 1997; **28**(6): 1208–1210.

22. Ringelstein EB, Droste DW, Babikian VL et al. Consensus on microembolus detection by TCD. International Consensus Group on Microembolus Detection. *Stroke* 1998; **29**(3): 725–729.

23. Lennard N, Smith J, Dumville J et al. Prevention of postoperative thrombotic stroke after carotid endarterectomy: the role of transcranial Doppler ultrasound. *J Vasc Surg* 1997; **26**(4): 579–584.

24. Levi CR, O'Malley HM, Fell G et al. Transcranial Doppler detected cerebral microembolism following carotid endarterectomy. High microembolic signal loads predict postoperative cerebral ischaemia. *Brain* 1997; **120**(Pt 4): 621–629.

25. Cantelmo NL, Babikian VL, Samaraweera RN, Gordon JK, Pochay VE, Winter MR. Cerebral microembolism and ischemic changes associated with carotid endarterectomy. *J Vasc Surg* 1998; **27**(6): 1024–1030.

26. Wardlaw JM, Offin R, Teasdale GM, Teasdale EM. Is routine transcranial Doppler ultrasound monitoring useful in the management of subarachnoid hemorrhage? *J Neurosurg* 1998; **88**(2): 272–276.

27. Hadani M, Bruk B, Ram Z, Knoller N, Bass A. Transiently increased basilar artery flow velocity following severe head injury: a time course transcranial Doppler study. *J Neurotrauma* 1997; **14**(9): 629–636.

28. Ries S, Schminke U, Fassbender K, Daffertshofer M, Steinke W, Hennerici M. Cerebrovascular involvement in the acute phase of bacterial meningitis. *J Neurol* 1997; **244**(1): 51–55.

29. Schmidt B, Klingelhöfer J, Schwarze JJ, Sander D, Wittich I. Noninvasive prediction of intracranial pressure curves using transcranial Doppler ultrasonography and blood pressure curves. *Stroke* 1997; **28**(12): 2465–2472.

30. Silvestrini M, Cupini LM, Placidi F, Diomedi M, Bernardi G. Bilateral hemispheric activation in the early recovery of motor function after stroke. *Stroke* 1998; **29**(7): 1305–1310.

31. Silvestrini M, Troisi E, Matteis M, Razzano C, Caltagirone C. Correlations of flow velocity changes during mental activity and recovery from aphasia in ischemic stroke. *Neurology* 1998; **50**(1): 191–195.

32. Knecht S, Deppe M, Ebner A et al. Noninvasive determination of language lateralization by functional transcranial Doppler sonography: a comparison with the Wada test. *Stroke* 1998; **29**(1): 82–86.

33. Klingelhöfer J, Matzander G, Sander D, Schwarze J, Boecker H, Bischoff C. Assessment of functional hemispheric asymmetry by bilateral simultaneous cerebral blood flow velocity monitoring. *J Cereb Blood Flow Metab* 1997; **17**(5): 577–585.

34. Matteis M, Silvestrini M, Troisi E, Cupini LM, Caltagirone C. Transcranial Doppler assessment of cerebral flow velocity during perception and recognition of melodies. *J Neurol Sci* 1997; **149**(1): 57–61.

35. Tiecks FP, Haberl RL, Newell DW. Temporal patterns of evoked cerebral blood flow during reading. *J Cereb Blood Flow Metab* 1998; **18**(7): 735–741.

36. Hamann GF, Schatzer KD, Frohlig G et al. Femoral injection of echo contrast medium may increase the sensitivity of testing for a patent foramen ovale. *Neurology* 1998; **50**(5): 1423–1428.

37. Schwarze JJ, Sander D, Kukla C, Wittich I, Babikian VL, Klingelhofer J. Methodological parameters influence the detection of right-to-left shunts by contrast transcranial Doppler ultrasonography. *Stroke* 1999; **30**(6): 1234–1239.

38. Anzola GP, Magoni M, Guindani M, Rozzini L, Dalla VG. Potential source of cerebral embolism in migraine with aura: a transcranial Doppler study. *Neurology* 1999; **52**(8): 1622–1625.

39. Knauth M, Ries S, Pohimann S et al. Cohort study of multiple brain lesions in sport divers: role of a patent foramen ovale. *BMJ* 1997; **314**(7082): 701–705.

40. Steventon DM, John PR. Power Doppler ultrasound appearances of neonatal ischaemic brain injury. *Pediatr Radiol* 1997; **27**: 147–149.

41. Guerriero S, Ajossa S, Mais V et al. Color Doppler energy imaging in the diagnosis of fetal intracranial hemorrhage in the second trimester. *Ultrasound Obstet Gynecol* 1997; **10**: 205–208.

42. Adams RJ, McKie VC, Hsu L et al. Prevention of a first stroke by transfusions in children with sickle cell anemia and abnormal results on transcranial Doppler ultrasonography. *N Engl J Med* 1998; **339**(1): 5–11.

43. Ophir J, Parker KJ. Contrast agents in diagnostic ultrasound. *Ultrasound Med Biol* 1989; **15**: 319–333.

44. Strandness DE, Eikelboom BC. Carotid artery stenosis—where do we go from here? *Eur J Ultrasound* 1998; 7(suppl 3) S17–S26.

45. Sitzer M, Furst G, Siebler M, Steinmetz H. Usefulness of an intravenous contrast medium in the characterization of high-grade internal carotid stenosis with color Doppler-assisted duplex imaging. *Stroke* 1994; **25**(2): 385–389.

46. Sitzer M, Rose G, Furst G, Siebler M, Steinmetz H. Characteristics and clinical value of an intravenous echo-enhancement agent in evaluation of high-grade internal carotid stenosis. *J Neuroimaging* 1997; 7(suppl 1): S22–S25.

47. Furst G, Saleh A, Wenserski F et al. Reliability and validity of noninvasive imaging of internal carotid artery pseudo-occlusion. *Stroke* 1999; **30**(7): 1444–1449.

48. Ries F, Honisch C, Lambertz M, Schlief R. A transpulmonary contrast medium enhances the transcranial Doppler signal in humans. *Stroke* 1993; **24**(12): 1903–1909.

49. Haggag KJ, Russell D, Brucher R et al. Contrast enhanced pulsed Doppler and colour-coded Duplex studies of the cranial vasculature. *Eur J Neurol* 1999; **6**(4): 443–448.

50. Otis S, Rush M, Boyajian R. Contrast-enhanced transcranial imaging. Results of an American phase-two study. *Stroke* 1995; **26**(2): 203–209.

51. Gerriets T, Seidel G, Fiss I, Modrau B, Kaps M. Contrast-enhanced transcranial color-coded duplex sonography: efficiency and validity. *Neurology* 1999; **52**(6): 1133–1137.

52. Murphy KJ, Bude RO, Dickinson LD, Rubin JM. Use of intravenous contrast material in transcranial sonography. *Acad Radiol* 1997; **4**(8): 577–582.

53. Stolz E, Kaps M, Kern A, Dorndorf W. Frontal bone windows for transcranial color-coded duplex sonography. *Stroke* 1999; **30**(4): 814–820.

54. Delcker A, Turowski B. Diagnostic value of three-dimensional transcranial contrast duplex sonography. *J Neuroimaging* 1997; **7**(3): 139–144.

55. Baumgartner RW, Arnold M, Gonner F et al. Contrast-enhanced transcranial color-coded duplex sonography in ischemic cerebrovascular disease. *Stroke* 1997; **28**(12): 2473–2478.

56. Nabavi DG, Droste DW, Kemeny V, Schulte-Altedorneburg G, Weber S, Ringelstein EB. Potential and limitations of echocontrast-enhanced ultrasonography in acute stroke patients: a pilot study. *Stroke* 1998; **29**(5): 949–954.

57. Nabavi DG, Droste DW, Schulte-Altedorneburg G et al. Diagnostic benefit of echocontrast enhancement for the insufficient transtemporal bone window. *J Neuroimaging* 1999; **9**(2): 102–107.

58. Droste DW, Nabavi DG, Kemeny V et al. Echocontrast enhanced transcranial colour-coded duplex offers improved visualization of the vertebrobasilar system. *Acta Neurol Scand* 1998; **98**(3): 193–199.

59. Postert T, Meves S, Bornke C, Przuntek H, Buttner T. Power Doppler compared to color-coded duplex sonography in the assessment of the basal cerebral circulation. *J Neuroimaging* 1997; **7**(4): 221–226.

60. Griewing B, Motsch L, Piek J, Schminke U, Brassel F, Kessler C. Transcranial power mode Doppler duplex sonography of intracranial aneurysms. *J Neuroimaging* 1998; **8**(3): 155–158.

61. Wardlaw JM, Cannon J, Statham PF, Price R. Does the size of intracranial aneurysms change with intracranial pressure? Observations based on color 'power' transcranial Doppler ultrasound. *J Neurosurg* 1998; **88**(5): 846–850.

62. Woydt M, Greiner K, Perez J, Krone A, Roosen K. Intraoperative color duplex sonography of basal arteries during aneurysm surgery. *J Neuroimaging* 1997; **7**(4): 203–207.

63. Mursch K, Schaake T, Markakis E. Using transcranial duplex sonography for monitoring vessel patency during surgery for intracranial aneurysms. *J Neuroimaging* 1997; **7**(3): 164–170.

64. Bailes JE, Tantuwaya LS, Fukushima T, Schurman GW, Davis D. Intraoperative microvascular Doppler sonography in aneurysm surgery. *Neurosurgery* 1997; **40**(5): 965–970.

65. Uggowitzer MM, Kugler C, Riccabona M et al. Cerebral arteriovenous malformations: diagnostic value of echo-enhanced transcranial Doppler sonography compared with angiography. *Am J Neuroradiol* 1999; **20**(1): 101–106.

66. Valdueza JM, Hoffmann O, Doepp F, Lehmann R, Einhaupl KM. Venous Doppler ultrasound assessment of the parasellar region. *Cerebrovasc Dis* 1998; **8**(2): 113–117.

67. Baumgartner RW, Nirkko AC, Muri RM, Gonner F. Transoccipital power-based color-coded duplex sonography of cerebral sinuses and veins. *Stroke* 1997; **28**(7): 1319–1323.

68. Ries S, Steinke W, Neff KW, Hennerici M. Echocontrast-enhanced transcranial color-coded sonography for the diagnosis of transverse sinus venous thrombosis. *Stroke* 1997; **28**(4): 696–700.

69. Berg D, Hoggenmuller U, Hofmann E et al. The basal ganglia in haemochromatosis. *Neuroradiology* 2000; **42**(1): 9–13.

70. Naumann M, Becker G, Toyka KV, Supprian T, Reiners K. Lenticular nucleus lesion in idiopathic dystonia detected by transcranial sonography. *Neurology* 1996; **47**(5) 1284–1290.

71. Berg D, Becker G, Zeiler B et al. Vulnerability of the nigrostriatal system as detected by transcranial ultrasound. *Neurology* 1999; **53**(5): 1026–1031.

72. Meairs S, Hennerici M. Four-dimensional ultrasonographic characterization of plaque surface motion in patients with symptomatic and asymptomatic carotid artery stenosis. *Stroke* 1999; **30**(9): 1807–1813.

73. Sobbe A, Stumpff U, Trubestein G, Figge H, Kozuschek W. Die Ultraschall-Auflosung von Thromben. *Klin Wochenschr* 1974; **52**(23): 1117–1121.

74. Lauer CG, Burge R, Tang DB, Bass BG, Gomez ER, Alving BM. Effect of ultrasound on tissue-type plasminogen activator-induced thrombolysis. *Circulation* 1992; **86**(4): 1257–1264.

75. Harpaz D, Chen X, Francis CW, Marder VJ, Meltzer RS. Ultrasound enhancement of thrombolysis and reperfusion in vitro. *J Am Coll Cardiol* 1993; **21**(6): 1507–1511.

76. Luo H, Nishioka T, Fishbein MC et al. Transcutaneous ultrasound augments lysis of arterial thrombi in vivo. *Circulation* 1996; **94**(4): 775–778.

77. Siegel RJ, Atar S, Fishbein MC et al. Noninvasive, transthoracic, low-frequency ultrasound augments

thrombolysis in a canine model of acute myocardial infarction. *Circulation* 2000; **101**(17): 2026–2029.

78. Francis CW, Blinc A, Lee S, Cox C. Ultrasound accelerates transport of recombinant tissue plasminogen activator into clots. *Ultrasound Med Biol* 1995; **21**(3): 419–424.

79. Behrens S, Daffertshofer M, Spiegel D, Hennerici M. Low-frequency, low-intensity ultrasound accelerates thrombolysis through the skull. *Ultrasound Med Biol* 1999; **25**(2): 269–273.

80. Tachibana K, Tachibana S. Albumin microbubble echo-contrast material as an enhancer for ultrasound accelerated thrombolysis. *Circulation* 1995; **92**(5): 1148–1150.

81. Nishioka T, Luo H, Fishbein MC et al. Dissolution of thrombotic arterial occlusion by high intensity, low frequency ultrasound and dodecafluoropentane emulsion: an in vitro and in vivo study. *J Am Coll Cardiol* 1997; **30**(2): 561–568.

82. Mizushige K, Kondo I, Ohmori K, Hirao K, Matsuo H. Enhancement of ultrasound-accelerated thrombolysis by echo contrast agents: dependence on microbubble structure. *Ultrasound Med Biol* 1999; **25**(9): 1431–1437.

83. Chang PH, Shung KK, Levene HB. Quantitative measurements of second harmonic Doppler using ultrasound contrast agents. *Ultrasound Med Biol* 1996; **22**(9): 1205–1214.

84. Mulvagh SL, Foley DA, Aeschbacher BC, Kiarich KK, Seward JB. Second harmonic imaging of an intravenously administered echocardiographic contrast agent: visualization of coronary arteries and measurement of coronary blood flow. *J Am Coll Cardiol* 1996; **22**(6): 1519–1525.

85. Porter TR, Xie F, Kricsfeld D, Armbruster RW. Improved myocardial contrast with second harmonic transient ultrasound response imaging in humans using intravenous perfluorocarbon-exposed sonicated dextrose albumin. *J Am Coll Cardiol* 1996; **27**(6): 1497–1501.

86. Postert T, Muhs A, Meves S, Federlein J, Przuntek H, Buttner T. Transient response harmonic imaging: an ultrasound technique related to brain perfusion. *Stroke* 1998; **29**(9): 1901–1907.

87. Seidel G, Algermissen C, Christoph A, Claassen L, Vidal-Langwasser M, Katzer T. Harmonic imaging of the human brain. Visualization of brain perfusion with ultrasound. *Stroke* 2000; **31**(1): 151–154.

88. Krishnan S, O'Donnell M. Transmit aperture processing for nonlinear contrast agent imaging. *Ultrason Imaging* 1996; **18**(2): 77–105.

89. Meairs S, Daffertshofer M, Neff W, Eschenfelder C, Hennerici M. Pulse-inversion contrast harmonic imaging: ultrasonographic assessment of cerebral perfusion. *Lancet* 2000; **355**(9203): 550–551.

51

Neurophysiology of inflammatory demyelinating disease

Kenneth J Smith

Diseases such as multiple sclerosis (MS) and Guillain–Barré syndrome (GBS) result in inflammatory demyelinating lesions within the central and peripheral nervous systems (CNS, PNS) respectively. The lesions cause a range of conduction abnormalities and these lead directly to the symptoms expressed. The nature of the particular symptoms expressed depends upon the pathway affected by the lesion.

RELAPSE—AXONAL CONDUCTION BLOCK

Demyelination

Perhaps the most prominent conduction deficit in inflammatory demyelinating disease is conduction block, and this is responsible for the most disabling, 'negative' symptoms such as blindness, paralysis and numbness. The most studied cause of conduction block is demyelination (Fig. 51.1), which will block conduction (initially at least; see below) even if only a single whole internode of myelin is lost. The block occurs specifically at the site of demyelination, irrespective of the direction of conduction: the morphologically unaffected portions of the axon appear to conduct normally.[1] In the author's experience, conduction block is the dominant electrophysiological feature of experimentally demyelinated axons at body temperature, in both the CNS and PNS, and it appears to be obligatory for at least the first few days following the loss of whole internodes (i.e. segmental myelin loss).[2–4] The initial failure of conduction is believed to arise primarily from an inadequate density of sodium channels in the newly exposed axolemma.[5]

Even partial loss of an internode can be sufficient to cause conduction block, especially if the loss is focused at the paranodes to cause nodal widening. Block due to nodal widening results primarily from

a reduction in the safety factor for conduction, due both to the dispersion of action currents from the excitable nodal membrane, and to the decreased internodal resistance and increased membrane capacitance of the demyelinated axolemma. (The safety factor for saltatory conduction is calculated by

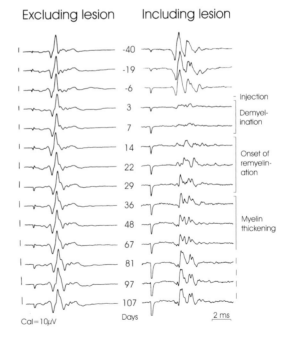

Figure 51.1 Records showing the changing pattern of conduction over an approximately 5-month period prior to, and during, the evolution of a central demyelinating and remyelinating lesion. Excluding the lesion (left), the records were quite stable, but through the lesion (right) conduction was blocked during the period of demyelination, and restored to the same axons during the period of remyelination. Modified from Smith et al,[2] and reproduced with permission. Cal, calibration.

dividing the current available to depolarize a node to its firing threshold, by the current necessary to do so.[6] Across normal internodes the safety factor is approximately 3–5, i.e. the local action current flowing from an active node to the next node is 3–5 times greater than is actually necessary to excite it.[7] In demyelinated axons the safety factor is much reduced,[8] and if it is reduced to less than unity, conduction fails.) These biophysical mechanisms are considered in more detail elsewhere.[9–15]

Inflammation

Although demyelination causes conduction deficits and will contribute directly to the symptoms of demyelinating disease, it is becoming clear that inflammation may also play an important role in symptom production. For example, there is evidence that inflammation contributes to visual loss in optic neuritis,[16] and that acute exacerbations in MS patients can be precipitated by a surge in circulating pro-inflammatory cytokines:[17,18] interferon gamma (IFN-γ) has been especially implicated. Cytokines are known to have both direct[19–21] and indirect effects on neural function,[22] and there is particular evidence that IFN-γ may act via the increased production of nitric oxide (NO). IFN-γ, particularly in combination with tumour necrosis factor alpha (TNF-α), is potent in stimulating the formation of the inducible form of the enzyme nitric oxide synthase (iNOS),[23–25] and this enzyme is prominent within MS lesions.[26–30] iNOS produces NO in sustained, high (i.e. low micromolar) concentrations, and the expression of the enzyme implies that NO production is raised in MS

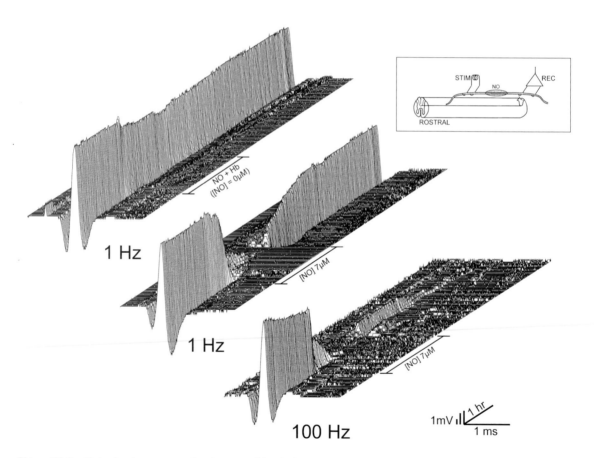

Figure 51.2 Plots showing compound action potentials obtained every 2 min from three spinal roots using the recording arrangement shown (inset): the earliest records are shown at the front. During the recording period, the roots were exposed for 2 h, either to a control solution in which NO was scavenged by the inclusion of haemoglobin (Hb) (left), or to a solution containing nitric oxide (NO) (centre and right). At 1 Hz stimulation (centre), the NO reversibly blocked conduction in all the axons, but if the axons were continuously stimulated at 100 Hz (right), the conduction block was rendered persistent. Reproduced with permission.[82]

lesions.[31] This production may be important, since there is experimental evidence that low micromolar concentrations of NO can block axonal conduction within minutes of NO exposure (Fig. 51.2),[32,33] especially in demyelinated axons.[32] NO might act via a direct effect on ion channels,[34-39] or perhaps by inhibition of mitochondrial energy production.[40-43] The role of reactive nitrogen and oxygen species in demyelinating disease has recently been reviewed.[44]

Blood–brain barrier/neuroelectric blocking factors

Apart from effects mediated by NO, it is also possible that inflammation may impair conduction by opening the blood–brain barrier,[45] thereby exposing axons to potentially deleterious factors in the vasculature. These might include putative 'neuroelectric blocking factors', although the identity of such factors, and their relevance to MS remains uncertain (reviews: Smith[8], Smith and McDonald[46]). Some evidence suggests that the factors may be antibodies,[47-50] and the possibility that antibodies may directly interact with ion channels has been reviewed.[51] Whether anti-ganglioside antibodies are involved remains unclear,[52-57] and some experiments suggest that serum blocking activity is not specific for demyelinating disease.[58] Apart from antibodies, there is evidence for the presence of unidentified, small molecular weight factors in the cerebrospinal fluid (CSF) of MS patients which may directly impair sodium channel function.[59-61]

Other factors

Inflammation might also affect conduction by modifying the properties of glial cells, particularly astrocytes and microglia.[62-65] Indeed, a functional coupling between neurons and astrocytes has recently been reported, perhaps involving gap junctions.[66] Also, since inflammation in MS occurs within the grey as well as the white matter, and since synaptic function can be disturbed by some inflammatory mediators,[67-71] especially NO,[72-76] it is possible that some neurological deficit may result from a disturbance in synaptic transmission. If so, the promptly beneficial effects of 4-aminopyridine (4-AP) in MS (review: Bever[77]) are easily explained, since this potassium channel blocking agent is a potent potentiator of synaptic transmission at therapeutic concentrations.[78,79] Recent reports indicate that inflammation may also result in an amplification of neurological deficit via the activation of glutamate receptors, especially AMPA/kainate (α-amino-3-

hydroxy-5-methyl-4-isoxazolepropionic acid/kainate) receptors.[80,81] These studies found that AMPA antagonists, such as NBQX, ameliorate the neurological deficit in experimental autoimmune encephalomyelitis (EAE).

REMISSION—RESTORATION OF CONDUCTION, ADAPTIVE MECHANISMS

Remissions arise primarily from the restoration of conduction to blocked axons, although adaptive 'plastic' changes also presumably play a role, as they do following other central damage such as that resulting from trauma. These adaptive changes are beyond the scope of this chapter, but they may help to compensate for both axonal loss and persistent conduction block.

There are at least three mechanisms underlying the restoration of conduction: the resolution of inflammation, the restoration of conduction to demyelinated axons, and repair by remyelination. These mechanisms can probably occur concurrently, perhaps even affecting different axons within the same lesion. It seems likely that the relative importance of each mechanism will vary between patients, and in individual patients at different times. It is widely accepted that the restoration of conduction will tend to reverse the neurological deficit caused by conduction block.

Inflammation

With regard to inflammation, it is reasonable to believe that the resolution of inflammation will relieve the conduction block arising from it, and certainly, in experimental lesions at least, conduction block mediated by NO is reversed within minutes of the removal of the NO, even when the conduction block has been imposed for some hours.[32,82] In agreement with this belief, clinical recovery in patients with MS tends to coincide with the resolution of inflammation (as judged by gadolinium diethylenetriaminepentaacetic acid (DTPA)-enhanced MRI), suggesting that this event permits the restoration of conduction.[16] Furthermore, the acute exacerbation of neurological deficit associated with a transient cytokine surge[83] tends to subside with the reduction in cytokine concentration, and it is prevented entirely by anti-inflammatory pretreatment with steroids.

Demyelination

The first conclusive evidence that conduction could be restored to segmentally demyelinated axons was provided by a sophisticated examination of conduction in spinal root axons demyelinated by the intrathecal injection of diphtheria toxin (Fig. 51.3a).[84] Conduction is restored by a process which includes the appearance of sodium channels along the demyelinated axolemma,[84,85] and these channels permit the transition from a saltatory to a more continuous mode of conduction across the demyelinated region. The mechanisms involved in the appearance of excitability along the demyelinated axolemma remain incompletely understood, but on physiological criteria both a seemingly continuous distribution of sodium channels (Fig. 51.3a),[84] and, in contrast, the aggregation of sodium channels into 'φ-nodes' (Fig. 51.3b) have been described.[85] φ-Nodes appear to be the precursors of the new nodes of Ranvier formed during remyelination, and it may be significant that the initial observation of a continuous distribution of sodium channels was made in a lesion (diphtheria toxin) in which repair by remyeli-

nation is only slowly achieved. A debate persists regarding the mechanism(s) involved in the aggregation of sodium channels at the new nodes of Ranvier formed during remyelination. Seemingly convincing evidence favours a view that the axon forms the channel aggregations and that the myelinating cells myelinate the gaps between them,[85–89] but also a view that the myelinating cells are primarily responsible for organizing the sodium channels.[90–94]

The likelihood that sodium channels appear along axons demyelinated by MS has been strengthened by the observation that the density of saxitoxin binding is increased within MS lesions.[95] However, these data are inconclusive, since although saxitoxin binds to sodium channels, the resolution of the study was insufficient to distinguish axonal from glial binding. A higher resolution was achieved in a more recent ultrastructural study of central axons experimentally demyelinated by ethidium bromide.[87]

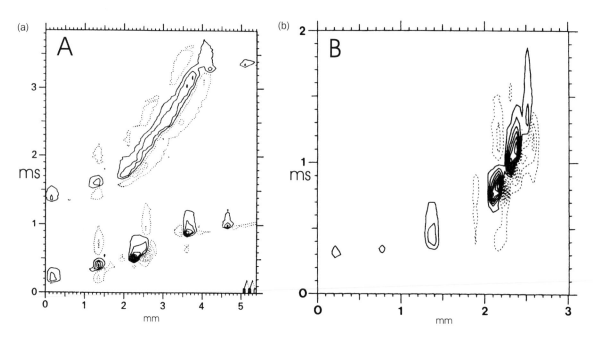

Figure 51.3 Contour maps showing conduction along axons experimentally demyelinated with diphtheria toxin (a) or lysophosphatidyl choline (LPC) (b). Inward currents (indicating the presence of sodium channels) are shown by solid lines, and outward currents (indicating the presence of potassium channels) by dashed lines. The axons can conveniently be imagined to lie along the bottom axis, with nodes spaced approximately every 1 mm: time progresses vertically. (a) shows conduction along two axons. The lower axon has been largely spared by the lesion, and the inward current occurs only at the nodes. The upper axon has a length of demyelination approximately two internodes in length, starting approximately 1.9 mm along the abscissa. The inward current along the demyelinated region is quite continuous in distribution, indicating a continuous distribution of sodium channels. In contrast, conduction along an internode demyelinated by LPC (from approximately 2.1 mm along the abscissa) indicates the presence of discrete foci of inward current, even though morphological examination established that the axon was demyelinated, i.e. remyelination had not started (b). Modified from Bostock et al[84] and Smith et al[85] and reproduced with permission.

Immunocytochemical techniques revealed node-like aggregations of sodium channels at locations along the demyelinated axolemma. Although the aggregations were present at a time when conduction had returned to some axons, the functional importance of the aggregations, and their possible relation to φ-nodes, remain uncertain.

Our understanding of the molecular constituents of myelinated and demyelinated axolemma is slowly increasing,[5,96] but data are still limited. It is clear that some degree of remodelling occurs in response to demyelination,[84,85] and it seems likely that the distribution and type of molecules expressed will vary over time,[97] perhaps under the influence of both neurotrophins[98–101] and the distribution and type of the surrounding glial and inflammatory cells. Certainly, ultrastructural membrane specializations have been described, particularly in patches of axolemma in contact with astroglial processes,[102–105] but not limited to such locations.[86,87] The presence of patches in association with glial cells increases the suspicion that the paucity of glial cells in many MS lesions[106] may have deleterious electrophysiological consequences.[107] However, central demyelinated axons have been proven to be able to conduct when at least 88% of their surface area is entirely devoid of glial contacts for several internodes.[108] Of particular interest will be data revealing the changes in the expression of the different types and sub-types of ion channels, exchangers and pumps.[5,97,109,110] It is particularly noteworthy, for example, that evidence for the presence of calcium channels along demyelinated axons has recently been presented.[111]

Following the demonstration that conduction could occur in demyelinated peripheral axons, nearly 20 years were to pass before there was proof that conduction could also occur in demyelinated central axons,[108] although evidence suggesting this possibility had accumulated.[1–3,112–117] In the author's experience, the restoration of conduction to central demyelinated axons is less promptly achieved than in peripheral axons, where conduction can be restored as early as 6 days after the induction of the demyelinating lesion.[85] However, in the CNS, conduction can be restored to many axons within 2 or 3 weeks of demyelination, even when several internodes have been demyelinated, and in the proven absence of any repair by remyelination.[108]

Factors favouring the restoration of conduction in a particular axon include a small diameter,[10,84,118] and either a short internode[10,14,84,107] or a widened node preceding the demyelinated region.[84] The first two of these factors characterize axons in the optic nerve, and they may contribute to the excellent recovery of vision which can follow optic neuritis. Since remyelinated internodes are shorter than normal, remyelination at the margins of lesions may also make a significant contribution to the restoration of conduction. However, axons as large as 5.5 μm in diameter have been proven to conduct in the absence of remyelination,[108] raising the possibility that most central axons might be able to conduct under ideal conditions. This possibility may help to explain the presence in some patients of clinically silent demyelinating lesions in pathways which are usually eloquent in symptom production.[119–124] Similarly silent lesions have been described in EAE when induced in mice deficient in the expression of major histocompatibility (MHC) class I,[125] although the reason for the absence of neurological deficit remains uncertain. Notwithstanding these considerations, readers are reminded that, in practice, conduction block is often the dominant feature of experimentally demyelinated lesions in the dorsal columns, spinal roots and sciatic nerve (K. J. Smith, unpublished observations), and this, together with other factors such as axonal loss (see below), may help to explain the fact that symptoms sometimes fail to undergo remission.

When conduction does occur in demyelinated axons, it is both much slower than normal, and also less secure. In the PNS, the velocity of conduction along the demyelinated region of rat ventral root axons is reduced 20–40-fold from normal to the range 0.7–2.3 m/s,[84,85] and it seems likely that similar values apply in the CNS. Even though the reduction in conduction velocity is apparent only along the demyelinated portion of the axon,[1] the slowing is sufficient in magnitude to result in a dispersion of the compound action potential, and, perhaps coupled with a reduction in the total number of axons conducting, it can result in diagnostically valuable delays in the visual,[126,127] somatosensory[128] and brainstem auditory[129,130] evoked potentials. The slowing can also disturb sensations dependent upon the precise timing of impulses in different axons, and so patients with unilateral optic neuritis may perceive the Pulfrich phenomenon without the normal need of a neutral density filter over one eye.[46]

Furthermore, auditory functions dependent upon precisely coordinated information may be distorted by a unilateral lesion in the auditory pathway.[131] However, since for most functions the nervous system is so much more dependent upon the presence or absence of action potentials than upon their precise timing, conduction delays are not usually manifest in the expression of symptoms. For example, normal visual acuity can be preserved in MS patients even when there are gross delays in the visual evoked potential.[126,127,130]

The relative insecurity of conduction in demyelinated axons is manifest in several ways, including an extraordinary dependence of conduction on body temperature, and a much reduced ability to conduct closely spaced impulses[1,108] and impulse trains.[1,46] These deficits can be expected to contribute to motor weakness and sensory disturbances, and they are discussed below.

Effects of temperature

The insecurity of conduction in demyelinated axons means that its success can be modulated by subtle influences in the environment of the axons. Temperature is one such influence, and the effects of temperature on conduction in demyelinated axons have often been demonstrated.[113,132–137] These changes have their parallels in the expression of clinical disease, and, particularly with lesions in the CNS, even subtle changes in body temperature can result in profound changes in the expression of symptoms (Uhthoff's phenomenon).[138] This effect has long been recognized,[139] and the effects can be dramatic. An improvement in vision upon drinking a glass of cold water has been described,[140,141] but even more striking can be the deleterious effects of body warming, such as during a hot shower or bath[142,143] or sunbathing.[144–146] Indeed, the deleterious effects of body warming are sufficiently common and robust to have underpinned the 'hot bath test' for multiple sclerosis.[147] The beneficial effects of body cooling have been considered for their therapeutic potential,[135,148,149] as have the (related) beneficial effects of action potential prolongation.[150–154] Interestingly, scorpion toxin markedly prolongs action potentials, and it has been shown to be effective in restoring conduction to demyelinated axons in the laboratory.[150] Field trials incorporating this therapy may inadvertently have been conducted, apparently with some favourable consequences, when MS patients have been travelling in the desert.[155] Based on related experimental observations, the potassium channel blocking agent 4-AP has also been examined in clinical trials in MS, and the drug is clearly beneficial in many patients[156] (review: Bever[77]). However, the widespread use of this therapy has been inhibited by the fact that the drug is potently proconvulsant at doses which are not much higher than the therapeutic dose.[157,158] Indeed, it is possible that the beneficial effects of the drug in patients owe more to its effects in potentiating synaptic transmission than to its effects in restoring conduction to demyelinated axons.[79]

Temperature can have such dramatic effects on conduction because demyelinated axons have an inherently low safety factor for conduction across the lesion.[8] In fact, the safety factor is typically reduced near to unity. The success of conduction in many demyelinated axons is therefore 'on a knife edge', since small changes in the safety factor can tip it either to just below unity, in which case conduction is blocked, or to just above unity, in which case conduction will succeed. Temperature changes have this property, since they affect the kinetics of the sodium channels in such a way that warming shortens the action potential,[148,159–161] thereby reducing the time for which current will be able to flow to depolarize the demyelinated region to its firing threshold. Cooling has the opposite effect. Since many demyelinated axons may be poised with safety factors near unity, even small temperature changes can effectively 'switch' conduction in large numbers of axons on or off, with corresponding changes in the expression of symptoms.

Conduction of pairs of impulses

A measure of the insecurity of conduction is provided by the refractory period for transmission (RPT) of an impulse through a demyelinated lesion.[1,4] In a study of central axons proven to be segmentally demyelinated, the absolute refractory period of the normal portion of the axons was 0.5–1.4 ms, but the RPT through the lesion in the same axons was 1.0–6.0 ms, with one axon having a RPT of 27 ms;[108] that is, conduction of the second impulse failed if the interval between the impulses was less than 27 ms. Since the RPT following the second impulse of a pair is even longer than after the first, it will be clear that demyelinated axons are unable faithfully to transmit trains of impulses at high frequency.

Conduction of impulse trains

Apart from having an inherently prolonged RPT, demyelinated axons also gradually accumulate refractoriness with repeated activation, and this further reduces their ability to conduct impulse trains.[1] Since certain impulses within a train (e.g. alternate impulses) will fail to be conducted across the demyelinated region, lesioned axons act as frequency filters, reducing an input frequency of, for example, 100 Hz to a much lower output frequency. The axon shown in Fig. 51.4 shows this property to a mild extent during the periods of conduction in record (d).

As well as filtering high-frequency trains of impulses into trains of lower frequency, demyelinated

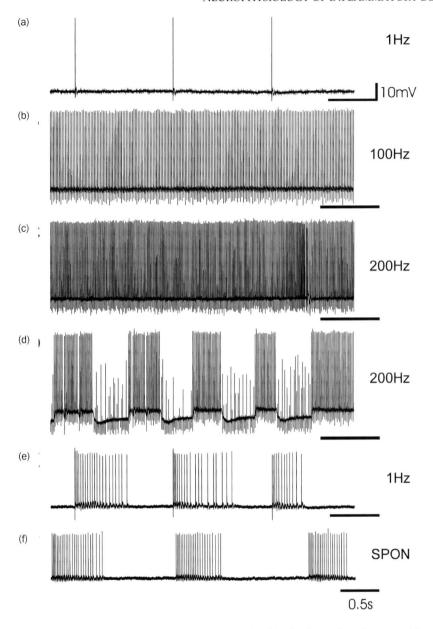

Figure 51.4 Segments of a continuous record obtained in vitro from a long, intra-axonal impalement of a central axon at or near a site of demyelination induced by the injection of ethidium bromide into the dorsal column 14 days previously (resting potential –60 mV). The RPT for this axon was prolonged from 0.77 ms in its unaffected portion to 1.32 ms through the lesion. The record illustrates several electrophysiological properties of demyelinated axons. For all the records shown, the recording site was on one side of the lesion, with the stimulating site on the other. Initially (a), the axon propagated a single action potential in response to each supramaximal electrical stimulus presented at 1 Hz (the stimulus artefacts are not distinguishable). The axon also faithfully propagated action potentials for 10 s at 100 Hz (b) and for 10 s at 200 Hz (c). However, the axon then entered intermittent periods of complete conduction block, and these were associated with periods of membrane hyperpolarization (d) (the irregular spikes during these periods represent stimulus artefacts occasionally captured by the analogue-to-digital converter). During the periods when the axon was conducting through the lesion, it was only able to transmit impulses in response to about 75% of the supramaximal stimuli. After 30 s of stimulation at 200 Hz, single impulses delivered at 1 Hz (as in (a)) now each evoked short bursts of impulses (e). If the axon was not stimulated (f), it now generated spontaneous bursts of impulses approximately every 2–3 s, even though the axon had been electrically silent before any stimulation had been applied. See Felts et al[204] for a more detailed description. Reproduced with permission.[46] Spon, spontaneous.

regions can also interpose periods of complete conduction block which may persist for approximately 0.2–2 s (Fig. 51.4d). Such periods can develop after just 1 s of stimulation at 500 Hz,[1] or after longer periods (e.g. 10–30 s) at more physiological frequencies (e.g. 100–200 Hz). A mechanism responsible for periodically 'turning an axon off' was revealed in elegant experiments to involve membrane hyperpolarization resulting from operation of the Na^+/K^+-ATPase (i.e. the sodium pump).[162] This pump is activated in response to a raised intra-axonal sodium ion concentration consequent upon the high-frequency impulse activity. The pump is electrogenic and so its activity results in membrane hyperpolarization (observable in Fig. 51.4d) which, in turn, reduces the safety factor by increasing the current necessary to depolarize the demyelinated axolemma. The resulting conduction block persists until the hyperpolarization subsides. Drugs which inhibit the Na^+/K^+-ATPase have been reported to improve conduction in both central[163] and peripheral[164,165] demyelinated axons, and some benefit was observed in three of seven MS patients in a small clinical trial of such drugs.[166]

The failure of demyelinated axons faithfully to conduct trains of impulses will obviously distort sensory information, and also contribute to weakness if the problem occurs in motor axons. The increasing failure of impulse transmission upon repeated activation may be an important factor contributing to the progressive weakness observed upon sustained muscular exertion in MS patients,[167] and it may also contribute to the 'fading' or blurring of vision sometimes described upon fixated gaze.[168,169]

Remyelination

Experimental studies have established that repair by remyelination is effective in restoring conduction in probably all affected axons, irrespective of whether the repair is effected primarily by oligodendrocytes (Fig. 51.1),[2,3] Schwann cells[4,107,170] (even within the CNS),[171,172] or transplanted olfactory ensheathing cells.[173–175] Remyelination also restores the security of conduction, inasmuch as the RPT of remyelinated axons is as short as normal,[2–4] and it restores the conduction velocity to near normal values. Axons repaired by remyelination are not noticeably hyperexcitable (see next section). Since repair by remyelination can occur in both GBS[176] and MS,[177–179] it is reasonable to believe that remyelination will play a major role in the remission of neurological deficit due to demyelination, and there is experimental evidence to support this view.[175,180]

In the PNS at least, it is known that each of the new nodes formed by remyelination is excitable,[85] and, indeed, new nodes in both the CNS[87] and PNS show aggregations of sodium channel immunoreactivity.[90,93]

POSITIVE SYMPTOMS—AXONAL HYPEREXCITABILITY

Apart from acquiring sufficient excitability to conduct, demyelinated regions can also become hyperexcitable (reviews: Smith et al,[181] Burke[182]), such that they can generate impulses ectopically for many hours, apparently spontaneously. The impulses can be generated in regular or bursting discharges, and they conduct away from their site of initiation in both directions along the axon.[183,184] Sensory axons are especially prone to such activity, and the ascending impulses can result in the expression of 'positive' symptoms such as tingling sensations and perhaps pain.

'Spontaneous' ectopic activity

As well as gaining the ability to conduct, demyelinated axons can also become hyperexcitable, so that they spontaneously generate trains of spurious impulses which arise at the demyelinated site and propagate away from it in both directions.[183–185] Both central[183,185] and peripheral[154,184,186–188] demyelinated axons can acquire this property, together with amyelinated axons.[189–191] Both continuous and bursting discharges have been observed, and each can persist for hours in the absence of any known external stimulus. Sensory axons are especially prone to hyperexcitability, and this doubtless contributes to the more frequent presence of positive sensory, rather than motor, phenomena in MS patients, although motor phenomena can also occur.[192–195] It has been suggested that when the ascending trains of sensory impulses arrive in the brain, generated concurrently in perhaps hundreds of different sensory axons, the brain may interpret the information as a tingling sensation referred to the body parts normally innervated by those axons,[183,185,196] and microneurographic examination supports this view.[188] Positive phenomena can also be enhanced in patients by measures to increase axonal hyperexcitability, such as hyperventilation, and treatment with bicarbonate or calcium chelators.[197,198]

Combined electrophysiological and pharmacological manipulations have provided evidence that spontaneous discharges can arise from inward sodium currents which develop along demyelinated axolemma,[109,199–202] and also from inward potassium currents which can result from the accumulation of potassium ions in a compartment around axons.[203,204] 'Spontaneous' discharges can sometimes be provoked in otherwise quiescent demyelinated axons by a period of sustained impulse activity (Fig. 51.4f),[204,205] and they can also sometimes be provoked by the propagation of single, normally evoked, impulses through the site of demyelination (Fig. 51.4e).[154,186,187,189,204] Impulses can also sometimes be 'reflected' from sites of demyelination;[10,187,206,207] that is, an impulse propagating through a demyelinated site can induce the formation of a second impulse which travels back along the same axon in the opposite direction. It is possible that a pair of reflecting sites could generate a train of apparently spontaneous impulses.

Ephaptic transmission between axons

Ephaptic interactions involving demyelinated axons are frequently invoked to explain otherwise puzzling clinical phenomena, but they have rarely been convincingly demonstrated. The best documented interaction occurred between normal and amyelinated (i.e. never myelinated, rather than demyelinated) axons in the spinal roots of the dystrophic mouse.[191,208] However, given the propensity of demyelinated axons to become hyperexcitable, it is reasonable to believe that ephaptic interactions can occur, and, indeed, that they may even be common. Certainly, some of the more complicated paroxysmal phenomena[195,209–211] are most easily explained by postulating the lateral spread of excitability across different, but anatomically adjacent, spinal tracts.

Massed synchronous discharges have on a few occasions been observed by the author arising from the spinal cord in animals with experimental demyelinating lesions in the dorsal columns. The discharges take the form of repeated bouts of high-frequency bursts of compound action potentials,[46] but their relevance to MS remains uncertain.

Mechanosensitivity

Demyelinated axons can become markedly mechanosensitive, so that they generate bursts of impulses in response to even mild deformation. Indeed, axons which are already spontaneously active can change their frequency of firing in response to exquisitely small distortions.[183,185] There is evidence[188] that mechanosensitivity of demyelinated axons underlies Lhermitte's phenomenon,[212,213]

namely the perception of 'electric shock' or tingling sensations which radiate down the limbs and body upon flexing the neck in patients with demyelinating lesions affecting the sensory axons in the cervical posterior columns. It is reasonable to suppose that a similar mechanism underlies the perception of flashes of light (phosphenes) upon eye movements in patients with demyelinating lesions of the optic nerve.[214] Stretch-sensitive ion channels[215] may underlie mechanosensitivity if they appear in the demyelinated membrane, but this possibility remains speculative at present.

Pain

It is possible that pain in inflammatory demyelinating disease may result, in part at least, from spontaneous activity arising in demyelinated axons, or from activity induced in nociceptive pathways by inflammatory mediators such as TNF-α.[216] At least some mechanisms of generation may involve sodium channels, since systemic injections of low concentrations of lignocaine typically provide an effective therapy.[217] However, although pain is a common complaint in MS patients,[218,219] the mechanisms responsible (which may be several) remain speculative, and poorly understood.

PROGRESSION—AXONAL LOSS AND PERSISTENT CONDUCTION BLOCK

It has long been suspected that the permanent neurological deficit associated with progressive MS may partly be due to persistent conduction block in demyelinated axons; the common presence of such conduction block has been mentioned above, and the phenomenon has also been described in chronic demyelinating peripheral neuropathy.[220] Apart from demyelination, it is now clear that axonal degeneration also plays an important role in the persistent loss of function which can occur in both MS[18,221–228] and GBS.[229,230] The mechanisms of axonal loss are largely beyond the scope of this chapter, but mention will be made of two observations that imply a role for axonal impulse activity. First, preliminary studies have revealed that sustained impulse activity at physiological frequencies (e.g. 4 h at 50 Hz or at 200 Hz) can cause axonal degeneration in central axons, if the activity occurs during the early period of repair by remyelination.[231] More mature remyelinated axons are resistant to degeneration caused in this way. The mechanisms responsible remain speculative, but may involve the configuration of ion channels at the new nodes of Ranvier, which may directly or indirectly put the axon at risk of excessive calcium accumulation during sustained activity. Interestingly, immunocytochemical evidence for calcium channels in demyelinated axons has recently been reported.[111] The second observation is that sustained impulse activity at physiological frequencies can induce axonal degeneration even in normal axons, if the activity occurs in conjunction with exposure to NO (Fig. 51.2).[82] NO is produced in raised concentrations in MS lesions,[26-31] and presumably also in the lesions of GBS. The combination of impulse activity and NO expression initiates a Wallerian-type degeneration at the site of NO exposure. It is interesting that it is the smallest axons which are most susceptible, since it is the smallest axons which are preferentially lost in MS.[232,233] Inflammatory concentrations of NO are known to inhibit mitochondrial energy production,[40,42,234-236] and it seems reasonable to hypothesize that the degeneration might result from the combination of an increased energy demand (from impulse activity) and a reduced capacity for energy production (from NO exposure). The consequent failure to maintain ion homeostasis would result in a raised intra-axonal calcium ion concentration, and the activation of intra-axonal degradative enzymes.

ACKNOWLEDGEMENTS

The author is currently supported by grants from the Multiple Sclerosis Society of Great Britain and Northern Ireland, and The Guy's and St. Thomas' Hospital Charitable Trust. Dr P. A. Felts is thanked for his expert comments on the manuscript.

REFERENCES

1. McDonald WI, Sears TA. The effects of experimental demyelination on conduction in the central nervous system. *Brain* 1970; **93**: 583–598.
2. Smith KJ, Blakemore WF, McDonald WI. Central remyelination restores secure conduction. *Nature* 1979; **280**: 395–396.
3. Smith KJ, Blakemore WF, McDonald WI. The restoration of conduction by central remyelination. *Brain* 1981; **104**: 383–404.
4. Smith KJ, Hall SM. Nerve conduction during peripheral demyelination and remyelination. *J Neurol Sci* 1980; **48**: 201–219.
5. Waxman SG, Ritchie JM. Molecular dissection of the myelinated axon. *Ann Neurol* 1993; **33**: 121–136.
6. Rushton WAH. Initiation of the propagated disturbance. *Proc R Soc Lond Biol* 1937; **124**: 210–243.
7. Tasaki I. *Nervous Transmission*. Springfield, Illinois: Charles C. Thomas, 1953.
8. Smith KJ. Conduction properties of central demyelinated and remyelinated axons, and their relation to symptom production in demyelinating disorders. *Eye* 1994; **8**: 224–237.
9. Bostock H. Impulse propagation in experimental neuropathy. In: Dyck PJ, Thomas PK, Griffin JW, Low PA, Poduslo JF, eds. *Peripheral Neuropathy*. Philadelphia: WB Saunders, 1993: 109–120.
10. Bostock H. The pathophysiology of demyelination. In: Herndon RM, Seil FJ, eds. *Multiple Sclerosis: Current Status of Research and Treatment*. New York: Demos Publications, 1994: 89–112.
11. Chiu SY, Ritchie JM. Evidence for the presence of potassium channels in the paranodal region of acutely demyelinated mammalian single nerve fibres. *J Physiol (Lond)* 1981; **313**: 415–437.
12. Stephanova DI, Chobanova M. Action potentials and ionic currents through paranodally demyelinated human motor nerve fibres: computer simulations. *Biol Cybern* 1997; **76**: 311–314.
13. Hille B. *Ionic Channels of Excitable Membranes*, 2nd edn. Sunderland, Massachusetts: Sinauer Associates Inc., 1992.
14. Waxman SG, Brill MH. Conduction through demyelinated plaques in multiple sclerosis: computer simulations of facilitation by short internodes. *J Neurol Neurosurg Psychiatry* 1978; **41**: 408–416.
15. Waxman SG, Foster RE. Ionic channel distribution and heterogeneity of the axon membrane in myelinated fibers. *Brain Res* 1980; **203**: 205–234.
16. Youl BD, Turano G, Miller DH et al. The pathophysiology of acute optic neuritis. An association of gadolinium leakage with clinical and electrophysiological deficits. *Brain* 1991; **114**: 2437–2450.
17. Moreau T, Coles A, Wing M et al. Transient increase in symptoms associated with cytokine release in patients with multiple sclerosis. *Brain* 1996; **119**: 225–237.
18. Coles AJ, Wing MG, Molyneux P et al. Monoclonal antibody treatment exposes three mechanisms underlying the clinical course of multiple sclerosis. *Ann Neurol* 1999; **46**: 296–304.
19. Mimura Y, Gotow T, Nishi T, Osame M. Mechanisms of hyperpolarization induced by two cytokines, hTNF alpha and hIL-1 alpha in neurons of the mollusc, *Onchidium*. *Brain Res* 1994; **653**: 112–118.
20. Hamm S, Rudel R, Brinkmeier H. Excitatory sodium currents of NH15-CA2 neuroblastoma x glioma hybrid cells are differently affected by interleukin-2 and interleukin-1β. *Pflugers Arch* 1996; **433**: 160–65.
21. Brinkmeier H, Kaspar A, Wietholter H, Rudel R. Interleukin-2 inhibits sodium currents in human muscle cells. *Pflugers Arch* 1992; **420**: 621–623.
22. Brosnan CF, Litwak MS, Schroeder CE, Selmaj K, Raine CS, Arezzo JC. Preliminary studies of cytokine-induced functional effects on the visual pathways in the rabbit. *J Neuroimmunol* 1989; **25**: 227–239.
23. Goureau O, Amiot F, Dautry F, Courtois Y. Control of nitric oxide production by endogenous TNF-alpha in mouse retinal pigmented epithelial and Muller glial cells. *Biochem Biophys Res Commun* 1997; **240**: 132–135.
24. Liu J, Zhao ML, Brosnan CF, Lee SC. Expression of type II nitric oxide synthase in primary human astrocytes and microglia: role of IL-1beta and IL-1 receptor antagonist. *J Immunol* 1996; **157**: 3569–3576.
25. Hu S, Sheng WS, Peterson PK, Chao CC. Differential regulation by cytokines of human astrocyte nitric oxide production. *Glia* 1995; **15**: 491–494.
26. Giovannoni G, Heales SJR, Land JM, Thompson EJ. The potential role of nitric oxide in multiple sclerosis. *Multiple Sclerosis* 1998; **4**: 212–216.

27. Oleszak EL, Zaczynska E, Bhattacharjee M, Butunoi C, Legido A, Katsetos CD. Inducible nitric oxide synthase and nitrotyrosine are found in monocytes/macrophages and/or astrocytes in acute, but not in chronic, multiple sclerosis. *Clin Diagn Lab Immunol* 1998; **5**: 438–445.

28. De Groot CJ, Ruuls SR, Theeuwes JW, Dijkstra CD, van der Valk P. Immunocytochemical characterization of the expression of inducible and constitutive isoforms of nitric oxide synthase in demyelinating multiple sclerosis lesions. *J Neuropathol Exp Neurol* 1997; **56**: 10–20.

29. Bagasra O, Michaels FH, Zheng YM et al. Activation of the inducible form of nitric oxide synthase in the brains of patients with multiple sclerosis. *Proc Natl Acad Sci USA* 1995; **92**: 12041–12045.

30. Bo L, Dawson TM, Wesselingh S et al. Induction of nitric oxide synthase in demyelinating regions of multiple sclerosis brains. *Ann Neurol* 1994; **36**: 778–786.

31. Cross AH, Manning PT, Keeling RM, Schmidt RE, Misko TP. Peroxynitrite formation within the central nervous system in active multiple sclerosis. *J Neuroimmunol* 1998; **88**: 45–56.

32. Redford EJ, Kapoor R, Smith KJ. Nitric oxide donors reversibly block axonal conduction: demyelinated axons are especially susceptible. *Brain* 1997; **120**: 2149–2157.

33. Shrager P, Custer AW, Kazarinova K, Rasband MN, Mattson D. Nerve conduction block by nitric oxide that is mediated by the axonal environment. *J Neurophysiol* 1998; **79**: 529–536.

34. Ahern GP, Hsu S-F, Jackson MB. Direct actions of nitric oxide on rat neurohypophysial K+ channels. *J Physiol (Lond)* 1999; **520**: 165–176.

35. Bielefeldt K, Whiteis CA, Chapleau MW, Abboud FM. Nitric oxide enhances slow inactivation of voltage-dependent sodium currents in rat nodose neurons. *Neurosci Lett* 1999; **271**: 159–162.

36. Chen C-H, Houchi H, Ohnaka M, Sakamoto S, Niwa Y, Nakaya Y. Nitric oxide activates Ca2+-activated K+ channels in cultured bovine adrenal chromaffin cells. *Neurosci Lett* 1998; **248**: 127–129.

37. Li Z, Chapleau MW, Bates JN, Bielefeldt K, Lee H-C, Abboud FM. Nitric oxide as an autocrine regulator of sodium currents in baroreceptor neurons. *Neuron* 1998; **20**: 1039–1049.

38. Erdemli G, Krnjevic K. Nitric oxide tonically depresses a voltage- and Ca-dependent outward current in hippocampal slices. *Neurosci Lett* 1995; **201**: 57–60.

39. Bolotina VM, Najibi S, Palacino JJ, Pagano PJ, Cohen RA. Nitric oxide directly activates calcium-dependent potassium channels in vascular smooth muscle. *Nature* 1994; **368**: 850–853.

40. Bolanos JP, Almeida A, Stewart V et al. Nitric oxide-mediated mitochondrial damage in the brain: mechanisms and implications for neurodegenerative diseases. *J Neurochem* 1997; **68**: 2227–2240.

41. Heales SJR, Barker JE, Stewart VC et al. Nitric oxide, energy metabolism and neurological disease. *Biochem Soc Trans* 1997; **25**: 939–943.

42. Bolanos JP, Heales SJ, Peuchen S, Barker JE, Land JM, Clark JB. Nitric oxide-mediated mitochondrial damage: a potential neuroprotective role for glutathione. *Free Rad Biol Med* 1996; **21**: 995–1001.

43. Bolanos JP, Peuchen S, Heales SJ, Land JM, Clark JB. Nitric oxide-mediated inhibition of the mitochondrial respiratory chain in cultured astrocytes. *J Neurochem* 1994; **63**: 910–916.

44. Smith KJ, Kapoor R, Felts PA. Demyelination: the role of reactive oxygen and nitrogen species. *Brain Pathol* 1999; **9**: 69–92.

45. Abbott NJ. Inflammatory mediators and modulation of blood–brain barrier permeability. *Cell Mol Neurobiol* 2000; **20**: 131–147.

46. Smith KJ, McDonald WI. The pathophysiology of multiple sclerosis: the mechanisms underlying the production of symptoms and the natural history of the disease. *Phil Trans R Soc Lond B* 1999; **354**: 1649–1673.

47. Schauf CL, Davis FA. Circulating toxic factors in multiple sclerosis: a perspective. *Adv Neurol* 1981; **31**: 267–280.

48. Schauf CL, Davis FA. The occurrence, specificity, and role of neuroelectric blocking factors in multiple sclerosis. *Neurology* 1978; **28**: 34–39.

49. Crain SM, Bornstein MB, Lennon VA. Depression of complex bioelectric discharges in cerebral tissue cultures by thermolabile complement-dependent serum factors. *Exp Neurol* 1975; **49**: 330–335.

50. Stefoski D, Schauf CL, McLeod BC, Haywood CP, Davis FA. Plasmapheresis decreases neuroelectric blocking activity in multiple sclerosis. *Neurology* 1982; **32**: 904–907.

51. Waxman SG. Sodium channel blockade by antibodies: a new mechanism of neurological disease? *Ann Neurol* 1995; **37**: 421–423.

52. Benatar M, Willison HJ, Vincent A. Immune-mediated peripheral neuropathies and voltage-gated sodium channels. *Muscle Nerve* 1999; **22**: 108–110.

53. Cavanna B, Carpo M, Pedotti R et al. Anti-GM2 IgM antibodies: clinical correlates and reactivity with a human neuroblastoma cell line. *J Neuroimmunol* 1999; **94**: 157–164.

54. Kaji R, Kimura J. Facts and fallacies on anti-GM1 antibodies: physiology of motor neuropathies. *Brain* 1999; **122**: 797–798.

55. Paparounas K, O'Hanlon GM, O'Leary CP, Rowan EG, Willison HJ. Anti-ganglioside antibodies can bind peripheral nerve nodes of Ranvier and activate the complement cascade without inducing acute conduction block in vitro. *Brain* 1999; **122**: 807–816.

56. Arasaki K, Kusunoki S, Kudo N, Tamaki M. The pattern of antiganglioside antibody reactivities producing myelinated nerve conduction block in vitro. *J Neurol Sci* 1998; **161**: 163–168.

57. Buchwald B, Weishaupt A, Toyka KV, Dudel J. Pre- and postsynaptic blockade of neuromuscular transmission by Miller–Fisher syndrome IgG at mouse motor nerve terminals. *Eur J Neurosci* 1998; **10**: 281–290.

58. Seil FJ, Leiman AL, Kelly JM. Neuroelectric blocking factors in multiple sclerosis and normal human sera. *Arch Neurol* 1976; **33**: 418–422.

59. Koller H, Buchholz J, Siebler M. Cerebrospinal fluid from multiple sclerosis patients inactivates neuronal Na+ current. *Brain* 1996; **119**: 457–463.

60. Brinkmeier H, Wollinsky KH, Seewald MJ, Hulser PJ, Mehrkens HH, Rudel R. Factors in the cerebrospinal fluid of multiple sclerosis patients interfering with voltage-dependent sodium channels. *Neurosci Lett* 1993; **156**: 172–175.

61. Aulkemeyer P, Hausner G, Brinkmeier H et al. The small sodium-channel blocking factor in the

cerebrospinal fluid of multiple sclerosis patients is probably an oligopeptide. *J Neurol Sci* 2000; **172**: 49–54.

62. Chao CC, Hu S, Peterson PK. Glia, cytokines, and neurotoxicity. *Crit Rev Neurobiol* 1995; **9**: 189–205.

63. Ridet JL, Malhotra SK, Privat A, Gage FH. Reactive astrocytes: cellular and molecular cues to biological function. *Trends Neurosci* 1997; **20**: 570–577.

64. Lee SC, Dickson DW, Brosnan CF. Interleukin-1, nitric oxide and reactive astrocytes. *Brain Behav Immun* 1995; **9**: 345–354.

65. Merrill JE, Benveniste EN. Cytokines in inflammatory brain lesions: helpful and harmful. *Trends Neurosci* 1996; **19**: 331–338.

66. Alvarez-Maubecin V, Garcia-Hernandez F, Williams JT, Van Bockstaele EJ. Functional coupling between neurons and glia. *J Neurophysiol* 2000; **20**: 4091–4098.

67. Yu B, Shinnick-Gallagher P. Interleukin-1 beta inhibits synaptic transmission and induces membrane hyperpolarization in amygdala neurons. *J Pharmacol Exp Therap* 1994; **271**: 590–600.

68. Martiney JA, Litwak M, Berman JW, Arezzo JC, Brosnan CF. Pathophysiologic effect of interleukin-1b in the rabbit retina. *Am J Pathol* 1990; **137**: 1411–1423.

69. Park HJ, Won CK, Pyun KH, Shin HC. Interleukin 2 suppresses afferent sensory transmission in the primary somatosensory cortex. *Neuroreport* 1995; **6**: 1018–1020.

70. Tancredi V, D'Arcangelo G, Grassi F et al. Tumor necrosis factor alters synaptic transmission in rat hippocampal slices. *Neurosci Lett* 1992; **146**: 176–178.

71. D'Arcangelo G, Grassi F, Ragozzino D, Santoni A, Tancredi V, Eusebi F. Interferon inhibits synaptic potentiation in rat hippocampus. *Brain Res* 1991; **564**: 245–248.

72. Kara P, Friedlander MJ. Dynamic modulation of cerebral cortex synaptic function by nitric oxide. *Prog Brain Res* 1998; **118**: 183–198.

73. Holscher C. Nitric oxide, the enigmatic neuronal messenger: its role in synaptic plasticity. *Trends Neurosci* 1997; **20**: 298–303.

74. Kilbinger H. Modulation of acetylcholine release by nitric oxide. *Prog Brain Res* 1996; **109**: 219–224.

75. Martinez-Serrano A, Borner C, Pereira R, Villalba M, Satrustegui J. Modulation of presynaptic calcium homeostasis by nitric oxide. *Cell Calcium* 1996; **20**: 293–302.

76. Wu SY, Dun NJ. Calcium-activated release of nitric oxide potentiates excitatory synaptic potentials in immature rat sympathetic preganglionic neurons. *J Neurophysiol* 1995; **74**: 2600–2603.

77. Bever CT, Jr. The current status of studies of aminopyridines in patients with multiple sclerosis. *Ann Neurol* 1994; **36**(suppl): S118–S121.

78. Felts PA, Smith KJ. The use of potassium channel blocking agents in the therapy of demyelinating diseases. *Ann Neurol* 1994; **36**: 454.

79. Smith KJ, Felts PA, John GR. Effects of 4–aminopyridine on demyelinated axons, synapses and muscle tension. *Brain* 2000; **123**: 171–184.

80. Pitt D, Werner P, Raine CS. Glutamate excitotoxicity in a model of multiple sclerosis. *Nature Med* 2000; **6**: 67–70.

81. Smith T, Groom A, Zhu B, Turski L. Autoimmune encephalomyelitis ameliorated by AMPA antagonists. *Nature Med* 2000; **6**: 62–66.

82. Kapoor R, Davies M, Smith KJ. Temporary axonal conduction block and axonal loss in inflammatory

neurological disease: a potential role for nitric oxide? *Ann NY Acad Sci* 1999; **893**: 304–308.

83. Moreau T, Coles A, Wing M et al. CAMPATH-IH in multiple sclerosis. *Multiple Sclerosis* 1996; **1**: 357–365.

84. Bostock H, Sears TA. The internodal axon membrane: electrical excitability and continuous conduction in segmental demyelination. *J Physiol (Lond)* 1978; **280**: 273–301.

85. Smith KJ, Bostock H, Hall SM. Saltatory conduction precedes remyelination in axons demyelinated with lysophosphatidyl choline. *J Neurol Sci* 1982; **54**: 13–31.

86. Deerinck TJ, Levinson SR, Bennett GV, Ellisman MH. Clustering of voltage-sensitive sodium channels on axons is independent of direct Schwann cell contact in the dystrophic mouse. *J Neurosci* 1997; **17**: 5080–5088.

87. Felts PA, Deerinck TJ, Ellisman MH, Levinson SR, Schwarz TL, Smith KJ. Sodium and potassium channel immunolocalization in demyelinated and remyelinated central axons. *Neuropathol Appl Neurobiol* 1998; **24**: 154–155.

88. Wiley-Livingston CA, Ellisman MH. Development of axonal membrane specializations defines nodes of Ranvier and precedes Schwann cell myelin elaboration. *Dev Biol* 1980; **79**: 70–91.

89. Kaplan MR, Meyer-Franke A, Lambert S et al. Induction of sodium channel clustering by oligodendrocytes. *Nature* 1997; **386**: 724–728.

90. Dugandzija-Novakovic S, Koszowski AG, Levinson SR, Shrager P. Clustering of Na+ channels and node of Ranvier formation in remyelinating axons. *J Neurosci* 1995; **15**: 492–503.

91. Rasband MN, Peles E, Trimmer JS, Levinson SR, Lux SE, Shrager P. Dependence of nodal sodium channel clustering on paranodal axoglial contact in the developing CNS. *J Neurosci* 1999; **19**: 7516–7528.

92. Vabnick I, Shrager P. Ion channel redistribution and function during development of the myelinated axon. *J Neurobiol* 1998; **37**: 80–96.

93. Novakovic SD, Deerinck TJ, Levinson SR, Shrager P, Ellisman MH. Clusters of axonal Na+ channels adjacent to remyelinating Schwann cells. *J Neurocytol* 1996; **25**: 403–412.

94. Vabnick I, Novakovic SD, Levinson SR, Schachner M, Shrager P. The clustering of axonal sodium channels during development of the peripheral nervous system. *J Neurosci* 1996; **16**: 4914–4922.

95. Moll C, Mourre C, Lazdunski M, Ulrich J. Increase of sodium channels in demyelinated lesions of multiple sclerosis. *Brain Res* 1991; **556**: 311–316.

96. Arroyo EJ, Scherer S. On the molecular architecture of myelinated fibers. *Histochem Cell Biol* 2000; **113**: 1–18.

97. Black JA, Waxman SG. Sodium channel expression: a dynamic process in neurons and non-neuronal cells. *Dev Neurosci* 1996; **18**: 139–152.

98. Fjell J, Cummins TR, Fried K, Black JA, Waxman SG. In vivo NGF deprivation reduces SNS expression and TTX-R sodium currents in IB4-negative DRG neurons. *J Neurophysiol* 1999; **81**: 803–810.

99. Dib-Hajj SD, Black JA, Cummins TR, Kenney AM, Kocsis JD, Waxman SG. Rescue of alpha-SNS sodium channel expression in small dorsal root ganglion neurons after axotomy by nerve growth factor in vivo. *J Neurophysiol* 1998; **79**: 2668–2676.

100. Black JA, Langworthy K, Hinson AW, Dib-Hajj SD, Waxman SG. NGF has opposing effects on Na+

channel III and SNS gene expression in spinal sensory neurons. *Neuroreport* 1997; **8**: 2331–2335.

101. Oyelese AA, Rizzo MA, Waxman SG, Kocsis JD. Differential effect of neurotrophins on injury-induced plasticity of GABA, receptors and sodium currents in cutaneous afferent DRG neurons. *Soc Neurosci Meeting Abstr* 1995; 4208.

102. Blakemore WF, Smith KJ. Node-like axonal specializations along demyelinated central nerve fibres: ultra-structural observations. *Acta Neuropathol* 1983; **60**: 291–296.

103. Rosenbluth J, Tao-Cheng J-H, Blakemore WF. Dependence of axolemmal differentiation on contact with glial cells in chronically demyelinated lesions of cat spinal cord. *Brain Res* 1985; **358**: 287–302.

104. Black JA, Felts P, Smith KJ, Kocsis JD, Waxman SG. Distribution of sodium channels in chronically demyelinated spinal cord axons: immuno-ultrastructural localization and electrophysiological observations. *Brain Res* 1991; **544**: 59–70.

105. Rosenbluth J, Blakemore WF. Structural specializations in cat of chronically demyelinated spinal cord axons as seen in freeze-fracture replicas. *Neurosci Lett* 1984; **48**: 171–177.

106. Barnes D, Munro PM, Youl BD, Prineas JW, McDonald WI. The longstanding MS lesion. A quantitative MRI and electron microscopic study. *Brain* 1991; **114**: 1271–1280.

107. Shrager P, Rubinstein CT. Optical measurement of conduction in single demyelinated axons. *J Gen Physiol* 1990; **95**: 867–890.

108. Felts PA, Baker TA, Smith KJ. Conduction in segmentally demyelinated mammalian central axons. *J Neurosci* 1997; **17**: 7267–7277.

109. Rizzo MA, Kocsis JD, Waxman SG. Mechanisms of paresthesiae, dysesthesiae, and hyperesthesiae: role of Na+ channel heterogeneity. *Eur Neurol* 1996; **36**: 3–12.

110. Dib-Hajj SD, Tyrrell L, Black JA, Waxman SG. NaN, a novel voltage-gated Na channel, is expressed preferentially in peripheral sensory neurons and down-regulated after axotomy. *Proc Natl Acad Sci USA* 1998; **95**: 8963–8968.

111. Kornek B, Djamshidian A, Storch MK et al. Distribution of calcium channel subunits in dystrophic axons of multiple sclerosis and experimental autoimmune encephalomyelitis. *J Neurol* 2000; **247**: 203.

112. Pender MP. The pathophysiology of acute experimental allergic encephalomyelitis induced by whole spinal cord in the Lewis rat. *J Neurol Sci* 1988; **84**: 209–222.

113. Pender MP, Sears TA. The pathophysiology of acute experimental allergic encephalomyelitis in the rabbit. *Brain* 1984; **107**: 699–726.

114. Pender MP. The pathophysiology of myelin basic protein-induced acute experimental allergic encephalomyelitis in the Lewis rat. *J Neurol Sci* 1988; **86**: 277–289.

115. Pender MP. Recovery from acute experimental allergic encephalomyelitis in the Lewis rat. Early restoration of nerve conduction and repair by Schwann cells and oligodendrocytes. *Brain* 1989; **112**: 393–416.

116. Kaji R, Suzumura A, Sumner AJ. Physiological consequences of antiserum-mediated experimental demyelination in CNS. *Brain* 1988; **111**: 675–694.

117. Chalk JB, McCombe PA, Pender MP. Conduction abnormalities are restricted to the central nervous system in experimental autoimmune encephalomyelitis induced by inoculation with proteolipid protein but not with myelin basic protein. *Brain* 1994; **117**: 975–986.

118. Waxman SG. Demyelination in spinal cord injury. *J Neurol Sci* 1989; **91**: 1–14.

119. Wisniewski HM, Oppenheimer D, McDonald WI. Relation between myelination and function in MS and EAE. *J Neuropathol Exp Neurol* 1976; **35**: 327.

120. Ghatak NR, Hirano A, Lijtmaer H, Zimmerman HM. Asymptomatic demyelinated plaque in the spinal cord. *Arch Neurol* 1974; **30**: 484–486.

121. Phadke JG, Best PV. Atypical and clinically silent multiple sclerosis: a report of 12 cases discovered unexpectedly at necropsy. *J Neurol Neurosurg Psychiatry* 1983; **46**: 414–420.

122. Ulrich J, Groebke-Lorenz W. The optic nerve in multiple sclerosis: a morphological study with retrospective clinico-pathological correlations. *Neuro-ophthalmology* 1983; **3**: 149–159.

123. Namerow NS. The pathophysiology of multiple sclerosis. In: Wolfgram F, Ellison GW, Stevens JG et al, eds. *Multiple Sclerosis: Immunology, Virology and Ultrastructure*. New York: Academic Press, 1972: 143–172.

124. O'Riordan JI, Losseff NA, Phatouros C et al. Asymptomatic spinal cord lesions in clinically isolated optic nerve, brain stem, and spinal cord syndromes suggestive of demyelination. *J Neurol Neurosurg Psychiatry* 1998; **64**: 353–357.

125. Rivera-Quinones C, McGavern D, Schmelzer JD, Hunter SF, Low PA, Rodriguez M. Absence of neurological deficits following extensive demyelination in a class I-deficient murine model of multiple sclerosis. *Nature Med* 1998; **4**: 187–193.

126. Halliday AM, McDonald WI, Mushin J. Delayed visual evoked response in optic neuritis. *Lancet* 1972; **1**: 982–985.

127. Halliday AM, McDonald WI, Mushin J. Visual evoked response in diagnosis of multiple sclerosis. *Br Med J* 1973; **4**: 661–664.

128. Small DG, Matthews WB, Small M. The cervical somatosensory evoked potential (SEP) in the diagnosis of multiple sclerosis. *J Neurol Sci* 1978; **35**: 211–224.

129. Robinson K, Rudge P. Abnormalities of the auditory evoked potentials in patients with multiple sclerosis. *Brain* 1977; **100**: 19–40.

130. Hume AL, Waxman SG. Evoked potentials in suspected multiple sclerosis: diagnostic value and prediction of clinical course. *J Neurol Sci* 1988; **83**: 191–210.

131. Levine RA, Gardner JC, Fullerton BC et al. Multiple sclerosis lesions of the auditory pons are not silent. *Brain* 1994; **117**: 1127–1141.

132. Davis FA, Jacobson S. Altered thermal sensitivity in injured and demyelinated nerve. A possible model of temperature effects in multiple sclerosis. *J Neurol Neurosurg Psychiatry* 1971; **34**: 551–561.

133. Davis FA, Schauf CL, Reed BJ, Kesler RL. Experimental studies of the effects of extrinsic factors on conduction in normal and demyelinated nerve. *J Neurol Neurosurg Psychiatry* 1975; **39**: 442–448.

134. Sears TA, Bostock H, Sheratt M. The pathophysiology of demyelination and its implications for the symptomatic treatment of multiple sclerosis. *Neurology* 1978; **28**: 21–26.

135. Sears TA, Bostock H. Conduction failure in demyelination: is it inevitable? *Adv Neurol* 1981; **31**: 357–375.

136. Rasminsky M. The effects of temperature on conduction in demyelinated single nerve fibers. *Arch Neurol* 1973; **28**: 287–292.

137. Pencek TL, Schauf CL, Low PA, Eisenberg BR, Davis FA. Disruption of the perineurium in amphibian peripheral nerve: morphology and physiology. *Neurology* 1980; **30**: 593–599.

138. Selhorst JB, Saul RF. Uhthoff and his symptom. *J Neuro-Ophthalmol* 1995; **15**: 63–69.

139. Uhthoff W. Untersuchungen über die bei der multiplen Herdsklerose vorkommenden Augenstörungen. *Arch Psychiatrie Nervenkrankheiten* 1890; **21**: 55–116.

140. Hopper CL, Matthews CG, Cleeland CS. Symptom instability and thermoregulation in multiple sclerosis. *Neurology* 1972; **22**: 142–148.

141. McDonald WI. The pathophysiology of multiple sclerosis. In: McDonald WI, Silberberg DH, eds. *Multiple Sclerosis*. London: Butterworth, 1986: 112–133.

142. Guthrie TC. Visual and motor changes in patients with multiple sclerosis. *Arch Neurol Psychiatry* 1951; **65**: 437–451.

143. Waxman SG, Geschwind N. Major morbidity related to hyperthermia in multiple sclerosis. *Ann Neurol* 1983; **13**: 348.

144. Berger JR, Sheremata WA. Reply to letter by F. A. Davis. *JAMA* 1985; **253**: 203.

145. Harbison JW, Calabrese VP, Edlich RF. A fatal case of sun exposure in a multiple sclerosis patient. *J Emerg Med* 1989; **7**: 465–467.

146. Avis SP, Pryse-Phillips WE. Sudden death in multiple sclerosis associated with sun exposure: a report of two cases. *Can J Neurol Sci* 1995; **22**: 305–307.

147. Malhotra AS, Goren H. The hot bath test in the diagnosis of multiple sclerosis. *JAMA* 1981; **246**: 1113–1114.

148. Davis FA, Schauf CL. Approaches to the development of pharmacological interventions in multiple sclerosis. *Adv Neurol* 1981; **31**: 505–510.

149. Waxman SG, Utzschneider DA, Kocsis JD. Enhancement of action potential conduction following demyelination: experimental approaches to restoration of function in multiple sclerosis and spinal cord injury. *Prog Brain Res* 1994; **100**: 233–243.

150. Bostock H, Sherratt RM, Sears TA. Overcoming conduction failure in demyelinated nerve fibres by prolonging action potentials. *Nature* 1978; **274**: 385–387.

151. Sherratt RM, Bostock H, Sears TA. Effects of 4-aminopyridine on normal and demyelinated mammalian nerve fibres. *Nature* 1980; **283**: 570–572.

152. Bostock H, Sears TA, Sherratt RM. The effects of 4-aminopyridine and tetraethylammonium ions on normal and demyelinated mammalian nerve fibres. *J Physiol (Lond)* 1981; **313**: 301–315.

153. Targ EF, Kocsis JD. 4-Aminopyridine leads to restoration of conduction in demyelinated rat sciatic nerve. *Brain Res* 1985; **328**: 358–361.

154. Bowe CM, Kocsis JD, Targ EF, Waxman SG. Physiological effects of 4-aminopyridine on demyelinated mammalian motor and sensory fibers. *Ann Neurol* 1987; **22**: 264–268.

155. Breland AE, Currier RD. Scorpion venom and multiple sclerosis. *Lancet* 1983; **2**: 1021.

156. Schwid SR, Petrie MD, McDermott MP, Tierney DS, Mason DH, Goodman AD. Quantitative assessment of sustained-release 4-aminopyridine for symptomatic treatment of multiple sclerosis. *Neurology* 1997; **48**: 817–821.

157. Bever CT, Jr., Young D, Anderson PA et al. The effects of 4–aminopyridine in multiple sclerosis patients: results of a randomized, placebo-controlled, double-blind, concentration-controlled, crossover trial. *Neurology* 1994; **44**: 1054–1059.

158. Blight AR, Toombs JP, Bauer MS, Widmer WR. The effects of 4-aminopyridine on neurological deficits in chronic cases of traumatic spinal cord injury in dogs: a phase I clinical trial. *J Neurotrauma* 1991; **8**: 103–119.

159. Paintal AS. The influence of diameter of medullated nerve fibres of cats on the rising and falling phases of the spike and its recovery. *J Physiol (Lond)* 1966; **184**: 791–811.

160. Schoepfle GM, Erlanger J. The action of temperature on the excitability, spike height and configuration and the absolute refractory period observed in the responses of single medullated nerve fibers. *Am J Physiol* 1941; **134**: 694–704.

161. Schauf CL, Davis FA. Impulse conduction in multiple sclerosis: a theoretical basis for modification by temperature and pharmacological agents. *J Neurol Neurosurg Psychiatry* 1974; **37**: 152–161.

162. Bostock H, Grafe P. Activity-dependent excitability changes in normal and demyelinated rat spinal root axons. *J Physiol (Lond)* 1985; **365**: 239–257.

163. Kaji R, Sumner AJ. Effect of digitalis on central demyelinative conduction block in vivo. *Ann Neurol* 1989; **25**: 159–165.

164. Kaji R, Sumner AJ. Ouabain reverses conduction disturbances in single demyelinated nerve fibers. *Neurology* 1989; **39**: 1364–1368.

165. Shrager P. Axonal coding of action potentials in demyelinated nerve fibers. *Brain Res* 1993; **619**: 278–290.

166. Kaji R, Happel L, Sumner AJ. Effect of digitalis on clinical symptoms and conduction variables in patients with multiple sclerosis. *Ann Neurol* 1990; **28**: 582–584.

167. McDonald WI. Mechanisms of functional loss and recovery in spinal cord damage. Outcome of severe damage to the central nervous system. *Ciba Found Symp* 1975; **34**: 23–33.

168. Waxman SG. Clinicopathological correlations in multiple sclerosis and related diseases. *Adv Neurol* 1981; **31**: 169–182.

169. McDonald I. Pathophysiology of multiple sclerosis. In: Compston A, Ebers G, Lassmann H, McDonald I, Matthews B, Wekerle H, eds. *McAlpine's Multiple Sclerosis*. London: Churchill Livingstone, 1998: 359–378.

170. Rubinstein CT, Shrager P. Remyelination of nerve fibers in the transected frog sciatic nerve. *Brain Res* 1990; **524**: 303–312.

171. Felts PA, Smith KJ. Conduction properties of central nerve fibers remyelinated by Schwann cells. *Brain Res* 1992; **574**: 178–192.

172. Honmou O, Felts PA, Waxman SG, Kocsis JD. Restoration of normal conduction properties in demyelinated spinal cord axons in the adult rat by transplantation of exogenous Schwann cells. *J Neurosci* 1996; **16**: 3199–3208.

173. Imaizumi T, Lankford KL, Waxman SG, Greer CA, Kocsis JD. Transplanted olfactory ensheathing cells

173. remyelinate and enhance axonal conduction in the demyelinated dorsal columns of the rat spinal cord. *J Neurosci* 1998; **18**: 6176–6185.

174. Utzschneider DA, Archer DR, Kocsis JD, Waxman SG, Duncan ID. Transplantation of glial cells enhances action potential conduction of amyelinated spinal cord axons in the myelin-deficient rat. *Proc Natl Acad Sci USA* 1994; **91**: 53–57.

175. Jeffery ND, Crang AJ, O'Leary MT, Hodge SJ, Blakemore WF. Behavioural consequences of oligodendrocyte progenitor cell transplantation into experimental demyelinating lesions in the rat spinal cord. *Eur J Neurosci* 1999; **11**: 1508–1514.

176. Prineas JW. Pathology of inflammatory demyelinating neuropathies. *Baillières Clin Neurol* 1994; **3**: 1–24.

177. Prineas JW, Connell F. Remyelination in multiple sclerosis. *Ann Neurol* 1979; **5**: 22–31.

178. Prineas JW, Kwon EE, Sharer LR, Cho E-S. Massive early remyelination in acute multiple sclerosis. *Neurology* 1987; **37**(suppl 1): 109.

179. Prineas JW, Barnard RO, Kwon EE, Sharer LR, Cho ES. Multiple sclerosis: remyelination of nascent lesions. *Ann Neurol* 1993; **33**: 137–151.

180. Jeffery ND, Blakemore WF. Locomotor deficits induced by experimental spinal cord demyelination are abolished by spontaneous remyelination. *Brain* 1997; **120**: 27–37.

181. Smith KJ, Felts PA, Kapoor R. Axonal hyperexcitability: mechanisms and role in symptom production in demyelinating diseases. *Neuroscientist* 1997; **3**: 237–246.

182. Burke D. Microneurography, impulse conduction, and paresthesias. *Muscle Nerve* 1993; **16**: 1025–1032.

183. Smith KJ, McDonald WI. Spontaneous and evoked electrical discharges from a central demyelinating lesion. *J Neurol Sci* 1982; **55**: 39–47.

184. Baker M, Bostock H. Ectopic activity in demyelinated spinal root axons of the rat. *J Physiol (Lond)* 1992; **451**: 539–552.

185. Smith KJ, McDonald WI. Spontaneous and mechanically evoked activity due to central demyelinating lesion. *Nature* 1980; **286**: 154–155.

186. Burchiel KJ. Abnormal impulse generation in focally demyelinated trigeminal roots. *J Neurosurg* 1980; **53**: 674–683.

187. Calvin WH, Devor M, Howe JF. Can neuralgias arise from minor demyelination? Spontaneous firing, mechanosensitivity, and afterdischarge from conducting axons. *Exp Neurol* 1982; **75**: 755–763.

188. Nordin M, Nystrom B, Wallin U, Hagbarth KE. Ectopic sensory discharges and paresthesiae in patients with disorders of peripheral nerves, dorsal roots and dorsal columns. *Pain* 1984; **20**: 231–245.

189. Huizar P, Kuno M, Miyata Y. Electrophysiological properties of spinal motoneurones of normal and dystrophic mice. *J Physiol (Lond)* 1975; **248**: 231–246.

190. Rasminsky M. Spontaneous activity and cross-talk in pathological nerve fibers. *Res Publ Assoc Res Nerv Ment Dis* 1987; **65**: 39–49.

191. Rasminsky M. Ectopic generation of impulses and cross-talk in spinal nerve roots of 'dystrophic' mice. *Ann Neurol* 1978; **3**: 351–357.

192. Andermann F, Cosgrove JBR, Lloyd-Smith DL, Gloor P, McNaughton FL. Facial myokymia in multiple sclerosis. *Brain* 1961; **84**: 31–44.

193. Hjorth RJ, Willison RG. The electromyogram in facial myokymia and hemifacial spasm. *J Neurol Sci* 1973; **20**: 117–126.

194. Jacobs L, Kaba S, Pullicino P. The lesion causing continuous facial myokymia in multiple sclerosis. *Arch Neurol* 1994; **51**: 1115–1119.

195. Kapoor R, Brown P, Thompson PD, Miller DH. Propriospinal myoclonus in multiple sclerosis. *J Neurol Neurosurg Psychiatry* 1992; **55**: 1086–1088.

196. Rasminsky M. Hyperexcitability of pathologically myelinated axons and positive symptoms in multiple sclerosis. *Adv Neurol* 1981; **31**: 289–297.

197. Davis FA, Becker FO, Michael JA, Sorensen E. Effect of intravenous sodium bicarbonate, disodium edetate (Na2EDTA), and hyperventilation on visual and oculomotor signs in multiple sclerosis. *J Neurol Neurosurg Psychiatry* 1970; **33**: 723–732.

198. Burchiel KJ. Ectopic impulse generation in demyelinated axons: effects of Pa_{CO_2}, pH, and disodium edetate. *Ann Neurol* 1981; **9**: 378–383.

199. Kapoor R, Li YG, Smith KJ. Slow sodium-dependent potential oscillations contribute to ectopic firing in mammalian demyelinated axons. *Brain* 1997; **120**: 647–652.

200. Honmou O, Utzschneider DA, Rizzo MA, Bowe CM, Waxman SG, Kocsis JD. Delayed depolarization and slow sodium currents in cutaneous afferents. *J Neurophysiol* 1994; **71**: 1627–1637.

201. Stys PK, Sontheimer H, Ransom BR, Waxman SG. Noninactivating, tetrodotoxin-sensitive Na+ conductance in rat optic nerve axons. *Proc Natl Acad Sci USA* 1993; **90**: 6976–6980.

202. Cummins TR, Waxman SG. Downregulation of tetrodotoxin-resistant sodium currents and upregulation of a rapidly repriming tetrodotoxin-sensitive sodium current in small spinal sensory neurons after nerve injury. *J Neurosci* 1997; **17**: 3503–3514.

203. Kapoor R, Smith KJ, Felts PA, Davies M. Internodal potassium currents can generate ectopic impulses in mammalian myelinated axons. *Brain Res* 1993; **611**: 165–169.

204. Felts PA, Kapoor R, Smith KJ. A mechanism for ectopic firing in central demyelinated axons. *Brain* 1995; **118**: 1225–1231.

205. Miller TA, Kiernan MC, Mogyoros I, Burke D. Activity-dependent changes in impulse conduction in normal human cutaneous axons. *Brain* 1995; **118**: 1217–1224.

206. Howe JF, Calvin WH, Loeser JD. Impulses reflected from dorsal root ganglia and from focal nerve injuries. *Brain Res* 1976; **116**: 139–144.

207. Calvin WH, Loeser JD, Howe JF. A neurophysiological theory for the pain mechanism of tic douloureux. *Pain* 1977; **3**: 147–154.

208. Rasminsky M. Ephaptic transmission between single nerve fibres in the spinal nerve roots of dystrophic mice. *J Physiol (Lond)* 1980; **305**: 151–169.

209. Matthews B. Symptoms and signs of multiple sclerosis. In: Compston A, Ebers G, Lassmann H, McDonald WI, Matthews B, Wekerle H, editors. *McAlpine's Multiple Sclerosis*. London: Churchill Livingstone, 1998: 145–190.

210. Matthews WB. Paroxysmal symptoms in multiple sclerosis. *J Neurol Neurosurg Psychiatry* 1975; **38**: 619–623.

211. Hartmann M, Rottach KG, Wohlgemuth WA, Pfadenhauer K. Trigeminal neuralgia triggered by auditory

stimuli in multiple sclerosis. *Arch Neurol* 1999; **56**: 731–733.

212. Lhermitte J, Bollack J, Nicholas M. Les douleurs à type de décharge électrique consécutives à la flexion céphalique dans la sclérose en plaques. *Rev Neurol* 1924; **2**: 56–62.

213. Kanchandani R, Howe JG. Lhermitte's sign in multiple sclerosis: a clinical survey and review of the literature. *J Neurol Neurosurg Psychiatry* 1982; **45**: 308–312.

214. Davis FA, Bergen D, Schauf C, McDonald I, Deutsch W. Movement phosphenes in optic neuritis: a new clinical sign. *Neurology* 1976; **26**: 1100–1104.

215. Yang XC, Sachs F. Mechanically sensitive, nonselective cation channels. *EXS* 1993; **66**: 79–92.

216. Sorkin LS, Xiao WH, Wagner R, Myers RR. Tumour necrosis factor-alpha induces ectopic activity in nociceptive primary afferent fibres. *Neuroscience* 1997; **81**: 255–262.

217. Petersen P, Kastrup J, Zeeberg I, Boysen G. Chronic pain treatment with intravenous lidocaine. *Neurol Res* 1986; **8**: 189–190.

218. Shibasaki H, McDonald WI, Kuroiwa Y. Racial modification of clinical picture of multiple sclerosis: comparison between British and Japanese patients. *J Neurol Sci* 1981; **49**: 253–271.

219. Rae-Grant AD, Eckert NJ, Bartz S, Reed JF. Sensory symptoms of multiple sclerosis: a hidden reservoir of morbidity. *Multiple Sclerosis* 1999; **5**: 179–183.

220. Lewis RA, Sumner AJ, Brown MJ, Asbury AK. Multifocal demyelinating neuropathy with persistent conduction block. *Neurology* 1982; **32**: 958–964.

221. Losseff NA, Webb SL, O'Riordan JI et al. Spinal cord atrophy and disability in multiple sclerosis. A new reproducible and sensitive MRI method with potential to monitor disease progression. *Brain* 1996; **119**: 701–708.

222. Truyen L, Van Waesberghe JHTM, Van Walderveen MAA et al. Accumulation of hypointense lesions ('black holes') on T1 spin-echo MRI correlates with disease progression in multiple sclerosis. *Neurology* 1996; **47**: 1469–1476.

223. Matthews PM. Axonal loss and demyelination in multiple sclerosis. *J Neurol Neurosurg Psychiatry* 1999; **67**: 708–709.

224. Trapp BD, Ransohoff R, Rudick R. Axonal pathology in multiple sclerosis: relationship to neurologic disability. *Curr Opin Neurol* 1999; **12**: 295–302.

225. De Stefano N, Matthews PM, Fu L et al. Axonal damage correlates with disability in patients with relapsing–remitting multiple sclerosis. Results of a longitudinal magnetic resonance spectroscopy study. *Brain* 1998; **121**: 1469–1477.

226. Matthews PM, De Stefano N, Narayanan S, Wolinsky JS, Arnold DL. Putting magnetic resonance spectroscopy studies in context: axonal damage and disability in multiple sclerosis. *Semin Neurol* 1998; **18**: 327–336.

227. Stevenson VL, Leary SM, Losseff NA et al. Spinal cord atrophy and disability in MS: a longitudinal study. *Neurology* 1998; **51**: 234–238.

228. Davie CA, Barker GJ, Webb S et al. Persistent functional deficit in multiple sclerosis and autosomal dominant cerebellar ataxia is associated with axon loss. *Brain* 1995; **118**: 1583–1592.

229. Giovannoni G, Hartung HP. The immunopathogenesis of multiple sclerosis and Guillain–Barre syndrome. *Curr Opin Neurol* 1996; **9**: 165–177.

230. Hughes RAC, Hadden RDM, Gregson NA, Smith KJ. Pathogenesis of Guillain–Barré syndrome. *J Neuroimmunol* 1999; **100**: 74–97.

231. Samtani V, Smith KJ. Sustained impulse activity can cause central remyelinated axons to undergo degeneration. *Neuropathol Appl Neurobiol* 2000; **26**: 186.

232. Lovas G, Szilagyi N, Majtenyi K, Palkovits M, Komoly S. Axonal changes in chronic demyelinated cervical spinal cord plaques. *Brain* 2000; **123**: 308–317.

233. McGavern DB, Murray PD, Rivera-Quinones C, Schmelzer JD, Low PA, Rodriguez M. Axonal loss results in spinal cord atrophy, electrophysiological abnormalities and neurological deficits following demyelination in a chronic inflammatory model of multiple sclerosis. *Brain* 2000; **123**: 519–531.

234. Brown GC, Bolanos JP, Heales SJ, Clark JB. Nitric oxide produced by activated astrocytes rapidly and reversibly inhibits cellular respiration. *Neurosci Lett* 1995; **193**: 201–204.

235. Zielasek J, Reichmann H, Kunzig H, Jung S, Hartung H-P, Toyka KV. Inhibition of brain macrophage/microglial respiratory chain enzyme activity in experimental autoimmune encephalomyelitis of the Lewis rat. *Neurosci Lett* 1995; **184**: 129–132.

236. Borutaite V, Brown GC. Rapid reduction of nitric oxide by mitochondria, and reversible inhibition of mitochondrial respiration by nitric oxide. *Biochem J* 1996; **315**: 295–299.

Index